ANTIBIOTIC RESISTANT BACTERIA – A CONTINUOUS CHALLENGE IN THE NEW MILLENNIUM

Edited by **Marina Pana**

Antibiotic Resistant Bacteria – A Continuous Challenge in the New Millennium
Edited by Marina Pana

Published by InTech

Janeza Trdine 9, 51000 Rijeka, Croatia

Publishing Process Manager Martina Blecic

Technical Editor Teodora Smiljanic

Cover Designer InTech Design Team

Additional hard copies can be obtained from orders@intechopen.com

Antibiotic Resistant Bacteria – A Continuous Challenge in the New Millennium,
Edited by Marina Pana
p. cm.
ISBN 978-953-51-0472-8

Meet the editor

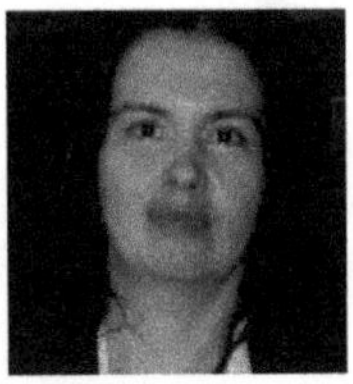

Dr. Marina Pana currently works at the National Institute of Research and Development for Microbiology and Immunology "Cantacuzino", in Bucharest, Romania. From 2008, she has been appointed as the National Contact Point for S.pneumoniae and N.meningitidis for European Centre for Disease Prevention and Control (ECDC). During her career, Dr. Pana has contributed to a number of workshops and medical seminars as their coordinator, as well as lecturer. She has attended numerous European Congresses (oral communications), especially those concerning bacterial antibiotic resistance. Dr. Pana is a reviewer of Romanian and international journals, and a member in ESCMID and European Society of Chemotherapy (ESC).

Contents

Preface

Antibiotic-resistant bacterial strains remain a major global threat, despite the prevention, diagnosis and antibiotherapy, which have improved considerably.

A better understanding of antibiotic resistant genes mechanisms and dissemination became an urgent need for advancing public health and clinical management, throughout Europe.

In this thematic issue, the scientists present their results of accomplished studies, in order to provide an updated overview of scientific information and also, to exchange views on new strategies for interventions in antibiotic-resistant bacterial strains cases and outbreaks.

As a consequence, the recently developed techniques in this field will contribute to a considerable progress in medical research.

However, the emergence of severe diseases caused by multi-drug-resistant microorganisms remains a public health concern, with serious challenges to chemotherapy and is open to scientific and clinical debate.

I take this occasion to thank so much, all contributors of this book, who demonstrated that always there is something in you that can rise above and beyond everything you think possible.

Dr. Marina Pana
National Contact Point for S.pneumoniae & N.meningitidis for ECDC,
Cantacuzino Institute,
Bucharest,
Romania

Part 1

Assessment of Antibiotic Resistance in Clinical Relevant Bacteria

1

Antibiotic Resistance: An Emerging Global Headache

Maimoona Ahmed
King Abdul Aziz University Hospital, Jeddah, Saudi Arabia

1. Introduction

The discovery of antibiotics was one of the greatest achievements of the twentieth century. The subsequent introduction of sulphonamides, penicillin and streptomycin, broad spectrum bacteriostatic antibiotics, bactericidal antibiotics, synthetic chemicals and highly specific narrow spectrum antibiotics to clinical medicine transformed the treatment of bacterial diseases (Baldry, 1976). However, due to the excessive and inappropriate use of antibiotics there has been a gradual emergence of populations of antibiotic -resistant bacteria, which pose a global public health problem (Komolafe, 2003).

According to the WHO, a resistant microbe is one which is not killed by an antimicrobial agent after a standard course of treatment (WHO, 1998). Antibiotic resistance is acquired by a natural selection process. Antibiotic use to combat infection, forces bacteria to either adapt or die irrespective of the dosage or time span. The surviving bacteria carry the drug resistance gene, which can then be transferred either within the species/genus or to other unrelated species (Wise, 1998). Clinical resistance is a complex phenomenon and its manifestation is dependent on the type of bacterium, the site of infection, distribution of antibiotic in the body, concentration of the antibiotic at the site of infection and the immune status of the patient (Hawkey, 1998).

Antibiotic resistance is a global problem. While several pathogenic bacteria are resistant to first line broad spectrum antibiotics, new resistant strains have resulted from the introduction of new drugs (Kunin, 1993, Sack *et al,* 1997, Rahal *et* al, 1997, Hoge, 1998). Penicillin resistant pneumococci initially isolated in Australia and Papua New Guinea is now distributed worldwide (Hansman *et al,* 1974, Hart and Kariuki, 1998). Similarly, multi-drug resistant *Salmonella typhi* was first reported in 1987 and has now been isolated throughout the Indian sub-continent, south-east Asia and sub-Saharan Africa. (Mirza *et al,* 1996) Komolafe *et al* (2003) demonstrated a general broad-spectrum resistance to panels of antibiotics in 20% of the bacterial isolates of burns patients. Multi -drug resistant tuberculosis poses the greatest threat to public health in the new millennium (Kraig, 1998).

2. Molecular epidemiology of resistance genes

Antibiotic resistance in bacteria may be intrinsic or acquired. Intrinsic resistance mechanisms are naturally occurring traits due to the genetic constitution of the organism.

These inherited properties of a particular species are due to lack of either the antimicrobial target site or accessibility to the target site (Schwarz *et al,* 1995). For example, obligate anaerobes are resistant to aminoglycosides as they lack the electron transport system essential for their uptake (Rasmussen, 1997). Gram -negative organisms are resistant to macrolides and certain ß-lactam antibiotics as the drugs are too hydrophobic to traverse the outer bacterial membrane (Nikaido, 1989). Acquired resistance is a trait that is observed when a bacterium previously sensitive to an antibiotic, displays resistance either by mutation or acquisition of DNA or a combination of the two (Tomasz and Munaz, 1995). The methods of acquiring antibiotic resistance are as follows:

- **Spontaneous mutations** - Spontaneous mutations or growth dependent mutations, that occur due to replication errors or incorrect repair of damaged DNA in actively dividing cells may be responsible for generating antibiotic resistance (Krasovec and Jerman, 2003). Point mutations that not only produce antibiotic resistance, but also permit growth are attributed to antibiotic resistance (Woodford and Ellington, 2007). For example, the quinolone resistance phenotype in *Escherichia coli* is due to mutations in seven positions in the *gyrA* gene and three positions in the *parC* gene (Hooper, 1999).
  As a bacterial cell has several targets, access and protection pathways for antibiotics, mutations in a variety of genes can result in antibiotic resistance. Studies showed that mutations in the genes encoding the targets of rifamicins and fluoroquinolones, i.e. RpoB and DNA-topoisomerases respectively, results in resistance to the compounds (Martinez and Baquero, 2000; Ruiz, 2003). Adewoye *et al* (2002) reported that mutation in *mexR,* in *P. aeruginosa* resulted in upregulation of the *mexA-mexB-oprM* operon, which was associated with resistance to ß-lactams, fluoroquinolones, tetracyclines, chloramphenicol and macrolides. Expression of antibiotic uptake and efflux systems may be modified by mutations in the regulatory gene sequence or their promoter region (Depardieu *et al.,* 2007; Piddock, 2006). Mutations in the *E. coli* mar gene results in up regulation of AcrAB, involved in the efflux of ß-lactams, fluoroquinolones, tetracyclines, chloramphenicol from the cell (Barbosa and Levy, 2000).
- **Hypermutation** - In the last few years, studies have focussed on the association between hypermutation and antibiotic resistance. In the presence of prolonged, non-lethal antibiotic selective pressure, a small population of bacteria enters a brief state of high mutation rate. When a cell in this 'hyper mutable' state acquires a mutation that relieves the selective pressure, it grows, reproduces and exits the state of high mutation rate. While the trigger to enter the hyper mutable state is unclear, it ahs been suggested that it is dependent on a special SOS -inducible mutator DNA polymerase (pol) IV (Krosovec and Jerman, 2003). Hypermutators have been found in populations of *E. coli, Salmonella enterica, Neisseria meningitidis, Haemophilus influenzae, Staphylococcus aureus, Helicobacter pylori, Streptococcus pneumoniae, P. aeruginosa* with frequencies ranging from 0.1 to above 60% (Denamur *et al.,* 2002; LeClerc *et al.,* 1996). It has been observed that the hypermutators isolated from the laboratory as well as from nature have a defective mismatch repair system (MMR) due to inactivation of the *mutS* or *mutL* genes (Oliver *et al,* 2002). The MMR system eliminates biosynthetic errors in DNA replication, maintains structural integrity of the chromosome and prevents recombination between non-identical DNA sequences (Rayssiguier *et al.,* 1989) Studies have shown that the hypermutators play a significant role in the evolution of antibiotic resistance and may also be responsible for the multiresistant phenotype (Martinez and Baquero, 2000; Giraud *et al.,* 2002; Chopra *et al.,* 2003; Blazquez, 2003, Macia *et al.,* 2005).

- **Adaptive mutagenesis** - Recent studies have demonstrated that in addition to spontaneous mutations, mutations occur in non-dividing or slowly dividing cells in the presence of non-lethal selective pressure. These mutations, known as adaptive mutations, have been associated with the evolution of antibiotic resistant mutants under natural conditions (Krasovec and Jerman, 2003; Taddei *et al.*, 1997; Bjedov *et al.*, 2003). Adaptive mutagenesis is regulated by the stress responsive error prone DNA polymerases V (*umuCD)* and IV (*dinB)* (Rosche and Foster, 2000; Sutton *et al.*, 2000). Piddock and Wise (1997) demonstrated that some antibiotics like quinolones induce a SOS mutagenic response and increase the rate of emergence of resistance in *E.coli.*
- **Horizontal gene transfer** - Transfer of genetic material between bacteria, known as horizontal gene transfer is responsible fro the spread of antibiotic resistance. Resistance genes, consisting of a single or multiple mutations, may be transferred between bacteria by conjugation, transformation or transduction, and are incorporated into the recipient chromosome by recombination. These genes may also be associated with plasmids and/or transposons. Simjee and Gill (1997) demonstrated high level resistance to gentamycin and other aminoglycosides (except streptomycin) in enteroccoci. The resistance gene was found to be associated with narrow and broad host range plasmids. Due to the conjugative nature of the plasmids, spread of the resistance gene to other pathogenic bacteria is likely.
- Horizontal transfer of resistance genes is responsible for the dissemination of multiple drug resistance. Gene cassettes are the smallest mobile genetic entities that carry distinct resistance determinants for various classes of antibiotics. Integrons are DNA elements, located on the bacterial chromosome or on broad host range plasmids, with the ability to capture one or more gene cassettes within the same attachment site. Movement of the integron facilitates transfer of the cassette-associated resistance genes from one DNA replicon to another. When an integron is incorporated into a broad host range plasmid, horizontal transfer of the resistance gene may take place. A plasmid with a pre-existing resistance gene cassette can acquire additional resistance gene cassettes from donor plasmids, thereby resulting in multiresistance integrons (Rowe-Magnus and Mazel, 1999; Ploy *et al.*, 2000). Over 40 gene cassettes and three distinct classes of integrons have been identified (Boucher *et al.*, 2007). Dzidic and Bedekovic (2003) investigated the role of horizontal gene transfer in the emergence of multidrug resistance in hospital bacteria and demonstrated the transfer of antibiotic resistance genes between Gram-positive and Gram negative bacilli from the intestine. The fact that bacteria that have been separately evolving for upto 150 million years can exchange DNA, has strong implications with regard to the evolution of antibiotic resistance in bacterial pathogens (Dzidic *et al.*, 2003; Vulic *et al.*, 1997; Normark and Normark, 2002).

3. Mechanisms of resistance

The mechanisms that bacteria exhibit to protect themselves form antibiotic action can be classified into the following types. Table 1 gives an overview of representative antibiotics and their mechanisms of resistance.

- **Antibiotic inactivation** - Inactivation of antibiotic could be a result of either inhibition of activation *in vivo* or due to modification of the parent antibiotic compound, resulting in loss of activity. Loss of enzymes involved in drug activation is a relatively new mechanism of drug resistance. Studies have demonstrated that mutations in the *nfsA* and *nfsB* genes, which encode cellular reductases that reduce members of the nitrofuran family (nitrofurantion, nitrofurazone, nitrofurazolidone, etc.), are associated with nitrofuran resistance (Kumar and Jayaraman, 1991; Zenno *et al.*, 1996; Whiteway *et al.*, 1998).

β-lactamase enzymes cleave the four membered β-lactam ring of antibiotic like penicillin and cephalosporin, thereby rendering the antibiotic inactive. The large number of β-lactamases identified have been classified based on their structure and function. (Bush *et al.*, 1995). The enzymes discovered early (the TEM-1, TEM-2 and SHV-1 β-lactamases) were capable of inactivating penicillin but not cephalosporin. However, subsequent variants with a variety of amino acid substitutions in and around their active sites were identified in many resistant organisms. These have been collectively called 'extended spectrum β-lactamases (ESBLs)' and act on later generation β-lactam antibiotics (Bradford, 2001).

While most of the ESBLs are derivatives of the early enzymes, newer families of ESBLs, like cefotaximases (CTM-X enzymes) and carbapenemases have been discovered recently (Bonnet, 2004; Walther-Ramussen, 2004; Canton and Coque, 2006, Livermore and Woodford, 2000; Nordman and Poirel, 2002; Queenan and Bush, 2007). The CTM-X genes are believed to have descended from progenitor genes present in *Klyuvera* spp. (Decousser *et al.*, 2001; Poirel *et al.*, 2002; Humeniuk *et al.*, 2002). These ESBLs pose a significant threat as they provide resistance against a broad antibacterial spectrum (Bradford, 2001).

Enzymatic acetylation of chloramphenicol is the most common mechanism by which pathogens acquire resistance to the antibiotic (Schwarz *et al.*, 2004). Mosher *et al.* (1995) established that O-phosphorylation of chloramphenicol affords resistance in *Streptomyces venezuelae* ISP 5230.

While the resistance to aminoglycosides due to inhibition of drug uptake in Gram negative organisms is well documented, aminoglycoside inactivating enzymes have been detected in many bacteria and plasmids. The presence of multiple NH_2 and OH groups enables inactivation of aminglycosides. Inactivation occurs through acylation of NH_2 groups and either phosphorylation or adenylation of the OH groups. (Azucena and Mobashery, 2001) Doi and Arakawa (2007) reported a plasmid-mediated mechanism of aminoglycoside resistance involving methylation of 16S ribosomal RNA.

Fluroquinolones (ciprofloxacin, norfloxacin, ofloxacin) inhibit DNA replication by targeting the enzymes, DNA gyrase and topoisomerase IV. Fluoroquinolone resistance occurs either through mutations in the genes coding for the subunits of DNA gyrase (*gyrA* and *gyrB*) and topoisomeraseIV (*parC* and *parE*), drug efflux, or a combination of both mechanisms. (Levy, 1992; Nikaido, 1996; Li and Nikaido, 2004; Ruiz, 2003; Oyamada *et al.*, 2006). However, Robiscek *et al* (2006) and Park *et al* (2006) demonstrated that a gene encoding an aminoglycoside-specific acetylase could mutate further to give an enzyme which could inactivate fluoroquinolones. This is an example to show that genes encoding minor and perhaps unrecognized activities, besides the major activity, could mutate further to gain extended activity and could be selected by appropriate selection pressures.

Type A and type B streptogramins bind to the 50S ribosomal subunit and inhibit translation (Wright, 2007). Resistance to type A streptogramin has been found to be mediated by an enzyme called VatD (virginiamycin acetyl transferase) acetylates the antibiotic (Seoane and Garcia-Lobo, 2000; Suganito and Roderick, 2002). Resistance to type B streptogramin is brought about by the product of the *vgb* gene, a C–O lyase (Mukhtar *et al.*, 2001). Homologues and orthologues of the genes encoding both the enzymes have been detected in a variety of nonpathogenic bacteria, environmental bacteria and plasmids (Wright, 2007).

- **Exclusion from the internal environment** - Alterations in permeability of the outer membrane of bacteria confers antibiotic resistance. This is commonly observed in Gram negative bacteria, such as *Pseudomonas aeruginosa* and *Bacteroides fragilis*. Reports have suggested that the loss or modification of, which are non-specific protein channels spanning the outer membrane, have resulted in antibiotic resistance. (Nikaido, 1989)

  Activation of efflux pump, which pump out the antibiotics that enter the cells thereby preventing intracellular accumulation, is also responsible for antibiotic resistance. (Nikaido, 1996; Li and Nikaido, 2004). The AcrAB/TolC system in *E. coli* is the best studied efflux system. The inner membrane protein, Acr B, and outer membrane protein, Tol C are linked by the periplasmic protein, Acr A. When activated, the linker protein is folds upon itself thereby, bringing the Acr B and Tol C proteins in close contact. This results in a channel from inside to the outside of the cell, through which antibiotics are pumped out. In antibiotic-sensitive cells, by the product of *acrR* gene, represses the AcrAB/TolC system. A mutation in *acrR*, causing an arg45cys change, activates expression of the system and consequent drug efflux. (Webber *et al*, 2005). Figure 1 shows the AcrAB/TolC efflux system in *E.coli*.

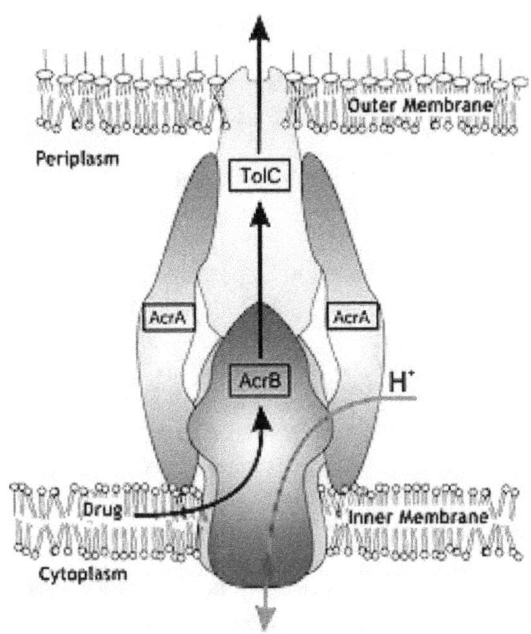

Fig. 1. Efflux system in E. coli (AcrAB/TolC) system (Pos, 2009)

Nine proton-dependent efflux pumps have been identified in *E. coli* so far. These cause the efflux of multiple antibiotics leading to multidrug resistance (Viveiros *et al.*, 2007). Ruiz (2003) demonstrated that although fluoroquinolone resistance occurred commonly due to target mutations, efflux mechanisms were also responsible for the phenomenon.

- **Target alteration** - Structural changes in the target site of the antibiotic prevent interaction of the antibiotic and its target, thus inhibiting the biological activity of the antibiotic. This is exemplified by penicillin resistance due to penicillin binding proteins (PBPs). PBPs are trans-peptidases which catalyse the crosslinking reaction between two peptides each linked to *N*-acetyl-muramic acid residues of the peptidoglycan backbone of the cell wall. Penicillin and other antibiotics which are structurally similar to the cross-linked dipeptide forma stable covalent complex with PBPs, inhibit the crosslinking reaction, resulting in weakening and lysis of the cell. Mutational changes in PBPs, which result in reduction in the affinity of PBPs to penicillin, over expression of endogenous, low-affinity PBPs encoding genes result in penicillin resistance (Zapun *et al.*, 2008).

  Vancomycin binds non-covalently to the cell-wall precursors of Gram-positive bacteria. The binding, which occurs through a set of five hydrogen bonds between the antibiotic and the *N*-acyl-D-ala–D-ala dipeptide portion of the stem pentapeptides linked to the *N*-acetyl muramic acid backbone, blocks the crosslinking transpeptidase reaction catalysed by the PBPs. As a result the cell walls are less rigid and more susceptible to lysis. In vancomycin-resistant organisms, the stem peptides terminate in D-lactate as against D-alanine in the sensitive strains. This eliminates the formation of the crucial hydrogen bond and results in a 1000-fold decrease in the affinity for vancomycin and consequent resistance to the same. This process is regulated by a two-component regulatory system involving a set of five genes (*vanR, vanS, vanH, vanA* and *vanX*). *Enterococci* as well as *Staphylococcus aureus* have been shown to acquire resistance to vancomycin by this mechanism, known as vancomycin evasion. (Walsh *et al.*, 1996; Arthur *et al.*, 1996; Courvalin, 2006)

  Ruiz (2003) reported that the eight amino acid substitutions in *gyrA* , which have been attributed to fluroquinolone resistance, are predominantly located in the quinolone resistance determining region (QRDR). Rifampicin resistance due to mutation in *rpoB*, the gene encoding the (R)-subunit of RNA polymerase has been observed in rifampicin resistant strains of Mycobacterium *tuberculosis,* laboratory strains of *E. coli,* other pathogens and non pathogens (Jin and Gross, 1988; Anbry-Damon *et al.*, 1998; Padayachee and Klugman, 1999; Somoskovi *et al.*, 2001).
- **Production of alternative target** - Bacteria may protect themselves from antibiotics, by production of an alternative target resistant to inhibition along with the original sensitive target. The alternative target circumvents the effect of the antibiotic and enables survival of the bacteria. In methicillin resistant *Staphylococcus aureus* (MRSA) alternative penicillin binding protein (PBP2a) is produced in addition to penicillin binding protein (PBP). As PBP2a is not inhibited by antibiotics the cell continues to synthesise peptidoglycan and has a structurally sound cell wall. It has been suggested that the evolution of vancomycin resistant enterococci may lead to transfer of genes to *S. aureus* resulting in vancomycin resistant MRSA (Michel and Gutmann, 1997).

Antibiotic Category	Examples	Mode of action	Major mechanisms of resistance
ß-lactams	Penicillin, Cephalosporin, Cetoximes, Carbapenems	Inhibition of cell wall synthesis	Cleavage by ß-lactamases, ESBLs, CTX-mases, Carbapenemases, altered PBPs
Aminoglycosides	Streptomycin, Gentamycin, Tobramycin, Amikacin	Inhibition of protein synthesis	Enzymatic modification, efflux, ribosomal mutations, 16S rRNA methylation
Quinolones	Ciprofloxacin, Ofloxacin, Norfloxacin	Inhibition of DNA	Efflux, modification, target mutations
Glycopeptides	Vancomycin	Inhibition of cell wall synthesis	Altered cell walls, efflux
Tetracyclines	Tetracycline	Inhibition of translation	Efflux
Rifamycins	Rifampicin	Inhibition of transcription	Altered ß-subunit of RNA polymerase
Streptogramins	Virginamycins, Quinupristin, Dalfoprisitin	Inhibition of cell wall synthesis	Enzymatic cleavage, modification, efflux
Oxazolidinones	Linezolid	Inhibition of formation of 70S ribosomal complex	Mutations in 23 S rRNA genes follwed by gene conversion.

Table 1. Representative antibiotics and their mechanisms of resistance. Adapted from Jayaraman, 2009

4. Conclusion

Emergence of antibiotic resistance is driven by repeated exposure of bacteria to antibiotics and access of bacteria to a large antimicrobial resistance pool. Pathogenic and non-pathogenic bacteria are becoming increasingly resistant to conventional antibiotics. While initial studies on antibiotic resistance investigated methicillin resistant *Staphylococcus aureus* and vancomycin resistant *Enterococcus spp.,* the focus has now shifted to multi drug resistant Gram -negative bacteria. The emergence of Gram negative *Enterobacteriaceae* resistant to carbapenem due to New Delhi metallo - ß -lactamase 1 (NDM-1) has been identified as a major global health problem. (Kumarasamy *et al,* 2010). However, it must be noted that resistance selected in non pathogenic or commensal bacteria could act as a reservoir of resistance genes, resulting in emergence of resistance in pathogens. There is a need to review the use and check the misuse of antibiotics and to adopt good infection control practices in order to control antibacterial resistance, since increasing antibiotic resistance has the potential to transport clinical medicine to the pre-antibiotic era.

5. References

Adewoye L, Sutherland A, Srikumar R and Poole K (2002). The *mexR* repressor of the mexAB-oprM multidrug efflux operon in *Pseudomonas aeruginosa*: Characterization of mutations compromising activity. *J. Bacteriol.* 184, 4308–4312.

Anbry-Damon H, Housy CJ and Courvalin P (1998) Characterisation of mutations in *rpo* B that confer rifampicin resistance in *Staphylococcus aureus. Antimicrob. Agents Chemother.* 42, 2590–2594

Arthur M, Reynolds PE, Depardieu F, Evers S, Dutka-Malen S, Quintillani Jr R and Courvalin P (1996) Mechanisms of glycopeptide resistance in enterococci. *J. Infect.* 32, 11–16.

Azucena E and Mobashery S (2001) Aminoglycoside-modifying enzymes: mechanisms of catalytic processes and inhibition. *Drug Res. Updates.* 4, 106–117.

Baldry, P. (1976). The battle against bacteria - a fresh look. Cambridge University Press; pp 156.

Barbosa TM and Levy SB (2000) Differential expression of over 60 chromosomal genes in *Escherichia coli* by constitutive expression of MarA. *J. Bacteriol.* 182, 3467–3474.

Bjedov I, Tenaillon O, Gerard B, Souza V, Denamur E, Radman M, Taddei F and Matic I (2003) Stress-induced mutagenesis in bacteria. *Science.* 300, 1404–1409.

Blazquez J (2003) Hypermutation as a factor contributing to the acquisition of antimicrobial resistance, *Clin. Infect. Dis.* 37, 1201–1209.

Bonnet R (2004) Growing group of extended spectrum β-lactamases: the CTX-M enzymes. *Antimicrob. Agents Chemother.* 48, 1–14.

Boucher Y, Labbate M, Koenig JE and Stokes HW (2007) Integrons: Mobilizable platforms that promote genetic diversity in bacteria. *Trends Microbiol.* 15, 301–309.

Bradford PA (2001) Extended spectrum β-lactamases (ESBL) in the 21st century: Characterisation, epidemiology and detection of this important resistance threat. *Clin. Microbiol. Rev.* 48, 933–951.

Bush K, Jacoby GA and Medeiros AA (1995) A functional classification of β-lactamases and its correlation with molecular structure. *Antimicrob. Agents Chemother.* 39, 1211–1233.

Canton R and Coque TM (2006) The CTX-M β-lactamase pandemic. *Curr. Opin. Microbiol.* 9, 466–475.

Chopra I, O'Neill AJ and Miller K (2003) The role of mutators in the emergence of antibiotic-resistant bacteria. *Drug Resist. Update.* 6, 137–145.

Courvalin P (2006) Vancomycin resistance in Gram-positive cocci. *Clin. Infect. Dis.* (*Suppl. 1*). 42, 25–34

Decousser JW, Poirel L and Nordman P (2001) Characterisation of chromosomally encoded, extended spectrum class 4, β-lactamase from *Kluyvera cryocrescens. Antimicrob. Agents Chemother.* 45, 3595–3598.

Denamur E, Bonacorsi S, Giraud A, Duriez P, Hilali F, Amorin C, Bingen E, Andremont A, Picard B, Taddei F and Matic I (2002) High frequency of mutator strains among human uropathogenic *Escherichia coli* isolates. *J. Bacteriol.* 184, 605–609

Depardieu F, Podglajen I, Leclercq R, Collatz E and Courvalin P (2007) Modes and modulations of antibiotic resistance gene expression. *Clin. Microbiol. Rev.* 20, 79–114.

Doi Y and Arakawa Y (2007) 16S ribosomal RNA methylation: emerging resistance mechanism against amino glycosides. *Clin. Infect. Dis.* 45, 88–94.

Dzidic S, Bacun-Druzina V and Petranovic M (2003) The role of mismatch repair in bacterial evolution. *Food Technol. Biotechnol.* 41, 177–182.

Dzidic S and Bedekovic V (2003) Horizontal gene transfer-emerging multidrug resistance in hospital bacteria. *Acta Pharmacol. Sin.* 24, 519–226.

Giraud A, Matic I, Radman M, Fons M and Taddei F (2002) Mutator bacteria as a risk factor in treatment of infectious diseases. *Antimicrob. Agents Chemother.* 46, 863–865

Hansman, D., Devitt, L., Miles, H. Riley, J. (1974). Pneumococci relatively unsusceptible to penicillin in Australia and New Guniea. *Medical Journal of Australia*; 2: 353 - 356.

Hart, C.A. and Kariuki, S. (1998). Antimicrobial resistance in developing countries. *British Medical Journal*; 317: 647 - 650.

Hawkey, P.M. (1998). The origins and the molecular basis of antibiotic resistance. *British Medical Journal*; 317: 657 - 660.

Hoge, C.W., Gambel, J.M., Srijan, A *et al.* (19980. Trends in antibiotic resistance among diarrheal pathogens isolated in Tailand over 15 years. *Clin. Infect. Disease,* 26: 341 - 345.

Hooper DC (1999) Mechanisms of fluoroquinolone resistance. *Drug Resist. Update.*, 2, 38–55.

Humeniuk C, Arlet G and Gautier V (2002) β-Lactamases of *Kluyvera ascorbita,* probable progenitors of some plasmid-encoded CTX-M types. *Antimicrob. Agents Chemother.* 46, 3045–3049.

Jayaraman R. (2009) Antibiotic resitance: an overview of mechanisms and a paradigm shift. *Current Science,* 96(11): 1475 - 1484.

Jin D and Gross C (1988) Mapping and sequencing of mutations in the *Escherichia coli rpo* B gene that lead to rifampicin resistance. *J. Mol. Biol.* 202, 45–58.

Komolafe, O.O. (2003) Antibiotic resistance in bacteria- an emerging public health problem. *Malawi Medical Journal,* 15(2): 63 - 67.

Kraig, E. (1998) Facing the microbial threat. *British Medical Journal,* 317 - 620.

Krasovec R and Jerman I (2003) Bacterial multicellularity as a possible source of antibiotic resistance. *Med. Hypotheses.* 60, 484–488.

Kumar AN and Jayaraman R (1991) Molecular cloning, characterization and expression of nitrofuran reductase gene of *Escherichia coli. J. Biosci.* 16, 145–159.

Kumarasamy KK, Toleman MA, Walsh TR, Bagaria J, Butt F, Balakrishnan R *et al.* (2010). Emergence of a new antibiotic resistance mechanism in India, Pakistan and the UK: a molecular, biological and epidemiological study. *Lancet;*

Kunin, C.M. (1993) Resistance to antimicrobial drugs - a worldwide calamity. *Annals of Internal Medicine,*118: 557 - 561.

LeClerc JE, Li B, Payne WL and Cebula TA (1996) High mutation frequencies among *Escherichia coli* and *Salmonella* pathogens. *Science.* 274, 1208–1211.

Li X and Nikaido H (2004) Efflux-mediated drug resistance in bacteria. *Drugs.* 64, 159–204.

Livermore DM and Woodford N (2000) Carbapenemases: a problem in waiting? *Curr. Opin. Microbiol.* 3, 489–495

Macia MD, Blanquer D, Togores B, Sauleda J, Perez JL and Oliver A (2005) Hypermutation is a key factor in development of multiple-antimicrobial resistance in *Pseudomonas aeruginosa* strains causing chronic lung infections. *Antimicrob. Agents Chemother.* 49, 3382–3386.

Martinez JL and Baquero F (2000) Mutation frequencies and antibiotic resistance. *Antimicrob. Agents Chemother.* 44, 1771–1777.

Matic I (2003) Stress-induced mutagenesis in bacteria. *Science.* 300, 1404–1409.

Michel M, Guttmann L (1997). Methicillin-resistant *Staphylococcus aureus* and vancomycin resistant enterococci: therapeutic realties and possibilities. *Lancet,* 349: 1901 - 1906

Mirza, S.H., Beeching, N.J., Hart, C.A. (1996) Multi-drug resistant typhoid: a global problem. *Journal of Medical Microbiology,* 44: 317 - 319.

Mosher RH, Camp DJ, Yang K, Brown MP, Shaw WV and Vining LC (1995) Inactivation of chloramphenicol by Ophosphorylation: A novel mechanism of chloramphenicol resistance in *Streptomyces venezuelae* ISP 5230, a CAM producer. *J. Biol. Chem.* 270, 27000–27006.

Mukhtar TA, Koteva KP, Hughes DW and Wright GD (2001) Vgb from *Staphylococcus aureus* inactivates streptogramin B antibiotics by an elimination mechanism, not hydrolysis. *Biochem.* 40, 8877–8886.

Nikaido, H. (1989) Outer membrane barrier as a mechanism of antimicrobial resistance. *Antimicrobial Agents and Chemotherapy,* 33: 1831 - 1836.

Nikaido H (1996) Multidrug efflux pumps of Gram-negative bacteria. *J. Bacteriol.* 178, 5853–5869.

Nordman P and Poirel L (2002) Emerging carbapenemases in Gramnegative aerobes. *Clin. Microbiol. Infect.* 8, 321–331.

Normark BH and Normark S (2002) Evolution and spread of antibiotic resistance. *J. Intern. Med.* 252, 91–106.

Oyamada Y, Ito H, Inoue M and Yamagashi J (2006) Topoisomerase mutations and efflux are associated with fluoroquinolone resistance in *Enterococcus faecalis. J. Med. Microbiol.* 55, 1395–1401.

Padayachee T and Klugman KP (1999) Molecular basis of rifampicin resistance in *Staphylococcus aureus. Antimicrob. Agents Chemother.* 43, 2361–2365.

Park CH, Robiscek A, Jacoby GA, Sahm D and Hooper DC (2006) Prevalence in the United States of a aac (6')-Ib-Cr encoding a ciprofloxacine modifying enzyme. *Antimicrob. Agents Chemother.* 50, 3953–3955.

Piddock LJ and Wise R (1987) Induction of the SOS response in *Escherichia coli* by 4-quinolone antimicrobial agents. *FEMS Microbiol. Lett.* 41, 289–294.

Ploy MC, Lambert T, Couty JP and Denis F (2000) Integrons: An antibiotic resistance gene capture and expression system. *Clin. Chem. Lab. Med.* 38, 483–487.

Poirel L, Kampfer P and Nordman P (2002) Chromosome encoded ambler class A β-lactamase of *Kluyvera georgiana,* a probable progenitor of a sub-group of extended spectrum β-lactamases. *Antimicrob. Agents Chemother.* 46, 4038–4040.

Pos KM (2009) Drug transport mechanism of the AcrB efflux pump. *Biochim Biophys Acta* 1794, 782-793.

Queenan AM and Bush K (2007) Carbapenemases: the versatile β-lactamases. *Clin. Microbiol. Rev.* 20, 440–458.

Rahal, K., Wang, F., Schindler, J *et al.* (1997). Reports on surveillance of antimicrobial resistance on individual countries. *Clin Infect. Disease,* 24(1): S69 - S 75.

Rasmussen, B.A., Bush, K., Tally, F.P. 1997. Antimicrobial resistance in anaerobes. *Clin Infect. Disease;* 24: S110- S120.

Rayssiguier C, Thaler DS and Radman M (1989) The barrier to recombination between *Escherichia coli* and *Salmonella typhimurium* is disrupted in mismatch-repair mutants. *Nature.* 342, 396–401.

Robiscek A *et al.* (2006) Fluoroquinolone-modifying enzyme: a new adaptation of a common aminoglycoside acetyl transferase. *Nature Med.* 12, 83–88.

Rosche WA and Foster P (2000) Mutation under stress: Adaptive mutation in *Escherichia coli.* In: *Bacterial stress responses,* G. Storz, R. Hengge-Aronis (Eds.), ASM press, Washington DC, USA.

Rowe-Magnus DA and Mazel D (1999) Resistance gene capture. *Curr. Opin. Microbiol.* 2, 483–488.

Ruiz J (2003) Mechanisms of resistance to quinolones: Target alteration, decrease accumulation and gyrase protection. *J. Antimicrob. Chemother.* 51, 1109–1117.

Sack, R.B., Rahman, M., Yunus, M., Khan, E.H. 1997. Antimicrobial resistance in organisms casuing diarrhoeal disease. *Clin. Infect. Disease;* 24(1): S102- S105.

Schwarz, S., Werckenthin, C., Pinter, L. *et al.* (1995) Chloramphenicol resistance in *Staphylococcus intermedius* from a single veterinary centre: Evidence for plasmid and chromosomal location of the resistance genes. *Veterinary Microbiology,,* 43: 151- 159.

Schwarz S, Kehrenberg C, Doublet B and Clockaart A (2004) Molecular basis of bacterial resistance to chloramphenicol and florphenicol. *FEMS Microbiol. Rev.* 28, 519–542.

Seoane A and Garcia-Lobo JM (2000) Identification of a streptogramin A acetyl transferase gene in the chromosome of *Yersinia enterocolitica. Antimicrob. Agents Chemother.* 45, 905–909.

Simjee S and Gill MJ (1997) Gene transfer, gentamicin resistance and *enterococci. J. Hosp. Infect.* 36, 249–259.

Somoskovi A, Parsons LM and Salfinger M (2001) The molecular basis of resistance to isoniazid, rifampin and pyrazinamide in *Mycobacterium tuberculosis. Respir. Res.* 2, 164–168.

Suganito M and Roderick SL (2002) Crystal structure of Vat D: an acetyl transferase that inactivates streptogramin A group of antibiotics. *Biochem.* 41, 2209–2216.

Sutton MD, Smith BT, Godoy VG and Walker GC (2000) The SOS response: Recent insights into *umuDC*-dependent mutagenesis and DNA damage tolerance, *Annu. Rev. Genet.* 34, 479–497.

Taddei F, Radman M, Maynard-Smith J, Toupance B, Gouyon PH, Godelle B (1997) Role of mutator alleles in adaptive evolution. *Nature.* 387, 700–702.

Tomasz, A., Munaz, R. 1995. ß-lactam antibiotic resistance in Gram-positive bacteria pathogens of upper respiratory tract: a brief overview of mechanism. *Microbial Drug Resistance;* 1:103 - 109

Viveiros M, Dupont M, Rodrigues L, Davin-Regli A, Martin M, Pages J and Amaral J (2007) Antibiotic stress, genetic response and altered permeability of *E. coli. PLoS One.* 2, e365.

Vulic M, Dionisio F, Taddei F and Radman M (1997) Molecular keys to speciation: DNA polymorphism and the control of genetic exchange in enterobacteria. *Proc. Natl. Acad. Sci. USA. 94* (1997) 9763–9767.

Walsh CT, Fisher SL, Park IS, Proholad M and Wu Z (1996) Bacterial resistance to vancomycin: five genes and one missing hydrogen bond tell the story. *Chem. Biol.* 3, 21–26.

Walther-Ramussen J and Hoiby N (2004) Cefotaximases (CTXMases), an extended family of extended spectrum β-lactamases. *Can. J. Microbiol.* 50, 137–165.

Whiteway J, Koziraz P, Veall J, Sandhu N, Kumar P and Hoecher B (1998) Oxygen insensitive nitroreductases: analysis of the roles of *nfs* A and *nfs* B in development of resistance to 5- nitrofuran derivatives in *Escherichia coli. J. Bacteriol.* 180, 5529–5539.

WHO fact sheet, Antimicrobial resistance, 1998; No. 194.

Wise, R. 1998. Antimicrobial resistance is a major threat to public health (Editorial). *British Medical Journal,;*

Wright GD (2007) The antibiotic resistome: the nexus of chemical and genetic diversity. *Nature Rev. Microbiol.* 5, 175–186.

Woodford N and Ellington MJ (2007) The emergence of antibiotic resistance by mutation. *Clin. Microbiol. Infect.* 13, 5–18.

Zapun A, Conters-Martel C and Vernet T (2008) Penicillin-binding proteins and β-lactam resistance. *FEMS Micribiol. Rev.* 32, 361–385.

Zenno S, Koike H, Kumar AN, Jayaraman R, Tanokura M and Saigo K (1996) Biochemical characterisation of Nfs A, the *Escherichia coli* major nitroreductase exhibiting a high amino acid sequence homology to Frp, a *Vibrio harveyi* flavin oxidoreductase. *J. Bacteriol.* 178, 4508–4514.

2

Antibiotic Resistance in Nursing Homes

Giorgio Ricci[1], Lucia Maria Barrionuevo[1], Paola Cosso[1],
Patrizia Pagliari[1] and Aladar Bruno Ianes[2]
[1]*Residenza Sanitaria Assistenziale Villa San Clemente, Segesta Group Korian, Villasanta (MB)*
[2]*Medical Direction, Segesta Group Korian, Milan*
Italy

1. Introduction

Until early 20th century, infectious diseases were primarily responsible for mortality in the United States; the average life expectancy were 47 years (US Department of Health and Human Services [DHHS], 1985).

The advent of antiseptic techniques, vaccinations, antibiotics and other public health measures, raised life expectancy. In the early 21st century life expectancy has risen to 76 to 80 years in most developed nations (Center for Diseases Control and Prevention, 2003). Therefore, it is estimated that, by the year 2030, in the United States, 70 million persons will be over 65 years old. (National Nursing Home Week, 2005)

This epidemiologic transition has shifted the burden of morbidity from infections and acute illness to chronic diseases and degenerative illness. (Centers for Diseases Control and Prevention, 2003)

Therefore, with multiple comorbid diseases, many older persons develop functional decline and dependency requiring institutionalization in nursing homes (Juthani-Mehta & Quagliariello, 2010). Nowadays there are over 16000 nursing homes in United States and approximately 1.5 million Americans reside in nursing homes. By 2050 the number of Americans requiring long-term care is expected to double, and this trend is expected in all developed nations (Jones AL & Al, 2009).

The patient population and environment of the nursing home, provide a milieu that permits the development of infections and promote transmission of infectious agents (Nicolle LE & Al, 2001; Juthani-Mehta M & Quagliariello VJ, 2010). This is because nursing home residents have a number of risk factors, including age-associated immunological changes (High K, 2007; van Duin D 2007a, 2007b), organ systems changes, multiple comorbid diseases (e.g dementias, diabetes mellitus, cardio-vascular diseases, chronic obstructive pulmonary disease, impaired dentition) (Bettelli G, 2011), and degenerative disease requiring the insertion of prosthetic devices (e.g. joint prostheses, implantable cardiac devices) that lead to frailty and disability with a high impact on development of infections (Jackson ML & Al, 2004; Curns AT & Al, 2005; Fry AM & Al, 2005).

1.1 Immunosenescence

A functional immune system is considered vital for the host's continued survival against onslaught of pathogens. In humans, as well as in many other species, it is becoming recognized that the immune system declines with age (immunosenescence), which leads to a higher incidence of infections, cancers and autoimmune diseases (Pawelec G, 1999). Immunosenescence involves both the host's capacity to respond to infections and the development of long-term immune memory, especially by vaccination (Muszkat M & Al, 2003; Aspinall R & Al, 2007; Jackson MI & Al, 2008; Boog CJP, 2009), therefore it is considered a major contributory factor to the increased frequency of morbidity and mortality among the elderly (Ginaldi, L & Al, 2001)

Immunosenescence is a multifactorial condition leading to many pathologically significant health problems in the aged population. Some of the age-dependent biological changes that contribute to the onset of immunosenescence are listed in Table 1.

Cells	Biological Changes	References
Hematopoietic stem cells	↓ Self-renewal capacity	Ito K & Al, 2004
Phagocytes	↓ Total number, ↓ Bactericidal activity	Lord JM & Al, 2001; Strout, R.D & Suttles J, 2005
Natural Killer (NK)	↓ Cytotoxicity	Bruunsgaard H & Al, 2001; Mocchegiani E & Malavolta M, 2004
Dendritic Cells	↓ Antigen-Presenting function	Uyemura K, 2002
B- lymphocytes	↓ Antibodies production ↑ AutoAntibodies	Han S & Al, 2003
Naïve lymphocytes	↓ Production	Hakim FT & Gress RE, 2007
Memory cells	↓ Functional competence	Ginaldi L & Al, 2001
Macrophages	Disregulation	Cambier J, 2005
Thymus	↓ Epithelial volume	Aspinall R & Andrew D, 2000
Thymocytes (i.e. premature T-cells)	Reduction/Exhausion on the number	Min H & Al, 2004
Lymphokines	↓ Production (e.g. IL-2)	Murciano C & Al, 2006; Voehringer D & Al, 2002; Ouyang Q & Al, 2003
T-cell receptor (TcR)	Shrinkage of antigen-recognition repertoire diversity	Naylor K & Al, 2005; Weng NP, 2006
Response to Antigenic stimulation	Impaired proliferation of T-cells	Murciano C & Al, 2006; Naylor K & Al, 2005; Weng NP, 2006; Voehringer DM & Al, 2006
Memory & Effector T-cells	Accumulation and Clonal expansion	Franceschi C & Al, 1999; Voehringer DM & Al, 2006
Changes in cytokine profile	e.g. ↑ Pro-inflammatory cytokines milieu	Suderkotter C & Kalden H, 1997

Table 1. Age-dependent biological changes of immunosenescence

At a glance, Hematopoietic stem cells (HSC), which provide the regulated lifelong supply of leukocyte progenitors that are in turn able to differentiate into a diversity of specialized immune cells (including lymphocytes, antigen-presenting dendritic cells and phagocytes) diminish in their self-renewal capacity. This is due to the accumulation of oxidative damage to DNA by aging and cellular metabolic activity and the shortening of telomeric terminals of chromosomes (Ito K & Al, 2004). There is a decline in the total number of phagocytes in aged hosts, coupled with an intrinsic reduction of their bactericidal activity (Lord JM & Al, 2001; Strout, R.D & Suttles J, 2005).

The cytotoxicity of Natural Killer (NK) cells and the antigen-presenting function of dendritic cells is known to diminish with old age (Bruunsgaard H & Al, 2001; Mocchegiani E & Malavolta M, 2004); the age-associated impairment of dendritic Antigen Presenting Cells (APCs) has profound implications as this translates into a deficiency in cell-mediated immunity and thus, the inability for effector T-lymphocytes to modulate an adaptive immune response (Uyemura K, 2002). There is a decline in humoral immunity caused by a reduction in the population of antibody producing B-cells along with a smaller immunoglobulin diversity and affinity (Han S & Al, 2003)

As age advances, there is a decline in both the production of new naive lymphocytes (Hakim FT & Gress RE, 2007), and the functional competence of memory cell populations, with increased frequency and severity of diseases such as cancer, chronic inflammatory disorders and autoimmunity (Ginaldi L & Al, 2001) .

A problem of infections in the elderly is that they frequently present with non-specific signs and symptoms, and clues of focal infection are often absent or obscured by underlying chronic conditions (Ginaldi L & Al, 2001). Ultimately, this provides problems in diagnosis and subsequently, treatment. In addition to changes in immune responses, the beneficial effects of inflammation devoted to the neutralisation of dangerous and harmful agents, early in life and in adulthood, become detrimental late in life in a period largely not foreseen by evolution, according to the antagonistic pleiotropy theory of aging (Franceschi C & Al, 2000a). It should be further noted that changes in the lymphoid compartment is not solely responsible for the malfunctioning of the immune system in the elderly. Although myeloid cell production does not seem to decline with age, macrophages become dysregulated as a consequence of environmental changes (Cambier J, 2005). The functional capacity of T-cells is most influenced by the effects of aging: the age-related alterations are evident in all stages of T-cell development, making them a significant factor in the development of immunosenescence (Linton P & Al, 2006). After birth, the decline of T-cell function begins with the progressive involution of the thymus, which is the organ essential for T-cell maturation following the migration of precursor cells from the bone marrow. This age-associated decrease of thymic epithelial volume results in a reduction/exhausion on the number of thymocytes (i.e. pre-mature T-cells), thus reducing output of peripheral naïve T-cells (Aspinall R & Andrew D, 2000; Min H & Al, 2004).

Once matured and circulating throughout the peripheral system, T-cells still undergo deleterious age-dependent changes. Together with the age-related thymic involution and the consequent age-related decrease of thymic output of new T cells, this situation leaves the body practically devoid of virgin T cells, which makes the body more prone to a variety of infectious and non-infectious diseases. (Franceschi C & Al 2000b)

T-cell components associated with immunosenescence include: deregulation of intracellular signal transduction capabilities (Fulop T & Al, 1999), diminished capacity to produce effector lymphokines (Murciano C & Al, 2006; Voehringer D & Al, 2002; Ouyang Q & Al, 2003), shrinkage of antigen-recognition repertoire of T-cell receptor (TcR) diversity (Naylor K & Al, 2005; Weng NP, 2006), cytotoxic activity of Natural Killer T-cells (NKTs) decreases (Mocchegiani E & Malavolta M, 2004), impaired proliferation in response to antigenic stimulation (Murciano C & Al, 2006; Naylor K & Al, 2005; Weng NP, 2006; Voehringer DM & Al, 2006), the accumulation and the clonal expansion of memory and effector T-cells (Franceschi C & Al, 1999; Voehringer DM & Al, 2006), hampered immune defenses against viral pathogens, especially by cytotoxic CD8+ T cells (Ouyang, Q & Al, 2003) and changes in cytokine profile e.g. increased pro-inflammatory cytokines milieu present in the elderly (Suderkotter C & Kalden H, 1997).

1.2 Organ system and aging

Alterations in organ systems occur with normal aging, and many of these physiologic alterations contribute to the development of infections (Vergese A & Berk S, 1990; Smith PW, 1994) (Table 2)

System	Aging changes
Skin	Epidermal thinning (Ghadially R & Al, 1995), ↓ elasticity, ↓ subcutaneous tissue, ↓ vascularity (Norman RA, 2003; Gilchrest BA, 1999)
Respiratory	↓ cough reflex, ↓ mucociliary transport, ↓ elastic tissue (Mittman C & Al, 1965), ↑ IgA/IgM in bronchoalveolar lavage and ↑ CD4+/CD8* lymphocytes (Meyer KC & Al, 1996) , ↓ antioxidant levels in epithelial lining fluid (Kelly FJ & Al, 2003)
Gastrointestinal	↓ motility, ↓ gastric acidity (Hall KE & Wiley JW, 1998)
Urinary	↓ urine osmolarity, ↑ perineal-vaginal colonization (women) (Farage MA & Maibach HI, 2011) ↑ prostate size and ↓ prostate secretion (men) (Nickel JC, 2003)

Table 2. Physiologic organ systems changes in the elderly

Although generally efficient defenses against infections are associated with the immune systems, many other elements have an important role.

Epithelia from skin, bladder, the bronchial and the digestive system, for a physical barrier and thereby play a key part in preventing bacteria from invading the human body (Ben-Yehuda A & Weksler ME, 1992). In particular, the skin changes, associated with aging lead to delayed wound healing (Ghadially R & Al, 1995).

Changes in respiratory tract function increase the likehood of aspiration and pneumonia. Apart for a decrease in immune function, various mechanisms are likely to contribute to the pneumonia risk of the elderly: blunting of protective reflexes in the airway, seen after stroke but also a part of normal ageing (Yamaya M & Al, 1991), decreased in mucociliary clearance (Incalzi RA & Al, 1989), loss of local immunity (decreased T-cell subsets and immunoglobulin in respiratory secretions) (Meyer KC, 2001).

Alterations in gastrointestinal tract physiology (e.g. decreased mobility and gastric acidity, decreased intestinal mobility, modifications of resident intestinal flora and intestinal mucus) increase the likelihood of infection after ingestion of a potential pathogen (Ben-Yehuda A & Weksler ME, 1992; Klontz KC & Al, 1997)

Moreover, the urinary tract is more vulnerable to infections in both elderly men and women even in absence of other diseases. Factors contributing to this vulnerability include mechanical changes (reduction in bladder capacity, uninhibited contractions, decreased urinary flow rate and post-void residual urine), urothelial change (enhanced bacterial adherence), prostatic hypertrophy in men (Ben-Yehuda A & Weksler ME, 1992) and hormonal changes (lack of estrogen in post menopausal women) (Yoshikawa TT & Al, 1996)

1.3 Chronic diseases and comorbility

The nursing home population has a high frequency if chronic diseases, many of which increase the likelihood of infections. These chronic diseases are often the major factor necessitating institutional care (Ouslander J, 1989; Hing F & Bloom B, 1990; Van Rensbergen G & Nawrot T, 2010). The most frequent diagnosed underlying chronic diseases include

dementia and neurologic diseases (Banaszak-Koll & Al, 2004; Bowman C & Al, 2004; Van Rensbergen G & Nawrot T, 2010), peripheral diseases (Chong WF & Al, 2011), cerebrovascular diseases (Bowman C & Al, 2004; Van Rensbergen G & Nawrot T, 2010; Chong WF & Al, 2011), chronic pulmonary conditions (Mc Nabney MK & Al, 2007; Van Rensbergen G & Nawrot T, 2010), hearth diseases (Chan KM & Al, 1998; Van Rensbergen G & Nawrot T, 2010; Chong WF & Al, 2011). The prevalence of diabetes mellitus varies from 10 to 30 per cent in the nursing home population (Garibaldi RA & Al, 1981; Nicolle LE & Al, 1984; Ahmed A & Al, 2003; Valiyeva E & Al, 2006; Mc Nabney MK & Al, 2007; IKED Report, 2007; Van Rensbergen G & Nawrot T, 2010).

Comorbidities contribute to the high frequency of infections in nursing homes because the high risk profile of nursing homes residents (Jette AM & Al, 1992): demented residents often have neurogenic bladder and inability to empty the bladder that results in an increased frequency of urinary tract infections (Nicolle LE, 2000; 2002). Patients with peripheral vascular disease have an high risk for skin and soft tissue infections because the impaired vascular supply to extremities and peripheral edema (Sieggreen MY & Kline RA, 2004; Ely JW & Al; 2006). Patients with chronic obstructive pulmonary disease are likely to have bacterial colonization of tracheobronchial tree and recurrent bronchopulmonary infections (Marin A & Al, 2010). Moreover, patients with diabetes mellitus, have increased prevalence of infections (Shah BR & Hux JE, 2003; Bertoni AG & Al, 2001): pneumonia (Valdez R & Al, 1999; Tan JS, 2000), lower urinary tract infections and pyelonephritis (Zhanel GG & Al, 1995; Stamm WE & Hooton TM, 1993), soft tissue infections, including the "diabetic foot", necrotizing fasciitis and mucocutaneous Candida infections (Votey SR & Peters Al, 2005; Fridkin SK & Al, 2005; Miller LG & Al, 2005). Others infections such as invasive (malignant) otitis externa, rhinocerebral mucormycosis (Durand M & Joseph M, 2005; Earhart KC, Baugh WP, 2005) and emphysematous infections (cholecystitis and pyelonephritis) (Votey SR & Al, 2005) occur almost exclusively in diabetics. The optimal management of infections in nursing homes residents includes ensuring optimal therapy of these associated diseases.

1.4 Functional impairment

Disability, functional dependence and deteriorating cognitive performance are strong predictors of nursing home admission among older adults (Jette AM & Al, 1992; Pourat N, 1995; Krauss NA & Altmann, 2004; Miller SC & Al, 1998; Gaugler JE & Al, 2007). On the other hand the chronic diseases affecting the elderly nursing home residents, lead to functional impairment and dependency in activity of daily living (Bajekal M , 2002; Flacker JM & Kiely DK, 2003; Sutcliffe C & Al, 2007; Andresen M & Puggaard L, 2009; Jones AL & Al, 2009).

Poor functional status in nursing home residents has been reported to be associated with increased occurrence of infections and high mortality rate (Curns AT & Al 2005; Jackson ML & Al, 2008; Juthani-Mehta M & Quagliariello VJ, 2010). Chair and bed-bound residents are at risk of pressure ulcers (Galvin J, 2002; Henoch I & Gustaffson M, 2003; Pressure Ulcer Advisory Panel/European Pressure Ulcer Advisory Panel Pressure Ulcer Prevention and Treatment Clinical Practice Guideline, 2009; Jankowski IM; 2010). Urinary incontinence is common, affecting as many as 50% of residents in nursing home and approaches to the management of incontinence (including indwelling bladder catheters and external collecting devices for elderly men), increase the incidence of urinary infections (Gammack JK, 2003; Richards CL. 2004; Eriksen HM & Al, 2007; Ricci G & Al, 2010). Fecal incontinence is also associated with an higher risk of urinary infection (Topinkovà E & Al, 1997;) and both urinary and fecal incontinence may contribute to extensive environmental contamination with pathogens and antimicrobial agent-resistant bacteria (Schnelle JF & Al, 1997; Leung FW & Schnelle JF, 2008; Pagliari P & Al, 2011).

1.5 Nutrition and malnutrition

There are a number of studies that document that 10 to 50% of nursing home residents are malnourished (Donini LM & Al, 2000; Saletti A & Al, 2000; Omran ML & Morley JE, 2000; Nakamura H & Al, 2006; Pauly L & Al, 2007). Over 50% of nursing home residents have reported to suffer from protein caloric malnutrition (Nakamura H & Al, 2006; Ordòñez J & Al, 2010). Vitamin, zinc and micronutrients deficiencies are also reported (Mandal SK & Ray AK, 1987; Girodon F & Al, 1997; Bates CJ & Al, 1999a; 1999b; Gosney MA & Al, 2008). The reasons for this high frequency of malnutrition might be comorbidities (Boström AM & Al, 2011; Shahin ES & Al, 2010), feeding difficulties (Hildebrandt GH & Al, 1997; Lamy M & Al, 1999; Lelovics Z, 2009; Chang CC & Roberts BL, 2011), impaired cognition (Blandford G & Al, 1998; Magri et Al, 2003; Bartholomeyczik S & Al, 2010; Boström AM & Al, 2011), bacterial overgrowth of the small bowel (e.g. Escherichia coli or anaerobic organisms) leading to malabsorption (Mc Evoy AJ & Al, 1983; Elphick HL & Al, 2006; Ziegler TR & Cole R, 2011) and poorer clinical outcomes (Kaganski N & Al, 2005; Stratton RJ & Al, 2006) .

1.6 Invasive devices

Because of multiple comorbidities and disabilities, nursing home residents are more likely to require invasive medical devices (e.g. indwelling urinary catheter, percutaneous and naso-gastric feeding tube, tracheostomy, intravenous catheter and cardiac device). Feeding tubes are present from 7 to 41% of cognitive impaired nursing homes residents and urinary catheterization rate range from 11 to 12%. (Warren JI & Al, 1989; Juthani-Mehta M & Quagliariello VJ, 2010)

Moreover the use of some devices, including tracheostomies and intravenous catheters, is increasing in the nursing homes, reflecting the increasing level of impairment among elderly patients admitted to these facilities.

Device use has been associated with both colonization and infection with antibiotic resistant organisms in nursing home residents (Mody L & Al, 2007; 2008; Rogers MA & Al, 2008; L, & Al, 2008; 2010): from 5 to 10% of nursing home residents have long-term indwelling urinary catheters with associated persistent polymicrobial bacteriuria, urinary tract infections (Warren JW & Al, 1982; Beck-Sague C & Al, 1993; Garibaldi RA, 1999; Ha US & Cho YH,

2006; Regal RE & Al, 2006;) and their complications (Ouslander J & Al, 1987; Warren JW & Al 1987; 1988), while enteral feeding solution given to patients with nasogastric and percutaneous feeding tubes, may be contaminated with bacteria of the family of Enterobacteriaceae, including Serratia spp and Enterobacter spp. (Freedland CP & Al, 1989; Greenow JE & Al, 1989). Moreover, nasogastric tubes have been reported to be associated with a greater occurrence of aspiration pneumonia (Fay DE & Al, 1991) which is one of factor promoting the use of percutaneous gastric or jejunal feeding tubes with subsequent complication of stomal site infections, peritonitis (Luman W & Al, 2001) and risk of developing Clostridium difficile antibiotic-associated diarrhea (AAD) (Asha NJ & Al, 2006).

Finally, intravenous peripheral line, peripherally inserted central catheter, tracheostomy and suprapubic urinary catheter are other commonly used devices in nursing home with an increasingly risk of developing sepsis, pneumonia, skin infections, soft tissue infections (Tsan L & Al, 2008). Device use has therefore associated with repeated courses of antimicrobial therapy foster the emergence of resistant pathogens. (Rogers MA & Al, 2008)

1.7 Drugs use in elderly nursing homes residents

Residents in nursing homes often have a complex and complicated illness profile ranging from simultaneous occurrence of several chronic diseases, depression, pain, sleep problems and dementia with the psychiatric and behavioral symptoms (Selbaek G & Al, 2007; Ricci G & Al, 2009) . Thus "polypharmacy" is the norm in nursing home population. The average nursing home resident receives from 5 to 10 different medications at any time (Beers MH & Al, 1992; Furniss L & Al, 1998; Doshi JA & Al, 2005; Kersten H & Al, 2009). Some of these medications may increase the likelihood of infections: atypical antipsychotics may impair consciousness and increase the frequency of aspiration (Knol W & Al, 2008; Gau JT & Al, 2010); H2 blockers and protonic pump inhibitors (PPI) lead to decreased gastric acidity and may contribute to increased gastrointestinal infections (Laheij RI & Al; 2004; Gulmez SE & Al, 2007;Eom CS & Al 2011; Laria A & Al, 2011). Oral and inhaled glucocorticoid therapy are associated with an increased dose-dependent risk of infections (Ernst P & Al, 2007; Calverley PM & Al, 2007; Kardos P & Al, 2007; Drummond MB & Al, 2008; Singh S & Al, 2009; Smitten AL, & Al 2008; Dixon WG & Al, 2011).

2. Management of infections in nursing homes

Clinical criteria used in the diagnosis and surveillance for infections in nursing homes, have generally been developed from observations in younger population with limited comorbidities. It was not until 2000 that the multifaceted nature of the evaluation of patients in long-term care facilities has led the Society for Healthcare Epidemiology of America and the American Geriatric Society to participation, review and support the Guidelines concerning the multidimensional assessment as part of the infectious disease evaluation in an older adult. (Bentley DW & Al, 2000; Kinsella K & Velkoff, VA , 2001; High KP & Al, 2005; Centre for Diseases Control and Prevention, 2003)

These guidelines are specifically intended to apply to older adult nursing home residents of the potential heterogeneity of conditions present in these facilities residents, suggests that the recommendations are intended to assist with the management of the majority of residents: older adults with multiple comorbidities and functional disabilities.

2.1 Clinical presentation of infections

Presentation of infections in nursing home residents are sometimes atypical (McGeer A & Al, 1991; Norman D & Toledo S, 1992; High K & Al, 2009). Several factors contribute to the difficulty of establishing a clinical diagnosis in these patients. Hearing and cognition are often impaired in nursing home patients: symptoms may not be expressed or correctly interpreted by caregivers. Chronic clinical conditions may obscure the sign of infection leading to misinterpretation or overlooking symptoms. For instance, urinary incontinence may mask symptoms of urinary infection, or congestive heart failure may mask symptoms of pulmonary infection. The presence of coexisting diseases such as chronic bronchitis, which may mask acute pneumonia, or rheumatoid arthritis, which can confound the presence of septic arthritis, may compound difficulties in making the diagnosis of infection. (Cantrell M & Norman DC, 2010)

Altered physiologic responses to infection, or for the manner to any acute illness, are due to man factors including the decremental biologic changes of normal aging, which may be exacerbated by lifestyle. For example, age-related changes in chest wall expansion and lung tissue elasticity, which may be made worse by smoking, contribute to a diminished cough reflex. A weakened cough has the double negative effect of contributing to a decline in pulmonary host defenses and making the diagnosis of respiratory infection more difficult.

Another example of an altered physiologic response to infection in older persons that deserves special mention is the often-observed blunted fever response (Harper C & Newton P, 1989; Wasserman M & Al, 1989; Norman D & Toledo S, 1992; Norman D & Yoshikawa TT, 1996) and increased frequency of afebrile infection (Gleckman B & Hibert D, 1982; Meyers B & Al, 1989)

Although fever is the cardinal sign of infection, the traditional definition of fever (oral temperature of 38° to 38.3°C) may not be sensitive enough to diagnose infection in elderly patients. Castle SC & Al (1991) found that, in a nursing home population, baseline body temperatures are approximately 0.5°C below those of a normal young person and that with infection, despite a rise in temperature comparable to that seen in the young, the maximum temperature may be below the traditional definition of fever. However, a temperature of 37.8°C coupled with a decline in functional status is highly indicative of infection in this population. (Castle SC & Al, 1991)

The presence or absence of fever—aside from facilitating or inhibiting the diagnosis of infection—has other implications. The presence of fever (as defined by an oral temperature of 38.3°C) is highly specific for the presence of a serious, usually bacterial, infection (Keating MJ III, & Al, 1984; Wasserman M & Al, 1989). Moreover, when the syndrome of fever of unknown origin (FUO) occurs in elderly persons, it typically signifies a treatable condition such as intra-abdominal infection, infective endocarditis, temporal arteritis, or other rheumatologic condition. (Knockaert DC & Al, 1993; Berland B & Gleckman RA, 1992).

A blunted fever response to infection frequently portends a poor prognosis (Weinstein MP & Al, 1983).

This may be relevant to the mounting evidence that fever may play an important role in host defenses (Kluger MJ & Al, 1996; Norman D & Yoshikawa TT, 1996). The peripheral leukocyte count in bacterial infection is not as high as that observed for younger population and leukocytosis is often absent. (Werner H & Kuntsche J, 2000). So, the elevation of acute phase protein may be a more reliable marker of infection than elevation of erythrocyte sedimentation rate.

In summary, an acute infection in the elderly may present with either typical clinical manifestations or subtle findings.

Signs and symptoms pointing to a specific organ system infection may be lacking. Thus, an infection should be sought in any elderly person with an unexplained acute to subacute (days to weeks) decline in functional status, falls, delirium, anorexia, weakness, disorientation (Gavazzi G, Krause KH, 2002)

2.2 Antimicrobial agent use in nursing homes

Antimicrobials agents are among the most frequently prescribed pharmaceutical agents in nursing homes; the account for approximately 40% of all systemic drugs used (Crossley K & Al, 1987; Wayne SJ & Al, 1992). It is estimated that two to four million courses of antibiotics are prescribed for residents of US nursing homes annually (Strausbaugh LJ & Joseph CL, 2000) . As a result, from 50 to 70% of residents receive at least one systemic antimicrobial agent during 1 year (Montgomery P & Al, 1995) and the prevalence of systemic antibiotic use is reported to be 8% (Crossley K & Al, 1987; Jacobson C & Strausbaugh LJ, 1990; Warren JW & Al, 1991; Montgomery P & Al, 1995; Lee YL & Al, 1996; Mylotte JM, 1996; Loeb M & Al, 2001a). In a 9-month surveillance study in a nursing home care unit (Jacobson C & Strausbaugh LJ, 1990), 51% of the 321 study patients received antimicrobial agents at some time during their stay. More than one agent was prescribed for 30% of these patients. In addition as many as 30% of nursing home residents receive at least one prescription for a topical antimicrobial agent each year (Yakabowich MR & Al, 1994; Montgomery P & Al, 1995).

A substantial proportion of antimicrobial treatment in nursing homes is considered inappropriate: from 30 to 75% of systemic antimicrobial agents (Zimmer JG & Al, 1986; Crossley K & Al 1987; Jones SR & Al, 1987; Katz PR & Al, 1990; Warren JW & Al, 1991; Yakabowich MR & Al, 1994; Pickering TD & Al, 1994; Montgomery P & Al, 1995) and up to 60% of topical antimicrobial agents (Montgomery P & Al, 1995) are inappropriately used.

The inappropriate use of antibiotics, especially in frail elderly nursing home residents, can be burdensome and harmful (Morrison RR & Al, 1998). From a broader public health perspective, antimicrobial use is the primary factor leading to the emergence of antimicrobial-resistant bacteria. Antibiotic resistance among bacteria implicated in the most common infections is rising exponentially throughout the word (D'Agata E & Mitchell SL, 2008). Infections caused by antimicrobial-resistant bacteria are associated with up to 5 times higher mortality rates and lead to more frequent and prolonged hospitalization compared with infections caused by antimicrobial-susceptible bacteria (Carmeli Y & Al, 2002; Cosgrove SE & Al, 2002; 2005). These issues are relevant for older patients who arbor relatively high of antimicrobial-resistant bacteria, and in nursing homes, where antimicrobials are the most frequently prescribed pharmaceutical agents (Crossley K & Al 1987; Warren JW & Al, 1991; Flamm RK & Al, 2004)

3. Infections in nursing homes

Infections are a frequent occurrence in nursing homes. The most important aspects are represented by endemic infections, epidemics and infections with resistant organisms

3.1 Endemic infections

The most frequent endemic infections are respiratory tract, urinary tract, skin and soft tissue, and gastrointestinal infections (primarily manifesting as diarrhea) (Strausbaugh LJ & Joseph CJ, 1999).

3.1.1 Occurrence of endemic infections

In United States nursing homes, 1.6 to 3,8 million infections occur (Strausbaugh LJ & Al, 2000). These infections are largely endemic and have an overall infection rate that ranges from 1,8 to 13,5 infections per 1000 resident care days (Strausbaugh LJ & Al, 2000). The variability of prevalence (Cohen E & Al, 1979; Garibaldi R & Al, 1981; Standfast SJ & Al, 1984; Setia U & Al, 1985; Scheckler W & Peterson P, 1986; Alvarez S & Al, 1988; Magaziner J & Al, 1991; Steinmiller A & Al, 1991; Eikelenboom-Boskamp A & Al, 2011) and incidence (Magnussen M & Robb S, 1980; Farber BF & Al, 1984; Nicolle LE & Al, 1984; Franson T & Al, 1986; Scheckler W & Peterson P, 1986; Viahov D & Al, 1987; Alvarez S & Al, 1988; Schicker JM & Al, 1988; Hoffman N & Al, 1990; Jacobson C & Strausbaugh LJ, 1990; Darnowsky S & Al, 1991; Jackson M & Al, 1992) rate of infections, reflects differences in patients populations in different study institutions, as well as differing surveillance definitions and methods for case ascertainment .

Many of these reports are from Veteran Administration facilities, where over 90% of the population are male and, thus, non representative of the general nursing home population, in which only 20 to 30% are male. The most frequent infections identified are usually respiratory tract infections, varying in rate from 0.46 to 4.4 per 1000 resident days. In most reports, this includes both upper and lower respiratory infections, because the difficulties in distinguishing the two diagnoses on the basis of clinical criteria alone (Cohen E & Al, 1979; Garibaldi R & Al, 1981; Standfast SJ & Al, 1984; Scheckler W & Peterson P, 1986; Magaziner J & Al, 1991). (Table 3)

The reported incidence of symptomatic urinary infections varies from 0,1 to 2,4 per 1000 resident days. (Nicolle LE, 2000)

The influence of different surveillance definition is notable in reports of incidence of febrile urinary infections. Symptomatic urinary infection may be defined permissively as a positive urine culture in a patient with fever and no other apparent source or, restrictively as a positive urine culture in a patient with fever and acute symptoms referable to the urinary tract (Schaeffer AJ & Schaeffer EM, 2007; High K & Al, 2009). Report using the permissive definition overestimate the occurrence of febrile urinary infection, while those using the restrictive definition certainly underestimate the incidence.

The clinical and economic impact of endemic infections in the nursing home residents is difficult to define, because these patients are highly chronic impaired, and additional morbidity from intercurrent infection is difficult to measure. Moreover, in case of fully dependent, non communicative, demented resident, mortality may not be considered an undesiderable outcome. Similarly, the prolongation of institutionalization may also not be meaningful as a measure of morbidity or cost in these permanently institutionalized elderly residents.

Reference	Incidence per 1000 resident days				
	All infections	Respiratory	Urinary	Skin & soft tissue	Gastrointest inal tract
Magnussen M & Robb S, 1980	3.4	0.46	2.4	0.3	0
Alvarez S & Al, 1988	2.7	0.7	1.2	0.5	Not stated
Nicolle LE & Al, 1984	4.1	1.8	0.1	1.0	0.9
Farber BF & Al, 1984	6.7	3.2	1.8	0.1	0
Franson T & Al, 1986	4.6	1.0	2.3	1.0	Not stated
Scheckler W & Peterson P, 1986	3.6	1.3	1.6	0.5	0.04
Vlahov D & Al, 1987	3.6	1.1	1.2	0.2	0.7
Schicker JM & Al, 1988	5.4	2.0	1.9	0.7	0.24
Jacobson C & Strausbaugh L, 1990	2.6	0.9	1.0	0.45	0.15
Hoffman N & Al, 1990	4.6	1.0	1.9	0.09	0
Darnowski S & Al, 1991	9.5	4.4	1.5	2.1	Not stated
Jackson M & Al, 1992	7.1	3.3	1.3	1.8	0.09
Brusaferro S & Moro ML, 2005	4.8	1.8	1.5	0.7	Not stated

Table 3. Incidence of infections in nursing homes (described in published studies)

Indices that may be used as measures of the impact of endemic infections include the volume of antimicrobial agent use (Warren JW & Al, 1982; Crossley K & Al, 1987; Montgomery P & Al, 1995), frequency of transfer to acute-care facilities for management of infection and infection-related mortality. Reports summarizing antimicrobial agent use consistently identify urinary infection as the most frequent diagnosis for which treatment is prescribed, with respiratory infections second in frequency (Zimmer JG & Al, 1986; Crossley K & Al, 1987; Warren JW & Al, 1991; Waine SJ & Al, 1992; Montgomery P & Al, 1995; Bentley DW & Al, 2000).

From 7 to 30% of elderly residents transferred from nursing homes to acute-care institutions, are transferred for management of infections (Irvine P & Al, 1984; Gordon WZ & Al, 1985; Jacobson C & Strausbaugh LJ, 1990; Kerr H & Byrd J, 1991); respiratory and urinary infections are the diagnoses that most commonly require transfer (Irvine P & Al, 1984; Gordon WZ & Al, 1985). One prospective study reported that 6,3% of all infectious episodes in nursing homes were associated with death, or 10,3 deaths per 100 residents per year (Nicolle LE & Al, 1984). However, overall mortality is reported to be similar in residents with and without infection (Jacobson C & Strausbaugh LJ, 1990). The only common infection with a high case/fatality ratio is pneumonia (Ahlbrecht H & Al, 1999). Autopsy series of elderly nursing home residents consistently fail to identify an infection other than pneumonia as an immediate cause of death (Nicolle LE & Al, 1987a; Gross JS & Al, 1988)

3.1.2 Respiratory tract infections

3.1.2.1 Upper respiratory tract infections

Upper respiratory infections in nursing home patients include sinusitis, otitis media, otitis externa and pharyngitis. Generally, the incidence of upper respiratory tract infections is reported to be less than that of lower respiratory tract infections: Scheckler and Peterson (1986) reported 1,1 upper respiratory tract infections per 100 resident months, compared with 1,9 pneumonia and bronchitis. The different clinical syndromes included as upper respiratory tract infections are usually reported as a single group, and the incidence of infection at each side is not known for nursing home residents. Group A streptococcus may cause pharyngitis, but most reports of streptococcal pharyngitis describe relatively uncommon episodes of epidemic infections (Schwartz B & Ussery X, 1992). Overall, these infections seem to have limited impact in the nursing home population.

3.1.2.2 Lower respiratory tract infections

Lower respiratory tract infections, including both pneumonia and bronchitis, are the most important infections occurring in nursing homes in both frequency and clinical consequences (Jackson M & Al, 1992; Beck-Sague C & Al, 1994). Increased aspiration of oropharyngeal contents and impairment pulmonary clearance mechanism resulting from physiologic aging changes, as well chronic pulmonary, cardiovascular and neurologic disease, contribute to the high incidence of pneumonia.

Pneumonia is the only infection that is an important contributor to mortality, in this population, with a reported case/fatality rate of 6 to 23% (Nicolle LE & Al, 1984; Scheckler W & Peterson P, 1986; Jackson M & Al, 1992; Jacobson C & Strausbaugh LJ, 1990).

Studies of the etiologies of nursing home-acquired pneumonia are generally flawed because they rely on expectorated sputum specimens to define bacteriology, and sputum specimens cannot differentiate oropharyngeal colonization from pulmonary infection.

Invasive methods to estabilish an etiologic cause (transtracheal or transthoracic aspiration, bronchoscopy) are infrequently performed in nursing home population. Bacteriemia occurs in less than 25% of cases, even if it would allow the identification of the causative agent.

With this limitations, streptococcus pneumoniae, remains the most important pathogen (Phair J & Al, 1978; Bentley DW, 1984; Farber BF & Al, 1984; Marrie TJ & Al, 1986; Peterson PK & Al, 1988). (Table 4)

Patients with chronic obstructive pulmonary disease have an increased frequency of bronchopneumonia, associated with Haemophilus influenzae and Moraxella catarrhalis. There is an increased occurrence of Gram-negative organism such Klebsiella pneumonia in the nursing home relative to other populations.

In at least one study in which specimen for culture were obtained through transtracheal aspiration, 37% of episodes were reported to have mixed respiratory flora (Bentley DW, 1984). Atypical pathogens such as Chlamydia pneumonia, Mycoplasma pneumonia and Legionella pneumophila may cause pneumonia in nursing home residents, but appear to be relatively infrequent.

Bacteria (percentage of total isolates)	Garb J & Al, 1978 (n=47)	Marrie TJ & Al, 1986 (n=12)	Peterson PK & Al, 1988 (n=129)	Bentley DW, 1984 (n=115)	Phillips SL & Brahaman-Phillips MA, 1993 (n=92)	Lim WS & Macfarlane JT, 2001 (n=22)	El-Sohl AA & Al, 2002 (n=21)	El-Sohl AA & Al, 2004 (n=93)	Carratala J & Al, 2007 (n=126)	Kothe H & Al, 2008 (n=1349)	Shindo Y & Al, 2009 (n= 141)
Streptococcus pneumoniae	19	17	30	32	34	55	0.04	25	27.8	43.3	13.5
Klebsiella pneumoniae	30	25	7.5	-	2.2	-	0.04	-	-	-	7.1
Hemophilus influentiae	4.3	-	23	5.2	23	-	-	-	11.9	3.4	-
Enterobacter spp	11	8.3	-	-	1.1	-	24	28	-	-	-
Escherichia coli	6.4	17	13	-	6.5	-	-	-	2.4	-	3.5
Serratia marcescens	4.3	-	-	-	-	-	-	-	-	-	-
Pseudomonas aeruginosa	4.3	-	2.5	-	6.5	-	14	-	1.6	-	5.7
Citrobacter spp	2.1	-	2.5	-	2.2	-	-	-	-	-	-
Proteus spp	-	-	2.5	-	2.2	-	-	-	-	-	2.8
Branhamella catarrhalis	-	-	13	-	4.3	-	-	-	-	-	-
Other Gram-	-	-	-	17	6.5	22	-	-	6.4	7.1	2.8
Staphylococcus aureus	19	8.3	7.5	1.7	12	-	33	31	2.4	2.2	9.9
Mixed	-	25	-	43	-	-	38	5	-	20.9	20.3

Table 4. Bacteria reported in published studies as a etiologic agents in subjects with nursing home-acquired pneumonia

3.1.2.3 Tuberculosis

The occurrence of Mycobacterium tuberculosis is variable among different institutions, although it is an important cause of infection in some nursing homes (Stead W, 1981; Stead W & Al, 1985; Brennen C & Al, 1988; Bentley DW, 1990a).

The prevalence of positive tuberculin skin test in nursing home residents has been reported to vary from 21 to 35% (Stead W & Al, 1985; Welty C & Al, 1985; Perez-Stable EJ & Al, 1988).

While active tuberculosis in nursing home residents is usually due to reactivation of latent infection, primary infection or reinfection may occur following exposure to an infectious case (Bentley DW, 1990a). Stead W (1985) reported that residents with negative skin test on admission to nursing homes, had a 5% year conversion rate in a home with a known infectious case, while the rate was 3,5% year in a home without a known case.

About 10% of skin test convertors who did not receive prophylactic isoniazid therapy developed active infection.

When an infectious case occurs, delay in diagnosis due to preexisting chronic pulmonary symptoms, or delay in obtaining a chest radiography, may lead to prolonged, extensive exposure of other residents and staff.

3.1.3 Urinary tract infections

3.1.3.1 Symptomatic urinary infections

In most survey the leading infection in nursing homes and in long-term care facilities is urinary tract infection (Bentley DW & Al, 2000; Philip W & Al, 2008) although with restrictive clinical definitions, symptomatic urinary infection is less frequent than respiratory infection (Stevenson KB & Al, 2005). Bacteriuria is very common in nursing home residents but, by itself, is not associated with adverse outcomes and does not affect survival (Eberle CM & Al 1993; Smith PW, 1985; Nicolle LE & Al, 2005a), therefore practitioners must distinguish symptomatic UTI from asymptomatic bacteriuria in making therapeutic decisions.

Diagnosing urinary tract infection in nursing home residents is problematic. Given the high incidence of asymptomatic bacteriuria and pyuria, a positive urine culture and pyuria on urinalysis are non-diagnostic (Nicolle LE, 2000). Practitioners utilize clinical criteria to differentiate symptomatic urinary tract infection from asymptomatic bacteriuria, but existing clinical criteria were developed by expert consensus (McGeer A & Al, 1991; Philip W & Al, 2008) . The McGeer consensus criteria for urinary tract infection are widely accepted as surveillance and treatment standards (Centers for Medicare and Medicaid (CMS) Manual System, 2005).

For residents without an indwelling catheter, three of the following criteria must be met to identify urinary tract infection : (1) fever ≥38°C; (2) new or increased burning on urination, frequency, or urgency; (3) new flank or suprapubic pain or tenderness; (4) change in character of urine; (5) worsening of mental or functional status (McGeer A & Al, 1991) The Loeb consensus criteria for urinary tract infection are minimum criteria necessary for empiric antibiotic therapy. For residents without an indwelling catheter, criteria include acute dysuria alone or fever (>37.9° or 1.5°C increase above baseline temperature) plus at least one of the following: new or worsening urgency, frequency, supra-pubic pain, gross hematuria, costovertebral angle tenderness, or urinary incontinence. (Loeb M & Al, 2001) The reliability, specifically inter-observer variability, for elements of these consensus criteria has not been determined.

If the typical symptoms of urinary tract infection are dysuria and frequency (cystitis) or fever and flank pain (pyelonephritis), the elderly may present with atypical or non-localizing symptoms. Chronic genitourinary symptoms are also common but are not attributable to bacteriuria (Nicolle LE & Al, 2005a; Ouslander JG & Schnelle JF, 2005). Because the prevalence of bacteriuria is high, a positive urine culture, with or without pyuria, is not sufficient to diagnose urinary infection (Nicolle LE & Al, 2005a). Clinical findings for diagnosis of urinary tract infection in non-catheterized residents must include some localization to the genitourinary tract (Mc Geer & Al, 1991). The diagnosis also requires a positive quantitative urine culture obtained by the clean-catch voided technique, by in and out catheterization, or by aspiration through a catheter system sampling port. A negative test for pyuria or a negative urine culture obtained prior to initiation of antimicrobial therapy, excludes urinary infection, while a positive urine culture is not helpful in defining a urinary source for symptoms. Given these provisos, rates of symptomatic urinary infection of 0,11 to 0,15 per bacteriuric year have been reported in studies with restrictive clinical definition, that require the presence of localizing genitourinary symptoms or signs (Nicolle LE, 1983; 1987). Moreover, symptomatic urinary infection is reported as the diagnosis necessitating transfer from a nursing home to an acute-care facility in 1 to 8% of such transfers (Irvine P, 1984; Gordon WZ, & Al, 1985). The urinary tract is the most common source of bacteriemia in the institutionalized elderly, contributing to over 50% of episodes (Setia U & Al, 1984; Rudman D & Al, 1988; Muder RR & Al, 1992; Nicolle LE & Al, 1994a) with a case/fatality ratio of 16 to 23% (Setia U & Al, 1985; Muder RR & Al, 1992; Nicolle LE & Al, 1994a). The prevalence of indwelling urethral catheters in the nursing homes is 7 to 10% (Ribeiro BJ & Smith SR, 1985; Warren JW & Al, 1989; Kunin CM & Al, 1992). Catheterization predisposes to clinical urinary tract infection and the catheterized urinary tract is the most common source of bacteriemia in nursing homes (Smith PW, 1985; Nicolle LE & Al, 1996). Bacteriemia occurs significantly more frequently in subjects with indwelling urinary catheters (Rudman D & Al, 1988; Muder RR & Al, 1992). Residents with long-time catheters often present with fever alone.

Nursing home residents with indwelling urinary catheters, are uniformly colonized with bacteria, largely attributable to biofilm on the catheter (Warren JW & Al, 1982). These organisms are often more resistant to oral antibiotics than bacteria isolated from elderly persons in the community (Gambert SR & Al, 1982; Daly PB & Al, 1991). Specimen collected through the catheter present for more than few days, reflect biofilm microbiology. For residents with chronic indwelling catheters and symptomatic infections, changing the catheter immediately prior to instituting antimicrobial therapy, allows collection of a bladder specimen, which is a more accurate reflection of infecting organisms (Raz R & Al, 2000). Catheter replacement immediately prior therapy is also associated with more rapid defervescence and lower risk of early symptomatic relapse post-therapy (Raz R & Al, 2000).

Guidelines for prevention of catheter-associated urinary tract infections in hospitalized patients (Wong ES & Hooden TM, 1981), are generally applicable to catheterized nursing home residents (Philip W & Al, 2008). Recommended measures include limiting use of catheters, insertion of catheters aseptically by trained personnel, use of as small diameter a catheter as possible, handwashing before and after catheter manipulation, maintenance of a closed catheter system, avoiding irrigation unless the catheter is obstructed, keeping the collecting bag below the bladder and maintaining good hydration in residents. Urinary catheters coated with antimicrobial materials have the potential to decrease urinary tract infections, but have not been studied in the nursing home setting (Ha US & Cho YH, 2006; Schumm K & Lam TB, 2008). For some residents with impaired voiding, intermittent catheterization is an option, and clean technique is as safe as sterile technique (Duffy LM & Al, 1995). External catheter are also a risk factor for urinary tract infections in male residents (Smith PW & Al, 1991), but are significantly more comfortable and associated with fewer adverse effects, including symptomatic urinary infection, than indwelling catheter (Saint S & Al, 2006). Local external care is required.

The reported microbiology of symptomatic urinary tract infections in nursing homes shows that E. coli in women, and Proteus Mirabilis in men are the most frequently isolated infecting organisms (Nicolle LE & Al, 1987; 1996; Ricci G & Al, 2010). Gram-negative organisms of increased antimicrobial resistance, including Klebsiella pneumoniae, Providencia spp, Morganella morganii, Enterobacter spp, Citrobacter spp and Pseudomonas aeruginosa are frequently isolated (Nicolle LE & Al, 1987; 1996; Ricci G & Al, 2010). Gram-positive organisms, including Enterococcus spp, coagulase-negative Staphylococci, and less frequently, Staphylococcus aureus, are also identified (Ricci G & Al, 2010). (Table 5)

Bacteria (percentage of total isolates)	Grude N & Al, 2001	Mathai D & Al, 2001	Nicolle LE, 2005	Das & Al, 2009	Ricci & Al, 2010
Escherichia coli	56.7%	46.9%	15%	53.6%	55,5%
Proteus Mirabilis	72%	5.0%	42%	14.6%	12.4%
Klebsiella pneumoniae	-	11%	8.2%	13.9%	11.8%
Providencia spp	-	-	22%	3.7%	0.26%
Morganella Morganii	-	-	-	1.5%	0.52%
Enterobacter cloacae	0.9%	-	7.1%	-	3.52%
Citrobacter spp	0.2%	-	-	-	0.26%
Pseudomonas aeruginosa	1.3%	7.5%	27%	2.6%	7.64%
Enterococcus faecalis	7.9%	12.8%	-	4.5%	2.35%
Coagulase-negative Staphylococci	12.5%	3.4%	2.4%	-	-
Staphylococcus aureus	2.2%	-	-	4.1%	-

Table 5. Bacteria reported in published studies as etiologic agents in urinary tract infections

Providentia stuartii, is an organism with a unique proclivity for causing infections in nursing homes (Flerer J & Ekstrom M, 1981; Muder RR & Al, 1992). The major site of isolation of the organism is the urinary tract of patients with long-term indwelling urinary catheters or external urine-collecting devices (Flerer J & Ekstrom M, 1981; Warren JW & Al, 1982). The occurrence of Providencia stuartii is highly variable among different facilities. When present, it is often identified in urine cultures from virtually all patients with long-term indwelling urinary catheters: this observation suggest that cross-infection either through the environment or on the hands of staff members is the major determinant of Providencia stuartii urinary infections in the nursing home setting (Nicolle LE & Al, 1983)

3.1.3.2 Asymptomatic bacteriuria

If the prevalence and the incidence of symptomatic urinary infection is high, the prevalence and the incidence of asymptomatic bacteriuria are also high (Table 6). In a male population from whom monthly urine cultures were obtained, the incidence of new episodes of bacteriuria was 45 per 100 patients/years (Nicolle LE & Al, 1983). In a female population, 1,2 infections per resident/year were identified (Nicolle LE & Al, 1987) and in a 58 month follow up of an Italian nursing home population, the rate of positive urine samples in asymptomatic subjects was higher than 45% (Ricci G & Al, 2010).

Early recurrence of bacteriuria following treatment is the norm, with as many as 50% of men or women experiencing recurrence within 6 weeks of therapy (Nicolle LE & Al, 1983; 1988). The 5 to 10% of nursing home residents managed with long-term indwelling catheters, have a 100% prevalence of asymptomatic bacteriuria, usually with three to five organism isolated at any time (Warren JW & Al, 1982). The reported microbiology of asymptomatic infections is summarized in Table 7 and is similar to that of symptomatic infections.

References	Prevalence (%)
Hedin K & Al, 2002	23
Hassanzadeh P & Motamedifar M, 2007	53
Lin YT & Al, 2007	57.8
Aguirre-Avalos G & Al 1999	24.7
Ouslander JG & Al, 1996	43
del Río G & Al, 1992	38.5
Kaye D & Al, 1989	23.5
Boscia JA, 1986	23.5
Rodhe N & Al 2006	14.8
Ricci G & Al, 2010	46,05

Table 6. The prevalence of asymptomatic bacteriuria (reported in published studies)

Bacteria (percentage of total isolates)	Hedding K & Al, 2002	Rahav G & Al, 2003	Lin YT & Al, 2006	Hassanzadeh P & Motamedifar M 2007	Ricci & Al, 2010
Escherichia coli	67.27	49.0	29.7	45.3	59.2
Proteus Mirabilis	9.09	2.0	-	13.2	14.11
Klebsiella pneumoniae	10.90	2.0	21.6	13.2	7.06
Providencia spp	-	-	16.2	-	-
Morganella Morganii	-	-	-	-	0.61
Enterobacter cloacae	1.81	2.0	-	3.8	0.31
Citrobacter spp	-	1.8	-		0.92
Pseudomonas aeruginosa	-	9.0	13.5	5.7	2.15
Enterococcus faecalis	7.27	8.0	-	-	2.15
Coagulase-neg Staphylococci	-	4.0	-	-	-
Staphylococcus aureus	-	6.0	-	5.7	-

Table 7. Bacteria reported in published studies as etiologic agents in asymptomatic bacteriuria

3.1.4 Skin and soft tissue infections in nursing homes

3.1.4.1 Pressure ulcers

The frequency of pressure ulcers (also termed "decubitus ulcers") in nursing homes patients reflects the quality of nursing home care (Shepard M & Al, 1987; Allman R, 1988). The reported prevalence of pressure ulcers, has varied from 1,6 to up of 20% in different institutions (Michocki RJ & Lamy PP, 1976; Spector WD & Al, 1988; Branders GH & Al, 1990; Young JB & Dobrzanski S, 1992; Nicolle LE & Al, 1994a; Berlowitz DR & Al, 1996; Coleman EA & Al, 2002; Zulkowski K & Al, 2005), with an incidence as high as 10 to 30% patient per year (Berlowitz DR & Wilking SVB, 1989; Branders GH & Al, 1990), and as low as 3,4 to 4,8 episodes per 100000 resident days (Nicolle LE & Al, 1994b). Pressure ulcers are associated with increased mortality (Branders GH & Al, 1990; Livesley NJ & Chow A, 2002; Garcia AD

& Thomas DR, 2006). Infected ulcers are reported to occur from 0,1 to 0,3 episodes per 1000 resident days (Farber BF & Al, 1984; Scheckler W & Peterson P, 1986) or 1,4 per 1000 ulcer days (Nicolle LE & Al, 1994b). Infected pressure ulcers often are deep soft tissue and may have underlying osteomyelitis, cellulitis and bacteremia. Muder RR & Al (1992) reported that 36% of bacteremic skin and soft tissue infections was due to infected decubiti with a case/fatality ratio of 14% for all skin infections, and Livesley NJ & Chow AW (2002) reported that secondary bacteremic infections have a 50% mortality.

Medical factors predisposing to pressure ulcers have been delineated (Berlowitz DR & Wilking SVB, 1989; Garcia AD & Thomas DR, 2006) and include immobility, pressure, friction, shear, moisture, steroids, incontinence, sensory impairment, malnutrition and infections; reduced nursing time can also increase the risk of developing pressure ulcers. Several of these factors may be partially preventable (i.e. malnutrition and fecal incontinence). Prevention of pressure ulcers involves developing a plan for turning, positioning, eliminating focal pressure, reducing shearing forces and keeping skin dry. Attention to nutrition, using disposable briefs and identifying residents at a high risk using prediction tools, can also prevent new pressure ulcers (Smith PW & Al, 2008). The goals are to treat infection, promote wound healing and prevent future ulcers. Many physical and chemical products are now available for the purpose of skin protection, debridement and packing, although controlled study are lacking in the area of pressure ulcer prevention and healing (Lyder CH, 2003) and a variety of products may be also used to relieve or distribute pressure, or to protect the skin (Smith PW & Al, 2008).

Because pressure ulcers, like the skin, are frequently colonized with several different bacteria, antibiotic therapy is not appropriate for a surface swab culture without sign and symptoms of infection (Smith PW & Al, 2008). Surface cultures yield a polymicrobial flora of gram positive and gram negative, aerobic and anaerobic species (Allman R, 1988; Nicolle LE & Al, 1994b). Therefore, surface cultures are not considered reliable to identify infection or, when infection is clinically present, in identify infecting organisms. Non intact skin is more likely to be colonized with pathogens; so some authors obtained positive results for 97% of cultures of superficial swab specimens (Rudelsky B & Al, 1992) even if there were a poor concordance between the different bacterial species identified by biopsy and those identified by aspiration (43% of positive specimens) and swab culture (63% of positive specimens). Another study compared deep-tissue biopsy with aspiration of draining pressure ulcers (Ehrenkranz NJ & Al, 1990). Compared with deep-tissue biopsy, this technique had a sensivity of 93% and a specificity of 99% Ehrenkranz NJ & Al, 1990). Similar species were identified by irrigation-aspiration and deep tissue biopsy. However, aspirates samples of clinically non infected ulcers have also been shown to contain bacteria in 30% of cases (Nicolle LE & Al, 1994b). Culture results must be interpreted with caution, because should not be used as the sole criterion for infections, without clinical or histopathological evidence of infection (Hirshberg J & Al, 2000). Despite the aforementioned information, there is agreement on the most frequently isolated bacteria, including Staphylococcus aureus, beta-Hemolytic Streptococci, Gram negative organisms (including Enterobacteriaceae and Pseudomonas spp, and other Gram positive organisms such Enterococcus spp) and Anaerobic organisms (Chow AW & Al, 1977; Sapico FI & Al, 1986; Muder RR & Al, 1992; Nicolle LE & Al, 1994b; Smith DM & Al, 2010; Lund-Nielsen B & Al, 2011). Colonization with Methicillin-Resistant Staphylococcus Aureus occurs frequently in institutions with

Endemic Methicillin-Resistant Staphylococcus Aureus (Bradley SF & Al, 1991; Strausbaugh LJ & Al, 1991)

3.1.4.2 Cellulitis

Cellulitis (infection of the skin and soft tissue) can occur either at the site of a previous skin break (pressure ulcer) or spontaneously. Skin infections generally are caused by group A Streptococci or Staphylococcus Aureus. However, in cases in which cellulitis is a complication of pressure ulcers or chronic foot ulcers in patients with diabetes or peripheral vascular impairment, infections with other agents, including members of the Enterobacteriaceae, anaerobes or polymicrobial flora are common. Outbreaks of group A streptococcal infections have been described, presenting as cellulitis, pharyngitis, pneumonia or septicemia (Auerbach SB & Al, 1992; Schwartz B & Ussery XT, 1992; Green CM & Al, 2005)

3.1.4.3 Conjunctivitis

Conjunctivitis in the adult presents as ocular pain, redness and discharge. Conjunctivitis has been reported frequently as a common infection in nursing home, but the frequency is variable in different institutions. A prevalence of 0.3 to 3.4% has been reported in different surveys (Garibaldi RA & Al, 1981; Schleckler W & Peterson P, 1986 ; Magaziner J & Al, 1991) while, the incidence of conjunctivitis on different units varied from 0.6 to 3.5 per 1,000 patient-days (Boustcha E & Nicolle LE, 1995). Conjunctivitis occurs more frequently in elderly residents with greater functional impairment (Garibaldi RA & Al, 1981; Boustcha E & Nicolle LE, 1995). It is likely that a high proportion of conjunctivitis cases are noninfectious but are due to irritative, viruses or other factors (Boustcha E & Nicolle LE, 1995). In the nursing homes cases may be sporadic or outbreak-associated (Garibaldi RA & Al, 1981). The batteriology of endemic conjunctivitis is not well studied, but Staphylococcus aureus appears to be the most frequent organism isolated (Boustcha E & Nicolle LE, 1995); infections with upper respiratory flora such as Moraxella catharralis and Haemophilus spp are also reported (Boustcha E & Nicolle LE, 1995). These organisms may be isolated, however, from the conjunctivae of patients without clinical conjunctivitis in the nursing home (Boustcha E & Nicolle LE, 1995). Conjunctivitis has been reported as a clinical presentation for some patients in outbreaks caused by group-A beta-Hemolytic Streptococcus and Methicillin-Resistant Staphylococcus aureus (Center for Disease Control, 1990a; Brennen C & Muder R, 1990). Epidemic conjunctivitis may spread rapidly through the nursing home. Transmission may occur by contaminated eye drops or hand cross contamination. Gloves should be worn for contact with eyes or ocular secretions, with hand hygiene performed immediately after removing gloves (Smith PW & Al, 2008)

3.1.5 Gastrointestinal infections

No surveys have identified either the incidence or the prevalence of infectious diarrhea in non epidemic setting. Most episodes of diarrhea in the nursing home patient are probably noninfectious in origin and are related to the patient's underlying disease, medications (including antibiotics) or diet, especially high protein supplements. Toxigenic Clostridium difficile has been reported to be endemic in some nursing homes (Bentley DW, 1990b; Thomas DB & Al, 1990): the prevalence of Clostridium difficile stool carriage has been reported to be 9 to 26%, with higher rates identified after antibiotic therapy. It is uncertain whether this phenomenon is limited to selected nursing homes or is generalizable. In those nursing homes with a high rates of colonization with endemic Clostridium difficile, most patients are asymptomatic, but carriage may persist for an extended time (Bentley DW, 1990b).

3.1.6 Bacteremia

Bacteremia in the nursing homes, although rarely detected, may be primary or secondary to an infection at another site: the most common source is urinary tract, with Escherichia coli being the culprit in over 50% of cases (Setia U & Al, 1984; Mylotte JM & Al, 2002). The majority of non urinary cases are secondary to skin or soft tissue infections or pneumonia. The incidence of bacteremia is reported to vary widely, from 4 to 39 episodes per 100000 resident days. The reported variation likely reflects differences in patient populations and interventions in different institutions. The case/fatality ratio for bacteremic patients is 21 to 35% (Setia U & Al, 1984; Rudman D & Al, 1988; Muder RR & Al, 1992; Nicolle LE & Al, 1994a) and is consistent with reports of mortality rates in other populations in which similar organisms have been isolated. (Table 8) From 9 to 22% of episodes are polymicrobial, with a soft tissue source most frequently associated with polymicrobial bacteremia.

Bacteria (percentage of total isolates)	Setia U & Al, 1984	Rudman D & Al, 1988	Muder RR & Al, 1992	Nicolle LE & Al, 1994	Siegman-Igra Y & Al, 2002	Mylotte JM & Al, 2002
Staphylococcus aureus	13	9.1	15	10	5	13
Methicillin-resistant S. aureus	-	7	5	-	9	5
Enterococcus spp	3.7	9.1	7.9	3.3	9	9
Coagulase-neg staphylococcus	0.9	-	3.9	-	-	-
ß-hemolitic streptococcus	3.7	-	4.4	6.7	-	-
Streptococcus pneumoniae	0.9	9.1	3.9	13	7	6
Other Gram-positive bacteria	2.8	-	0.5	-	-	-
Escherichia coli	32	15	13	37	24	27
Providencia stuartii	5.6	24	13	-	-	1
Proteus spp	14	18	8.9	10	21	13
Klebsiella pneumoniae	10	-	5.4	6.7	12	3
Pseudomonas aeruginosa	7.4	6.1	3	-	-	3
Morganella morganii	-	-	3.9	-	-	-
Other gram-negative bacteria	1.9	9.1	4.4	3.3	-	-
Anaerobes	3.7	-	-	10	-	-
Mortality (% subjects)	35	21	21	24	35	18

Table 8. Bacteria reported in published studies as etiologic agents in bloodstream infections and mortality rate

In recent years, the acuity of illness in nursing home residents has risen with a most frequent use of central/peripheral venous catheters and an increased of related bacteremic complications. The CDC Guidelines for prevention of intravascular catheter-related infections is a useful resource and generally applicable to nursing homes (O'Grady NO & Al, 2002). Relevant points include aseptic insertion of the intravascular cannula, daily inspection of the intravascular catheter for complications such as phlebitis, and quality control of intravascular fluids and administration sets.

3.2 Outbreaks of bacterial infections in nursing homes

Most of nursing homes infections are sporadic; many are caused by colonizing organism with relatively low virulence. However the nursing home, provides a milieu that is conductive in outbreaks of infectious diseases due to close proximity of susceptible patients in the institutional setting and subsequent cross-transmission of organisms among patients through contact with staff members or environmental contamination. An outbreak or transmission within facility may occur explosively, with many clinical cases appearing within a few days, or may, for example, involve an unusual clustering of Methicillin-Resistant Staphylococcus Aureus clinical isolates on a single nursing unit over several months. On the other hand, a case of Methicillin-Resistant Staphylococcus Aureus infection may follow a prolonged period of asymptomatic colonization after an aspiration event or development of a necrotic wound (Drinka PJ & Al, 2005). Tissue invasion may also be facilitated by the presence of a urinary catheter or chronic wounds. Outbreaks in nursing homes, accounted for a substantial proportion (15%) of reported epidemics (Centers for Disease Control and Prevention, 1989a). Clustering of urinary tracts infections, diarrhea, skin and soft tissue infection, conjunctivitis, and antibiotic resistant bacteriuria have been noted (Strausbaugh, L.J., & Al, 2003). Major outbreak of bacterial infection have also been ascribed to Clostridium difficile (Bentley DW, 1990b; Simor AE & Al, 2002;), Salmonella spp. (Standaert SM & Al, 1994), Escherichia coli (Ryan CA & Al, 1986; Carter AO & Al, 1987), group A Streptococcus (Center for Disease Control, 1990a; Auerbach SB & Al, 1992; Harkness GA & Al, 1992; Schwartz B & Ussery XT, 1992; Arnold KE & Al, 2006), Chlamydia pneumoniae (Troy CJ & Al, 1997; Nakashima K & Al, 2006), Staphylococcus aureus (Bradley SF & Al, 1991; Hsu CCS, 1991) and other pathogens (Table 9).

Nursing homes accounted for 2% of all foodborne disease outbreaks reported to the Centers for Disease Control (1975-1987) and 19% of outbreak associated death (Levine WJ & Al, 1991). Transmissible gastrointestinal pathogens may be introduced to the facility by contaminated food or water or infected individuals. High rate of fecal incontinence, as well as gastric hypochlorhydria, make the nursing home ideal for secondary fecal-oral transmission, underscoring the vulnerability of elderly to infections, as well as the role of cross infection in residents with devices, open wounds or incontinence. In addition, mobile residents with poor hygiene, may interact directly facilitating the spread of infections (Standaert SM & Al, 1994; Musher DM & Al, 2004)

3.2.1 Gastrointestinal infections

Bacterial gastroenteritis (caused by Clostridium difficile, Bacillus cereus, Escherichia coli, Campylobacter spp, Clostridium perfrigens or Salmonella spp) as well as viral and parasitic gastroenteritis are well-known causes of diarrhea outbreaks in nursing homes (Carter OA & Al, 1987; White KE & Al, 1989; Slotwiner-Nie PK & Brandt LI, 2001; Olsen SJ & Al, 2001; Winquist AG & Al, 2001; Simor AF & Al, 2002).

Bacteria	Reference(s)
Staphylococcus aureus	Johnson ET, 1983; Storch GA & Al, 1987; Thomas JC & Al, 1989; Bradley SF & Al, 1991; Hsu CCS, 1991; Levine WJ & Al, 1991; Muder RR, 1991; Strausbaugh LJ & Al, 1991
Group A Streptococcus	Reid RT & Al, 1983; Ruben FC & Al, 1984; Center for Disease Control, 1990a; Auerbach SB & Al, 1992; Harkness GA & Al, 1992; Schwartz B & Ussery XT, 1992; Arnold KE & Al, 2006
Escherichia coli O157:H7	Ryan CA & Al, 1986; Carter AO & Al, 1987
Salmonella spp.	Baine WE & Al, 1973; Levine WJ & Al, 1991; Jackson M, 1992; Standaert SM & Al, 1994
Shigella spp.	Levine WJ & Al, 1991
Bordetella pertussis	Addis DG & Al, 1991
Haemophilus influenzae	Smith PF & Al, 1988
Campylobacter jejuni	Levine WJ & Al, 1991
Aeromonas hydrophila	Bloom H & Bottone E, 1990
Antimicrobial agent-resistant gram-negative bacilli	Shlaes DM & Al, 1986; Rice LB, 1990; John JE & Ribner B 1991; Wingard F & Al, 1993
Clostridium perfrigens	Levine WJ & Al, 1991
Clostridium difficile	Bentley DW, 1984; 1990b; Simor AE & Al, 2002
Bacillus cereus	Levine WJ & Al, 1991
Mycobacterium tuberculosis	Stead W, 1981; Narain JJ & Al, 1985; Bentley D, 1990a; Stead W & Al, 1985
Chlamydia pneumoniae	Troy CJ & Al, 1997; Nakashima K & Al, 2006
Legionella spp	Seenivasan MH & Al, 2005

Table 9. Bacteria reported to have caused outbreaks in nursing homes (published studies)

The elderly are at increased risk of infectious gastroenteritis due to age-related decrease in gastric acid. In fact, while food products are usually the vehicle for introduction of the organism, subsequent person to person spread often occurs, prolonging the duration of the outbreak.

In a population with high prevalence of incontinence, the risk of cross infections is substantial, particularly due to shared bathroom, dining and rehabilitation facilities (Bennet RG, 1993). Foodborne disease outbreaks are very common in this setting, most often caused by Salmonella spp or Staphylococcus aureus (Levine W & Al, 1991; Centre for Diseases Control and Prevention, 2004).

E coli 0157:H7 and Giardia also may cause foodborne outbreaks, underscoring the importance of proper food preparation and storage. Some gastroenteritis outbreaks due to Salmonella spp and enterohemorragic E coli, have had a reported case/fatality ratios up to 12% (Levine W & Al, 1991); by contrast, the case/fatality ratio for most other pathogens is low.

3.2.2 Group-A Streptococcus

Outbreak of Group-A Streptococcal infection (Streptococcus pyogenes) have been frequently reported in nursing homes (Center for Disease Control, 1990a; Reid RT & Al, 1983; Ruben FC & Al, 1984; Auerbach SB & Al, 1992; Schwartz B & Ussery XT, 1992). Infected patients may present with bacteremia, pneumonia, cellulitis, wound infection, pharyngitis or conjunctivitis (Schwartz B & Ussery XT, 1992). Rarely, a toxic shock-like syndrome occurs.

Residents with skin ulcers and wounds are at greater risk of invasive infection. In most outbreaks, geographic localization to a floor or wing of the nursing home occurs (Schwartz B & Ussery XT, 1992).

3.2.3 Others outbreaks

A recent paper by Utsumi and co-workers (2010) identified between 1966 and 2008, six hundred and one articles or reports in English, dealing with outbreaks in nursing homes.

Thirty-seven pathogens (21 types of bacteria) were associated with 206 outbreaks. In addition to the above mentioned bacteria, were involved Chlamydia Pneumoniae , Haemophilus Influentiae, Bordetella Pertussis, Neisseria Meningitidis, Aeromonas Hydrophila, and Bacillus Cereus.

The reported median attack rate (proportion of persons who developed infection among those exposed) and their reference lists were reported in Table 10.

Bacteria	Attack rate	References
Chlamydia Pneumoniae	46%	Rice LB & Al, 1990; Miyashita N & Al, 2005; Nakashima K & Al, 2006
Haemophilus Influentiae	11%	Smith PF & Al, 1988
Bordetella Pertussis	36%	Addis DG & Al, (1991)
Neisseria Meningitidis	3%	Anonymus, 1998
Aeromonas Hydrophila	17%	McAnulty JM & Al, 2000
Bacillus Cereus	24%	Halvorsrud J & Orstavik I , 1980

Table 10. Attack rate of outbreaks as reported in published studies

Mycobacterium tuberculosis is responsible for outbreaks spreading from one facility to another (Ijaz, K & Al, 2002). The high frequency of prior infection with Mycobacterium tuberculosis in the elderly population, coupled with the immunological decline, characteristic of elderly persons, foments higher rates of tuberculosis in the nursing home setting. A survey of 15379 reported cases in 29 state indicated that the incidence of tuberculosis among nursing home residents was 39,2 cases per 100000 population, compared with 21,5 cases per 100000 population among elderly persons living in community (Center for Disease Control, 1990b). Residents who develop reactivated disease and residents who develop active tuberculosis after exposure to those with reactivated disease, constitute the source for facility-wide outbreaks. Because many infected older residents do not present with the classic features of tuberculosis (Rajagopalan S & Yoshikawa TT, 2000), infection in residents may remain unrecognized for prolonged period of time, which sustains transmission. Accordingly, a number of tuberculosis outbreaks involving both residents and staff have been reported (Centers for Disease Control, 1990b; Rajagopalan S & Yoshikawa TT, 2000; Kashef I & Al, 2002). The Centers for Disease Control (1990b) has published specific guidelines for the prevention of tuberculosis in nursing homes.

Since 1990, ten reports have described outbreaks of Streptococcus pneumoniae in nursing homes (Gleinch S & Al, 2000). These have frequently occurred in facilities with low pneumococcal vaccination rates. Multidrug-resistant strains of Streptococcus pneumonia accounted for 4 of these outbreaks. The largest, involved a 100-bed nursing home in Oklahoma (Nuorti JP, 1998). Eleven of 84 residents (13%) developed pneumonia, and 3 residents died. The outbreak strain, serotype "23F", exhibited resistance to penicillin, other ß-lactam antibiotics, trimethoprim-sulfamethoxazole, erythromycin, clindamycin and tetracycline.

Additional reports besides that of Loeb and colleagues (2000) document the occurrence of outbreaks caused by Chlamydia pneumoniae. The attack rate for 3 outbreaks caused by Chlamydia pneumoniae in Ontario nursing homes ranged from 44% to 68% among residents and it was 34% among the staff of one nursing home (Troy CJ & Al, 1997). Of the 302 residents affected, 16 developed pneumonia and 6 died.

Single report identify 5 other respiratory tract pathogens that have caused outbreak in nursing home residents: Chlamydia psittaci (Smith PW, 1994), Legionella pneumophila (Stout JE & Al, 2000), Haemophilus influenza type B (Smith PF, 1988) and Bordetella pertussis (Addis DG & Al, 1991).

4. Antibiotic resistance

Because infections occur frequently in nursing homes, residents are exposed to antimicrobial agents (Nicolle LE & Al, 1984, 1996; Finnegan TP & Al, 1985; Magaziner J & Al, 1991; Jackson M & Al, 1992). With mostly broad-spectrum antibiotics available and in wide use, resistance problems has been repeatedly documented since the early 1970s.

Indeed, numerous studies based on routine surveillance data, indicate a strong relationship between use and resistance (van de Sande-Bruinsma N & Al, 2008) but, nowadays, the epidemiology of antimicrobial resistance in nursing homes remains poorly understood (Lautenbach E & Al, 2009).

4.1 Sources of antibiotic resistance

Antimicrobial agent-resistant bacteria may be introduced into nursing homes by two different routes. They may emerge endogenously in patient flora during courses of antimicrobial therapy, or they may enter with new residents who are already colonized or infected (Bradley SF & Al, 1991; Mulhausen PL & Al, 1996; Muder RR & Al, 1999). Emergence may reflect selection of resistant strains or acquisition of genetic determinants that confer resistance by either spontaneous mutation or gene transfer. Spontaneous mutations that confer resistance are thought to be rare, but two studies have suggested that gene transfer plays a an important role in long-term care facilities. In an outbreak caused by ceftazidime-resistant bacteria in a chronic-care facility in Massachusetts, Rice and colleagues (1990) reported that the outbreak arose from plasmid transmission among different species and genera of Enterobacteriaceae, and not from dissemination of a single resistant isolate. The outbreak, which involved 29 patients, was caused by strains of Klebsiella pneumonia, Enterobacter cloacae, Escherichia coli, Serratia spp., Enterobacter agglomerans and Citrobacter diversus, that produced similar extended-spectrum ß-lactamases whose genes were located on closely related plasmids. The outbreaks had followed the introduction of ceftazidime into the facility, and its widespread empiric use. Similar observation were reported in a study of gentamicin-resistant gram negative bacilli in a Veterans' Administration nursing home care unit (Shlaes DM & Al, 1990). One Escherichia coli plasmid, which conferred resistance to ampicillin, carbenicillin, tetracycline and sulfonamides, proved identical to plasmids from two Citrobacter freundii strains and a Providencia stuartii strain isolated from three different patients. The introduction of resistant strain by colonized or infected patients who are admitted from other facilities has also been documented: one study reported the entry of an Methicillin-Resistant Staphylococcus aureus strain into the nursing home by a patient who was colonized at the referring hospital (Strausbaugh LJ & Al, 1991). Another study, revealed that 8 of 10 patients admitted to an intermediate-care ward were already colonized with strains of members of the Enterobacteriaceae carrying a plasmid encoding a novel ß-lactamase (Shlaes DM & Al, 1988). Regarding of the route of entry for resistant pathogens into the nursing home, antimicrobial use drives selection pressure for new acquisitions. Bjork and colleagues (1984) reported that in 10 patients with chronic indwelling urinary catheters residing in a Veterans' Administration nursing home care unit in North Dakota over 30 months, 70% of 63 antibiotic courses resulted in bacteriuria with organism resistant to the antibiotic that had been administred. As 40% of the positive urine cultures were polymicrobial, it is likely that antimicrobial therapy merely selected out the more resistant strains. The authors identified cross-infection in only one case and a greater percentage of Escherichia coli strains isolated from nursing home residents were resistant to ampicillin, tetracycline and trimethoprim-sulfamethoxazole, than Escherichia coli strains isolated from patients in the adjoining hospital.

4.2 Risk factors for acquisition of antibiotic resistance

Few studies have examined risk factors for infection with antimicrobial pathogens in nursing home patients. Infections with antibiotic resistant bacteria appears to occur most often in nursing home patients with antecedent colonization (Bradley SF & Al, 1991; Muder RR & Al, 1991; Mulhausen PL & Al, 1996). However, risk factors for colonization and infection are not necessarily the same. Overall infection with resistant bacteria was more likely to occur in nursing home residents who had been hospitalized recently or who a substantial decline in functional status (Terpenning MS & Al, 1994). Muder and colleagues (1991) reported risk factors for Methicillin-Resistant Staphylococcus Aureus (MRSA) infection in residents of their intermediated-care ward and nursing home care unit. In a stepwise logistic regression analysis, both persistent Methicillin-Resistant Staphylococcus Aureus colonization and dialysis were independent risk factor for Methicillin-Resistant

Staphylococcus Aureus infection. Terpenning and colleagues (1994) in an Ann Arbor, Michigan, identified risk factors for infection caused by both Methicillin-Resistant Staphylococcus Aureus and resistant Gram negative bacilli. By stepwise logistic regression analysis, diabetes mellitus and peripheral vascular disease were significant independent risk factors for Methicillin-Resistant Staphylococcus Aureus infection. Moreover, the presence of an indwelling urinary catheter or intermittent urinary catheterization, pressure ulcers and prior antibiotic use were significant independent risk factors for infection caused by resistant Gram-negative bacilli (Terpenning MS & Al, 1994; Muder & Al, 1997) . In a cross-sectional survey among 1,215 residents of long-term care facilities in Jerusalem, the Vancomycin-Resistant Enterococci (VRE) carriage rate was 9.6%. Previous hospitalization and antibiotic treatment were associated with elevated Vancomycin-Resistant Enterococci colonization rate. In contrast, moderate and severe levels of dependency and prolonged stay in a nursing home were associated with a decrease in the Vancomycin-Resistant Enterococci colonization rate. (Benenson S & Al, 2009).

In a prospective cohort study a total of 3339 patients with invasive pneumococcal infection were identified between 1995 and 2002. Multivariate modeling revealed that risk factors for infection with penicillin-resistant as opposed to penicillin-susceptible pneumococci were year of infection, absence of chronic organ system disease and previous use of penicillin, trimethoprim-sulfamethoxazole and azithromycin. Infection with trimethoprim-sulfamethoxazole-resistant pneumococci was associated with absence of chronic organ system disease and with previous use of penicillin, trimethoprim-sulfamethoxazole, and azithromycin. Infection with macrolide-resistant isolates was associated with previous use of penicillin, trimethoprim-sulfamethoxazole, clarithromycin, and azithromycin. Infection with fluoroquinolone-resistant pneumococci was associated with previous use of fluoroquinolones, current residence in a nursing home, and nosocomial acquisition of pneumococcal infection (Vanderkooi OG, 2005).

4.3 Risk factors for colonization

Given the high prevalence of colonization with antibiotic-resistant strains in nursing homes, why do some patients never become colonized and others become persistent carriers? When colonized nursing home residents have been compared with non carriers, underlying illness, presence of intravenous, urinary or enteral feeding devices, antibiotic use, presence of wounds, decline in functional status and increased intensity of nursing care have been associated to various degrees with High-level Gentamicin-Resistant Enterococci, Vancomycin-Resistant Enterococci, Drug-Resistant Streptococcus Pneumoniae and Methicillin-Resistant Staphylococcus Aureus (Zervos MJ & Al, 1987; Bradley SF & Al, 1991; Chenoweth CE & Al, 1994; Terpenning MS & Al, 1994; Brennen C & Al, 1998). Similar risk factors for the carriage of resistant Gram Negative Bacilli have been found. Nursing home residents colonized with resistant Gram Negative Bacilli were significantly more likely to have lived in a large skilled nursing facility, have had prior antibiotic treatment, or have had urinary incontinence or a catheter, than non colonized persons in nursing homes or the community (Gaynes RP & Al, 1985). Colonization with Gram Negative Bacilli resistant to Gentamicin, trimethoprim or cefriaxone, has been associated to varying degrees with increased length of stay, increased debility, need for a urinary device, prior pneumonia, presence of wound or chronic disease (Huovinen P, 1984; Shlaes DM, 1986; MacArthur RD

& Al, 1988; Bradley SF & Al, 1991; Wingard E & Al, 1993; Terpenning MS & Al, 1994). Given the overlap in risk factors, it is not surprising to find that many nursing home residents are colonized with more than one antibiotic-resistant pathogen (Chenoweth CE & Al, 1994; Terpenning MS & Al, 1994; Brennen C & Al, 1998)

4.4 Occurrence: organisms and antibiotic resistance

Even though interest in the epidemiology of antibiotic resistance in healthcare setting outside hospital is on the increase, the extend of antibiotic resistance in nursing home is still relatively unknown. Most information is derived from surveillance studies of infections in nursing home residents or outbreak investigations. No studies have defined the overall magnitude of this problem in a systematic manner, but available data suggest that antimicrobial agent resistant pathogens are frequently encountered in this setting. In fact nursing homes residents have an high frequency of colonization with antimicrobial-resistant organisms, including Methicillin-Resistant Staphylococcus Aureus, Vancomycin-Resistant Enterococci, Enterococci with high-level Gentamicin-Resistance, Extended-Spectrum ß-Lactamase-Fluoroquinolone-Resistant Gram-Negative Pathogens, Gram-Negative Uropathogens, , Penicillin-Resistant Pneumococci.

4.4.1 Methicillin-Resistant Staphylococcus Aureus (MRSA)

Methicillin-Resistant Staphylococcus Aureus was first described in 1961, and since then it has become a worldwide problem (Jevons MP, 1961; Tansel & Al, 2003; Diekema DJ & Al, 2004; Corrente M & Al, 2005). The presence of Methicillin-Resistant Staphylococcus Aureus in nursing homes was first reported in 1970 by O'Tool (O'Toole & Al, 1970). Methicillin-Resistant Staphylococcus Aureus is a frequent colonizer of debilitated patients; on this point, Bradley observed that the rate of colonization with Methicillin-Resistant Staphylococcus Aureus was <25% (Bradley SF & Al, 1991). The same Author showed that in two of the most common sites of colonization, nares and wound, colonization rates range from 8 to 53% and from 30 to 82% respectively (Bradley SF, 1999). Lee YL and colleagues (1997) reported a one-year prospective surveillance study of Staphylococcus Aureus colonization and infection. Nasal and stool or rectal screening cultures were done on admission, and all patients underwent screening on at least a quarterly basis for one year. Overall, 35% of patients were colonized at least once with Staphylococcus Aureus (72% Methicillin-Susceptible; 25% Methicillin-Resistant; 3% mixed phenotype). Mendelson evaluated the rate of colonization by Staphylococcus Aureus, especially Methicillin-Resistant Staphylococcus Aureus, in 270 elderly residents of a large long-term care facility. The Authors showed that 23,3% of residents were carriers of Staphylococcus Aureus and 27% of those had Methicillin-Resistant Staphylococcus Aureus (Mendelson G & Al, 2003). It is estimated that residents of nursing homes who are colonized with Methicillin-Resistant Staphylococcus Aureus have a 4 to 6 fold increase in infection rate. In a study by Muder RR and colleagues (1991), 25% of Methicillin-Resistant Staphylococcus Aureus carriers had an episode of staphylococcal infection, versus only 4% of Methicillin-Susceptible Staphylococcus Aureus carriers.

In a retrospective cohort study, Capitano showed that the median infection management cost of a Methicillin-Resistant Staphylococcus Aureus infection was six times greater than that of a Methicillin-Susceptible Staphylococcus Aureus infection, whereas the median associated nursing care cost was two times greater. The median overall infection cost associated with Methicillin-Resistant Staphylococcus Aureus was 1,95 times greater than that associated with Methicillin-Susceptible Staphylococcus Aureus. Nursing care cost constituted the major portion of the overall infection cost for both groups (Methicillin-Susceptible Staphylococcus Aureus = 51%; Methicillin-Resistant Staphylococcus Aureus = 48%) (Capitano B & Al, 2003).

Risk factors for Methicillin-Resistant Staphylococcus Aureus colonization include: residence in a medical ward or medical intensive care unit or prolonged hospitalization (13 weeks), advanced age and a history of invasive procedures (Asensio A & Al, 1996). In a study by O'Sullivan, the risk factors significantly associated with Methicillin-Resistant Staphylococcus Aureus colonization were male sex, age over 80 years, residence in the nursing home for more than six months, hospitalization during the previous six months, peripheral vascular disease, pressure ulcers, steroid therapy, poor general skin condition, antibiotic therapy during the previous three months and a mental test score of less than 14. Multivariate analysis identified male sex and pressure ulcers as independent variables (O'Sullivan NP & Keane CT, 2000). In a case control study conducted in a community nursing home, Thomas reported that nasogastric intubation and antibiotic therapy in the previous 6 months were the most important factors associated with Methicillin-Resistant Staphylococcus Aureus colonization (Thomas JC & Al, 1989). Other risk factors are indwelling urinary catheters and urinary incontinence (Terpenning MS & Al, 1994).

4.4.2 Vancomycin-Resistant Enterococci (VRE)

First described in 1987 in Europe Vancomycin Resistant Enterococci have recently emerged as important nosomial pathogens and in the last years have become among the most feared pathogens in US hospitals. Studies dealing with the emergence of Vancomycin-Resistant Enterococci in the United States, revealed that most patients with Vancomycin-Resistant Enterococci were in Intensive Care Units (Clark NC & Al, 1993). Colonization with Vancomycin-resistant Enterococcus has been reported from community settings in the United States, including, to a limited extend, long-term care facilities (Coque TM & Al, 1996; Bonten MJ & Al, 1998). Bonilla showed that prevalence of Vancomycin-Resistant Enterococcus colonization among patients in the long-term care facilities at the Ann Arbor Department of Veterans Affairs Medical Center, exceeded the prevalence in the intensive care unit and in the general medical wards (Bonilla HF & Al, 1997). Brennan decribed the epidemiology of Vancomycin-Resistant Enterococcus colonization in a 400 bed long-term care facility for veterans. The author observed that 24 of 36 patients were colonized with Vancomycin-Resistant Enterococcus that persisted for 67 days and were associated with antibiotic administration (Brennan C & Al, 1998). In a prospective cohort study, 45% (45 of 100 patients) were colonized with Vancomycin-Resistant Enterococcus. The risk factors identified by univariate analysis were: hospitalization in the prior 60 days, an admission diagnosis of infection, inability to ambulate, presence of a feeding tube or urinary catheter or decubitus ulcer and documented more probable antibiotic use in the previous 60 days (particularly the use of Vancomycin and third generation cephalosporins). Stepwise logistic regression analysis identified the presence of decubitus ulcer or hospital admission, and documented a probable antibiotic use in the 60 days before admission, as significant risk factors for colonization with Vancomycin-Resistant Enterococcus at the time of admission (Elizaga ML & Al, 2002).

4.4.3 Enterococci with high-level gentamicin resistance

Two studies, both from the Ann Arbor Veterans Administration nursing home care unit have identified risk factors for colonization with Gentamicin-Resistant Strains of Enterococci. In the first study a one-day prevalence survey reported by Zervos and colleagues, the need for advanced nursing care and antibiotic therapy in the prior 3 months were independent risk factors for colonization (Zervos MJ & Al, 1987). In the second study, presence of wounds, renal failure, intermittent catheterization, low Katz functional status and low serum albumin were independent risk factors for colonization with strains possessing high-level resistance to gentamicin (Terpenning MS & Al, 1994).

4.4.4 Extended-spectrum ß-lactamase gram-negative pathogens (ESBLs)

The first report of Extended-Spectrum ß-Lactamase Gram-Negative bacilli, came from Europe and were quickly followed by reports in the United States. This type of antimicrobial resistance is now recognized worldwide. The prevalence of Extended-Spectrum ß-Lactamase Gram-Negative Pathogens in long-term care facilities is becoming alarming. The first reported outbreak of bacteria resistant to ceftazidime in the United States occurred in 1990 among patients in a chronic care facility in Massachusetts (Rice LB & Al, 1990). In a study of ceftazidime-resistant Escherichia coli and Klebsiella pneumonia in Chicago, 31 of 35 patients from 8 nursing facilities harboured an Extended-Spectrum ß-Lactamase producing enteric pathogen. (Weiner J & Al, 1999). Weiner reported that prior exposure to ciprofloxacin or trimethoprim-sulfamethoxazole was an independent predictor of colonization with Escherichia coli resistant to ceftazidime among nursing home residents. Molecular analysis of isolates, showed that a particular resistance-conferring plasmid appeared frequently, thus supporting the growing concern that long-term facilities may act a reservoir for antimicrobial drug-resistant organisms. Several studies have evaluated the risk factors for colonization or infections with Extended-Spectrum ß-Lactamase-producing organisms in the hospitalized patients. Reported risk factors include the presence of intravascular catheters, emergency intra-abdominal surgery, gastrotomy or jejunostomy tube, gastrointestinal colonization, length of hospital or intensive care unit stay, prior antibiotics (including third generation cephalosporins), severity of illness, presence of an urinary catheter, and ventilator assistance (Schiappa DA & Al, 1996). In a case-control study, Sandoval and colleagues (2004) showed that exposure to any cephalosporin and percentage of residents using gastrotomy tubes within the nursing home, were associated with having a clinical isolate resistant to third-generation cephalosporin (Sandoval C & Al, 2004). Nursing home residents would appear to have several additional risk factors for infection with Extended-Spectrum ß-Lactamase- Gram-Negative producing organisms. It has been well documented that hand-washing rates are low among nursing home personnel (Denman SJ & Burton JR, 1992). Urinary catheterization and decubitus ulcers are frequent, and have been associated with colonization of non- Extended-Spectrum ß-Lactamase producing, antibiotic-resistant gram negative bacilli (Muder RR & Al, 1991; SmithPW & Al, 2000).

4.4.5 Fluoroquinolone-resistant gram-negative pathogens

Resistance in fluoroquinolones has been increasing over time in long-term care facilities. In a correlational longitudinal survey study, Viray showed that Escherichia Coli fluoroquinone-resistance rates was high but variable, and were generally increasing over time (Viray M &

Al, 2005). In a case control study, Cohen showed that Fluoroquinone-Resistant Escherichia coli urinary tract infection was more common with prior fluoroquinolone use (Cohen AE & Al, 2006). Maslow conducted a cross-sectional study to determine the prevalence of, and risk factors for colonization with Fluoroquinone-Resistant Escherichia coli in residents of a long-term care facility. Fluoroquinone-Resistant Escherichia coli were identified from rectal swabs for 25 of 49 (51%) partecipants at study entry. On multivariate analyses, prior fluoroquinolone use was the only independent risk factor for Fluoroquinone-Resistant Escherichia coli carriage and was consistent for fluoroquinolone exposures in the previous 3, 6, 9 or 12 months. Pulsed-field gel electrophoresis of Fluoroquinone-Resistant Escherichia coli identified clonal spread of one strain among 16 residents (Maslow JN & Al, 2005).

4.4.6 Gram-negative uropathogens

Shlaes and colleagues identified risk factors for urinary colonization with Gentamicin-Resistant Gram-negative Bacilli in patients of a Veteran Administration nursing home care unit near Cleveland, Ohio, using stepwise logistic regression (Shlaes DM & Al, 1986). Perineal or rectal colonization with Gentamicin-Resistant strains and presence of a urinary catheter were significant independent risk factors. Another study at the same institution by Wingard and colleagues, examined carriage of Trimethoprim-Resistant Gram-negative Bacilli (Wingard E & Al, 1993). Functional status and length of stay were significant independent risk factors for colonization: functional status was the most important risk factor for acquiring Trimethoprim-Resistant strains by cross-colonization. Gaynes, studying colonization with multiply resistant Gram-negative bacilli in patients admitted to the hospital from community nursing homes, reported that bladder dysfunction, residence in large nursing homes, age and prior antibiotic use were independent risk factors (Gaynes RP & Al, 1985). Terpenning identified intermittent catheterization, inflammatory bowel disease, chronic renal disease, presence of wounds and prior pneumonia, to be independent risk factors for colonization with Gentamicin and/or Ceftriaxone-Resistant Gram-negative Bacilli in a stepwise regression analysis (Terpenning MS & Al, 1994).

4.4.7 Penicillin-Resistant Pneumococci

Penicillin resistance is common in Streptococcus Pneumoniae and is a problem all over the world, both in the community and in hospital setting. In 2002, the European Antimicrobial Resistance Surveillance project (http://www.earss.rivm.nl) reported five countries with a prevalence of Penicillin-Resistant Pneumococci of greater than or equal to 30%. Overall, in 2002, the European Antimicrobial Resistance Surveillance Project reported 11% of Streptococcus Pneumoniae strains as non susceptible to penicillin and 17% non susceptible to erythromycin. Two events have occurred since 2000 that may have reduce the selective pressure driving antimicrobial resistance: the more appropriate use of antimicrobial and the pneumococcal conjugate vaccine (Klugman KP, 2004).The earlier study reports by Millar and Denton were among the first to describe Penicillin-Resistant Pneumococcal infection in elderly institutionalized and debilitated patients (Denton M & Al, 1993; Millar MR & Al, 1994). Nuorti reported a significant outbreak of Penicillin-Resistant Pneumococci in a long-term care facility in rural Oklaoma. The Author observed that 13% of the residents developed pneumonia, and that the mortality rate was 23%. Resistant isolates were recovered from 64% of residents with pneumonia and from 23% of non infected residents (Nuorti JP & Al, 1998).

4.4.8 Others organisms

In addition to those listed above, there are other kinds of antimicrobial-resistant pathogens. Smith and colleagues described an outbreak caused by an Ampicillin-Resistant strain of Haemophilus influenzae, involving six patients in a nursing home and adjoining hospital during a 1-month period (Smith PF & Al, 1988). Two patients were bacteremic and one died. All patients had personal contact with at least one other case patient, suggesting person-to-person spread. Sturm and colleagues reported a similar outbreak involving 15 subjects in a pulmonary rehabilitation centre in the Netherlands (Sturm AW & Al, 1990). The outbreak strain of Haemophilus influenza was resistant to amoxicillin, thrimethoprim-sulfamethoxazole, chloramphenicol and tetracycline. Choi described a nursing home outbreak caused by Salmonella Heidelberg serotype, frequently expressing multiple resistance (Choi AT & Al, 1990). Forty-four (22%) of the 199 residents were affected. Patients treated with antibiotics excreted the outbreak strain for a median duration of 14 weeks, prolonging the presence of a potential source for additional cases.

Although Acinetobacter infections in long-term care facilities and nursing homes are not well described, during the last decade, increasingly resistant strains of Acinetobacter, necessitating greater use of broad-spectrum antibiotics, such imipenem and ampicillin-sulbactam (Jain R & Danziger LH, 2004; Bassetti M & Al, 2008).

Sengstock and colleague in a six-year period reported in an increase of Multi-Drug-Resistant Acinetobacter baumannii, a link between increasing antibiotic-resistance, morbidity and mortality, and a transfer between hospital and nursing home and viceversa (Sengstock DM & Al, 2010). The article demonstrated that Acinetobacter baumannii is widespread including hospitals, long-term acute-care and nursing homes, and that the transfer of multidrug-resistant strains among health care facilities is bidirectional. These data confirm previous report (Gould CV & Al, 2006; Saeed S & Al, 2006; Stephens C & Al, 2007; Furuno JP & Al, 2008)

5. Conclusions

In the nursing home setting, antimicrobial use is an important issue, relevant to antimicrobial resistance. Previous study have found relatively high rates of antimicrobial use and substantial inappropriate use of antimicrobial agents in nursing homes and long-term care facilities (Zimmer JG & Al, 1986; Crossley K & Al 1987; Jones SR & Al, 1987; Katz PR & Al, 1990; Warren JW & Al, 1991; Yakabowich MR & Al, 1994; Pickering TD & Al, 1994; Montgomery P & Al, 1995). In addition to increasing the risk of colonization or infection with antimicrobial-resistant organisms, inappropriate antimicrobial use adds cost to resident care and may place the patient at increased risk for drug adverse reactions (Mylotte JM, 1999). Recommendations for improving antimicrobial use have included development of a formulary and continuing review of antimicrobial use and prevalence of antimicrobial resistance in cultures obtained from patients with suspected infections. In the last decades, an increasing number of nursing homes have developed infections control programs with surveillance and control activities (Smith PW, 1999). A major contribution to this development was the publication of guidelines by the Association for Professional in Infection Control and Epidemiology (APIC) - Society for Healthcare Epidemiologists of America (SHEA) in 1997 (Smith PW & Rusnak PG, 1997), revisited in 2008 (Smith PW & Al, 2008).

5.1 Prevention and control of infections in nursing homes

Most nursing homes have infection control programs, even if the components of these programs vary among different institutions and countries. (Garibaldi RA & Al, 1981; Crossley K & Al, 1985; Kabbuz RF & Tenney JH, 1988; Campbell B, 1991). The overall goal of the infection control program is to prevent infections and, when that is not possible, to limit interpatient transmission of potential pathogens (Nicolle LE & Garibaldi RA, 1995). Surveillance for infections in the nursing home is integral to the program (Smith PW, 1987). Valid infection surveillance requires the use of standard definitions, appropriate for the nursing home (McGeer AB & Al, 1991), effective case finding measures, systematic analysis and reporting of data, and an awareness to identify potential outbreaks as easy as possible. The optimal method for surveillance in nursing home is not identified, because it differs depending on the characteristics of each nursing home, staffing and patients populations.

Infection prevention and control is important for continuum of care and their main functions are (a) to obtain and manage clinical data, including surveillance information for endemic and epidemic infections; (b) to develop and recommend policies and procedures; (c) to intervene directly to prevent infections and (d) to educate and train health care workers, patients and caregivers. (Table 11)

An effective infection control program includes a method of surveillance for infections and antimicrobial-resistant pathogens, an outbreak control plan for epidemics, isolation and standard precautions, hand hygiene, staff education, an employee health program, a resident health program, policy formation and periodic review with audits, and a policy to communicate reportable diseases to public health authorities.

Infection surveillance in nursing homes involves collection of data on nursing home-acquired infections (Do AM & Al, 1999). Surveillance can be limited to a particular objective or may be a facility-wide goal. Surveillance often is based on individual patient risk factors, focused on a unit or based on a particular pathogen or infection type.

Surveillance may be either passive or active; in passive surveillance ("routine surveillance"), an infection control professional uses data collected for routine patient care. Although less costly in term of resources, passive surveillance is inherently biased. It may underestimate the magnitude of outcomes measured and delay detection of outbreaks. The feasibility of passive surveillance has been demonstrated and has led to continuing education opportunities.

Active surveillance uses multiple data sources to detect infections and antimicrobial resistance early, but data in nursing homes are lacking. Hospital definitions may not be applicable in nursing home setting; modified nursing home specific criteria were developed by a Canadian Consensus Conference, which took into account the unique limitations of the nursing home setting (McGeer A & Al, 1991). These criteria have been used widely but not uniformly (Danzig LE & Al, 1995). In addition a facility must have clear goals and aims for setting up a surveillance program. These goals, like other elements of an infection control program have to be reviewed periodically to reflect changes in the facility's population, pathogens of interest and changing antimicrobial resistance patterns. In addition, plans to analyse the data and use them to design and implement proven preventive measures, must be made in advance. The analysis and reporting of infection rates in nursing homes must be conducted monthly, quarterly and annually to detect trends. Because the length of stay in nursing home is long, and each resident is at risk for a prolonged duration, infection rates (infections/1000 resident days) can be calculated by using resident days or average resident census for the surveillance period as the denominator. These data can be used to estabilish endemic baselines rates and recognize variations from the baseline that could represent an outbreak. Feed back to the nursing home staff is critical to the success of the surveillance program, and this information should lead to specific infection control initiatives and follow up surveillance.

The Centers for Disease Control and Prevention's Healthcare Infection Control and Prevention Advisory Committee (HICPAC) proposes use of "Standard Precautions" which have been designed for the care of all patients in hospitals (Garner JS, 1996). "Standard Precautions" apply to blood, all body fluids, secretions and excretions regardless of whether they contain visible blood, skin that is not intact, or mucous membrane material. Designed to reduce the risk of transmission of pathogens from apparent and ambiguous source of infection, these precautions include hand hygiene compliance, glove use, masks, eye protection, gown and avoidance of injuries from sharp materials. Transmission-based precautions are intended for use with patients who may be infected with highly transmissible or epidemiologically significant pathogens. These include airborne precautions, droplet precautions and contact precautions.

Although these guidelines were designed for acute care setting, several of them, especially the universal precautions, apply to nursing home setting as well. However, facilities should evaluate these guidelines and individualize the plan to obtain cultures based on the population they serve.

Healthcare workers may play an important role in the dissemination of antibiotic-resistant bacteria in nursing homes (Thomas JC & Al, 1989): contamination of the hand of healthcare workers has been recognized as playing a role in the transmission of pathogenetic bacteria to patients since the observations of Holmes, Semmelweis and other, more than 100 years ago (Otherson MJ & Otherson HB, 1987). Hand antisepsis remains the most effective and last expansive measure to prevent transmission of nosocomial infections. However, compliance with hand washing recommendations among healthcare workers averages only 30-50% and improves only modestly following educational interventions (Mody L & Al, 2003). Healthcare workers frequently reported poor compliance with hand hygiene measures because of skin irritation from frequent washing, too little time because of a heavy workload, and simply forgetting. Introduction of alcohol-based hand rubs have been shown to enhance compliance with hand hygiene in the nursing home setting, and should be used to complement educational initiatives (Mody L & Al, 2003).

While the cost of introducing alcohol-based hand rubs could be a concern of nursing homes, recent data in acute care have shown that the total costs of a hand hygiene promotion campaign, including alcohol-based hand rubs, corresponded to less than 1% of costs that could be attributed to nosocomial infections (Pittet D & Al, 2004). Introducing the alcohol-based hand rubs must take into account some problems: alcohol-based hand rubs should not be used if hands are visibly soiled, in which case hand hygiene with antimicrobial soup and water is recommended. Alcohol-based hand rubs can cause dry skin; however recent data on rubs containing emollients have shown to cause less skin irritation and dryness (Centers for Disease Control , 2002).

Strategy	Measures
Management strategies	
Infection control program	
Surveillance	• Review microbiology data • Maintain line listing of cases • Prevalence surveys of residents, staff or new admissions • Identify readmission cases
Outbreak investigation	
Policies, isolates, environment	
Staff education	
Antimicrobial utilization program	
Employee health program	
Patient care strategies	
Optimal management of comorbidities	
Optimal nutrition	
Avoidance of invasive devices	
Vaccination	• Influenza • Pneumococcus • Tetanus
Screening	• Hepatitis B and C virus • Tuberculosis (selected cases)
Precautions	• Hand-washing, antimicrobial soaps • Environment decontamination • Private room for colonized/infected residents • Barrier precautions for colonized/infected residents • Strict isolation for colonized/infected residents • Isolation of new admission • Special placement colonized/infected residents • Cohort colonized/infected residents • Cohort colonized personnel • Establish isolation ward
Reduction of reservoir	• Exclusion of colonized/infected residents from facility • Rapid discharge of colonized/infected residents • Decolonization therapy of residents, personnel o new admissions
Outbreak management	
Mechanism for early identification	
Policies for laboratory utilization	
Case finding and analysis	
Isolation and cohorting	
Specific therapy	

Table 11. Recommended approaches to the prevention and minimization of infections and outbreaks in nursing home

Another key point of the infection control program is staff education. Ongoing staff education is critical in health care setting, because of the plethora of literature published every year, advancements in technology and regulatory demands. The infection control program plays a vital role in educating nursing home personnel on various infection control measures, particularly in view of rapid staff turnover. Informal education and quality improvement meeting should be complemented with in-service education on various topics, including hand hygiene compliance, antimicrobial usage and antimicrobial resistance, appropriate and early diagnosis of infections, infection control and prevention measures, isolation precautions and policies.

5.1.2 Patient care practices

Patient-specific strategies to prevent infection are targeted to increase general and specific immunity and, hence, limit susceptibility to infection. These include maintenance of adequate nutrition and optimal management of associated chronic diseases. For example, nursing care practices should attempt to minimize or prevent the occurrence of aspiration in patients with neurologic impairment, avoid trauma to neuropathic feet, and prevent the occurrence of pressure ulcers in patients with limited mobility. Ensuring optimal use of immunizing agents is important, including pneumococcal vaccination (Center for Disease Control, 1989b). Use of invasive devices should be limited to those situations in which they are essential for patient care. When tube feeding is necessary to maintain nutritional status, percutaneous gastrostomy or jejunostomy feeding tubes may be preferred over nasogastric tubes because of a reported decreased occurrence of aspiration pneumonia (Fay DE & Al, 1991), even if other studies have not supported this observation (Clocon JO & Al, 1988; Peak A & Al, 1990). It has been suggested that use of external condom catheters for incontinence in men may be associated with a lower incidence of invasive urinary tract infections compared with long-term indwelling catheters, but this, too, is controversial, because of reported increased incidence of phimosis and skin irritation that predisposes to urinary infections (Flerer J & Ekstrom M, 1981).

5.1.3 Outbreaks management

Outbreaks of infection should be anticipated in the nursing home setting and policies to respond to a suspected or proven outbreak must be developed prior to occurrence. Such policies should include general aspects of outbreak management including identification, communication and authority, as well as specific issues related to the most frequent organisms likely to occur. Adequate management requires ongoing surveillance for infection to ensure early identification, specific criteria to identify a potential outbreak, case finding strategies and laboratory backup to identify the etiologic agent and plan appropriate interventions. Authority within the facility to initiate appropriate measures to control an outbreak should be clearly defined. Early notification and ongoing communication within the institution and with appropriate public health authorities must be outlined clearly prior to the crisis of an epidemic.

The response to the outbreak must include immediate control measures to identify and isolate cases, as appropriate, and limit patient and staff exposure. Control measures will include use of patient isolation, limitations in patient movement and interaction with the facility and, frequently, specific therapy. Compliance with isolation practices leads to special problems in nursing homes. As patients' room are their permanent residence, transfer within the institution for isolation purposes is disruptive for patients and family. Cognitive impaired residents will not be able to understand the reasons for and practices of isolation and it may be difficult to restrict movement for some of these patients. Policies developed, should acknowledge these potential problems and identify the methods by which they will be addressed. An integral part of outbreak management is a review and analysis of the course of the outbreak, impact and potential problem areas that may be changed to improve management in the future.

6. References

Addis, D.G., Davis, J.P., Meade, R.D., Burstyn, D.G., Meissner, M., Zastrow, J.A., Berg, J.L., Drinka, P., & Phillips, R. (1991) A pertussis outbreak in a WInsconsin nursing home. *J Infect Dis* 164: 704-710

Aguirre-Avalos, G., Zavala-Silva, M.L., Díaz-Nava, A., Amaya-Tapia, G., Aguilar-Benavides, S. (1999) Asymptomatic bacteriuria and inflammatory response to urinary tract infection of elderly ambulatory women in nursing homes. *Arch Med Res* 30 (1): 29-32

Ahlbrecht, H., Shearen, C., Degelau, J., & Guay, D.R. (1999) Team approach to infection prevention and control in nursing home setting. *Am J Infect Control* 27: 64-70

Ahmed, A. ,Allman, R.M., & DeLong, J.F. (2003) Predictors of nursing home admission for older adults hospitalized with heart failure. *Arch Gerontol Geriatr* 36 (2): 117-126

Allman, R. (1988) Pressure ulcers among the elderly. *N Engl J Med* 320: 850-853

Alvarez, S., Shell, C., Woolley, T., Berk, S., & Smith, J. (1988) Nosocomial infections in long-term care facilities. *J Gerontol* 43: M9-M17

Andresen, M. & Puggaard, L. (2009) Autonomy among physically frail older people in nursing home settting: a study protocol for an intervention study. *BMC Geriatrics* 8:32

Anonymus (1998) Outbreaks of group B Meningococcal disease - Florida, 1995 and 1997. *Morbil Mortal Weekly Rep* 47: 833-837

Arnold, K.E., Schweitzer, J.L., Wallace, B, Salter, M., Neeman, R., & Hlady, W.G (2006) Tightly clustered outbreak of group A streptococcal disease at a long term care facility. *Infect Control Hosp Epidemiol* 27: 1377-1384

Asensio, A., Guerriero, A., Quereda, C., Lizan, M., & Martinez-Ferrer, M. (1996) Colonization and infection with Methicillin-Resistant Staphylococcus Aureus: associated factors and eradication. *Infect Control Hosp Epidemiol* 17: 20-28

Asha NJ Tompkins, D., & Wilcox, M.H. (2006) Comparative analysis of prevalence, risk factors, and molecular epidemiology of antibiotic-associated diarrhea due to Clostridium difficile, Clostridium perfringens, and Staphylococcus aureus. *J Clin Microbiol* 2006 Aug; 44(8): 2785-2791.

Aspinall, R. & Andrew, D. (2000) Thymic involution in aging. *J Clin Immunol* 20 (4): 250–256

Aspinall, R. Del Giudice, G., Effros, R.B., Grubeck-Loebenstein, B., & Sambhara, S. (2007) Challenges for vaccination in the elderly. *Immun Ageing* 4; 9-18

Auerbach, S.B., Schwartz, B., Williams, D., Fiorilli, M.G., Adimora, A.A., & Breiman, R.F.Al (1992) Outbreak of invasive group A streptococcal infections in a nursing home: leson on prevention and control. *Arch Intern Med* 152: 1017-1022

Baine, W.E., Gagarosa, J., Bennet, J & Barker, W.Jr. (1973) Institutional salmonellosis. *J Infect Dis* 128: 357-360

Bajekal, M. (2002) Survey for England 2000: Characteristics of care homes and their residents. London: the Stationery Office, 2002

Banaszak-Koll, Fendrick, A. Mark., Foster., N.L., Herzog, A.R., Kabeto, M.U., Kent, D.M., Straus, W. L, & Langa, K.M. (2004) Predicting nursing home admission: estimates from a 7-year-follow up of a nationally representative sample o folder Americans. Alzh Dis Assoc Disord 18 (2): 83-89

Bartholomeyczik, S., Reuther, S., Luft, L., van Nie, N., Meijers, J., Schols, J., & Halfens, R. (2010) Prevalence of malnutrition, interventions and quality indicators in German nursing homes - first results of a nationwide pilot study. *Gesundheitswesen* 2010 Dec; 72(12): 868-74.

Bassetti, M., Righi, E., Esposito, S., Petrosillo, N., & Nicolini, L. (2008) Drug treatment for multidrug treatment-resistant Acinetobacter baumannii. *Future Microbiol* 3: 649-660

Bates ,C.J. Prentice, A., Cole, T.J., van der Pols, J.C., Doyle, W., Finch, S., Smithers, G., & Clarke, P.C. (1999a) Micronutrients: highlights and research challenges from the 1994-1995 National Diet and Nutrition Survey of people aged 65 years and over. *Br J Nutr* 82: 7-15

Bates, C.J., Prentice, A., & Finch, S. (1999b) Gender differences in food and nutrient intakes and status indices from the National Diet and Nutrition Survey of people aged 65 years and over. *J Clin Nutr* 53: 694-699

Beck-Sague, C., Banerjee, S., & Jarvis, W.R. (1993) Infectious diseases and mortality among US nursing home residents. *Am J Public Health*. 1993 Dec; 83(12): 1739-1742.

Beck-Sague, C., Villarino, E., Giuliano, D., Welbel, S., Latts, L., Manangan L.M., Sinkowitz, R.L. & Jarvis, W.R. (1994) Infectious diseases and death among nursing home residents: results of surveillance in 13 nursing homes. Infect *Control Hosp Epidemiol* 15: 494-496

Beers, M.H., Ouslander, J.G., Fingold, S.F., Morgenstern, H., Reuben, D.B., Rogers, W., Zeffren, M.J., & Beck, J.C. (1992) Inappropriate medication prescribing in skilled-nursing facilities. *Ann Intern Med* 117: 684-689

Benenson, S., Cohen, M.J., Block, C., Stern, S., Weiss, Y., Moses, A.E. & JIRMI Group (2009) Vancomycin-resistant enterococci in long-term care facilities. I*nfect Control Hosp Epidemiol.* 30(8): 786-789

Bennet, R.G. (1993) Diarrhea among residents of long-term care facilities. *Infect Control Hosp Epidemiol* 14: 397-404

Bentley, D,W., (1984) Bacterial pneumonia in the elderly: clinical features, diagnosis, etiology and treatment. *Gerontology*30: 297-307

Bentley, D.W., (1990a) Tuberculosis in long-term care facilities. *Infect Control Hosp Epidemiol* 11: 42-46

Bentley, D.W., (1990b) Clostridium difficile-associated disease in long-term care facilities. *Infect Control Hosp Epidemiol* 11:434-438

Bentley, D.W., Bradley, S., High, K., Schoenbaum, S., Taler, G., & Yoshinawa, T.T. (2000) Practice guideline for evaluation of fever and infection in long-term care facilities. *Clin Infect Dis* 31: 640-653

Ben-Yehuda, A., & Weksler, M.E. (1992) Host resistance and the immune system. *Clin Geriatr Med* 8:701-711

Berland, B. & Gleckman, R.A. (1992): Fever of unknown origin in the elderly: A sequential approach to diagnosis. *Postgrad Med* 92:197–210.

Berlowitz, D.R. & Wilking, S.V.B. (1989) Risk factors for pressure sores. . *J Am Geriatr Soc* 37: 1043-1050

Berlowitz, D.R., Brandeis, G.H., Brand, H.K., Halpern, J., Ash, A.S., & Moskowitz, M.A. (1996) Evaluating pressure ulcer occurrence in long term care. Pitfalls in interpreting administrative data. *J Clin Epidemiol* 49: 289-292

Bertoni, A.G., Saydah, S., & Brancati, F,L. (2001) Diabetes and the risk of infection-related mortality in the United States. *Diabetes Care.* 24:1044-1049

Bettelli, G. (2011) Preoperative evaluation in geriatric surgery: comorbidity, functional status and pharmacological history. Minerva *Anestesiol 77: 1-2*

Bjork, D.T., Pelletler, L.L., & Tight, R.R. (1984) Urinary infections with antibiotic resistant organisms in catheterized nursing home patients. *Infect Control* 5: 173-176

Blandford, G., Watkins, L.B., & Mulvihill, M.N. (1998) Assessing abnormal feeding behavior in dementia: a taxonomy and initial finding. In: *Weight Loss and Eating Behavior in Alzheimer's Patients. Research and Practice in AD.* Eds Vellas B, Riviere S, Fitte J. New York: Serdi Publishing Company

Bloom, H., & Bottone, E. (1990) Aeromonas hydrphila diarrhea in a long-term care setting. *J Am Geriatr Soc* 38: 804-806

Bonilla, H.F., Zervos, M.A., Lyons, M.J., Bradley, S.F., Hedderwick, S.A:, Ramsey, M.A., Paul, L.K., & Kauffman, C.A. (1997) Colonization with Vancomycin-resistant Enterococcus faecium: comparison of a long-term care unit with an acute-care hospital. *Infect Control Hosp Epidemiol* 18: 333-339

Bonten, M.J., Slaughter, S., Hayden, M.K., Nathan, C., Van Voorhis, J., & Weinstein, R.A. (1998) External sources of Vancomycin-resistant Enterococci for intensive care units. *Crit Care Med* 26: 2001-2004

Boog, C.J.P. (2009) Principles of vaccination and possible development strategies for rational design. *Immunol Lett* 122: 104-107

Boscia, J.A., Kobasa, W.D., Knight, R.A., Abrutyn, E., Levison, M.E., Kaye, D. (1986) Epidemiology of bacteriuria in an elderly ambulatory population. *Am J Med* 80 (2): 208-214

Boström, A.M., Van Soest, D., Kolewaski, B., Milke, D.L., & Estabrooks, C.A. (2011) Nutrition Status Among Residents Living in a Veterans' Long-Term Care Facility in Western Canada: A Pilot Study. *J Am Med Dir Assoc* 12 (3): 217-225

Boustcha, E. & Nicolle, L.E. (1995) Conjunctivitis in a long-term care facility. *Infect Control Hosp Epidemiol* 16(4): 210-6.

Bowman, C., Whistler, J., & Ellerby, M. (2004) A national census of care home residents. *Age Ageing* 33: 561-566

Bradley, S.F. (1999) Methicillin-resistant Staphylococcus Aureus long-term concerns. *Am J Med* 106: 2-10

Bradley, S.F., Terpenning, M.S., Ramsey, M.A., Zarins, L.T., Jorgensen, K.A., Sottile, W.S., Scheberg. D.R., & Kauffman, C.A. (1991) Methicillin-resistant Staphylococcus Aureus: colonization and infection in a long-term care facility. *Ann Intern Med* 115: 417-422

Branders, G.H., Norris, J.N., Nash, D.V., & Lipsitz, L.A. (1990) The epidemiology and natural history of pressure ulcers in elderly nursing home residents. *J Am Med Assoc* 264: 2905-2909

Brennan, C., Wagner, M.M., & Muder, R.R. (1998) Vancomycin-resistant Enterococcus faecium in a long-term care facility. *J Am Geriatr Soc* 46: 157-160

Brennen, C. & Muder, R. (1990) Conjunctivitis associated with methicillin-resistant staphylococcus aureus in a long-term care facility. *Am J Med* 88 (suppl 5): 14N-17N

Brennen, C., Muder, R.R., & Muraca, P. (1988) Occult endemic tuberculosis in a chronic care facility. *Infect Control Hosp Epidemiol* 9: 548-552

Brennen, C.,Wagener, M.M., & Muder, R.R. (1998) Vancomycin-resistant Enterococcus faecium in a long-term care facility. *J Am Geriatr Soc* 46: 157-160

Brusaferro, S. & Moro, M.L. (2005) Le residenze assistenziali per anziani: una nuova sfida per il controllo delle infezioni correlate alle pratiche assistenziali. *Giorn It Inf Osp* Gennaio- Marzo 2005; 12: 8-21

Bruunsgaard, H., Pedersen, A.N., Schroll, M., & Skinhøj, P., Pedersen, BK. (2001). "Decreased natural killer cell activity is associated with atherosclerosis in elderly humans". *Exp Gerontol* 37 (1): 127–136

Calverley, P.M., Anderson, J.A., Celli, B., Ferguson, G.T., Jenkins, C., Jones, P.W., Yates, J.C., & Vestbo, J., TORCH investigators. (2007) Salmeterol and fluticasone propionate and survival in chronic obstructive pulmonary disease. *N Engl J Med* 356: 775-789

Cambier, J. (2005). Immunosenescence: a problem of lymphopoiesis, homeostasis, microenvironment, and signaling. *Immunological Reviews* 205: 5–6.

Campbell, B. (1991) Surveillance and control of infections in long-term care: the Canadian experience. *Am J Med* 91 (Suppl 3B): 3B - 286S-288S

Cantrell, M. & Norman, D.C. (2010) Practice of Geriatrics Chapter 38 Infections in "Free Medical Textbook" October 5, 2010. Avaible at: *http://medtextfree.wordpress.com/2010/10/05/chapter-38-infections/*

Capitano, B., Leshem, O.A., Nightingale, C.H., & Nicolau, D.P. (2003) Cost effect of managing Methicillin-Resistant Staphylococcus Aureus in a long-term care facility. *J Am Geriatr Soc* 51: 10-16

Carmeli, Y., Eliopoulous, G.M., Mozaffari, E., & Samore, M. (2002) Health and economic outcomes of vancomycin-resistant enterococci. *Arch Intern Med* 162(19): 2223-2228

Carratalà, J., Mykietiuk, A., Fernandez-Sabé, N., Suàrez, C., Dorca, J., Verdaguer, R., Manresa, F., & Gudiol, F. (2007) Health care-associated pneumonia requiring hospital admission. Epidemiology, antibiotic therapy and clinical outcomes. *Arch Intern Med* 167: 1393-1399

Carter, A.O., Borczyk, A.A., Carlson, J.A.K., Harvey, B., Hockin, J.C., Karmali, M.A., Kriehan, C., Korn, D.A., & Lior, H. (1987) A severe outbreak of Escherichia coli O157:H7 associated hemorrhagic colitis in a nursing home. *N Engl J Med* 317; 1496-1500

Carter, O.A., Borcyk, A.A., Carlson, J.A., Harvey, B., Hockin, J.C., & Karmali, M.A. (1987) Infectious diarrhea in the elderly. *N Engl J Med* 317: 1495-1500

Castle, S.C., Norman, D., Yeh, M., Miller, D., & Yoshikawa, T. (1991): Fever response in elderly nursing home residents: Are the older truly colder? *J Am Geriatr Soc* 39: 853–857.

Centers for Disease Control and Prevention (1989a) Surveillance for epidemics. *Morbid Mortal Weekly Rep* 38: 694-696

Centers for Disease Control and Prevention (1989b) Recomendations of the Immunization Practices Advisory Committee. Pneumococcal polysaccharide vaccine. *Morbid Mortal Weekly Rep* 38: 64-67

Centers for Disease Control and Prevention (1990a) Nursing home outbreaks of invasive group-A streptococcal infections - Illinois, Kansas, Noth Carolina and Texas. *Morbid Mortal Weekly Rep* 39: 577-579

Centers for Disease Control and Prevention (1990b) Prevention and control of tuberculosis in facilities providing long-term care to the elderly: recommendations of the Advisory Committee for Elimination of Tuberculosis. *Morb Mortal Wkly Rep* 39 (RR-10): 7-20

Centers for Diseases Control and Prevention (2004) Diagnosis and management of foodborne illnesses. A primer for physicians and other health care professionals. *Morbid Mortal Weekly Recomm Rep* 53: 1-33

Centers for Diseases Control and Prevention. (2002) Guidelines for hand hygiene in healthcare settings: recommendation of the health infection control practices advisory committee and the HICPAC/SHEA/APIC/IDSA hand hygiene task force. *Morbid Mortal Weekly Recomm Rep* 21: S3-S40

Centers for Diseases Control and Prevention. (2003) Public Health and Aging - United States and worldwide. *MMWR Morb Mortal Wkly Rep* 2003 february 14; 52(6):101-106

Centers for Medicare and Medicaid (CMS) Manual System, State Operations Manual. *Appendix.* 2005. pp. 183–4

Chan, K.M., Wong, S.F., & Yoong, T. (1998) Nursing home applications: reason and possible interventions. *Singapore Med J* 39(10): 451-455

Chang, C.C. & Roberts, B.L. (2011) Malnutrition and feeding difficulty in Taiwanese older with dementia. *J Clin Nurs* 2011 apr 26; doi: 10.1111/j.1365-2702.2010.03686.x.

Chenoweth, C.E., Bradley, S.F., Terpenning, M.S., Zarins, L.T., Ramsey, M.A., & Schaberg, D.R. (1994) Colonization and transmission of high level gentamicin-resistant enterococci in a long-term care facility. *Infect Control Hosp Epidemiol* 15: 703-709

Choi, A.T., Yoshikawa, T., Bridge, J., Schlaffer, A., Osterwell, D., Reid, D., & Norman, D.C. (1990) Salmonella outbreak in a nursing home. *J Am Geriatr Soc* 38: 531-534

Chong, W.F., Ding, Y. Y., & Heng, B.H. (2011) A comparison of comorbidities obtained from hospital administrative data and medical chart in older patients with pneumonia. *BMC Health Serv Res* 11: 105

Chow, A.W., Galpin, J.E., & Guze, L.B. (1977) Clindamycin for treatment of sepsis caused by decubitus ulcers. *J Infect Dis* 735: 565-568

Clark, N.C., Cooksey, R.C., Hill, B.C., Swenson, J.M., & Tenover, F.C. (1993) Characterization of glycopeptides-resistant enterococci from US hospitals. *Antimicrob Agents Chemiother* 37: 2311-2317

Clocon, J.O., Silverstone, F.A., Graver, L.M., & Foley, C.J. (1988) Tube feedings in elderly patients: indications, benefits and complications. *Arch Intern Med* 148: 429-433

Cohen, E., Hierholzer, W., Schilling, C., & Snydman, D. (1979) Nosocomial infections in skilled nursing facilities: a preliminary survey. *Public Health Rep* 94: 162-165

Cohen, E., Lautenbach, E., Morales, K.H., & Linkin, K.H. (2006) Fluoroquinolone-resistant Escherichia coli in the long-term care setting. *Am J Med* 119: 958-963

Coleman, E.A., Martau, J.M., Lin, M.K., & Kramer, A.M. (2002) Pressure ulcers prevalence in long-term nursing home residents since the implementation of OBRA '87. Omnibus Budget Reconciliation Act (comment). . *J Am Geriatr Soc* 50: 728-732

Coque, T.M., Tomayko, J.F., Ricke, S.C., Okhyusen, P.C., & Murray, B.E. (1996) Vancomycin-Resistant Enterococci from nosocomial, community and animal sources in the United States. *Antimicrob Agents Chemiother 40: 2605-2609*

Corrente, M., Monno, R., Totaro, M., Martella, V., Buonavoglia, D., Rizzo, C., Ricci, D., Rizzo, G., & Buonavoglia C (2005) Characterization of methicillin-resistant Staphylococcus Aureus (MRSA) isolated at the Policlinico Hospital fo Bary (Italy). *New Microbiol* 28 (1): 57-65

Cosgrove, S.E., Kaye, K.S., Eliopoulous, G.M., & Carmeli, Y. (2002) Health and economic outcomes of the emergence of third-generation cephalosporin resistance in Enterobacter Species. *Arch Intern Med* 162(2): 185-190

Cosgrove, S.E., Kaye, K.S., Harbarth, S., Karchmer, A.W., & Carmeli, Y. (2005) The impact of methicillin resistance in Staphylococcus aureus bacterieremia on patients outcome: mortality, length of stay and hospital charges. *Infect Control Hosp Epidemiol* 26 (2) : 166-174

Crossley, K., Henry, K., Irvine, P., & Willenbring, K. (1987) Antibiotic use in nursing homes: prevalence, cost and utilization review. *Bull NY Acad Med* 63: 510-518

Crossley, K., Irvine, P., Kaszar, D.J. & Loewenson, R.B. (1985) Infection control practices in Minnesota nursing homes. *J Am Med Assoc* 254: 2918-2921

Curns, A.T., Holman, R.C., Sejvar, J.J., Owing, M.F., & Schonberger, L.B. (2005) Infectious disease hospitalizations among older adults in the United States from 1990 to 2002. *Arch Intern Med* 165 (21); 2005 nov 28: 2514-2520

D'Agata, E. & Mitchell, S.L. (2008) Pattern of antimicrobial use among nursing home residents with advanced dementia. *Arch Intern Med* 2008 Febbruary 25; 168 (4): 357-362

Daly, P.B., Smith, P.W., Rusnak, P.G., & Woods, G.L. (1991) A microbiologic survey of long-term care facilities. *Nebr Med J* 76: 161-165

Danzig, L.E., Short, L.J. & Collins, K. (1995) Bloodstream infections associated with a needless intravenous infusion system in patients receiving home infusion therapy. *J Am Med Assoc* 273: 1862-1864

Darnowsky, S., Gordon, M., & Simor, A. (1991) Two years infection surveillance in a geriatric long-term care facility. *Am J Infect Control 19: 185*-190

Das, R., Perrelli, E., Towle, V., van Ness, P.H., & Juthani-Meta, M. (2009) Antimicrobial susceptibility of bacteria isolated from urine sample obtained from nursing home residents. *Infect Control Hosp Epidemiol* 30 (11): 116-119

del Río, G., Mestre, J., & Dalet, F. (1992) Prevalence and treatment of bacteriuria in the geriatric population. *Enferm Infecc Microbiol Clin* 10(10): 602-606

Denman, S.J., & Burton, J.R. (1992) Fluid intake and urinary tract infection in the elderly. *J Am Med Assoc* 267: 2245-2249

Denton , M., Hawkey, P.M., Hoy, C.M., & Porter, C (1993) Co-existent cross-infection with Streptococcus pneumonia and Group B Streptococci on an adult oncology unit. *J Hosp Infect* 23: 271-278

Diekema, D.J., Bootsmiller, B.J., Vaughn, T.E., Woolson, R.F., Yankey, J.W., Ernst, E.J., Flach, S.D., Ward, M.M., Franciscus, C.L., Pfaller, M.A., & Doebbeling, B.G.N. (2004) Antimicrobial resistance trends and outbreak frequency in United States Hospitals. *Clin Infect Dis* 38: 78-85

Dixon, W.G., Kezouh, A., Bernatsky, S., & Suissa, S. (2011) The influence of systemic glucocorticoid therapy upon the risk of non-serious infection in older patients with rheumatoid arthritis: a nested case-control study. *Ann Rheum Dis.* 2011 Jun; 70(6): 956-960.

Do, A.N., Ray, B.J., & Banerjee, S.N. (1999) Bloodstream infection associated with needless device use and importance of infection control practices in the home health setting. *J Infect Dis* 179: 442-448

Donini, L.M., DeFelice, R., Tagliaccica, A., Palazzotto, A., De Bemardini, L., & Cannella, C. (2000) MNA predictive value in long-term care. *Age & Nutrition* 11:2–5

Doshi, J.A., Shaffer, T., Briesacher, B.A. (2005) National estimates of medication use in nursing homes: findings from the 1997 Medicare Current Beneficiary Survey and the 1996 Medical Expenditure Survey. *J Am Geriatr Soc* 53: 438-443

Drinka, P.J., Stemper, M.E., Gauerke, C.D., Miller, J.E., Goodman, B.M., & Reed, K.D. (2005) Clustering of multiple endemic strins of methicillin-resistant Staphylococcus aureus in a nursing home: an 8-year study. *Infect Control Hosp Epidemiol* 26: 215-218

Drummond, M.B., Dasenbrook, C.E., Pitz, N.W., Murphy, D.J., & Fan, E. (2008) Inhaled corticosterois in patients with stable chronic obstructive pulmonary disease: a systematic review and meta-analysis. *J Am Med Assoc* 300: 2407-2416

Duffy, L.M., Cleary, J., Ahern, S., Kuskowski, M.A., West, M., & Wheeler, L. (1995) Clean intermittent catheterization: safe, cost-effective bladder management for male residents of VA nursing homes. *J Am Geriatr Soc* 43: 865-870

Durand, M., & Joseph, M. (2005) Infections of the upper respiratory tract. Available at: *http: //www.mheducation.com/HOL2_chapters/HOL_chapters/chapter30.htm* Accessed July 12, 2005

Earhart, K.C. & Baugh, W.P., (2005) Rhinocerebral mucormycosis. Available at: *http: //www.emedicine.com/med/topic2026.htm* Accessed July 12, 2005

Eberle, C.M., Winsemius, D., Garibaldi, R.A. (1993) Risk factors and consequences of bacteriuria in non-catheterized nursing home residents. *J Gerontol.* 48(6): M266–M271.

Ehrenkranz, N.J., Alfonso, B., & Nerenberg, D. (1990) Irrigation-aspiration for culturing draining decubitus ulcers: correlation of bacteriological findings with a clinical inflammatory scoring index. *J Clin Microbiol* 28: 2389-2393

Eikelenboom-Boskamp, A., Cox-Claessens, J.H., Boom-Poels, P.G., Drabbe, M.I., Koopmans, R.T, & Voss, A. (2011) Three-year prevalence of healthcare-associated infections in Dutch nursing homes. *J Hosp Infect* 78 (1): 59-62

Elizaga, M.L., Weinstein, R.A., & Hayden, M.K. (2002) Patients in long-term care facilities: a reservoir for Vancomycin Resistant Enterococci. *Clin Infect Dis* 34: 441-446

Elphick, H.L., Elphick, D.A., & Sanders, D.S. (2006) Small bowel bacterial overgrowth. An unrecognized cause of malnutrition in older adults. *Geriatrics* 2006 sept; 61 (9): 21-26

El-Sohl, A.A., Aquilina, A.T., Dhillon, R.S., Ramadan, F., Nowak, P., & Davies, N. (2002) Impact of invasive strategy on management of antimicrobial treatment failure in institutionalized older people with severe pneumonia. *Am J Resp Crit Care Med* 166: 1038-1043

El-Sohl, A.A., Pietrantoni, C., Bhat, A., Bhora, M., & Berbary, E. (2004) Indicators of potentially drug-resistant bacteria in severe nursing home-acquired pneumonia. *Clin Infect Dis* 39: 474-480

Ely, J.W., Osheroff, J.A., Chambliss, M.L., & Ebell, M.H. (2006). Approach to leg edema of unclear etiology. *J Am Board Fam Med* 19(2):148–160.

Eom, C.S., Jeon, C.Y., Lim, J.W., Cho, E.G., Park, S.M., & Lee, K.S. (2011) Use of acid-suppressive drugs and risk of pneumonia: a systematic review and meta-analysis. *Can Med Assoc J* 2011 Feb 22; 183(3): 310-319

Eriksen, H.M., Koch, A.M., Elstrøm, P., Nilsen, R.M., Harthug, S., & Aavitsland, P. (2007) Healthcare-associated infection among residents of long term care facilities: a cohort and nested case-control study. *Journal of Hospital Infection* 65 (4): 334-340

Ernst, P., Gonzalez, A.V., Brassard, P., & Suissa, S. (2007) Inhaled corticosterois use in chronic obstructive pulmonary disease and the risk of hospitalization for pneumonia. *Am J Respir Crit Care Med* 176: 162-166

Farage, M.A. & Maibach, H.I. (2011) Morphology and physiological changes of genital skin and mucosa. *Curr Probl Dermatol.* Febb, 10, 2011; 40:9-19

Farber, B.F., Poplausky, M., Gruber, M., & Brody, J.P. (1984) A prospective study of nosocomial infections in a chronic care facility. *J Am Geriatr Soc* 32: 499-502

Fay, D.E., Poplausky, M., Gruber, M., & Lance, P. (1991) Long term enteral feeding: a retrospective comparison of delivery via percutaneous endoscopic gastrostomy and nasoenteric tubes. *Am J Gastroenterol* 86: 1604-1609

Finnegan, T.P., Austin, T.W., & Cape, R.D. (1985) A 12-month fever surveillance study in a veterans' long-stay institution. *J Am Geriatr Soc* 33: 590-594

Flacker, J.M. & Kiely, D.K. (2003) Mortality-related factors and 1-year survival in nursing home residents. *J Am Geriatr Soc* 51: 213-221

Flamm, R.K., Weaver, M.K., Thornsberry, C., Jones, M.E., Karlowsky, J.A. & Sahm, D.F. (2004) Factors associated with relative rate of antibiotic resistance in Pseudomonas aeruginosa isolated tested in clinical laboratories in the United States from 1999 to 2002. *Antimicrob Agents Chemiother* 48 (7): 2431-2436

Flerer, J. & Ekstrom, M. (1981) An outbreak of Providencia stuartii urinary tract infections: patients with condom catheters are a reservoir of the bacteria. *J Am Med Assoc* 245: 1553-1555

Flournoy, D.J. (1994) Antimicrobial susceptibilities of bacteria from nursing home residents in Oklahoma. *Gerontology* 40: 53-56

Franceschi, C., Bonafè, M., & Valensin, S. (2000b) Human immunosenescence: the prevailing of innate immunity, the failing of clonotypic immunity, and the filling of immunological space. *Vaccine* 18 (16): 1717–1720

Franceschi, C., Bonafè, M., Valensin, S., Olivieri, F., De Luca, M., Ottaviani, E., & De Benedictis, G. (2000a) Inflamm-aging: An Evolutionary Perspective on Immunosenescence". *Ann N Y Acad Sci* 908: 244–254

Franceschi, C., Valensin, S., Fagnoni, F., Barbi, C., & Bonafè, M. (1999) Biomarkers of immunosenescence within an evolutionary perspective: the challenge of heterogeneity and the role of antigenic load. *Experimental Gerontolgy* 34: 911–921

Franson, T., Duthie, E., Cooper Jr.J., van Oudenhove, G., & Hoff, R. (1986) Prevalence survey of infections and their predisposing factors at a hospital-based nursing home care unit. *J Am Geriatr Soc* 34: 95-100

Freedland, C.P., Roller, R.D., Wolfe, B.M., & Flynn, N.M. (1989) Microbial contamination of continuous drip feeding. *J Parenter Enter Nutr* 13: 18-22

Fridkin, S.K., Hageman, J.C., Morrison, M., Sanza, L.T., Como-Sabetti, K., Jernigan, J.A., Harriman, K., Harrison, L.H., Lynfield, R., & Farley, M.M., Active Bacterial Core Surveillance Program of the Emerging Infections Program Network. (2005). Methicillin-resistant Staphylococcus aureus disease in three communities. *N Engl J Med* 352:1436-1444

Fry, A.M., Shay, D.K., Holman, R.C., Curns, A.T., & Anderson, L.J. (2005) Trends in hospitalizations for pneumonia among persons aged 65 years or older in the United States, 1988-2002. *J Am Med Assoc* 294 (21); 2005 Dec 7: 2712-2719

Fulop, T., Gagné, D., Goulet, A.C., Desgeorges, S., Lacombe, G., Arcand, M., & Dupuis, G. (1999) Age-related impairment of p56lck and ZAP-70 activities in human T lymphocytes activated through the TcR/CD3 complex. *Exp Gerontol* 34 (2): 197–216.

Furniss, L., Craig, S.K., Burns, A. (1998) Medication use in nursing homes for the elderly. *Int J Geriatr Psychiatry* 13: 433-439

Furuno, J.P., Hebden, J.N., & Standiford, H.C. (2008) Prevalence of methicillin-resistant Staphylococcus aureus and Acinetobacter baumannii in long-term acute care facility. *Am J Infect Control* 36: 468-471

Galvin, J. (2002) An audit of pressure ulcer incidence in a palliative care setting. Int J Palliat Nurs 8(5):214-221

Gambert, S.R., Duthie, E.H. Jr., Priefer, B., & Rabinovitch, R.A. (1982) Bacterial infections in hospital-based skilled nursing facility. *J Chron Dis* 35: 781-786

Gammack, J.K. (2003) Use and management of chronic urinary catheters in long term care: much controversy, little consensus. *J Am Med Dir Assoc* 4(2 Suppl) S52-S59

Garb, J., Brown, R., Garb, J., & Tuthill, R. (1978) Differences in etiology of pneumonias in nursing home and community patients. *J Am Med Assoc* 240: 2169-2172

Garcia, A.D. & Thomas, D.R. (2006) Assessmet and management of chronic pressure ulcers in the elderly. *Med Clin North Am* 90: 925-944

Garibaldi, R.A. (1999) Residential care and the elderly: the burden of infection. J *Hosp Infect* 1999 Dec; 43 Suppl: S9-18.

Garibaldi, R.A., Brodine, S., & Matsumiya, S. (1981) Infections among patients in nursing homes. Policies, prevalence and problems. *N Eng J Med* 305: 731-735

Garner, J.S. (1996) The Hospital Infection Control Practices Advisory Committee, guideline for isolation precautions in hospitals. *Infect Control Hosp Epidemiol* 17: 53-80

Gau, J.T., Acharya, U., Khan, S., Heh, V., Mody, L., & Kao, T.C. (2011) Pharmacotherapy and the risk for community-acquired pneumonia. *BMC Geriatrics* 10: 45

Gaugler, J.E., Duval, S., Anderson, K.A., & Kane, R.L. (2007) Predicting nursing home admission in U.S.: A meta-analysis. *BMC Geriatrics* 7: 13

Gavazzi, G., Krause, K.H. (2002) Ageing and infection. *Lancet Infect Dis* 2(11): 659-666

Gaynes, R.P., Weinstein, R.A., Chamberlain, W., & Kabins, S.A. (1985) Antibiotic resistant flora in nursing home patients admitted to the hospital. *Arch Intern Med* 145: 1804-1807

Ghadially, R., Brown, B.E., Sequeira-Martin, S.M., Feingold, K.R., & Elias, P.M. (1995). The aged epidermal permeability barrier. Structural, functional, and lipid biochemical abnormalities in humans and a senescent murine model. J *Clin Invest.* 95:2281–2290

Gillchrest, B.A. (1999) Aging of the skin. In: *Principles of geriatric medicine and gerontology.* Hazard WR, Blass JP, Ettinger WH, Halter JB, Ouslander JG (eds.) 4th edition, Mc Graw Hill: 1999;573-590

Ginaldi, L., Loreto, M.F., Corsi, M.P., Modesti, M., & De Martinis, M. ,(2001). Immunosenescence and infectious diseases. *Microbes and Infection* 3 (10): 851–857

Girodon, F., Lombard, M., Galan, P., Brunet-Lecomte, P., Monget, A.L., Arnaud, J., Preziosi, P., & Hercberg, S. (1997) Effect of micronutrient supplementation on infection in institutionalized elderly subjects: a controlled trial. *Ann Nutr Metab* 41: 98-107

Gleckman, B. & Hibert, D. (1982) Afebrile bacteriemia: a phenomenon in geriatric patients. *J Am Med Assoc* 248: 1478-1481

Gleich, S., Morad, Y., & Echague, R (2000) Streptococcus pneumonia serotype 4 outbreaks in a home for the aged: report and review of recent outbreaks. *Infect Control Hosp Epidemiol* 21: 711-717

Gordon, W.Z., Kane, R.L., & Rothemberg, R. (1985) Acute hospitalization in a home for the aged. *J Am Geriatr Soc* 35: 519-523

Gosney, M.A., Hammond, M.F., Shenkin, A., & Allsup, S. (2008) Effect of micronutrient supplementation on mood in nursing home residents. *Gerontology* 54: 292-299

Gould, C-V-, Rothemberg, R., & Steinberg, J.P. (2006) Antibiotic resistance in long-term acute care hospitals: the perfect storm. *Infect Control Hosp Epidemiol* 27: 920-925

Green, C.M., van Beneden, C:A., Javadi, M., Skoff, T.H., Beall, B., & Facklam, R. (2005) Cluster of death from Group A streptococcus in a long-term care facility - Georgia 2001. *Am J Infect Control* 33: 108-113

Greenow, J.E., Christenson, E.J., & Montos, P. (1989) Contamination of enteral nutrition system during prolonged use. J Parenter Enter Nutr 13: 23-25

Gross, J.S., Neufeld, R.R., Libow, L.S., Gerber, I., & Rodstein, M. (1988) Autopsy study of the elderly institutionalized patient. *Arch Intern Med* 148: 173-176

Grude, N., Tveten, Y & Kristiansen, B.E. (2001) Urinary tract infections in Norway: bacterial etiology and susceptibility. A retrospective study of clinical isolates. *Clin Microbiol Infect* 7: 543-547

Gulmez, S.E., Holm, A., Frederiksen, H., Jensen, T.G., Pedersen, C., & Hallas, J. (2007) Use of proton pump inhibitors and the risk of community-acquired pneumonia: a population-based case-control study. *Arch Intern Med* 167: 950-955

Ha, U.S. & Cho, Y.H. (2006) Catheter-associated urinary tract infections: new aspects of novel urinary catheters. *Int J Antimicrob Agents.* 2006 Dec; 28(6): 485-90.

Hakim, F.T. & Gress, R.E. (2007) Immunosenescence: deficits in adaptive immunity in elderly. *Tissue antigens* 70 (3): 179–189

Hall, K.E. & Wiley, J.W. (1999) Age-associated changes in gastrointestinal function. In: *Principles of geriatric medicine and gerontology.* Hazard, W.R., Blass, J.P., Ettinger, W.H., Halter, J.B., Ouslander, J.G. (eds.) 4th edition, Mc Graw Hill: 1999; 835-842

Halvorsrud, J., & Orstavik, I. (1980) An epidemic of rotavirus-associated gastroenteritidis in a nursing home for te elderly. *Scand J Infect Dis* 12: 161-164

Han, S., Yang, K., Ozen, Z., Peng, W., Marinova, E., Kelsoe, G., & Zheng, B. (2003). "Enhanced differentiation of splenic plasma cells but diminished long-lived high-affinity bone marrow plasma cells in aged mice". *J Immunol* 170 (3): 1267–1273

Harkness, G.A., Bentley, D.W., Mottley, M., & Lee, J. (1992) Streptococcus pyogenes outbreak in a long term care facility. *Am J Infect Control* 20: 142-148

Harper, C. & Newton, P. (1989) Clinical aspects of pneumonia in the elderly veterans. *J Am Geriatr Soc* 37:867-872

Hassanzadeh, P., & Motamedifar, M. (2007) The prevalence of asymptomatic bacteriuria in long term care facility residents in Shiraz, Southwest Iran: a cross-sectional study. *Pak J Biol Sci* 10 (21): 3890-3894

He, Z., Sun, Z., Liu, S., Zhang, Q., & Tan, Z. (2009) Effect of early malnutrition on mental system, metabolic syndrome and immunity and the gastrointestinal tract. *J Vet med Sci* 71 (9): 1143-1150

Hedin, K., Petersson, C., Wideback, K., Kahlmeter, G., & Mölstad, S. (2002) Asymptomatic bacteriuria in a population of elderly in municipal institutional care. *Scand J Prim Health Care* 20 (3): 166-168

Henoch, I. & Gustaffson, M. (2003) Pressure ulcers in palliative care: development of a hospice pressure ulcer risk assessment scale. *Int J Palliat Nurs* 9(11):474-484

High, K. (2007) Immunization in older adults. *Clin Geriatr Med* 2007; August; 23 (3): 669-685. Viii-ix

High, K., Bradley, S., Gravenstein, S., Mehr, D.R., Quagliariello, V.J., Richards, C., & & Yoshinawa, T.T. (2009) Clinical practice guideline for the evaluation of fever and infection in older adult residents of long-term care facilities: 2008 Update by the Infectious Disease Society of America. *Clin Infect Dis* 48: 149-171

High, K., Bradley, S., Loeb, M., Palmer, R., Quagliariello, V., & Yoshinawa, T.T. (2005) A new paradigm for clinical investigation of infectious syndromes in older adults: assessment of functional status as a risk factor and outcome measure. *Clin Infect Dis* 40: 114-122

Hildebrandt, G.H., Dominguez, B.L., Schork, M.A., Loesche, W.J. (1997) Functional units, chewing, swallowing and food avoidance among elderly. *J Prosthet Dent* 77: 588-595

Hing, E. & Bloom, B. (1990) Long-term care for the functionally dependent elderly. *Vital Health Stat* n°104, 1990

Hirshberg, J., Rees, R.S., Marchant, B., & Dean, S. (2000) Osteomyelitis related to pressure ulcers: the cost of neglect. *Adv Skin Wound Care* 13: 25-29

Hoffman, N., Jenkins, R., & Putney, K. (1990) Nosocomial infection rates during a one-year period in a nursing home care unit of a Veterans Administration hospital. *Am J Infect Control* 18: 55-63

Hsu, C.C:S. (1991) Serial survey of Methicillin-resistant Staphylococcus aureus nasal carriage among residents in a nursing home. *Infect Control Hosp Epidemiol 12: 416-421*

Huovinen, P. (1984) Trimethoprim-resistant Escherichia coli in a geriatric hospital. *J Infect* 8: 145-148

Ijaz, K., Dillaha, J.A, & Yang, Z (2002) Unrecognized tuberculosis in a nursing home causing death with spread of tuberculosis to the community. J Am Geriatr Soc (2002) 50; 1213-1218

IKED (Initiative for quality improvement and Epidemiology of Diabetes) Report, 2007. National Public Health Institute, Brussel, Belgium 2007

Incalzi, R.A., Maini, C.L., Fuso, L., Giordano, A., Carbonin, P.U., Galli, G. (1989) Effect of aging on mucociliary clearance. *Compr Gerontol* [A] 3: 65-68

Irvine, P., van Buren, N., & Crossley, K. (1984) Causes for hospitalization of nursing homes residents. *J Am Geriatr Soc* 32: 103-105

Ito, K Hirao, A., Arai, F., Matsuoka, S., Takubo, K., Hamaguchi, I., Nomiyama, K., Hosokawa, K., Sakurada, K., Nakagata, N., Ikeda, Y., Mak, T.W., & Suda, T. (2004) Regulation of oxidative stress by ATM is required for self-renewal of haematopoietic stem cells". *Nature* 431 (7011): 997–1002

Jackson, M., Fierer, J., Barrett-Connor, E., Fraser, D., Klauber, M.R., Hatch, R., Burkhart, B., & Jones, M. (1992) Intensive surveillance for infections in a three-year study of nursing home patients. *Am J Epidemiol* 135: 685-696

Jackson, M.L., ., Neuzil, K.M., & Thompson, W.W. (2004) The burden of community acquired pneumonia in seniors: results of a population-based study. *Clin Infect Dis* 39 (11); 2004 Dec: 1642-1650

Jackson, M.L., Nelson, J.C., Weiss, N.S., Neuzil, K.M., Barlow, W., & Jackson, L.A. (2008) Influenza vaccination and risk of community-acquired pneumonia in immunocompetent elderly people: population-based, nested case-control study. *Lancet* 372: 398-405

Jacobson, C. & Strausbaugh, L.J. (1990) Incidence and impact of infection in a nursing home care unit. *Am J Infect Control 18: 151-159*

Jain, R., & Danziger, L.H. (2004) Multidrug-resistant Acinetobacter infections: an emerging challenge to clinician. *Ann Pharmacother* 38: 1449-1459

Jankowski, I.M. (2010) Tips for protecting critically ill patients from pressure ulcers. *Crit Care Nurse* 30 (2): S7-S9

Jette, A.M., Branch, L.G., Sleeper, L.A., Feldman, H., Sullivan, L.M. (1992) High risk profile for nursing home admission. *The Gerontologist* 32(5): 634-640

Jevons, M.P. (1961) "Celbein-resistant" staphylococci. *Br Med J* 1: 124-125

John, J.E., & Ribner, B.S. (1991) Antibiotic resistance in long-term care facilities. *Infect Control Hosp Epidemiol* 12: 245-250

Johnson, E.T. (1983) The condom catheter: urinary tract infection and other complications. *South Med J* 76: 579-582

Jones, A.L., Dwyer, L.L., Bercovitz, A.R., & Strahan, G.W. (2009) The National Nursing Home Survey: 2004 overview. *Vital Health Stat* 2009; 167: 1–155

Jones, S.R., Parker, D.F., Kiebow, E.S., Kimbrough, R.C., & Freur R.S. (1987) Appropriateness of antimicrobial therapy in long-term care facilities. *Am J Med* 83: 499-502

Juthani-Mehta, M. & Quagliariello, V.J., (2010) Infectious diseases in the Nursing Home setting: challenges and opportunities for clinical investigation. *Clin Infect Dis* 15; 51(8) 2010 October: 931-938

Kabbuz, R.F., & Tenney, J.H., (1988) Infection control in Maryland nursing homes. *Infect Control Hosp Epidemiol* 9: 159-162

Kaganski, N., Berner, Y., Koren-Morag, N., Perelman, L., Knobler, H., & Levy, S. (2005) Poor nutritional habits are predictors of poor outcome in very old hospitalized patients. *Am J Clin Nutr* 82: 784-791

Kardos, P., Wencker, M., Glaab, T., & Vogelmeier, C. (2007) Impact of salmeterol/fluticasone propionate versus salmeterol on exacerbations in severe chronic obstructive pulmonary disease. *Am J Respir Crit Care Med* 175: 144-149

Kashef, I., Dillaha, J.A., Yang, Z., Cave, M.D., & Bates, J.H. (2002) Unrecognized tuberculosis in a nursing home causing death with spread of tuberculosis to the community. *J Am Geriatr* Soc 50: 1213-1218

Katz, P.R., Beam, T.R., Brand, F., & Boyer, K (1990) Antibiotic use in the nursing home. Physician practice patterns. *Arch Intern Med* 150: 1465-1468

Keating, M.J. 3rd., Klimek, J.J., Levine, D.S., & Kiernan, F.J. (1984): Effect of aging on the clinical significance of fever in ambulatory adult patients. *J Am Geriatr Soc* 32: 282–287

Kelly, F.J., Dunster, C., & Mudway, I. (2003) Air pollution and the elderly oxidant/antioxidant issues with consideration. *Eur Resp J* Suppl. 40: 70S-75S

Kerr, H. & Byrd, J. (1991) Nursing home patients transferred by ambulance to a VA emergency department. *J Am Geriatr Soc* 39: 132-136

Kersten, H., Ruths, S., & Wyller TB (2009) Pharmacotherapy in nursing homes. *Tidsskr Nor Laegeforen* 2009 Sep 10; 129(17): 1732-1735

Kinsella, K., & Velkoff, V.A. (2001) International population report (series P95/01-1) Washington DC. US Government Printing Office, 2001

Klontz, K.C., Adler, W.H., & Potter, M. (1997) Age-dependent resistance factors in the pathogenesis of foodborne infectious disease. *Aging* (Milano) 9: 320-326

Kluger, M.J., Kozak, W., Conn, C.A., Leon, L.R., & Soszynski, D. (1996): The adaptive value of fever. *Infect Dis Clin North Am* 10: 1–20

Klugman, K.P. (2004) Vaccination: a novel approach to reduce antibiotic resistance. *Clin Infect Dis* 39: 649-651

Knockaert, D.C., Vanneste, L.J., & Bobbaers, H.J. (1993): Fever of unknown origin in elderly patients. *J Am Geriatr Soc* 32: 282–287.

Knol, W., van Marum, R.J., Jansen, P.A., Souverein, P.C., Schobben, A.F., & Egberts, A.C. (2008) Antipsychotic drug use and risk of pneumonia in elderly people. *J Am Geriatr Soc* 56: 661-666

Kothe, H., Bauer, T., Marre, R., Suttorp, N., Welte, T., Dalhoff, K., & The Competence Network for Community-Acquired Pneumonia study group (2008) Outcome of community-acquired pneumonia: influence of age, residence status and antimicrobial treatment. *Eur Respir J* 32: 139-146

Krauss, N.A. & Altman, B.M. (2004) Research findings *5: Characteristics of nursing home residents, 1996. December 2004. Agency for Healthcare Research and Quality, Rockville, MD. Available at: *http:// www.meps.ahrq.gov/mepsweb7data_file7pubications7rf57rf5.shtml*

Kunin, C.M., Douthitt, S., Dancing, J., Anderson, J., & Moeschberger, M. (1992) The association between the use of urinary catheters and morbidity and mortality among elderly patients in nursing homes. *Am J Epidemiol* 135: 291-301

Laheji, R.J., Sturkenboom, M.C., Hassing, R.J., Dieleman, J., Stricker, B.H., & Jansen, J.B. (2004) Risk of community-acquired pneumonia and use of gastric acid-suppressive drugs. *J Am Med Assoc* 292: 1955-1960

Lamy, M., Mojon, P., Kalykakis, G., Legrand, R., & Butz-Jorgensen, E. (1999) Oral status and nutrition in the institutionalized elderly. *J Dent* 27: 443-448

Laria, A., Zoli, A., Gremese, E., & Ferraccioli, G.F. (2011) Proton pump inhibitors in rheumatic diseases: clinical practice, drug interactions, bone fractures and risk of infections. *Reumatismo* 2011 Mar;63(1):5-10.

Lautenbach, E., Marsicano, R., Tolomeo, P., Heard, M., Serrano, S., & Stieritz, D.D. (2009) Epidemiology of Gram negative antimicrobial resistance in a multi-state network of long-term care facilities. Infect Control Hosp Epidemiol 30 (8): 790-793

Lee, Y.L., Cesario, T., Gupta, G., Flionis, L., Tran, C., Decker, M., & Thrupp, L.D. (1997) Surveillance of colonization and infection with Staphylococcus Aureus susceptible or resistant to Methicillin in a community skilled-nursing facility. *Am J Infect Control* 25: 312-321

Lee, Y.L., Thrupp, L.D., & Nothvogel, S. (1996) Infection surveillance and antibiotic utilization in a community-based skilled nursing facility. *Aging Clin Exp Res* 8: 113-122

Lelovics, Z. (2009) Nutritional status and nutritional rehabilitation of elderly people living in long-term care institutions. *Orv Hetil* 2009 Nov 1; 150(44): 2028-2036.

Leung, F.W. & Schnelle, J.F. (2008) Urinary and fecal incontinence in nursing home residents. *Gastroenterol Clin North Am 37(3) 697*

Levine, W.J., Smart, J., Archer, D., Bean, N., & Tauxe, R. (1991) Foodborne disease outbreaks in nursing homes, 1975 trough 1987. J. Am. Med. Assoc. 266: 2105-2109

Lim, W.S. & Macfarlane, J.T. (2001) A prospective comparison of nursing home acquired pneumonia with community acquired pneumonia. *Eur Resp J* 18: 362-368

Lin, Y.T., Chen, L.K., Lin, M.H., & Hwang, S.J. (2006) Asymptomatic bacteriuria among the institutionalized elderly. *J Chin Med Assoc* 69 (5): 213-217

Linton, P., Lustgarten, J., & Thoman, M. (2006) T cell function in the aged: Lessons learned from animal models. *Clinical and Applied Immunology Reviews* 6: 73–97

Livesley, N.J. & Chow, A.W. (2002) Infected pressure ulcers in elderly individuals. *Clin Infect Dis* 35: 1390-1396

Loeb, M., , McGeer, A., McArthur, M., Peeling, R.W., Petric, M., & Simor, A.E. (2000) Surveillance for outbreaks of respiratory tract infections in nursing homes. Can Med Assoc J 162: 1113-1117

Loeb, M., Bentley, D.W., Bradley, S., Crossley, K., Garibaldi, R., Gantz, N., McGeer, A., Muder, R.R., Mylotte, J., Nicolle, L.E., Nurse, B., Paton, S., Simor, A.E., Smith, P., & Strausbaugh, L. (2001b) Development of minimum criteria for the initiation of antibiotics in residents of long-term-care facilities: results of a consensus conference. *Infect Control Hosp Epidemiol* 22(2): 120–124

Loeb, M., Simor, A.E., & Walter, S. (2001a) Antibiotic use in Ontario facilities that provide chronic care. *J Gen Intern Med* 16: 376-383

Lord, J,M., Butcher, S., Killampali, V., Lascelles, D., & Salmon, M. (2001) Neutrophil ageing and immunesenescence. *Mech Ageing Dev* 122 (14): 1521–1535

Luman, W., Kwek, K.R., Loi, K.L., Chiam, M.A., Cheung, W.K., & Ng, H.S. (2001) Percutaneous endoscopic gastrostomy--indications and outcome of our experience at the Singapore General Hospital. Singapore Med J. 2001 Oct; 42(10): 460-465.

Lund-Nielsen, B., Adamsen, L., Gottrup, F., Rorth, M., Tolver, A., & Kolmos, H.J. (2011) Qualitative bacteriology in malignant wounds. A prospective, randomized, clinical study to compare the effect of honey and silver dressings. Ostomy Wound Manag 57(7): 28-36

Lyder, C.H. (2003) Pressure ulcer prevention and management. *J Am Med Assoc* 289: 223-226

MacArthur, M.D., Lehman, M.H., Currie-McCumber, C.A., & Shlaes, D.M. (1988) The epidemiology of gentamicin-resistant Pseudomonas aeruginosa on an intermediate care unit. *Am J Epidemiol* 128: 821-827

Magaziner, J., Tenney, J.H., DeForge, B., Hebel, R., Muncie, H.L., & Warren, J.W. (1991) Prevalence and characteristics of nursing home-acquired infection in the aged. *J Am Geriatr Soc* 39: 1071-1078

Magnussen, M. & Robb, S. (1980) Nosocomial infections in a long-term care facility. *Am J Infect Control* 8: 12-17

Magri, F., Borza, A., del Vecchio, S., Chytiris, S., Cuzzoni, G., Busconi, L., Rebesco, A., & Ferrari, E. (2003) Nutritional assessment of demented patients: a descriptive study. *Aging Clin Exp Res* 15: 148-153

Mandal, S.K., & Ray, A.K., (1987) Vitamin C status of elderly patients on admission into an assessment geriatric ward. *J Int Med Res* 15: 96-98

Marin, A., Monsó, E., Garcia-Nuñez, M., Sauleda, J., Noguera, A., Pons, J., Agustí, A., & Morera, J. (2010) Variability and effects of bronchial colonization in patients with moderate COPD. *Eur Respir J* 35: 295-302

Marrie, T.J., Durant, H., & Kwan, C. (1986) Nursing home-acquired pneumonia: a case-control study. *J Am Geriatr Soc* 34: 697-702

Maslow, J.N., Lee, B., & Lautenbach, E. (2005) Fluoroquinone-resistant Escherichia coli carriage in long term care facility. *Emerg Infect Dis* 11: 889-894

Mathai, D., Jones, R.N., Pfaller, M-A- & the SENTRY Partecipant Group North America (2001) Epidemiology and frequency of resistance among pathogens causing urinary tract infections in 1510 hospitalized patients: a report from the SENTRY Antimicrobial Surveillance Program (North America). Diagnostic Microbiol Infect Dis 40 (3): 129-136

Mc Evoy, A.J., Dutton, A.J., & James, O.F.W. (1983) Bacterial contamination of the small intestine is an important cause of occult malasorption in the elderly. *Br Med J* 287: 789-793

Mc Geer, A., Campbell, A.B., Eckert, D.G., Emori, T.G., Hierholzer, W.J., Jackson, M.M., Nicolle, L.E., Peppler, C., Rivera, A., Simor, A.E., Smith, P.W., & Wang, E. (1991) Definitions of infections for surveillance in long-term care facilities. *Am J Infect Control* 19: 1-7

Mc Nabney, M.K., Wolff, J.L., Semanick, L.M., Kasper, J.D., & Boult, C. (2007) Care needs of higher functioning nursing home residents. *J Am Med Dir Assoc* 8(6): 409-412

McAnulty, J.M., Keene, W.E., & Leland, D. (2000) Contaminated drinking water in one town manifesting as an outbreak of cryptosporidiosis in another. *Epidemiol Infect* 125: 79-86

Mendelson, G., Yearmack, Y., Granot, E., Ben-Israel, J., Colodner, R., & Raz, R. (2003) Staphylococcus Aureus carrier state among elderly residents of a lont-term care facility. *J Am Med Assoc* 4: 125-127

Meyer, K.C. (2001) The role of immunity in susceptibility to respiratory infection in the aging lung. *Respir Physiol* 1: 23-31

Meyer, K.C., Ershler, W., & Rosenthal, N.S. (1996) Immune dysregulation in the aging human lung. *Am J Respir Crit Care Med* 153: 1072-1079

Meyers, B., Sherman, E., Mendelson, M., Velasquez, G., Srulevitch-Chin, E., & Hubbard, M. (1989) Bloodstream infection in the elderly. *Am J Med* 86; 379-384

Michocki, R.J. & Lamy, P.P. (1976) The problem of pressure sores in a nursing home population: statistical data. *J Am Geriatr Soc* 24: 323-328

Millar,M.R., Brown, N.M., Tobin, G.W., Murphy, P.J., Winsdor, A.C.M., & Speller, D.C.E. (1994) Outbreak of infection with penicillin-resistant Streptococcus pneumonia in a hospital for the elderly. *J Hosp Infect* 27: 99-104

Miller, L.G., Perdreau-Remington, F., Rieg, G., Mehdi, S., Perlroth, J., Bayer, A.S., Tang, A.W., Phung, T.O.,& Spellberg, B. (2005) Necrotizing fasciitis caused by community-associated methicillin-resistant Staphylococcus aureus in Los Angeles. *N Engl J Med* 352:1445-1453

Miller, S.C., Prohaska, T.R., Furner, S.E., Freels, S., Brody, J.A., & Levy, P.S. (1998) Time to nursing home admission for persons with Alzheimer's disease: the effect of health care systems characteristics. *J Gerontol B Psychol Sci Soc Sci* 53B: S341-S353

Min, H., Montecino-Rodriguez, E., Dorshkind, K. (2004) Reduction in the developmental potential of intrathymic T cell progenitors with age". *J Immunol* 173 (1): 245–250

Mittman, C., Edelman, N.H., & Norris, A.H. (1965) Relationship between chest wall and pulmonary compliance with age. *J Appl Physiol* 20; 1211-1216

Miyashita, N., Ouch, K., & Shoji H. (2005) Outbreak of Chlamydophila pneumonia infection in long-term care facilities and an affiliated hospital. *J Med Microbiol* 54: 1243-1247

Mocchegiani, E. & Malavolta, M. (2004). NK and NKT cell functions in immunosenescence. *Aging Cell* 3 (4): 177–1

Mocchegiani, E., Costarelli, L., Giacconi, R., Piacenza, F., Basso, A., & Malavolta, M. (2011) Zinc, metallothioneins and immunosenescence: effect of zinc supply as nutrigenomic approach. *Biogerontology* 2011 Apr 19; DOI: 10.1007/s10522-011-9337-4

Mody, L., Kaufman, S.R., Donabedian, S., Zervos, M., & Bradley, S.F. (2008) Epidemiology of staphylococcus aureus colonization in nursing home residents. *Clin Infect Dis* 2008 may 1st; 46 (9): 1368-1373

Mody, L., Maheshwari, S., Galecki, A., Kauffman, C.A., & Bradley, S.F. (2007) Indwelling device use and antibiotic resistance in nursing homes: identifying a high-risk group. *J Am Geriatr Soc* 2007 Dec; 55(12): 1921-1926

Mody, L., McNeil, S.A., & Sun, R. (2003) Introduction of a waterless alcohol-based hand rub in a long-term care facility. *Infect Control Hosp Epidemiol* 24: 165-171

Montgomery, P., Semenchuk, M., & Nicolle, L.E. (1995) Antimicrobial use in nursing homes in Manitoba. *J Geriatr Drug Ther* 9: 55-74

Morrison, R.R., Ahronheim, J.C., & Morrison, G.R. (1998) Pain and discomfort associated with common hospital procedures and experiences. *J Pain Symptom Manage* 15 (2): 61-101

Muder, R.R., Brennen, C., Drennings, S.D., Stout, J.E., Wagener, M.M. (1997) Multiply antibiotic-resistant Gram negative bacilli in a long-term care facility: a case-control study of patient risk factors and prior antibiotic use. *Infect Control Hosp Epidemiol* 18: 809-813

Muder, R.R., Brennen, C., Wagener, M.M., & Goetz, A.M. (1992) Bacteriemia in long-term care facility: a five year prospective study of 163 consecutive episodes. *Clin Infect Dis* 14: 647-654

Muder, R.R., Brennen, C., Wagener, M.M., Vickers, R.M., Rihs, J.D., Hancock, G.A., Yee, Y.C., Miller, J.M. & Yu, V.L. (1991) Methicillin-resistant Staphylococcal colonization and infection in a long-term care facility. *Ann Intern Med* 114: 107-112

Mulhausen, P.L., Harrell, I.J., Weinberger, M., Kochersberger, G.G., & Feusser, J.R. (1996) Contrasting methicillin-resistant Staphylococcus aureus colonization in Veterans' Affairs and community nursing homes. AM J Med 100: 24-31

Murciano, C., Villamón, E., Yáñez, A., O'Connor, J.E., Gozalbo, D., & Gil, ML. (2006). Impaired immune response to Candida albicans in aged mice. *J Med Microbiol* 55 (Pt 12): 1649–1656

Musher, D.M., & Musher B.L. (2004) Contagious acute gastrointestinal infections. *N Engl J Med* 351: 2417-2427

Muszkat, M., Greenbaum, E., Ben-Yehuda, A., Oster, M., Yeu'l, E., Heimann, S., Levy, R., Friedman, G., & Zakay-Rones, Z. (2003) Local and systemic immune response in nursing-home elderly following intranasal or intramuscular immunization with inactivated influenza vaccine. *Vaccine* 21 (11-12): 1180–1186

Mylotte, J.M., Tayara, A., & Goodnough, S. (2002) Epidemiology of bloodstream infection in nursing home residents: evaluation in a large cohort from multiple homes. *Clin Infect Dis* 35: 1484-1490

Mylotte, J.M. (1996) Measuring antibiotic use in a long-term care facility. *Am J Infect Control* 24: 174-179

Mylotte, J.M. (1999) Antimicrobial prescribing in long-term care facilities. *Infect Control Hosp Epidemiol* 27: 10-19

Nakamura, H., Fukushima, H., Miwa, Y., Shiraki, M., Gomi, I., Saito, M., Mawatari, K., Kobayashi, H., Kato, M., & Moriwaki, H. (2006) A longitudinal study on the nutritional state of elderly women at a nursing home in Japan. *Intern Med* DOI:10.2169/internalmedicine.45.1743

Nakashima, K., Tanaka, T., Kramer, M.H., Takahashi, H., Ohyama, T., & Kishimoto, T. (2006) Outbreak of Chlamydia pneumonia infection in a Japanese nursing home, 1999-2000. *Infect Control Hosp Epidemiol* 27: 1171-1177

Narain, J.J., Lofgren, J., Warren, E & Stead, W. (1985) Epidemic tuberculosis in a nursing home: a retrospective cohort study. *J Am Geriatr Soc* 33: 258-263 & Al, 1985;

Naylor, K., Li, G., Vallejo, A.N., Lee, W.W., Koetz, K., Bryl, E., Witkowski, J., Fulbright, J., Weyand, C.M., & Goronzy, J.J. (2005) The influence of age on T cell generation and TCR diversity. *J Immunol* 174 (11): 7446–7452

Nickel, J.C. (2003) Benign prostatic hyperplasia: does prostate mass matter? *Rev Urol* 5 (suppl 4); S12-S17

Nicolle, L.E. (2000) Urinary tract infections in long-term-care facility residents. *Clin Infect Dis* 31: 757-761

Nicolle, L.E. (2001) Preventing infection in non hospital settings: Long-term care. *Emerging Infect Dis* 2001; 7 (2), march-april 2001: 205-207

Nicolle, L.E. (2002) Urinary tract infections in geriatric and institutionalized patients. *Curr Opin Urol* 12: 51-55

Nicolle, L.E., Evans, G., Laverdieve, M., Phillips, P., Quan, C., & Rotstein, C. (2005b) Complicated urinary tract infection in adults Can J Infect Dis Med Microbiol 16: 349-360

Nicolle, L.E., & Garibaldi, R.A. (1995) Infection control in long-term care facilities. *Infect Control Hosp Epidemiol* 16: 348-353

Nicolle, L.E., Bjornson, J., Harding, G., & Mac Donell, J. (1983) Bacteriuria in elderly institutionalized men. *New Engl J Med* 309: 1420-1425

Nicolle, L.E., Bradley, S., Colgan, R., Rice, J.C., Schaeffer, A., & Hooton, T.M. (2005) Infectious diseases Society of America Guidelines for the diagnosis and treatment of asymptomatic bacteriuria in adults. *Clin Infect Dis* 40: 643-654

Nicolle, L.E., Henderson, E., Bjornson, J., McIntyre, M., Harding, G., & Mac Donell, J. (1987a) The association of bacteriuria with resident characteristics and survival in elderly institutionalized med. *Arch Intern Med* 106: 682-686

Nicolle, L.E., Mayhew, W.J., & Bryan, L. (1987b) Prospective, randomized comparison of therapy and no therapy for asymptomatic bacteriuria in institutionalized elderly women. *Am J Med* 83: 27

Nicolle, L.E., Mayhew, W.J., & Bryan, L. (1988) Outcome following antimicrobial therapy for asymptomatic bacteriuria. *Age Ageing* 17: 187-192

Nicolle, L.E., McIntyre, M., Hoban, D., & Murray, D. (1994a) Bacteriemia in a long-term care facility. *Can J Infect Dis* 5: 130

Nicolle, L.E., McIntyre, M., Zacharias, I.L., & Mac Donell, J. (1984) Twelve month surveillance of infections in institutionalized elderly men. *J Am Geriatr Soc* 32: 513-519

Nicolle, L.E., Orr, P., Duckworth, H., Brunks, J., Kennedy, J., Urias, B., Murray, D., & Al Harding, G. (1994b) Prospective study of decubitus ulcers in two long term care facilities. *Can J Infect Control* 9: 35-38

Nicolle, L.E., Strausbaugh, L.J., & Garibaldi, R.A. (1996) Infections and antibiotic resistance in nursing homes. *Clin Microbiol Rev* 9: 1-7

Norman, D. & Yoshikawa, T.T. (1996) Fever in the elderly. *Infect Dis Clin North Am* 10: 93–100

Norman, D. & Toledo, S. (1992) Infections in elderly persons: an altered clinical presentation. *Clin Geriatr Med* 8: 713-719

Norman, R.A. (2003) Geriatric dermatology. *Dermatol Ther* 16:260–268

Notice to readers: National Nursing Home Week - May 8-14, 2005. *MMWR Morb Mortal Wkly Rep* 2005 May 6; 54(17): 438

Nuorti, J.P., Butler, J.C. & Crutcher, J.M. (1998) An outbreak of multidrug-resistant pneumococcal pneumonia and bacteria among unvaccinated nursing home residents. *N Engl J Med* 338: 1861-1868

O'Grady, N.O., Alexander, M., Dellinger, E.P., Gerberding, J.L., Heard, S.O., & Maki, D.G. (2002) Guidelines for prevention of intravascular catheter-related infections. Centers for Disease Control and Prevention. *MMWR Recomm Rep* 51: 1-29

O'Sullivan, N.P., Keane, C.T. (2000) Risk factors for colonization with Methicillin-Resistant Staphylococcus Aureus among nursing home residents. *J Hosp Infect* 45: 206-210

O'Toole, R.D., Drew, W.L., Dahlgren, B.J. & Beaty, H.N. (1970) An outbreak of methicillin resistant Staphylococcus aureus infection. Observation in hospital and in nursing home. *J Am Med Associa* 213: 257-263

Olsen, S.J., DeBess, E.E., McGivern, T.E., Marano, N., Eby, T., & Mauvais, S. (2001) Noscomial outbreak of fluoroquinolone-resistant Salmonella infection. *N Engl J Med* 344: 1572-1579

Omran, M.L. & Morley, J.E. (2000) Assessment of protein energy malnutrition in older persons. Part I: history, examination, body composition, and screening tools. *Nutrition* 16: 50-63

Ordòñez, J., De Antonio Veira, J.A., Pou Soler, C., Navarro Calero, J, Rubio Navarro, J., Marcos Olivares, S., López Ventura, M. (2010) Efecto de un suplemento nutricional oral hiperproteico en pacientes desnutridos ubicados en residencias geriátricas. *Nutr Hosp* July-Aug. 2010; 25 (4): 549-554

Otherson, M.J., & Otherson, H.B. (1987) A history of handwashing seven hundred years at a snail's pace. *The Pharos* 50: 23-27

Ouslander, J. & Schnelle, J.F. (1995) Incontinence in the nursing home. *Ann Intern Med* 122: 438-449

Ouslander, J. (1989) Medical care in the nursing home. *J Am Med Assoc* 262: 2582-2590

Ouslander, J., Greengold, B., & Chen, S. (1987) Complication of chronic indwelling urinary catheters among male nursing home patients: a perspective study. *J Urol* 138: 1191-1195

Ouslander, J.G., Schapira, M., Schnelle, J.F., Fingold, S. (1996) Pyuria among chronically incontinent but otherwise asymptomatic nursing home residents. *J Am Geriatr Soc* 44(4): 420-423

Ouyang, Q., Wagner, W.M., Voehringer, D., Wikby, A., Klatt, T., Walter, S., Müller, C.A., Pircher, H., & Pawelec, G. (2003) Age-associated accumulation of CMV-specific CD8+ T cells expressing the inhibitory killer cell lectin-like receptor G1 (KLRG1). *Exp Gerontol* 38 (8): 911–920.

Pagliari, P., Cosso, P., Ricci, G., & Ianes, A.B. (2011) Quale antibiotico per la terapia delle cistiti nell'anziano in RSA? *G Gerontol* 57: 498

Pauly., L., Stehle, P., & Volkert, D. (2007) Nutritional situation of elderly nursing home residents. *Z Gerontol Geriatr.* 40 (1): 3–12.

Pawelec, G. (1999). Immunosenescence: impact in the young as well as the old? *Mech Ageing Dev 108: 1-7*

Peak, A., Cohen, C.E., & Mulvihill, M.N. (1990) Long-term enteral feeding of aged demented nursing home patients. *J Am Geriatr Soc* 38: 1195-1198

Perez-Stable, E.J., Flaherty, D., Schecter, G., Slutkin, G., & Hopewell, D.C. (1988) Conversion and reversion of tuberculin reaction in nursing home residents. *Am Rev Respir Dis* 137: 801-804

Peterson, P.K., Stein, D., Guay, D.R.P., Logan, G., Obald, S., Gruninger, R., Davies, S., & Breitenbucher, R. (1988) Prospective study of lower respiratory tract infections in an extended-care nursing home program: potential role of oral ciprofloxacin. *Arch Intern Med* 85: 164-171

Phair, J., Kauffman, C.A., Bjorson, A., Adams, L., & Linuetmann, C. Jr. (1978) Failure to respond to influenza vaccine in the aged: correlation with B-cell number and function. *J Lab Clin Med* 92: 822-828

Philip, W., Bennett, G., Bradley, S., Drinka, P., Lautenbach, E., Marx, J., Mody, L., Nicolle, L.E. & Stevenson, K. (2008) SHEA/APIC Guideline: Infection prevention and control in the long-term care facility, July 2008. *Infect Control Hosp Epidemiol* Sept. 2008; 29 (9): 785-814

Phillips, S.K. & Branaman-Phillips, M.A. (1993) The use of intramuscular cefoperazone versus intramuscular ceftriaxone in patients with nursing home acquired pneumonia. *Am J Med* 41: 1071-1074

PHS D. (Ed.) US Department of Health and Human Services (DHHS) PHS. National Center for Health Statistics. Health United States 1985. Hyattsville, MD: 1985 p. 86-1232

Pickering, T.D., Gurwitz, J.H., Zaleznik, D., Noonan, J. P., & Avorn, J. (1994) The appropriateness of oral fluoroquinolone prescribing in long-term care setting. *J Am Geriatr Soc* 42: 28-32

Pittet, D., Sax, H., & Hugonnet, S. (2004) Cost implications of successful hand hygiene promotion. *Infect Control Hosp Epidemiol* 25: 264-266

Pourat, N. (1995) Ethnic/racial differences in the use of nursing home services among the elderly. *Annual Research Meeting of the Academy for Health Service Research and Health Policy.* Abstract Book, Chicago, IL, June 4-6 1995

Pressure Ulcer Advisory Panel/European Pressure Ulcer Advisory Panel Pressure Ulcer Prevention and Treatment Clinical Practice Guideline. Washington, DC: National Pressure Ulcer Advisory Panel; 2009

Rajagopalan, S., & Yoshikawa, TT. (2000) Tuberculosis in long-term care facilities. *Infect Control Hosp Epidemiol* 21: 611-615

Raz, R., Schiller, D., & Nicolle, L.E. (2000) Chronic indwelling catheter replacement before antimicrobial therapy for symptomatic urinary tract infection. *J Urol* 164: 1254-1258

Regal, R.E., Pham, C.Q., & Bostwick, T.R. (2006) Urinary tract infections in extended care facilities: preventive management strategies. Consult Pharm. 2006 May; 21(5): 400-409.

Reid, R.T., Briggs, R.S., Seal, D.V., & Pearson, A.D. (1983) Virulent Streptococcus pyogenes outbreak and spread in a geriatric unit. *J Infect* 6: 219-225

Ribeiro, B.J. & Smith, S.R. (1985) Evaluation of urinary catheterization and urinary incontinence in a general nursing home population. *J Am Geriatr Soc* 33: 479-482

Ricci, G., Cosso, P., Leonetti, A., Pagliari, P., & Ianes, A.B. (2009) I disturbi psicocomportamentali nella demenza: studio di un campione di soggetti anziani residenti in Residenza Sanitaria Assistenziale. *G Gerontol* 57: 70-77

Ricci, G., Cosso, P., Pagliari, P., & Ianes, A.B. (2010) Le infezioni delle basse vie urinarie nell'anziano in residenza sanitaria assistenziale: studio osservazionale di 54 mesi. *G Gerontol* 58: 270-278

Rice, L.B., Willey, S.H., Papanicolaou, G.A., Medeiros, A.A., Eliopoulos, G.M., Moellering, R.C., & Jacoby, G.A. (1990) Outbreak of ceftazidime resistance caused by estende-spectrum-ß-lactamases at a Massachusetts chronic-care facility. *Antimicrob Agents Chemiother* 34: 2193-2199

Richards, C.L. (2004) Urinary tract infections in the frail elderly: issues for diagnosis, treatment and prevention. *Int Urol Nephrol* 36(3): 457-63

Rodhe, N., Mőlstad , S., Englund, L., & Svärdsudd, K. (2006) Asymptomatic bacteriuria in apopulation of elderly resident living in a community setting: prevalence characteristics and associated factors. *Fam Pract* doi:10-1093/fampra/cml007

Rogers, M.A., Mody, L., Chenoweth, C., Kaufman, S.R. & Saint, S. (2008) Incidence of antibiotic resistant infection in long-term residents of skilled nursing facilities. *Am J Infect Control* 2008 sept; 36 (7): 472-475

Ruben, F.C:, Norden, B., Heisler, B., & Korica, Y (1984) An outbreak of Streptococcus pyogenes infections in a nursing home. *Ann Intern Med* 101: 494-496

Rudelsky, B., Lipschits, M., Isaacsohn, M., & Sonnenblick, M. (1992) Infected pressure sores: comparison of methods for bacterial identification. *South Med J* 85: 901-903

Rudman, D., Hontanosas, A., Cohen, C., & Mattson, D. (1988) Clinical correlates of bacteriemia in a Veterans Administration extended care facility. *J Am Geriatr Soc* 36: 726-732

Ryan, C.A., Tauxe, R.V., Hosek, G.W., Wells, J.G., Stoesz, P.A., & McFadden, H.W.Jr. (1986) Escherichia coli O157:H7 diarrhea in a nursing home: clinical, epidemiological and pathological findings. *J Infect Dis* 154: 631-638

Saeed, S., Fakih, M.G., Riederer, K., Shah, A.R., & Khatib, R. (2006) Interinstitutional and intrainstitutional transmission of a strain of Acinetobacter Baumannii detected by molecular analysis: comparison of pulsed-field gel electrophoresis and repetitive sequence-based polymerase chain reaction. *Infect Control Hosp Epidemiol* 27: 981-983

Saint, S., Kaufman, S.R., Rogers, M.A., Baker, P.D., Ossenkop, K., & Lipsky, B.A. (2006) Condom versus indwelling urinary catheters: a randomized trial. *J Am Geriatr Soc* 54: 1055-1061

Saletti, A., Lindgren, E.Y., Johansson, L., & Cederholm, T. (2000) Nutritional status according to mini nutritional assessment in an institutionalized elderly population in Sweden. *Gerontology* 46(3):139–145

Sandoval, C., Walter, S.D., MCGeer, A., Simor, A.E., Bradley, S.F., Moss. L.M., & Loeb, M.B. (2004) Nursing home residents and Enterobacteraceae Resistant to third-generation Cephalosporins. *Emerg Infect Dis* 10: 1050-1055

Sapico, F.I., Ginunas, V.J., & Thornhill-Joynes, M.T. (1986) Quantitative microbiology of pressure sores in different stages of healing. *Diagn Microbiol Infect Dis* 5: 31-38

Schaeffer, A.J., & Schaeffer, E.M. (2007) Infections of the urinary tract. In: Wein, A.J., et Al. Campbell-Walsh *Urology. 9th ed.* Philadelphia, Pa.: Saunders; 2007. *http://www.mdconsult.com/das/book/body/202281144-2/0/1445/0.html.*

Scheckler, W. & Peterson, P. (1986) Infections and infections control among residents of eight rural Wisconsin nursing homes. *Arch Intern Med* 146: 1981-1984

Schiappa, D.A:, Hayden, M.J., Matushek, M.G., Hashemi, F.N., Sullivan, J., Smith, K.Y., Miyashiro, D., Quinn, J.P., Weinstein, R.A., & Trenholme, G.M. (1996) Ceftazidime-resistant Klebsiella pneumoniae and Escherichia coli bloodstream infection: a case-control and molecular epidemiology investigation. *J Infect Dis* 174: 529-536

Schicker, J.M., Franson, T.R., Duthie, Jr., E.H., & LeClair, S.M. (1988) Comparison of methods for calculation and depiction of incidence infection rates in long-term care facilities. *J Clin Epidemiol* 41: 757-761

Schnelle, J.F., Adamson, G.M., Cruise, P.A., al-Samarrai, N., Sarbaugh, F.C., Uman, G., & Ouslander, J.G. (1997) Skin disorders and moisture in incontinent nursing home resident: intervention implications. *J Am Geriatr Soc* 45 (10) 1182.1188

Schumm, K. & Lam, T.B. (2008) Types of urethral catheters for management of short-term voiding problems in hospitalized adults: a short version Cochrane review. *Neurourol Urodyn* 27(8): 738-746

Schwartz, B. & Ussery, X. (1992) Group A streptococcal outbreaks in nursing homes. *Infect Control Hosp Epidemiol* 13: 742-747

Seenivasan, M.H., Yu, V.L., & Muder, R.R. (2005) Legionnaires' disease in long-term care facilities: overview and proposed solutions. *J Am Geriatr Soc* 53: 875-880

Selbaek, G., Kirkevold, Ø., & Engedal, K. (2007) The prevalence of psychiatric symptoms and behavioural disturbances and the use of psychotropic drugs in Norwegian nursing homes. *Int J Geriatr Psychiatry* 22: 843-849

Sengstock, D.M., Thyagarajan, R., Apalara, J., Mira, A., Chopra, T., & Kaye, K.S. (2010) Multi-drug resistant Acinetobacter baumannii: an emerging pathogen among older adults in community hospital and nursing homes. *Clin Infect Dis* 50 (12) 1611-1616

Setia, U., Serventi, I., & Lorenz, P. (1984) Bacteremia in a long-term care facility: spectrum and mortality. *Arch Intern Med* 144: 1633-1635

Setia, U., Serventi, I., & Lorenz, P. (1985) Nosocomial infections among patients in long-term care facility: spectrum, prevalence, and risk factors. *Am J Infect Control* 13: 67-62

Shah, B.R. & Hux, J.E. (2003) Quantifying the risk of infectious diseases for people with diabetes. *Diabetes Care.* 26:510-513

Shahin, E.S., Meijers, J.M., Schols, J.M., Tannen, A., Halfens, R.J., & Dassen, T. (2010) The relationship between malnutrition parameters and pressure ulcers in hospital and nursing homes. *Nutrition* 2010 sept; 26 (9): 886-889

Shepard, M., Parker, D., & DeClerque, N. (1987) The underreporting of pressure sores in patients transferred between hospital and nursing home. *J Am Geriatr Soc* 35: 159-160

Shindo, Y., Sato, S., Maruyama, E., Ohashi, T., Ogawa, M., Hashimoto, N., Imaizumi, K., Sato, T., & Hasegawa, Y. (2009) Health-care-associated pneumonia among hospitalized patients in a Japanese community hospital. *Chest* 135: 633-640

Shlaes, D.M., Currie-McCumber, C.A., & Lehman, M.H. (1988) Introdution of a plasmid encoding the OHIO-1 ß-lactamase to an intermediate care ward by patient transfer. *Infect Control Hosp Epidemiol* 9: 317-319

Shlaes, D.M., Lehman, M.H., Currie-McCumber, C.A., Kim, C.H., & Floyd, R. (1986) Prevalence of colonization with antibiotic resistant gram-negative bacilli in a nursing home care unit: the importance of cross-colonization as documented by plasmid analysis. *Infect Control* 7: 538-545

Shlaes, D.M., Lehman, M.H., Currie-McCumber, C.A., Kim, C.H., & Floyd, R. (1986) Prevalence of colonization with antibiotic resistant gram-negative bacilli in a nursing home care unit: the importance of cross-colonization as documented by plasmid analysis. *Infect Control* 7: 538-545

Sieggreen, M.Y. & Kline, R.A. (2004) Arterial insufficiency and ulceration: diagnosis and treatment options. *Nurs Pract.* 29 (9): 46–52.

Siegman-Igra, Y., Fourer, B., & Orni-Wasserlauf, R (2002) Reappraisal of community-acquired bacteremia: a proposal of a new classification for the spectrum of acquisition of bacteremia. *Clin Infect Dis* 34: 1431-1439

Simor, A.F., Bradley, S.F., Strausbaugh, L.J., Crossley, K., & Nicolle, L.E., SHEA Long-Term Care Commitee (2002) Clostridium difficile in long-term care facilities for the elderly. *Infect Control Hosp Epidemiol* 23: 696-703

Singh, S., Amin, A.V., & Loke, Y.K. (2009) Long-term use of inhaled corticosteroids and the risk of pneumonia in chronic obstructive pulmonary disease: a meta-analysis. *Arch Intern Med* 169: 219-229

Slotwiner-Nie, P.K. & Brandt, L.I. (2001) Infectious diarrhea in the elderly. *Gastroenterol Clin North Am* 30: 625-635

Smith, D.M., Snow, D.E., Rees, E., Zischkau, A.M., Hanson, J.D., Walcott, R.D., Sun, Y., White, J., Kumar, S., & Dowd, S.E. (2010) Evaluation of the bacteria diversity of pressure ulcers using bTEFAP pyro-sequencing. *BMC Med Genomics* 3: 41

Smith, P.F., Stricof, R.L., Shayegani, M., & Morse, D.L. (1988) Cluster of Haemophilus influenza type B infection in adults. *J Am Med Assoc* 260: 1446-1448

Smith, P.W. (1985) Infections in long-term care facilities. *Infect Control* 6: 435-436

Smith, P.W. (1987) Consensus conference on nosocomial infections in long-term care facilities. *Am J Infect Control* 15: 97-100

Smith, P.W. (1999) Development of nursing home infection control. *Infect Control Hosp Epidemiol* 20: 303-305

Smith, P.W. (Ed) (1994) *Infections control in long term care facilities*, 2nd ed. Delmar Publisher Inc., Albany, NY, pp 131-146

Smith, P.W., & Rusnak, P.G. (1997) Infection prevention and control in the long-term care facility. SHEA long-term-care Committee and APIC Guidelines Committee. *Infect Control Hosp Epidemiol* 18; 831-849

Smith, P.W., Bennett, G., Bradley, S., Drinka, P., Lautenbach, E., Marx, J., Mody, L., Nicolle, L.E., & Stevenson, K. (2008) SHEA/APIC Guidelines: Infection prevention and control in the long-term care facility, July 2008. *Infect Control Hosp Epidemiol* 29 (9): 785-814

Smith, P.W., Daly, P.B., & Roccaforte, J.S. (1991) Current status of nosocomial infection control in extended care facilities. *Am Med J* 91: S281-S285

Smith, P.W., Seip, C.W., Schaefer, S.C:, & Bell-Dixon, C (2000) Microbiologic survey of long-term care facilities. *Am J Infect Control* 28: 8-13

Smitten, A.L., Choi, H.K., Hochberg, M.C., Suissa, S., Simon, T.A., Testa, M.A., & Chan, K.A. (2008) The risk of hospitalized infection in patients with rheumatoid arthritis. *J Rheumatol* 35:387–93

Spector, WD., Kapp, W.D., Tucker, R.J., & Sternberg, J. (1988) Factors associated with presence of decubitus ulcers at admission to nursing homes. *Gerontologist* 28: 830-834

Stamm, W.E. & Hooton, T.M. (1993) Management of urinary tract infections in adults. *N Engl J Med* 329:1328-1334

Standaert, S.M., Hutcheson, R.H., Schaffener, W. (1994) Nosocomial transmission of Salmonella gastroenteritis to laundry workers in a nursing home. *Infect Control Hosp Epidemiol 15: 22-26*

Standfast, S.J., Michelsen, P.B., Baltch, A.I., Smith, R.P., Latham, F.K., Spellacy, A.B., Venezia, R.A., & Andritz, M.H. (1984) A prevalence survey of infections in a combined acute and long-term care hospital. *Infect Control* 5: 177-184

Stead, W. (1981) Tuberculosis among elderly persons: an outbreak in nursing home. *Ann Intern Med* 94: 606-610

Stead,W., Lofgren, J., Warren, E., & Thomas, C. (1985) Tuberculosis as an endemic and nosocomial infection among the elderly in nursing homes. *N Engl J Med* 312: 1483-1487

Steinmiller, A., Robb, S., & Muder, R. (1991) Prevalence of nosocomial infections in long-term care Veterans medical centers. *Am J Infect Control* 19: 143-146

Stephens, C., Franceis, S.J., Abell, V., DiPersio, J.R., & Wells, P. (2007) Emergence of Acinetobacter baumannii in critically ill patients within an acute care teaching hospital and a long-term acute care hospital. *Am J Infect Control* 35: 212-215

Stevenson, K.B., Moore, J., Colwell, H., & Sleeper, B. (2005) Standardized infection surveillance in long-term care: interfacility comparison from a regional cohort facilities. *Infect Control Hosp Epidemiol* 26: 231-238

Storch, G.A., Radcliff, J.L., Meyer, P.L. & Hirinchs, J,H. (1987) Methicillin-resistant Staphylococcus aureus in a nursing home. *Infect Control* 8: 24-29

Stout, J.E., Brennen, C., & Muder, R.R. (2000) Legionnaires' disease in a newly constructed long-term care facility. *J Am Geriatr Soc* 48: 1589-1592

Stratton, R.J., King, C.L., Stroud, M.A., Jackson, A.A., & Elia, M. (2006) "Malnutrition Universal Screening Tool' predicts mortality and length of hospital stay in acutely ill elderly. *Br J Nutr* 95(2): 325-330

Strausbaugh, L.J. & Joseph, C.J. (1999) Epidemiology and prevention of infections in residents of long term care facilities. In: Mayhall, C.G., editor. *Hospital epidemiology and infection control.* 2nd ed. Philadelphia: Lippincott Williams & Wilkins; 1999. p. 1461

Strausbaugh, L.J., & Joseph, C.J. (2000) The burden of infection in long-term care. *Infect Control Hosp Epidemiol* 21: 674-679

Strausbaugh, L.J., Jacobson, C., Sewell, D.L., Potter, S., & Ward, T.T. (1991) Methicillin-resistant Staphylococcus Aureus in extended care facilities: experiences in a Veteran's Affairs Nursing Home and review of the literature. *Infect Control Hosp Epidemiol* 12: 151-159

Strausbaugh, L.J., Sukumar, S.R., Joseph, C.L. (2003) Infectious disease outbreaks in nursing homes: an unappreciated hazard for frail elderly persons. *Clin Infect Dis* 36: 36: 870-876

Strout, R.D. & Suttles, J. (2005) Immunosenescence and macrophage functional plasticity: dysregulation of macrophage function by age-associated microenvironmental changes". *Immunol Rev* 205: 60–71

Sturm, A.W., Monstert, R., Roning, P.J.E., van Klingeren, B., & van Alphen, L. (1990) Outbreak of multiresistant nonencapsulated Haemophilus influenza infection in a pulmonary rehabilitation centre. *Lancet* 335: 214-216

Suderkotter, C. & Kalden, H. (1997) Aging and the skin immune system. *Arch Dermatol* 133 (10): 1256–1262

Sutcliffe, C., Burns, A., Challis, D., Mozley, C.G., Cordingley, L., Bagley, H.,& Huxley, P. (2007) Depressed mood, cognitive impairment, and survival in older people admitted to care homes in England. *Am J Geriatr Psychiatry* 15: 708-715

Tan, J.S. (2000) Infectious complications in patients with diabetes mellitus. *Int Diabetes Monitor* 12: 1-7

Tansel, O., Kugoglu, F., Mutlu, B., Anthony, R.M., Uyar, A., Vahaboglu, H., & French, G.L. (2003) A methicillin-resistant staphylococcus aureus outbreak in a new University hospital due to a strain transferred with an infected patient from another city, six month previously. *New Microbiol* 26 (2): 175-180

Terpenning, M.S., Bradley, S.F., Wan, J.Y., Chenoweth, C.E., Jorgenson, K.A. & Kauffman, C.A. (1994) Colonization and infection with antibiotic-resistant bacteria in a long-term care facility. *J Am Geriatr Soc* 42: 1062-1069

Thomas, D.B., Bennett, R.G., Laughon, B.E., Greenough, W.B., & Barlett, J.G. (1990) Post-antibiotic colonization with Clostridium difficile in nursing home patients. *J Am Geriatr Soc* 38: 415-420

Thomas, J.C., Bridge, J., Waterman, S., Vogt, J., Kilman, L., & Hancock, G. (1989) Transmission and control of methicillin-resistant Staphylococcus aureus in a skilled nursing facility. *Infect Control Hosp Epidemiol* 10: 106-110

Thomas, J.C., Bridge, J., Waterman, S., Vogt, J., Kilman, L., & Hancock, G. (1989) Transmission and control of methicillinn-resistant Staphylococcus aureus in a skilled nursing facility. *Infect Control Hosp Epidemiol* 10: 106-110

Topinkovà, E., Neuwirth, J., Stankovǻ, M., Mellanovǻ, A., & Haas, T. (1997) Urinary and fecal incontinence in geriatric facilities in the Czech Republic. *Cas Lek Cesk* 136 (18): 573-577

Troy, C.J., Peeling, R.W., Ellis, A.G., Hockin, J.C., Bennet, D.A., & Murphy, M.R. (1997) Chlamydia pneumoniae as a new source of infectious outbreaks in nursing homes. *J Am Med Assoc* 277: 1214-1218

Tsan, L., Langberg, R., Davis, C., Phillips, Y., Pierce, J., Hojlo, C., Gibert, C., Gaynes, R., Montgomery, O., Bradley, S., Danko, L., & Roselle, G. (2008) Prevalence of nursing home-associated infections in the Department of Veterans Affairs nursing home care units. Am J Infect Control. 2008 Apr; 36(3): 173-9.

Tsan, L., Langberg, R., Davis, C., Phillips, Y., Pierce, J., Hojlo, C., Gibert, C., Gaynes, R., Montgomery, O., Bradley, S., Danko, L., & Roselle, G. (2010) Nursing home-associated infections in Department of Veterans Affairs community living centers. *Am J Infect Control*. 2010 Aug; 38(6): 461-466

Utsumi, M., Makimoto, K., Quroshi, N., & Ashida N. (2010) Types of infectious outbreaks and their impact in elderly care facilities: a review of the literature. *Age Ageing* 39: 299-305

Uyemura, K., Castle, S.C., & Makinodan, T. (2002) The frail elderly: role of dendritic cells in the susceptibility of infection. *Mech Ageing Dev* 123 (8): 955–962

Valdez, R., Narayan, K.M., Geiss, L.S., & Engelgau, M.M. (1999). Impact of diabetes mellitus on mortality associated with pneumonia and influenza among non-Hispanic black and white US adults. *Am J Public Health* 89:1715-1721.

Valiyeva, E.,. Russell, L.B., Miller ,J.E., & Safford, M.M. (2006) Lifestyle-related risk factors and risk of future nursing home admission. *Arch Intern Med* 166(9): 985-990

van de Sande-Bruinsma, N., Grundmann, N., Verloo, D., Tiemersma, E., Monen, J., & Goossens H. (2008) Antimicrobial use and resistance in Europe. *Emerg Infect Dis* 14: 1722-1730

Van Duin, D., Mohanty, S., & Thomas, V. (2007b). Age-associated deficits in human TLR-1/2 function. *J Immunol* 178 (2), 2007 Jan 15: 970-975

Van Duin, D., Allore, H.G. & Mohanty, S. (2007a). Prevaccine determination of the expression of costimulatory B7 molecules in activated monocytes predicts influentia vaccine responses in young and older adults. *J Infect Dis* 195 (11) june 2007; 1590-1597

Van Rensbergen, G. & Nawrot, T. (2010) Medical conditions of nursing homes admission. *BMC Geriatrics* 10:46

Vanderkooi, O.G., Low, D.E., Green, K., Powis, J.E., McGeer, A. & Toronto Invasive Bacterial Disease Network. (2005) Predicting antimicrobial resistance in invasive pneumococcal infections. *Clin Infect Dis* 40(9):1288-1297.

Vergese, A. & Berk, S. (Eds) (1990) *Infections in nursing homes and long-term care facilities.* Karger, Basel, 1990

Viahov, D., Tenney, J., Cervino, K., & Shamer, D. (1987) Routine surveillance for infections in nursing homes: experience at two facilities. *Am J Infect Control* 15: 47-53

Viray, M., Linkin, D., Maslow, J.N., Stieritz, D.D., Carson, L.S., Bilker, W.B., & Lautenbach, E. (2005) Longitudinal trends in antimicrobial susceptibilities across long-term care facilities: emergence of fluoroquinolone resistance. *Infect Control Hosp Epidemiol* 26: 56-62

Voehringer, D., Koschella, M., Pircher, H. (2002) Lack of proliferative capacity of human effector and memory T cells expressing killer cell lectin-like receptor G1 (KLRG1) *Blood* 100 (10): 3698–3702

Votey, S.R. & Peters, A.L. (2005) Diabetes mellitus, type 2 - a review. Available at: *http:// www.emedicine.com /emerg/topic134.htm* Accessed July 12, 2005

Warren, J.W., Tenney, J., Hoopes, J.M., Muncie, H.L., & Antony, W.C. (1982) A prospective microbiologic study of bacteriuria in patients with chronic indwelling catheters. *J Infect Dis* 146: 719-723

Warren, J.W., Damron, D., Tenney, J., Hoopes, J.M., Deforge, R., & Muncie, H.Jr. (1987) Fever, bacteriemia and death as complications of bacteriuria in women with long-term urethral catheters. *J Infect Dis* 155: 1151-1158

Warren, J.W., Muncie, H.Jr. & Hall-Craggs, M. (1988) Acute pyelonephritis associated with bacteriuria during long-term catheterization: a prospective clinico-pathological study. *J Infect Dis* 158: 1341-1346

Warren, J.W., Palumbo, F.B., Fitterman, L., & Speedle, S.M. (1991) Incidence and characteristics of antibiotic use in aged nursing home patients. *J Am Geriatr Soc* 39: 963-972

Warren, J.W., Steinberg, L., Uebel, R., & Tenney, J. (1989) The prevalence of urethral catheterization in Maryland nursing homes. *Arch Intern Med* 149: 1535-1537

Wasserman, M., Levinstein, M., Keller, E., Lee, S., & Yoshikawa, T. (1989): Utility of fever, white blood cell, and differential count in predicting bacterial infections in the elderly. *J Am Geriatr Soc* 37: 534–543

Wayne, S.J., Rhyne, R. L., & Stratton, M. (1992) Longitudinal prescribing patterns in a nursing home population. *J Am Geriatr Soc* 40: 53-56

Weiner, J., Quinn, J.P., Bradford, P.A., Goering, R.V., Nathan, C., Bush, K., & Weinstein, R.A. (1999) Multiple antibiotic resistant Klebsiella and E. Coli in nursing homes. *J Am Med Assoc* 281: 517-523

Weinstein, M.P., Towns, M.L, Quartey, S.M., Mirrett, S., Reimer, L.G., Parmigiani, G., Reller, L.B. (1983): The clinical significance of positive blood cultures: A comprehensive analysis of 500 episodes of bacteremia and fungemia II. Clinical observations with special reference to factors influencing prognosis. *Rev Infect Dis* 5:54–70

Welty, C., Burstin, S., Muspratt, S., & Tager, I.B. (1985) Epidemiology of tuberculosis infections in chronic care population. *Am Rev Respir Dis* 132: 133-136

Weng, N.P. (2006) Aging of the immune system: how much can the adaptive immune system adapt?. *Immunity* 24 (5): 495–499

Werner, H. & Kuntsche, J. (2000) Infection in the elderly--what is different? *Z Gerontol Geriatr.* 2000 Oct; 33(5): 350-356.

White, K.E., Hedberg, C.W., Edmonson, L.M., Jones, D.B., Osterholm, M.T. & MacDonald, K.L. (1989) An outbreak of Giardiasis in a nursing home with evidence for multiple modes of transmission. *J Infect Dis* 160: 298-304

Wingard, F., Shlaes, J., Mortimer, E., & Shlaes, D (1993) Colonization and cross-colonization of nursing home patients with thrimetoprim-resistant gram-negative bacilli. *Clin Infect Dis* 16: 75-81

Winquist, A.G., Roome, A., Mshar R, Fiorentino, T, Mshar, P., & Hadler, J. (2001) Outbreak of campylobacteriosis at a senior center. *J Am Geriatr Soc* 49: 304-307

Wong, E.S. & Hooten, T.M. (1981) Guideline for prevention of catheter-associated urinary tract infections. *Infect Control* 2: 125-130

Yakabowich, M.R., Keeley, G.,& Montgomery, P.R. (1994) Impact of a formulary on personal care homes in Manitoba. *Can Med Assoc J* 150: 1601-1607

Yamaya, M., Yanai M, Ohrui, T., Arai, H., & Sasaki, H. (1991) Interventions to prevent pneumonia among older adults. *J Am Geriatr Soc* 49: 85-90

Yoshikawa, T.T., Nicolle, L.E., & Norman, D.C. (1996) Management of complicated urinary tract infections in older patients. *J Am Geriatr Soc* 44: 1235-1241

Young, J.B. & Dobrzanski, S. (1992) Pressure sores epidemiology and current management concepts. *Drugs Aging* 2: 42-57

Zervos, M.J., Terpenning, M.S., Schaberg, D.R., Therasse, P.M., Mendendorp, S.V., & Kauffman, C.A. (1987) High-level aminoglycoside-resistant enterococci: colonization of nursing home and acute care hospital patients. *Arch Intern Med* 147: 1591-1594

Zhanel, G.G., Nicolle, L.E., & Harding, G.K.M. (1995) Prevalence of asymptomatic bacteriuria and associated host factors in women with diabetes mellitus. *Clin Infect Dis* 21: 316-322

Ziegler, T.R., Cole, C.R. (2007) Small bowel bacterial overgrowth in adults: a potential contributor to intestinal failure. *Curr Gastroenterol Rep* 2007 Dec; 9(6): 463-467

Zimmer, J.G., Bentley, D.W., Valenti, W.M. & Watson, N.M. (1986) Systemic antibiotic use in nursing homes. A quality assessement. *J Am Geriatr Soc* 34: 703-710

Zulkowski, K., Langemo, D., & Posthauer, M. (2005) NUAP. Coming to Consensus on Deep Tissue Injury. *Adv Skin Wound Care* 18: 28-29

3

The Natural Antibiotic Resistances of the Enterobacteriaceae *Rahnella* and *Ewingella*

Wilfried Rozhon, Mamoona Khan and Brigitte Poppenberger
Max F. Perutz Laboratories, University of Vienna, Austria

1. Introduction

The antibiotic resistance genes present in clinical isolates are usually acquired and located on mobile elements allowing their horizontal transfer to other strains or even across bacterial species. Consequently, resistance genes with 100% sequence identity may be found in otherwise unrelated genera while the occurrence of such an acquired resistance within a certain species is highly variable.

In contrast, a number of bacteria are naturally resistant against some antibiotics. The molecular basis for natural resistance may be a general factor like the lack of the targeted pathway, a variant of the targeted molecule that is not inhibited by the antibiotic or a membrane limiting entry of the antibiotic into the cell. In addition natural resistance may also be mediated by a resistance gene belonging to the cell's core genes. Such resistance genes are vertically inherited, shared by (nearly) all isolates of a species and co-evolve with their hosts. They are often encoded by the chromosome, are usually immobile and their expression level is tightly regulated or very low. The establishment of such a resistance requires a long lasting, usually mild selection pressure as it may be present in the soil, which contains many microorganisms producing antibiotics. Examples for this type of natural resistance are the chromosomally encoded β-lactamases found in several species of the Enterobacteriaceae (Naas et al., 2008), many of them colonising plants and soil.

Although these environmental microorganisms pose a low risk to human health, concerns about the spread of their antibiotic resistance genes to pathogens have arisen. Their resistance genes are usually non-mobile, but inclusion into mobile genetic elements may allow the spread to unrelated bacteria. In the last two decades the CTX-M type enzymes have become the most prevalent extended-spectrum β-lactamases (EBSLs) in pathogenic Enterobacteriaceae (Canton & Coque, 2006). The CTX-M enzymes are believed to originate from *Klyvera ascorbata* and *Klyvera georgiana* chromosomal β-lactamases (Olson et al., 2005; Rodriguez et al., 2004). The inclusion of these genes in integrons located on large conjugative plasmids has likely facilitated their spread among the Enterobacteriaceae. Such plasmids contain frequently multiple resistance genes, which might have further enhanced spread of the CTX-M genes in microbial communities by co-selection (Canton & Coque, 2006). Once established in pathogens the spectrum of the resistance genes may be increased by point mutations further impeding treatment of infections with antibiotics. Thus improved understanding of natural resistance, conditions favouring transfer of resistance genes to pathogens and the underlying molecular mechanisms are important areas of research.

Rahnella and *Ewingella,* two closely related genera of the Enterobacteriaceae, are naturally resistant to several β-lactam antibiotics. *Rahnella* is widespread in nature and routinely present in the daily human diet but also *Ewingella* may be present at high titers in some kinds of food. Both microorganisms have been infrequently isolated from clinical specimens. Here the biology, natural habitats, clinical significance and antibiotic susceptibility patterns of *Ewingella* and *Rahnella* will be addressed. Novel results about their resistance genes will be presented and the evolution of these genes and the potential for their transfer to other bacteria will be discussed.

2. Biology, clinical significance and antibiotic resistances of *Rahnella* and *Ewingella*

In 1976 a new class of Enterobacteriaceae was defined during a numerical taxonomy study and provisionally named 'group H2' (Gavini et al., 1976). Based on DNA relatedness studies this group was later proposed as a new species, *Rahnella aquatilis* (Izard et al., 1979). In the following years strains belonging to this novel genus were infrequently isolated from water and clinical specimens and *Rahnella* was thought to be a rare microorganism (Farmer et al., 1985) until it was found to be frequent in plant and soil specimens. Also *Ewingella* was recognised as a separate group of the Enterobacteriaceae in a phenotypical study, which was subsequently confirmed by DNA-DNA hybridisation experiments (Grimont et al., 1983). Based on current reports *Ewingella* is believed to be a rare member of the Enterobacteriaceae (Brenner & Farmer 2005) but some studies indicate that it might be common in some ecological niches. Investigations of clinical isolates revealed that *Rahnella* and *Ewingella* are resistant to several antibiotics, mainly β–lactams. The susceptibility patterns suggested the presence of an extended spectrum Ambler class A β-lactamase (ESBL) in *Rahnella* (Stock et al., 2000), which could be confirmed by cloning and sequencing of the resistance gene (Bellais et al., 2001). The susceptibility pattern and detection of the enzyme by SDS-PAGE/nitrocefin staining suggested an Ambler class C β-lactamase (AmpC) for *Ewingella* (Stock et al., 2003). Here we report for the first time a DNA sequence-based phylogenetic analysis confirming that the *Ewingella* β-lactamase belongs to the AmpC class.

2.1 Biology, habitat and possible applications of *Rahnella* and *Ewingella*

The genus *Rahnella* comprises three genomospecies, *Rahnella aquatilis* (= genomospecies 1), *Rahnella* genomospecies 2 and *Rahnella* genomospecies 3 (Brenner et al., 1998), while the genus *Ewingella* consists of only one species: *Ewingella americana.* Based on phenotypical tests two biogroups of *Ewingella americana* have been defined, which show differences in L-rhamnose and D-xylose fermentation (Grimont et al., 1983). Strains belonging to *Rahnella* and *Ewingella* have no special nutritional requirements and can use a number of carbon sources. They are able to grow in the temperature range from close to 0°C to approximately 40°C, although many strains show a reduced biochemical activity at elevated temperatures (Brenner & Farmer 2005; Brenner et al., 1998; Davis & Eyles, 1992; Jensen et al., 2001; McNeil et al., 1987).

Rahnella is widely distributed and has been isolated from many types of samples. It is frequently found in the rhizosphere and tightly associated with roots and tubers of plants (Berge et al., 1991; Heulin et al., 1994; Jafra et al., 2009; Rozhon et al., 2010) but is also present on other parts of plants including leaves (Hamilton-Miller & Shah, 2001; Hashidoko et al., 2002), fruits (Lindow et al., 1998) and seeds (Cankar et al., 2005; Iimura & Hosono, 1996). Other sources are water (Brenner et al., 1998; Gavini et al., 1976; Niemi et al., 2001), soil (Martinez et al., 2007) and the intestine of snails, slugs (Brenner et al., 1998) and even American mastodon remains (Rhodes et al., 1998). Recently, *Rahnella* was also found at a high frequency in the gut of ghost moths (Yu et al., 2008) and to be associated with larvae and adults of the mountain pine beetle (Winder et al., 2010). *Rahnella* is frequently present in the human diet and has been isolated from different types of food including vegetables (Hamilton-Miller & Shah, 2001; Raphael et al., 2011; Rozhon et al., 2010; Ruimy et al., 2010a), sprouts (Cobo Molinos et al., 2009), fruits (Rozhon et al., 2006), meat (Brightwell et al., 2007; Lindberg et al., 1998) and beverages (Hamze et al., 1991; Jensen et al., 2001). In contrast to its wide distribution in nature *Rahnella* is rarely isolated from clinical specimens.

Ewingella has also been isolated from vegetables (Hamilton-Miller & Shah, 2001) and vacuum-packaged meat (Brightwell et al., 2007), but seems to be significantly less frequent than *Rahnella* in such samples. In contrast, *Ewingella* is very common on mushrooms including button mushroom, shiitake and oyster mushroom (Reyes et al., 2004). Importantly, *Ewingella* is the causative agent of a browning disorder of button mushroom called 'internal stipe necrosis' (Inglis & Peberdy, 1996), which causes significant economic loss. In addition, *Ewingella* has also been isolated from molluscs (Müller et al., 1995). Clinical specimens tested positive for *Ewingella* were mainly blood and swabs from the respiratory tract and wounds.

Rahnella and *Ewingella* have some interesting properties for agronomic and industrial applications. Both seem to promote plant growth and *Rahnella* may be useful as antagonist for controlling plant pathogens including *Erwinia amylovora*, causing fire blight of pear and apple trees (Laux et al., 2002), and *Xanthomonas campestris*, the causative agent of black rot (El-Hendawy et al., 2005). In addition, *Rahnella* might improve the supply of plants with nutrients like phosphate (Kim et al., 1997) and it is able to fix nitrogen (Heulin et al., 1994). The polysaccharides levan and lactan produced by different strains of *Rahnella* have interesting properties for industrial processes (Kim et al., 2003; Matsuyama et al., 1999; Pintado et al., 1999; Seo et al., 2002). The high uranium(VI) resistance of *Rahnella* and its ability to bind this toxic heavy metal is currently intensively investigated and its potential for bioremediation is studied (Beazley et al., 2007; Geissler et al., 2009; Martinez et al., 2007). Because of the increasing interest a project for sequencing of the *Rahnella* genome was launched and recently finished. The sequence of environmental strain *Rahnella aquatilis* Y9602 is available from the genbank database (www.ncbi.nlm.nih.gov) under accession number NC_015061.

2.2 Clinical significance

Rahnella and *Ewingella* are only occasionally isolated from clinical specimens and the clinical significance of both microorganisms is still under debate. Both are believed to be opportunistic pathogens. The pathogenic potential of *Rahnella* seems to be relatively low while a few fatal outcomes of infections caused by *Ewingella* have been reported.

2.2.1 Clinical significance of *Rahnella*

Several reports describe the isolation of *Rahnella* in a clinical context (Table 1). However, in some cases the clinical significance is difficult to assess particularly because many patients had some underlying conditions including haematologic and solid organ malignancy, diabetes and AIDS or had undergone surgery. The age of the patients ranged from 11 months to 78 years and an, although statistically insignificant, male predominance has been recognised among them (Gaitán & Bronze, 2010). Typical sites of isolation were blood, wounds and urine. Interestingly, a significant number of patients developed symptoms during hospitalisation suggesting nosocomial infections.

The first description of *Rahnella* in a clinical context dates back to 1985, where it was isolated from a burn wound (Farmer et al., 1985). In another case *Rahnella* was isolated from a surgical wound that had persisted for more than eight months and was repeatedly tested negative for bacteria before a purulent exudate appeared. At that time pure cultures of *Rahnella* could be isolated from the wound exudate (Maraki et al., 1994). Since *Rahnella* is easy to cultivate and previous efforts to detect bacteria in the wound were negative it seems most likely that the wound was infected recently before the exudate appeared, for instance during the daily wound cleansing procedure. In a further case *Rahnella* was isolated from a diabetes mellitus associated foot wound. Although the infection reacted well to treatment with ampicillin-sublactam the toe and the second digit of the foot had to be amputated because of severe necrosis. This course of disease belongs to the most severe described for an infection with *Rahnella*. However, the ulceration of the wound had begun two month before any medical treatment was started and a co-infection with *Candida sp.* was diagnosed.

While, in a clinical context, *Rahnella* was first isolated from a wound swab, its most frequent site of isolation was blood. *Rahnella* bacteraemia was associated with fever and in two cases with septic shock (Chang et al., 1999; Gaitán & Bronze, 2010). Most patients showed *Rahnella* bacteraemia during hospitalisation (9 of 15 cases) and venous catheters, surgery and drug abuse seem to pose risk factors for infection with this bacterium (Funke & Rosner, 1995; Gaitán & Bronze, 2010; Hoppe et al., 1993; Oh & Tay, 1995). In two epidemiologically related cases a parenteral nutrition fluid was identified as the most probable source of *Rahnella* (Caroff et al., 1998). Both cases appeared in the same hospital within three days and the bacterial strains isolated from the blood of both patients showed identical biochemical profiles and antibiograms and shared the same macrorestriction and ribotyping profiles. Also other patients who had received the same batch of the parenteral nutrition fluid experienced episodes of shivers but blood cultures were not taken impeding further analysis (Caroff et al., 1998). In one very unusual case a contaminated intravenous infusion fluid that a patient had self-administrated could be identified as the source of *Rahnella* (Chang et al., 1999). Thus in a number of cases *Rahnella* cells were directly introduced into the blood circulation. Under certain circumstances *Rahnella* may also be able to spread from the urinary tract to the blood system. Blood cultures of a febrile 76-year old man complaining of nausea and vomiting grew *Rahnella*. The patient had a history of a benign prostatic hypertrophy and the analysis of his urine revealed "many" bacteria. Because of these results and the underlying conditions pyelonephritis was suggested as a possible source of the patient's bacteraemia (Tash, 2005). Since the bacteria isolated from blood and urine of this patient were not compared by biochemical and molecular methods a causal link between the urinary tract infection and bacteraemia remains speculative. With respect to that it is important to note that *Rahnella* was isolated from urine in some other cases but no signs for bacteraemia were reported (Alballaa et al., 1992; Domann et al., 2003; O'Hara et al., 1998).

Case	Year, country	Age, sex	Signs and symptoms	Site	Underlying condition(s)	Treatment	Outcome	Reference
1	1985[a], USA	NA	NA	Burn wound	Burn	NA	NA	(Farmer et al., 1985)
2	1986, USA	37 y, M	Cough, fever, night sweats, diarrhoea	Bronchial washings	AIDS; co-infection with *Cryptococcus neoformans*	Ampicillin, gentamycin	Cure	(Harrell et al., 1989)
3	1987, Belgium	79 y, M	Fever, expectoration	Sputum, bronchial aspirate	Chronic lymphocytic leukaemia emphysema, bronchopulmonary infection with *Pneumococcus*	Trimethoprim-sulfamethoxazole	Cure	(Christiaens et al., 1987)
4	1988, France	42 y, F	Septicaemia, leukaemic relapse	Blood	Acute lymphocytic leukaemia, diabetes mellitus, bronchial asthma, Hickman catheter	Vancomycin, ceftazidime	NA	(Goubau et al., 1988)
5	1991, Saudi Arabia	40 y, M	Dysuria	Urine	Renal transplant (status post)	Amoxicillin; ciprofloxacin	Cure	(Alballaa et al., 1992)
6	1992, Greece	63 y, F	Purulent exudate	Surgical wound	Osteoporosis, alcoholism, operation at the left knee	Trimethoprim-sulfamethoxazole	Cure	(Maraki et al., 1994)
7	1992, Germany	7 y, M	Fever (39.5°C)	Blood	Bone marrow transplant recipient; Hickman catheter	Gentamycin, azlocillin, flucloxacllin; amikacin, ceftriaxone, vancomycin	Cure	(Hoppe et al., 1993)
8	1994[a], Italy	59 y, F	Fever	Blood	Chronic renal failure, parenteral nutrition via a Hickman catheter	Ciprofloxacin	Cure	(Caraccio et al., 1994)
9	1994, Switzerland	21 y, M	Fever (39°C)	Blood	AIDS, positive for HBV, HCV and HDV antibodies, recent infection with *Staphylococcus aureus*, intravenous drug abuse	Ciprofloxacin	Cure	(Funke & Rosner, 1995)
10	1995[a], Singapore	48 y, M	Fever (38.2°C)	Blood	Diabetes mellitus (for 2 y), pulmonary tuberculosis, appendicular abscess	Ampicillin, gentamycin, amoxicillin-clavulanate, gentamycin	Cure	(Oh & Tay, 1995)
11	1995[a], Singapore	57 y, M	Fever	Blood	Laryngeal carcinoma, total laryngectomy	Metronidazole, ceftriaxone; gentamycin	Cure	(Oh & Tay, 1995)
12	1996[a], Spain	2 y, F	Acute gastroenteritis	Faeces	None	None	Cure	(Reina & Lopez, 1996)
13	1996[a], Spain	2 y, M	Acute gastroenteritis	Faeces	AIDS	None	Cure	(Reina & Lopez, 1996)

Case	Year, country	Age, sex	Signs and symptoms	Site	Underlying condition(s)	Treatment	Outcome	Reference
14	1996[a], Japan	11 m, F	Fever (39.7°C), cough	Blood	Congenital heart disease	Cefpodoxime-proxetil; cefotaxime; cefazolin, netilmicin, ceftazidime	Cure	(Matsukura et al., 1996)
15	1997, France	32 y, F	Fever (>38°C)	Blood	Ingestion of a caustic product, parenteral nutrition via a catheter	Removal of the catheter	Cure	(Caroff et al., 1998)
16	1997, France	61 y, M	Fever (40°C)	Blood	Relapse from a renal carcinoma (status post), parenteral nutrition via a catheter	Ticarcillin-clavulanate, vancomycine	Cure	(Caroff et al., 1998)
17	1998[a,b], Japan	NA	NA	Urine	Chronic urinary tract infection	NA	NA	(O'Hara et al., 1998)
18	1999, Korea	26 y, M	Fever (38.2°C), septic shock	Blood	Contaminated intravenous fluid; healthy individual	Ceftriaxone, imipenem	Cure	(Chang et al., 1999)
19	1999[a], Tunisia	65 y, F	Fever (38.5°C), ketosis	Blood	Diabetes mellitus for 5 y	Cefotaxime, trimethoprim-sulfamethoxazole	Cure	(Boukadida et al., 1999)
20	2000, USA	46 y, M	Fever	Blood	B-cell lymphoblastic leukaemia, immunosuppressive medication, Hickman catheter	Piperacillin-tazobactam, gentamycin	Cure	(Carinder et al., 2001)
21	2000, Spain	63 y, M	Fever (37.8°C), excessive exudate	Trache-ostomy exudate	Laryngeal carcinoma (status post)	Amoxicillin-clavulanic acid; cefotaxime, amikacin	Cure	(Fajardo & Bueno, 2000)
22	2003[a], NA	NA, F	NA	Urine	Co-infection with *Candiada albicans*	None	NA	(Domann et al., 2003)
23	2004[a], USA	76 y, M	Fever (39.8°C)	Blood	Benign prostatic hypertrophy, bacteria in urine	Tracheostomy tube Levofloxacin	Cure	(Tash, 2005)
24	2009[a], Turkey	57 y, F	Ulcerated foot wound	Wound	Diabetes mellitus for 20 years, co-infection with *Candida* sp.	Ampicillin-sublactam; Amputation of a toe	Cure	(Aktaş et al., 2009)
25	2009, Italy	78 y, M	Fever, sepsis	Blood	hospitalised at an intensive care unit, co-infection with *Candida famata* and *Pantoea agglomerans* [c]	Meropenem	NA	(Liberto et al., 2009)
26	2011, USA	27 y, F	Septic shock, fever (38.1°C)	Blood	Sickle cell disease, central venous catheter	Ciprofloxacin, removal of the catheter	Cure	(Gaitán & Bronze, 2010)

Table 1. Infections caused by *Rahnella*. All cases we could find in the literature are included. [a] Year of report (the year of isolation is not available); [b] The isolates were obtained in the 1990s; [c] *Pantoea agglomerans* is considered as the reason for the sepsis.

Rahnella was also isolated from the faeces of two children with acute diarrhoea. In both cases typical enteropathogenic bacteria, parasites and viruses could not be detected. However, the detection of *Rahnella* in the faeces of patients with diarrhoea is not a sufficient reason for the conclusion that this microorganism is the true cause of the infectious process (Reina & Lopez, 1996). It seems indeed unlikely that *Rahnella* is an enteropathogen since this organism is frequently present in food, particularly vegetables which are frequently eaten raw, while the isolation of *Rahnella* from faeces from patients suffering acute gastroenteritis seems to be a rare exception.

Infections with *Rahnella* reacted very well to treatment with antibiotics and most patients recovered rapidly, though even many of them were immunocompromised. Some patients recovered even without antibiotic treatment (Caroff et al., 1998; Reina & Lopez, 1996). Importantly, no deaths were reported as outcome of an infection with *Rahnella*. These data and the fact that *Rahnella* is a frequent microorganism routinely present in the human diet suggest that it has only a slight pathogenic capacity and its ability to infect humans may be highly dependent on their immunological status.

Currently few data about the pathogenic capacities of the three genomospecies of *Rahnella* are available. The routinely used phenotypic tests allow identification of *Rahnella* only at the genus level. Thus the genomospecies of the isolates of the cases summarised in Table 1 is unknown. A study using DNA-DNA hybridisation revealed that three clinical isolates belonged to *Rahnella aquatilis* (= genomospecies 1) and three were identified as *Rahnella* genomospecies 2 (Brenner et al., 1998) indicating that both genomospecies may act as opportunistic pathogens. However, a study including more strains is highly demanded to assess any potential differences of the pathogenic potential of the *Rahnella* genomospecies.

2.2.2 Clinical significance of *Ewingella americana*

Ewingella americana has been isolated from a variety of clinical specimens, particularly blood and wound swabs and less frequently from sputum (Brenner & Farmer 2005). Typical underlying conditions were surgeries, injuries from accidents, drug abuse and renal failure (Table 2). Some patients had diabetes, received immunosuppressive therapy, were HIV positive or suffered from other chronic infections. However, in contrast to infections with *Rahnella*, a significant number of patients were fully immunocompetent.

Most patients had undergone surgery prior development of bacteraemia, suggesting nosocomial infections. Pien and Bruce (1986) described a nosocomial outbreak of *Ewingella* bacteraemia. Six cases of *Ewingella* bacteraemia appeared in an intensive care unit of a hospital within six weeks. All infected patients had high fever or leukocytosis and had undergone either cardiovascular or peripheral vascular surgery. A careful environmental culturing study identified a contaminated ice bath used to cool syringes for cardiac output determinations as most likely source for the bacteria. *Ewingella americana* was cultured from the bath and its removal from the intensive care unit terminated the outbreak (Pien & Bruce, 1986). In another hospital *Ewingella americana* was diagnosed in blood drawn from 20 patients (Gardner et al., 1985). None of the patients had symptoms typical for *Ewingella americana* sepsis. An environmental investigation revealed that the bacteria were present in a citric buffer anticoagulant used to fill coagulation tubes. Review of blood drawing procedures showed that the non-sterile coagulation tubes were frequently filled first

Case	Year, country	Age, sex	Signs and symptoms	Site	Underlying condition(s)	Treatment	Outcome	Reference
1	1982-1983, USA	55 y, F	Postoperative fever, sepsis	Blood	Aortoiliac graft bypass, aorta occlusion, diabetes	Ampicillin, carbenicillin, gentamicin	Cure	(Pien & Bruce, 1986)
2	1982-1983, USA	57 y, M	Postoperative fever	Blood	Ventricular aneurysmetomy, lower extremity thrombectomy	Cefotaxime, gentamicin, mezlocillin	Cure	(Pien & Bruce, 1986)
3	1982-1983, USA	58 y, M	Postoperative fever	Blood	Coronary artery bypass surgery	Gentamicin, mezlocillin, trimethoprim-sulfamethoxazole	Cure	(Pien & Bruce, 1986)
4	1982-1983, USA	54 y, F	Postoperative fever	Blood	Aorta-iliac artery bypass	Gentamicin, trimethoprim-sulfamethoxazole, doxycycline	Cure	(Pien & Bruce, 1986)
5	1983[a], USA	41 y, M	Postoperative fever (39.2°C)	Blood	Bypass surgery; atherosclerosis, diabetes mellitus; intravascular catheters; co-infection with *Pseudomonas* sp.	Gentamicin, trimethoprim-sulfamethoxazole	Cure	(Pien et al., 1983)
6	1985 , South Africa	46 y, M	Wound (traffic accident)	Wound swab	Wounds originating from a traffic accident; co-infection with *Staphylococcus aureus*	None	Cure	(Bear et al., 1986)
7	1989, Germany	30 y, F	adhesive eyelids, itching	Conjuncti-vae (swab)	None	Amoxicillin-clavulanate	Cure	(Heizmann & Michel, 1991)
8	1991, Belgium	75 y, M	Cholecystis, fever (39.4°C)	Blood	Surgery of the gallbladder; also *Pseudomonas aeruginosa, Candida albicans* and *Serratia marcescens* were isolated from the patient	Temocillin	Cure	(DeVreese et al., 1992)
9	1991[a], Spain	31 y, M	Balanitis	Penile exudate	HIV, intravenous drug abuse, several opportunistic infections	Tobramycin	Cure	(Sanmartin Jimenez et al., 1991)
10	1995[a], Spain	18 m, M	Acute gastroenteritis	Faeces	None	None	Cure	(Reina et al., 1995)
11	1999[a], Greece	70 y, F	Peritonitis, fever (37.4°C)	Peritoneal dialysate	End-stage renal disease , ambulatory dialysis for 5 years	Amikacin, vancomycin	Cure	(Kati et al., 1999)

Case	Year, country	Age, sex	Signs and symptoms	Site	Underlying condition(s)	Treatment	Outcome	Reference
12	1999, France	38 y, M	Fever (39°C)	Blood	AIDS, intravenous drug abuse (a syringe used was rinsed with water from a fountain), co-infection with *Candida sp.*	Ceftriaxone, amikacin	Cure	(Le Gall et al., 2000)
13	2000, Belgium	57 y, F	Fever (38.8°C)	Blood	Peripheral blood progenitor cell transplantation, treatment with cyclosporine A; Hickman catheter	Removal of the catheter	Cure	(Maertens et al., 2001)
14	2000[a], Brasilia	38 y, F	Kerato-conjunctivitis	Conjuncti-vae (swab)	Soft contact lens	Ciprofloxacin	Cure	(Da Costa et al., 2000)
15	2003[a], Germany	74 y, F	Waterhouse–Friderichsen syndrome	Blood from heart and spleen	Pain in the left leg; otherwise healthy	Tramadol (for treatment of pain)	Death	(Tsokos, 2003)
16	2004[a], Greece	72 y, M	Fever (38.5°C), diffuse abdominal pain	Peritoneal effluent	end-stage renal failure, dialysis for 3 years	Ceftazidime, tobramycin	Cure	(Papaefstathiou et al., 2004)
17	2003[a], Korea	35 y, M	Pneumonia, fever (38.2°C)	Sputum	Chronic renal failure for 7 y; rejection of the transplanted kidney; coinfection with alpha-haemolytic streptococci	Ceftriaxone, isepamicin	Cure	(Ryoo et al., 2005)
19	2007[a], USA	77 y, F	Shortness in breath	Sputum	Infection with *Mycobacterium tuberculosis* and *M. avium* (status post); Cohen's disease	Trimethoprime-sulfamethoxazole	Cure	(Pound et al., 2007)
20	2007, Saudi Arabia	30 y, M	Pneumonia	Tracheal aspirate	Multiple severe injuries from a traffic accident, coma, contusion on the right upper lung, multiple organ failure	No treatment with antibiotics is described	Death	(Bukhari et al., 2008)

Table 2. Infections caused by *Ewingella*. All cases we could find in the literature are included. [a] Year of report (the year of isolation is not available).

allowing contamination of the subsequently filled culture tubes (McNeil et al., 1985). At least some of the patients received inappropriate, unnecessary antimicrobial therapy, incurring the risk of adverse drug reactions and the selection of drug-resistant bacteria (McNeil et al., 1987).

A fatal case of Waterhouse–Friderichsen syndrome was associated with an *Ewingella* infection of a previously healthy 74-year-old women (Tsokos, 2003). She experienced dragging pain in her left leg. Since the physical examination was unremarkable except for restricted mobility caused by the painful leg and her temperature was normal, just an analgetic was administered and bed rest ordered. On the next morning she was found dead in her bed. An autopsy revealed intraparenchymal haemorrhages in both adrenal glands, the heart showed granulocytic infiltration, clots were present in the larger arterial vessels and her brain and lungs were oedematous. *Ewingella americana* could be isolated from heart and spleen blood obtained during autopsy. In agreement with a suspected sepsis a highly increased level of procalcitonin was measured. Death was attributed to acute adrenal insufficiency due to Waterhouse–Friderichsen syndrome caused by *Ewingella americana* (Tsokos, 2003). In a second case the death of a 30-year-old man was associated with pneumonia caused by *Ewingella americana* (Bukhari et al., 2008). In this case the patient was admitted deeply comatose with multiple severe injuries caused by a road traffic accident to hospital. His brain showed oedema, intercerebral haemorrhage in basal ganglia to the right thalamus and subarachnoid haemorrhage along with the fracture of the frontal bone. The upper part of his right lung showed contusion. *Ewingella americana* was identified in his tracheal aspirate but not from any other sample of the patient. The isolated strain exhibited multiple antibiotic resistances but it was not reported whether the patient received any antibiotic treatment. On the eighth day of admission he went to a stage of multiple organ failure and died. It was hypothesised that the cause of death may be pneumonia associated with brain damage (Bukhari et al., 2008). However, because of the underlying conditions it is difficult to rate whether the infection with *Ewingella* was indeed the cause of death. Only two other cases of respiratory infection caused by *Ewingella* have been reported. In both cases the patients recovered quickly after treatment with antibiotics. However, it is important to note that in one of these cases the isolated strain was multidrug resistant (Pound et al., 2007).

In two cases *Ewingella* was associated with eye infection (Da Costa et al., 2000; Heizmann & Michel, 1991). Swabs of the conjunctivae grew the microorganism. Symptoms were keratoconjunctivitis, adhesive eyelids, itching and impaired secretion of tears. In both cases the infection reacted well to antibiotic treatment and the symptoms were relieved in a few days. One report describes also the isolation of *Ewingella* from faeces of a patient with diarrhoea. However, like in the cases of isolation of *Rahnella* from faeces, the clinical significance of this finding is unclear. Since *Ewingella* may be present on some kinds of food, isolated bacteria may originate from the ingested food and be unrelated to diarrhoea. Studies on the frequency of *Ewingella* in the human diet and additional case reports are necessary to rate the enteropathogenic potential of this microorganism.

Taken together these reports suggest that *Ewingella* has a higher pathogenic capacity than *Rahnella*. Several cases of infection in immunocompetent patients were reported. *Ewingella* may also cause infections with fatal outcome. Furthermore, while all *Rahnella* strains isolated so far are susceptible to most antibiotics, two multiple drug resistant isolates of *Ewingella* have been reported. The origin of these resistances, their molecular basis and capacity to spread to other genera are intriguing questions to be addressed in the future.

2.3 Identification of *Rahnella* and *Ewingella*

Reliable identification of strains is crucial for determining appropriate treatments of infections, hygiene monitoring in medical centres and industry and for basic research studies investigating the biology and ecology of microorganisms. In the past *Rahnella* strains were often identified as *Enterobacter agglomerans*, which may also explain that *Rahnella* was thought to be a rare genus while it is now considered as a relatively frequent bacterium.

Rahnella and *Ewingella* can be isolated using media not inhibitory for Enterobacteriaceae such as MacConkey agar or Bromothymol blue lactose agar. Levine EMB agar is especially suitable for *Rahnella*, which forms dark colonies on this medium (Rozhon et al., 2010). *Ewingella* was successfully isolated from mushrooms using VRBG agar (Reyes et al., 2004) or LB agar plates. The latter were anaerobically incubated to suppress growth of *Pseudomonas* (Inglis & Peberdy, 1996). Since a single phenotypic test allowing identification of *Rahnella* or *Ewingella* is lacking, a complete set of biochemical tests is necessary for identification. *Rahnella* is often described to be phenylalanine deaminase positive, which is a very rare characteristic among the Enterobacteriaceae, and to be motile at 25°C but not at 37°C. However, it must be emphasised that *Rahnella* shows only a very weak positive reaction for phenylalanine deaminase and some isolates react negative. Similarly, some strains are also immotile at 25°C. Thus the results of these two tests should be interpreted with care. It is important to note that the three *Rahnella* genomospecies can not be differentiated by biochemical tests (Brenner et al., 1998). Nevertheless, in many reports strains are claimed to be identified as '*Rahnella aquatilis*' although only phenotypic tests were performed. Such classifications should be evaluated very critically. The three *Rahnella* genomospecies were originally identified by DNA-DNA hybridisation experiments (Brenner et al., 1998). With the rapid development of molecular techniques in the last decades DNA sequencing of housekeeping genes is now the method of choice for identification of *Rahnella* at the genomospecies level and for confirmation of the identification of *Ewingella*. For sequencing

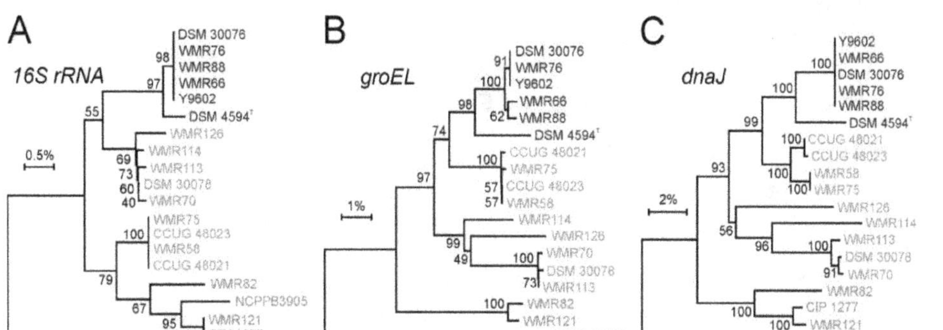

Fig. 1. Neighbour-joining trees based on partial *16S rRNA* (A), *groEL* (B) and *dnaJ* (C) gene sequences of *Rahnella* and *Ewingella*. The trees were constructed with MEGA4 (Tamura et al., 2007) using the p-distance model. Percentage bootstrap values of 1000 replicates are indicated at the corresponding nodes. The scale bars represents the indicated sequence difference. *Erwinia amylovora* ATCC 49946 was used as outgroup. Strains belonging to *Rahnella aquatilis*, *Rahnella* genomospecies 2, *Rahnella* genomospecies 3 and *Ewingella americana* are shown dark blue, light blue, green and red, respectively.

of the (partial) *16S rRNA* gene the primer pair 16S-3/16S-5 can be employed (sequences: 5´-ATATTGCACAATGGGCGC-3´ and 5´-GCCATTGTAGCACGTGTGTAG-3´, respectively; amplicon: 881 bp) (Rozhon et al., 2011). For verification a part of the *groEL* gene can be sequenced using the primer pair groEL-fwd/groEL-rev (sequences: 5´-ATGGCAGCTAAAGACGTAAAATT-3´ and 5´- TTACGACGRTCGCCRAAGC-3´, respectively; amplicon: 857 bp) (Rozhon et al., 2011). In addition a part of the *dnaJ* gene can be sequenced using the primer pair dnaJ-fwd/dnaJ-rev (sequences: 5´-CAGTATGGTCATGCAGCCTTTGAACA-3´ and 5´-TCAAAGAACTTTTTCACGCCGTC-3´, respectively; amplicon: 917 bp). Neihgbour-joining trees constructed with such sequences are shown in Figure 1. The genbank database contains numerous *Rahnella* and *Ewingella 16S rRNA* and several *groEL* and *dnaJ* gene sequences. Since little is known about the identification of most of these strains only sequences of strains deposited to strain collections should be used for analysis of the obtained data (Table 3).

Strain	Synonyms	*16S rRNA*	*groEL*	*dnaJ*
Rahnella aquatilis DSM 4594[T]	CCUG 14185[T]	FM876214	FM877005	HE577308
Rahnella aquatilis DSM 30076		FM876215	FM877006	HE577309
Rahnella genomospecies 2 CCUG 48021 [a]		U88434	FM877008	HE577311
Rahnella genomospecies 2 CCUG 48023		U88438	FM877009	HE577312
Rahnella genomospecies 2 CCUG 21213		FM876216	FM877007	NA
Rahnella genomospecies 3 DSM 30078 [b]	LMG 2640	U90758	FM877012	HE577310
Ewingella americana GTC 1277	DSM 4560, CCUG 14506	AB273745	NA	AB272652
Ewingella americana NCPPB 3905		X88848	NA	NA

Table 3. Accession numbers of *16S rRNA*, *groEL* and *dnaJ* gene sequences of *Rahnella* and *Ewingella* strains. Abbreviations: CCUG: Culture Collection, University of Göteborg (www.ccug.se); DSM: Deutsche Sammlung von Mikroorganismen (www.dsmz.de); GTC: Gifu Type Culture Collection; LMG: BCC/LMG Belgian Co-ordinated Collection of Microorganisms (bccm.belspo.be); NCPPB: National Collection of Plant Pathogenic Bacteria (www.ncppb.com); NA: not available. [a] Reference strain for genomospecies 2. [b] Reference strain for genomospecies 3.

2.4 Antibiotic resistance of *Rahnella* and *Ewingella*

2.4.1 Susceptibility patterns

The susceptibility patterns of more than 180 *Rahnella* strains have been described in the literature (Table 4). Many of these strains were isolated from clinical specimens but more than 75 originate from environmental samples (most of them were obtained in the study of Ruimy et al. (2010b) and in this study). *Rahnella* was found to be resistant to narrow spectrum penicillins, aminopenicillins, carboxypenicillins and most strains showed a low-level resistance to ureidopenicillins with MICs below 16 mg/l (Stock et al., 2000). Resistance was also observed for 1st and 2nd generation cephalosporins while most strains were sensitive or at least intermediate for 3rd and all strains were sensitive to 4th generation cephalosporins and carbapenems. Addition of β-lactamase inhibitors including clavulanic acid, sublactam and tazobactam decreased the MICs of all β-lactams tested. This pattern suggests the presence of a cavulainc acid-sensitive extended spectrum Ambler class A β-lactamase (Ambler, 1980) resembling the chromosomally encoded class A β-lactamase of *Klebsiella* sp. (Labia et al., 1979; Sykes & Matthew, 1976), *Escherichia hermanii* (Stock &

Antibiotic [a]	Class[b]	(Christiaens et al., 1987)	(Freney et al., 1988)	(Goubau et al., 1988)	(Harrell et al., 1989)	(Hohl et al., 1990)	(Alballaa et al., 1992)	(Hoppe et al., 1993)	(Maraki et al., 1994)	(Oh & Tay, 1995)	(Funke & Rosner, 1995)	(Matsukura et al., 1996)	(Caroff et al., 1998)	(O'Hara et al., 1998)	(Chang et al., 1999)	(Stock et al., 2000)	(Fajardo & Bueno, 2000)	(Bellais et al., 2001)	(Carinder et al., 2001)	(Tash, 2005)	(Aktaş et al., 2009)	(Ruimy et al., 2010b)	(Gaitán & Bronze, 2010)	This study
No. of strains tested		1	12	1	1	6	1	1	1	2	1	1	2	1	1	72	1	2	1	1	1	55	1	20
Amikacin	AMG						S	S	S		S					S				S	S			
Amoxicillin	APEN	R						R			R		R			R	R	R				R		R
Amoxicillin + In	APEN	S	S			SIR		S	R		S		S			S	R	S		S	S	S		S
Ampicillin	APEN	R	R	I	R		R		R	R	R	I			R				R	R	R		R	IR
Ampicillin + In	APEN															R			S	S				
Azlocillin	UPEN								S							IR								
Aztreonam	MOB								S	S								S		S	S	S	S	
Benzylpenicillin	NPEN															R								R
Carbenicillin	CPEN													S										R
Cefaclor	CEF2															SIR								IR
Cefamandole	CEF2	S							S															
Cefazolin	CEF1			R	R		R	R				S				SIR			R	S	R		S	
Cefepime	CEF4															S		S			S	S		
Cefotaxime	CEF3								S			S			S	S		I		S	S	SI		SI
Cefoxitin	CEF2		S						R				S		S	SIR		S		S	S			
Ceftazidime	CEF3								S	S			S			S		S	S	S	S	S		
Ceftriaxone	CEF3					S	S	S	S	I						SIR		S	S	S			S	
Cefoperazone	CEF3											S				SIR				S				
Cefuroxime	CEF2	S		R				R			I		I			IR		R		S				
Cephalothin	CEF1	S	R		R				R	R	R		R		R		R	R		S				IR
Chloramphenicol	O	S			S			R		S	S			S		SI					S			
Ciprofloxacin	FQU					S	S		S	S	S					S			S	S	S		S	
Fosfomycin	O							R						R		R								
Gentamycin	AMG	S			S		S	S	S	S	S	S		S	S	S			S	S	S		S	
Imipenem	CARB							S	S	S	S	S	S		S	S	S	S	S	S	S	S		
Meropenem	CARB															S		S						S
Netilmicin	AMG								S	S		S				S								
Piperacillin	UPEN								S		S		S			SIR		I	S	S	R	R	S	
Piperacillin + In	UPEN															S		S			S	S		
Tetracycline	TET			S	S				S	S	S					SIR					S			
Ticarcillin	CPEN		R							S			R			R		R		R		R	R	
Ticarcillin + In	CPEN																	S		S		S		
TMP/SMX	SUL			S	S	S	R	S	S	S		S			S	S			S	S	S		S	
Tobramycin	AMG							S	S		S					S				S			S	

Table 4. Susceptibility pattern of *Rahnella*. [a] In: β-lactamase inhibitor (clavulanic acid, sublactam or tazobactam); TMP/SMX: trimethoprim/sulfamethoxazole. [b] Classes of antibiotics: AMG: aminoglucosides; APEN: aminopenicillins; CARB: carbapenems; CEF1-4: 1st to 4th generation cephalosporins; CPEN: carboxybenicillins; FQU: flouroquinolons; MOB: monobactams; NPEN: narrow spectrum penicillins; O: other; SUL: sulfonamides; TET: tetracyclines; UPEN, ureidopenicillins. S: susceptible; I: intermediate; R: resistant.

Antibiotic [a]	Class[b]	(Pien et al., 1983)	(Bear et al., 1986)	(Pien & Bruce, 1986)	(Freney et al., 1988)	(Hohl et al., 1990)	(Heizmann & Michel, 1991)	(DeVreese et al., 1992)	(Reina et al., 1995)[c]	(Kati et al., 1999)	(Da Costa et al., 2000)[c]	(Maertens et al., 2001)	(Stock et al., 2003)	(Papaefstathiou et al., 2004)	(Ryoo et al., 2005)	(Pound et al., 2007)	(Bukhari et al., 2008)	This study
No. of strains tested		1	1	4	8	3	1	1	1	1	1	1	20	1	1	1	1	2
Amikacin	AMG	R	S	S						S			S		S	R	R	
Amoxicillin	APEN												SIR					R
Amoxicillin + In	APEN		R		SIR	IR			R	S		S	SIR	S			I	R
Ampicillin	APEN	S		S	SIR		S	S	R	S	R	S		S	S	R		R
Ampicillin + In	APEN						S				R		SI		S	R	R	
Aztreonam	MOB							S					S	S	S	R	R	
Benzylpenicillin	PEN									R	R		R					R
Carbenicillin	CPEN	S		S				S		S								R
Cefaclor	CEF2												R					R
Cefamandole	CEF2	S		S														
Cefazolin	CEF1											R	SIR			R	R	
Cefepime	CEF4									S			S		S	R	R	
Cefotaxime	CEF3	S	S	S	SI		S			S		S	S		S	I	R	S
Cefoxitin	CEF2	S	S	R	R								SIR		S	R		
Ceftazidime	CEF3		S					S		S			S			I	R	
Ceftriaxone	CEF3					S				S			S			R	R	
Cefuroxime	CEF2							S		I		I	SR			R	R	
Cephalothin	CEF1	S		R	R				R	R				R	R		R	R
Cephradine	CEF1		R															
Chloramphenicol	O	S	S	S									S	S				
Ciprofloxacin	FQU					S							S	S	S	R		
Ertapenem	CARB															R		
Fosfomycin	O												SIR					
Gentamycin	AMG	R					S			S		S				R	R	
Imipenem	CARB			S				S					S	S	S	R	R	
Levofloxacin	FQU															R		
Meropenem	CARB												S					S
Netilmicin	AMG		S					S										
Ofloxacin	FQU									S		S	S					
Piperacillin	UPEN	S		S								S	S	S	S			
Piperacillin + In	UPEN		S				S	S					S		S	I	R	
Tetracycline	TET	S	S	S							R		SI	R	S	R	R	
Ticarcillin	CPEN				R								S				R	
Ticarcillin + In	CPEN															S	R	
TMP/SMX	SUL	S		S		S		S					S	S		S	R	
Tobramycin	AMG	R	S					S				S				R	R	

Table 5. Susceptibility pattern of *E. americana*. [a, b] For codes see Table 4. [c] Only resistance information was published.

Wiedemann, 1999) and *Serratia fonticola* (Peduzzi et al., 1997). In contrast to *Rahnella*, *Escherichia hermanii* and the *Klebsiella* isolates were sensitive to 1st and 2nd generation cephalosporins while the *Serratia fonticola* β-lactamase showed activity even against 3rd generation cephalosoprins. The unique susceptibility pattern of *Rahnella* indicates an enzyme distant from the other Ambler class A β-lactamases.

Also most *Ewingella* strains are resistant to several β-lactamases, mainly 1st and 2nd generation cephalosporins, while they were sensitive to 3rd and 4th class cephalosporins. In contrast to *Rahnella* only a low or medium-level resistance for penicillins could be observed. The distribution of the MICs of these antibiotics showed a peak at the concentration range clinically defined as 'intermediate' resulting in strains that were sensitive, intermediate or resistant (Stock et al., 2003). This overlap is likely the reason that the phenotypes of ampicillin and amoxicillin resistance seem to be inconsistent in the literature (see Table 4). The β-lactamase of *Ewingella* is insensitive to inhibitors, which is typical for class C β-lactamases.

Apart from β-lactams the most remarkable resistance of *Rahnella* and *Ewingella* was for fosfomycin. The MICs of most strains exceeded 64 mg/l and often reached 512 mg/l (Stock et al., 2000; Stock et al., 2003). Also one highly resistant *Rahnella* isolate with a MIC exceeding 1600 mg/l was reported (O'Hara et al., 1998). Other resistances shared by most strains included only such to which other species of the Enterobacteriaceae are also intrinsically resistant, for instance macrolides, lincosamides and glycopeptides.

Remarkably, two multidrug resistant strains of *Ewingella* were reported. Based on an antibiogram a successful treatment with cefotetan and trimethoprim/sulfamethoxazole was initiated in one case (Pound et al., 2007), while no information about antibiotic therapy was reported in the second case (Bukhari et al., 2008). Further reports of strains with unusual susceptibility patterns are rare and usually only one or two additional resistances were observed (Table 4 and 5). Thus treatment of infections is usually simple. In several cases trimethoprim/sulfamethoxazole, ciprofloxacin, gentamycin and 3rd generation cephalosporins were successfully used. For *Rahnella* also combinations of penicillins with β-lactamase inhibitors may be an option, while this is inappropriate for *Ewingella* infections.

2.4.2 Antibiotic resistance genes and their evolution

Cloning and sequencing of the *Rahnella* β-lactamase (bla_{RAHN-1}) confirmed that it belongs to the Ambler group C (Bellais et al., 2001). The bla_{RAHN-1} gene comprises 888 bp and its translated amino acid sequence shows 75%, 71% and 67% identity to the chromosomally encoded β-lactamases of *Serratia fonticola, Kluyvera cryocrescens* and *Citrobacter sedlakii* and approximately 70% identity to plasmid encoded CTX-M type ESLBs found in isolates of *Klebsiella pneumoniae, Escherichia coli, Acinetobacter baumanii* and other species (Figure 2B). Currently the sequences of the complete bla_{RAHN} loci of four different strains are available. They show a similar pattern: bla_{RAHN} and its surrounding genes have the same transcriptional orientation. An upstream transcriptional regulator that may regulate bla_{RAHN} expression is lacking (Figure 2A). The expression of many chromosomally encoded class A β-lactamases including that of *Citrobacter diversus* (Jones & Bennett, 1995) and *Proteus vulgaris* (Ishiguro & Sugimoto, 1996) is regulated by LysR-type transcription factors but also some examples lacking such a control system, for instance bla_{KLUC-1} of *Kluyvera cryocrescens* (Decousser et al., 2001), are known. A recent phylogenetic study using partial β-lactamase gene sequences of *Rahnella* strains isolated from different vegetables and fruits revealed two

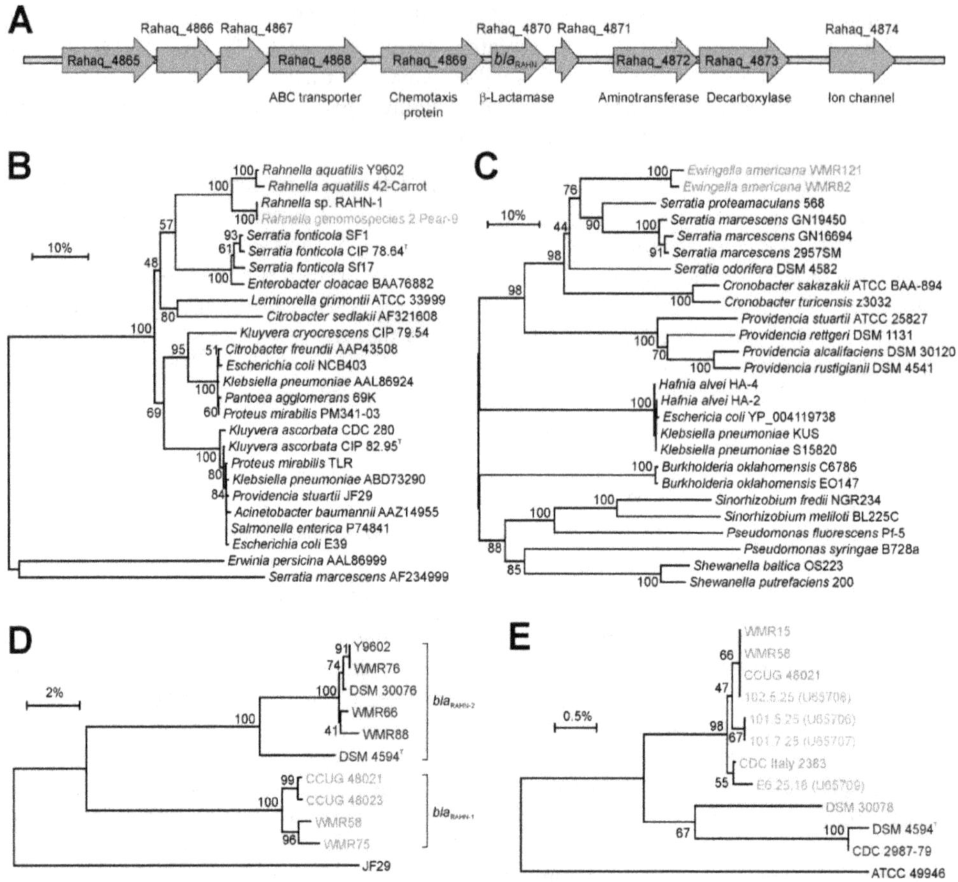

Fig. 2. The antibiotic resistance genes of *Rahnella* and *Ewingella*. (A) The bla$_{\mathrm{RAHN}}$ locus and its surrounding genes from strain *Rahnella aquatilis* Y9602 are shown. (B) Phylogentic trees of class A β-lactamases related to *bla*$_{\mathrm{RHAN}}$ and (C) class C enzymes related to AmpC of *Ewingella americana*. (D) β-lactamases of *Rahnella aquatilis* and *Rahnella* genomospecies 2 cluster in two different clades. *Providencia stuartii* JF29 was used as outgroup. (E) *Rahnella* isolates obtained from 12,000 year old mastodon remains (shown in orange; the accession numbers are given in brackets) cluster with recent strains belonging to *Rahnella* genomospecies 2. The tree shown is based on partial *16S rRNA* gene sequences. The same methods and colour codes like in Figure 1 were used.

clusters (Ruimy et al., 2010b). A similar dichotomy was also observed for a phlyogenetic tree based on partial *16S rRNA* and *rpoB* sequences (Ruimy et al., 2010a). The originally described *bla*$_{\mathrm{RHAN\text{-}1}}$ gene (Bellais et al., 2001) clustered with the sequences obtained from *Rahnella* genomospecies 2. The variant found in *Rahnella aquatilis* was named *bla*$_{\mathrm{RHAN\text{-}2}}$ (Ruimy et al., 2010b). Here we provide data confirming the results of these studies: we sequenced the (partial) *bla* gene of a number of reference strains and environmental isolates. The obtained phylogenetic tree (Figure 2D) is in agreement with that obtained for the *16S rRNA, groEL* or *dnaJ* gene (Figure 1). These data clearly suggest that *bla*$_{\mathrm{RHAN}}$ was present in the ancestor before the divergence in genomospecies. Previously the isolation of *Rahnella* strains from 12,000 year old American mastodon remains was reported. We used the partial *16S rRNA* gene sequence of these isolates and of recent reference strains to construct a phlyogenetic tree (Figure 2E). The four prehistoric strains cluster clearly with genomospecies 2. This indicates that divergence in genomospecies occured significantly more than 12,000 years ago. Thus the bla_{RHAN} seems to be present in *Rahnella* for a long time and thus represents a natural resistance of this microorganism.

However, we were unable to obtain any PCR product for strains belonging to *Rahnella* genomospecies 3 although these strains were intermediate or resistant to amoxicillin and cephalothin. Thus *Rahnella* genomospecies 3 may either possess a β-lactamase resistance gene unrelated to $bla_{RAHN\text{-}1}$ and $bla_{RAHN\text{-}2}$ or the primer binding sites may be different. Since the β-lactam susceptibility pattern of the three *Rahnella* genomospecies is very similar, the latter explanation seems more plausible.

Based on the susceptibility pattern an Abler class C β-lactamase was suggested for *Ewingella americana* (Stock et al., 2003). Using different primer combinations we could amplify and sequence the (partial) *ampC* gene of the strains WMR82 and WMR121. The amino acid sequence shows 72% identity to AmpC of *Serratia proteamaculans* and approximately 67% and 59% to AmpC of other *Serratia* species and to the *Providencia* cluster, respectively (Figure 2C). It is interesting to note that the AmpC sequences of the two *Ewingella* isolates share only 96.3% sequence identity. In contrast the plasmid encoded mobile β-lactamases found in some *Klebsiella pneumoniae* and *Escherichia coli* isolates exceed 98% identity (Figure 2C). It is believed that they originate from the chromosomally encoded *ampC* gene of *Hafnia alvei* (Girlich et al., 2000). This result and the observation that the vast majority of *Ewingella americana* strains have a similar susceptibility pattern suggest natural rather than acquired β-lactam resistance for this microorganism.

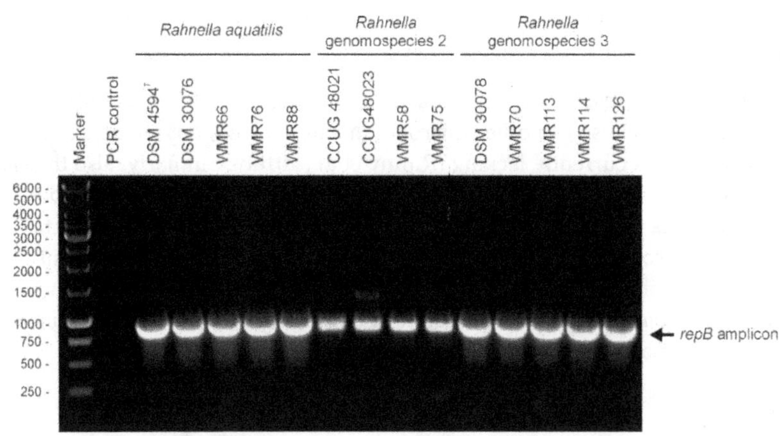

Fig. 3. The plasmid pRAHAQ01 is ubiquitously present in *Rahnella*. The (putative) replication gene *repB* of plasmid pRAHAQ01 could be detected by PCR in all strains tested.

While the molecular basis of β-lactam resistance is well known, the genotype of the fosfomycin resistance remains elusive. The high level of fosfomycin resistance observed in several strains and the report of successful transfer of the fosfomycin resistance to *Serratia marcescens* (O'Hara et al., 1998) rather suggest the presence of a specific fosfomycin:glutation-S-transferase than mutations in the GlpT, a transporter necessary for entry of fosfomycin into the cell.

2.4.3 The plasmid complement of *Rahnella*

Originally bla_{RAHN-1} was thought to be chromosomally encoded, since transfer experiments to *Escherichia coli* failed (Bellais et al., 2001). The recently completed *Rahnella* genome sequencing project showed unambiguously that the β-lactamase gene of strain Y9602 is located on a 617 kb megaplasmid, pRAHAQ01. The bla_{RAHN-2} locus and the surrounding genes of pRAHAQ01 share striking homology to three previously reported bla_{RAHN-1} and bla_{RAHN-2} sequences (Bellais et al., 2001; Ruimy et al., 2010b), indicating that they may also be plasmid born. To investigate this in more detail we analysed the sequence of pRAHAQ01 for putative plasmid replication genes and found only one candidate: Rahaq_4731 or *repB*. RepB shares 82% amino acid sequence identity with the replication protein of pEA29, a large plasmid of the plant pathogen *Erwinia amylovora* (McGhee & Jones, 2000). PCR analysis using primers for a conserved part of the *repB* gene showed a positive result for all strains tested (Figure 3). Moreover, in a previous study the presence of 400 kb to 700 kb megaplasmids in *Rahnella* soil isolates has been described (Evguenieva-Hackenberg & Selenska-Pobell, 1995). This substantiates that bla_{RAHN} may be commonly plasmid encoded. pRAHAQ01 and a second large plasmid found in strain Y9602 seem to be immobile since no known transfer system could be found on their backbones. Furthermore, no evidence could be found that bla_{RAHN} is located on a transposon or an integron.

A number of *Rahnella* strains possess also small plasmids. The majority of them were found to belong to the ColE1 family but also some ColE2 and rolling circle plasmids were isolated. Interestingly, the *Rahnella* ColE1 plasmids formed a distinct cluster in the ColE1 family and lacked any mobilisation system, suggesting that they rarely spread by horizontal gene transfer events. The ColE2 and the rolling circle plasmids possessed mobilisation systems but, like the ColE1 plasmids, were cryptic and did not encode any resistance gene (Rozhon et al., 2010).

Taken together these results suggest that the *Rahnella* β-lactamase, although plasmid encoded, is hardly mobilised to other microorganisms. Indeed, any evidence for its spread to human pathogens is currently lacking (Ruimy et al., 2010b). Similarly, also the *ampC* gene of *Ewingella* has so far remained restricted to its natural host but further experiments are necessary to rate its ability for mobilisation. Such studies would be important because previous reports provide evidence that *Ewingella americana* may be present in clinical environments (McNeil et al., 1987; Pien & Bruce, 1986) and the appearance of multiple drug resistant *Ewingella americana* strains (Bukhari et al., 2008; Pound et al., 2007) indicates that this micoorganism may exchange genetic information with human pathogens.

3. Conclusion

Rahnella is commonly associated with plants and *Ewingella* has been found at high titers in cultured mushrooms. Thus these two Enterobacteriaceae may be frequent in some types of food. Both may appear as infrequent human opportunistic pathogens. Infections are easy to treat if the specific antibiotic resistance patterns of these bacteria are considered. *Rahnella* and *Ewingella* are naturally resistant to several β-lactams, which is mediated by an Ambler class A and an Ambler class C β–lactamase, respectively. The β-lactam resistance gene of *Rahnella*, bla_{RAHN}, is located on the large non-mobile plasmid pRAHAQ01. This plasmid belongs to the pEA29 family, which is commonly found in plant associated bacteria. *Rahnella* acquired *bla*$_{RAHN}$ presumably in prehistoric times before the divergence into genomospecies. Since then *bla*$_{RAHN}$ has co-evolved with its host and diverged to *bla*$_{RAHN-1}$ and *bla*$_{RAHN-2}$ found in *Rahnella* genomospecies 2 and in *Rahnella aquatilis*, respectively. The variant present in *Rahnella* genomospecies 3 remains to be identified. Although *bla*$_{RAHN}$ is located on a plasmid it is not per se mobile and so far no hint for its mobilisation to other species has been found. However, since several examples of chromosomal resistance genes that were transferred into pathogens have been documented, it can not be excluded that also *bla*$_{RAHN}$ may spread to other bacteria in the future. Based on the suceptibility pattern it was previously hypothesised that the β-lactamase of *Ewingella americana* is an Ambler class C enzyme. Here we have provided compelling data confirming this assumption. However, further studies are necessary to assess whether the *Ewingella ampC* gene is chromosome or plasmid born and its potential for transfer needs to be investigated. *Rahnella* and *Ewingella* are also naturally resistant to fosfomycin. The molecular basis of this resistance remains elusive. Other resistances were rarely reported for *Rahnella*, while recently two multidrug resistant strains of *Ewingella* were described. These characteristics should be considered for treatment of infections and for potential applications of *Rahnella* and *Ewingella*.

4. Acknowledgment

We would like to thank Harald Preßlmayer for translation of French, Spanish and Italian manuscripts. This work was supported by the Austrian Science Fund.

5. References

Aktaş, E.; Külah, C.; Cömert, F.; Bektaş, Z. & Kargi, E. (2009). Isolation of *Rahnella aquatilis* from bone and soft tissue of a foot of a patient with diabetes (case report). *Türk Mikrobiyoloji Cemiyeti Dergisi*, Vol.39, No.1-2, (January 2009), pp. 54-57, ISBN 0258-2171

Alballaa, S.R.; Qadri, S.M.; al-Furayh, O. & al-Qatary, K. (1992). Urinary tract infection due to *Rahnella aquatilis* in a renal transplant patient. *Journal of clinical microbiology*, Vol.30, No.11, (November 1992), pp. 2948-2950, ISBN 0095-1137

Ambler, R.P. (1980). The structure of beta-lactamases. *Philosophical transactions of the Royal Society of London, Series B*, Vol.289, No.1036, (May 1980), pp. 321-331, ISBN 0962-8436

Bear, N.; Klugman, K.P.; Tobiansky, L. & Koornhof, H.J. (1986). Wound colonization by *Ewingella americana*. *Journal of clinical microbiology*, Vol.23, No.3, (March 1986), pp. 650-651, ISBN 0095-1137

Beazley, M.J.; Martinez, R.J.; Sobecky, P.A.; Webb, S.M. & Teillefert, M. (2007). Uranium biomineralization as a result of bacterial phosphatase activity: Insights from bacterial isolates from a contaminated subsurface. *Environmental science and technology*, Vol.41, No.16, (August 2007), pp. 5701-5707, ISBN 0013-936X

Bellais, S.; Poirel, L.; Fortineau, N.; Decousser, J.W. & Nordmann, P. (2001). Biochemical-genetic characterization of the chromosomally encoded extended-spectrum class A beta-lactamase from *Rahnella aquatilis*. *Antimicrobial agents and chemotherapy*, Vol.45, No.10, (October 2001), pp. 2965-2968, ISBN 0066-4804

Berge, O.; Heulin, T.; Achouak, W.; Richard, C.; Bally, R. & Balandreau, J. (1991). *Rahnella aquatilis*, a nitrogen-fixing enteric bacterium associated with the rhizosphere of wheat and maize. *Canadian journal of microbiology*, Vol.37, No.3, (March 1991), pp. 195-203, ISBN 0008-4166

Boukadida, J.; Maaroufi, A. & Chaib, A. (1999). Septidmie à *Rahnella aquatilis*. *Médecine et maladies infectieuses*, Vol.29, No.11, (November 1999), pp. 718-720, ISBN 0399-077X

Brenner, D.J. & Farmer , J.J. (2005). Order XIII. "Enterobacteriales", In: *Bergey´s Manual of Systematic Bacteriology, Volume 2, Part B*, D.J. Brenner, N.R. Krieg, J.T. Staley, (Eds.). *Springer*, pp. 587-850, ISBN 978-0387-24144-9, New York, USA

Brenner, D.J.; Muller, H.E.; Steigerwalt, A.G.; Whitney, A.M.; O'Hara, C.M. & Kampfer, P. (1998). Two new *Rahnella* genomospecies that cannot be phenotypically differentiated from *Rahnella aquatilis*. *International journal of systematic bacteriology*, Vol.48, No.1, (January 1998), pp. 141-149, ISBN 0020-7713

Brightwell, G.; Clemens, R.; Urlich, S. & Boerema, J. (2007). Possible involvement of psychrotolerant Enterobacteriaceae in blown pack spoilage of vacuum-packaged raw meats. *International journal of food microbiology*, Vol.119, No.3, (November 2007), pp. 334-339, ISBN 0168-1605

Bukhari, S.Z.; Hussain, W.M.; Fatani, M.I. & Ashshi, A.M. (2008). Multi-drug resistant *Ewingella americana*. *Saudi medical journal*, Vol.29, No.7, (July 2008), pp. 1051-1053, ISBN 0379-5284

Cankar, K.; Kraigher, H.; Ravnikar, M. & Rupnik, M. (2005). Bacterial endophytes from seeds of Norway spruce (*Picea abies* L. Karst). *FEMS microbiology letters*, Vol.244, No.2, (March 2005), pp. 341-345, ISBN 0378-1097

Canton, R. & Coque, T.M. (2006). The CTX-M beta-lactamase pandemic. *Current opinion in microbiology*, Vol.9, No.5, (October 2006), pp. 466-475, ISBN 1369-5274

Caraccio, V.; Rocchetti, A. & Garavelli, P. (1994). *Rahnella aquatilis* bacteremia in a patient with chronic renal failure. *Giornale di malattie infettive e parassitarie*, Vol.46, No.5, (May 1994), pp. 330-331, ISBN 0017-0321

Carinder, J.E.; Chua, J.D.; Corales, R.B.; Taege, A.J. & Procop, G.W. (2001). *Rahnella aquatilis* bacteremia in a patient with relapsed acute lymphoblastic leukemia. *Scandinavian journal of infectious diseases*, Vol.33, No.6, (June 2001), pp. 471-473, ISBN 0036-5548

Caroff, N.; Chamoux, C.; Le Gallou, F.; Espaze, E.; Gavini, F.; Gautreau, D.; Richet, H. & Reynaud, A. (1998). Two epidemiologically related cases of *Rahnella aquatilis* bacteremia. *European Journal of Clinical Microbiology and Infection Diseases*, Vol.17, No.5, (May 1998), pp. 349-352, ISBN 0934-9723

Chang, C.L.; Jeong, J.; Shin, J.H.; Lee, E.Y. & Son, H.C. (1999). *Rahnella aquatilis* sepsis in an immunocompetent adult. *Journal of clinical microbiology*, Vol.37, No.12, (December 1999), pp. 4161-4162, ISBN 0095-1137

Christiaens, E.; Hansen, W. & J., M. (1987). Isolement des expectorations d'un patient atteint de leucemie lymphoide chronique et de broncho-emphyseme d'une

Enterobacteriaceae nouvellement decrite: *Rahnella aquatilis. Médecine et maladies infectieuses*, Vol.17, No.12, (December 1987), pp. 732-734, ISBN 0399-077X

Cobo Molinos, A.; Abriouel, H.; Ben Omar, N.; Lopez, R.L. & Galvez, A. (2009). Microbial diversity changes in soybean sprouts treated with enterocin AS-48. *Food microbiology*, Vol.26, No.8, (December 2009), pp. 922-926, ISBN 1095-9998

Da Costa, P.S.; Tostes, M.M. & de Carvalho Valle, L.M. (2000). A case of keratoconjunctivitis due to *Ewingella americana* and a review of unusual organisms causing external eye infections. *Braz J Infect Dis*, Vol.4, No.5, (October 2000), pp. 262-267, ISBN 1413-8670

Davis, J.A. & Eyles, M.J. (1992). Discolouration of cottage cheese caused by *Rahnella aquatilis* in the presence of gluco delta-lactone. *Australian journal of diary technology*, Vol.47, No.1, (January 1992), pp. 62-63, ISBN 0004-9433

Decousser, J.W.; Poirel, L. & Nordmann, P. (2001). Characterization of a chromosomally encoded extended-spectrum class A beta-lactamase from *Kluyvera cryocrescens. Antimicrobial agents and chemotherapy*, Vol.45, No.12, (December 2001), pp. 3595-3598, ISBN 0066-4804

DeVreese, K.; Claeys, G. & Verschraegen, G. (1992). Septicemia with *Ewingella americana. Journal of clinical microbiology*, Vol.30, No.10, (October 1992), pp. 2746-2747, ISBN 0095-1137

Domann, E.; Hong, G.; Imirzalioglu, C.; Turschner, S.; Kuhle, J.; Watzel, C.; Hain, T.; Hossain, H. & Chakraborty, T. (2003). Culture-independent identification of pathogenic bacteria and polymicrobial infections in the genitourinary tract of renal transplant recipients. *Journal of clinical microbiology*, Vol.41, No.12, (December 2003), pp. 5500-5510, ISBN 0095-1137

El-Hendawy, H.H.; Osman, M.E. & Sorour, N.M. (2005). Biological control of bacterial spot of tomato caused by *Xanthomonas campestris* pv. *vesicatoria* by *Rahnella aquatilis. Microbiological research*, Vol.160, No.4, pp. 343-352, ISBN 0944-5013

Evguenieva-Hackenberg, E. & Selenska-Pobell, S. (1995). Genome analysis of five soil bacterial isolates named formerly *Enterobacter agglomerans. Journal of Applied Bacteriology*, Vol.79, No.1, (July 1995), pp. 49-60, ISBN 1365-2672

Fajardo, M. & Bueno, M.J. (2000). Isolation of *Rahnella aquatilis* in the tracheostomy exudate from a patient with laryngeal cancer. *Enfermedades infecciosas y microbiologia clinica*, Vol.18, No.5, (May 2000), pp. 251, ISBN 0213-005X

Farmer, J.J.; R., D.B.; Hickman-Brenner, F.W.; McWhorter, A.; Huntleycarter, G.P.; Asbury, M.A.; Riddle, C.; Wathen-Grady, H.G.; Elias, C.; Fanning, G.R.; Steigerwalt, A.G.; O'Hara, C.M.; Morris, G.K.; Smith, P.B. & Brenner, D.J. (1985). Biochemical identification of new species and biogroups of Enterobacteriaceae isolated from clinical specimens. *J Cin Microb*, Vol.21, No.1, (January 1985), pp. 46-76, ISBN 0095-1137

Freney, J.; Husson, M.O.; Gavini, F.; Madier, S.; Martra, A.; Izard, D.; Leclerc, D. & Fleurette, D. (1988). Susceptibilities to antibiotics and antiseptics of new species of the family Enterobacteriaceae. *Antimicrobial agents and chemotherapy*, Vol.62, No.6, (June 1988), pp. 873-876, ISBN 0066-4804

Funke, G. & Rosner, H. (1995). *Rahnella aquatilis* bacteremia in an HIV-infected intravenous drug abuser. *Diagnostic microbiology and infectious disease*, Vol.22, No.3, (July 1995), pp. 293-296, ISBN 0732-8893

Gaitán, J.I. & Bronze, M.S. (2010). Infection caused by *Rahnella aquatilis*. *The American journal of the medical sciences*, Vol.339, No.6, (June 2010), pp. 577-579, ISBN 1538-2990

Gardner, S.; Kabat, K. & Shulman, S.T. (1985). An outbreak of pseudobacteremia caused *by Ewingella americana*. *Pediatric Research*, Vol.19, No.4/2, (April 1985), pp. 200, ISBN 0031-3998

Gavini, F.; Ferragut, C.; Lefebvre, B. & Leclerc, H. (1976). Étude taxonomique d'entérobactéries appartenant ou apparentés au genre Enterobacter. *Annales de microbiologie*, Vol.127, No.B, (February 1976), pp. 317-335, ISBN 0300-5410

Geissler, A.; Merroun, M.; Geipel, G.; Reuther, H. & Selenska-Pobell, S. (2009). Biogeochemical changes induced in uranium mining waste pile samples by uranyl nitrate treatments under anaerobic conditions. *Geobiology*, Vol.7, No.3, (June 2009), pp. 282-294, ISBN 1472-4669

Girlich, D.; Naas, T.; Bellais, S.; Poirel, L.; Karim, A. & Nordmann, P. (2000). Biochemical-genetic characterization and regulation of expression of an ACC-1-like chromosome-borne cephalosporinase from *Hafnia alvei*. *Antimicrobial agents and chemotherapy*, Vol.44, No.6, (June 2000), pp. 1470-1478., ISBN 0066-4804

Goubau, P.; Van Aelst, F.; Verhaegen, J. & Boogaerts, M. (1988). Septicaemia caused by *Rahnella aquatilis* in an immunocompromised patient. *European Journal of Clinical Microbiology Infection Diseases*, Vol.7, No.5, (October 1988), pp. 697-699, ISBN 0934-9723

Grimont, P.A.; Farmer, J.J.; Grimont, F.; Asbury, M.A.; Brenner, D.J. & Deval, C. (1983). *Ewingella americana* gen.nov., sp.nov., a new Enterobacteriaceae isolated from clinical specimens. *Annales de microbiologie*, Vol.134A, No.1, (January 1983), pp. 39-52, ISBN 0300-5410

Hamilton-Miller, J.M. & Shah, S. (2001). Identity and antibiotic susceptibility of enterobacterial flora of salad vegetables. *International journal of antimicrobial agents*, Vol.18, No.1, (July 2001), pp. 81-83, ISBN 0924-8579

Hamze, M.; Mergaert, J.; van Vuuren, H.J.; Gavini, F.; Beji, A.; Izard, D. & Kersters, K. (1991). *Rahnella aquatilis*, a potential contaminant in lager beer breweries. *International journal of food microbiology*, Vol.13, No.1, (May 1991), pp. 63-68, ISBN 0168-1605

Harrell, L.J.; Cameron, M.L. & O'Hara, C.M. (1989). *Rahnella aquatilis*, an unusual gram-negative rod isolated from the bronchial washing of a patient with acquired immunodeficiency syndrome. *Journal of clinical microbiology*, Vol.27, No.7, (July 1989), pp. 1671-1672, ISBN 0095-1137

Hashidoko, Y.; Itoh, E.; Yokota, K.; Yoshida, T. & Tahara, S. (2002). Characterization of five phyllosphere bacteria isolated from *Rosa rugosa* leaves, and their phenotypic and metabolic properties. *Bioscience, biotechnology, and biochemistry*, Vol.66, No.11, (November 2002), pp. 2474-2478, ISBN 0916-8451

Heizmann, W.R. & Michel, R. (1991). Isolation of *Ewingella americana* from a patient with conjunctivitis. *European Journal of Clinical Microbiology and Infection Diseases*, Vol.10, No.11, (November 1991), pp. 957-959, ISBN 0934-9723

Heulin, T.; Berge, O.; Mavingui, P.; Gouzou, L.; Hebbar, K.P. & Balandreau, J. (1994). *Bacillus polymyxa* and *Rahnella aquatilis*, the dominant N_2-fixing bacteria associated with wheat rhizosphere in French soils. *European Journal of Soil Biology*, Vol.30, No.1, (January 1994), pp. 35-42, ISBN 1164-5563

Hohl, P.; Lüthy-Hottenstein, J.; Zollinger-Iten, J. & Altwegg, M. (1990). *In vitro* activities of fleroxacin, cefetamet, ciprofloxacin, ceftriaxone, trimethoprim-sulfamethoxazole, and amoxicillin-clavulanic acid against rare members of the family Enterobacteriaceae primarily of human (clinical) origin. *Antimicrobial agents and chemotherapy*, Vol.34, No.8, (August 1990), pp. 1605-1608, ISBN 0066-4804

Hoppe, J.E.; Herter, M.; Aleksic, S.; Klingebiel, T. & Niethammer, D. (1993). Catheter-related *Rahnella aquatilis* bacteremia in a pediatric bone marrow transplant recipient. *Journal of clinical microbiology*, Vol.31, No.7, (July 1993), pp. 1911-1912, ISBN 0095-1137

Iimura, K. & Hosono, A. (1996). Biochemical characteristics of *Enterobacter agglomerans* and related strains found in buckwheat seeds. *International journal of food microbiology*, Vol.30, No.3, (July 1996), pp. 243-253, ISBN 0168-1605

Inglis, P.W. & Peberdy, J.F. (1996). Isolation of *Ewingella americana* from the cultivated mushroom, *Agaricus bisporus*. *Current microbiology*, Vol.33, No.5, (November 1996), pp. 334-337, ISBN 0343-8651

Ishiguro, K. & Sugimoto, K. (1996). Purification and characterization of the *Proteus vulgaris* BlaA protein, the activator of the beta-lactamase gene. *Journal of biochemistry*, Vol.120, No.1, (July 1996), pp. 98-103, ISBN 0021-924X

Izard, D.; Gavini, F.; Trinel, P.A. & Leclere, H. (1979). *Rahnella aquatilis*, nouveau membre de la famille des Enterobacteriaceae. *Annales de microbiologie*, Vol.130, No.2, (February 1979), pp. 163-177, ISBN 0300-5410

Jafra, S.; Przysowa, J.; Gwizdek-Wisniewska, A. & van der Wolf, J.M. (2009). Potential of bulb-associated bacteria for biocontrol of hyacinth soft rot caused by *Dickeya zeae*. *Journal of applied microbiology*, Vol.106, No.1, (January 2009), pp. 268-277, ISBN 1365-2672

Jensen, N.; Varelis, P. & Whitfield, F.B. (2001). Formation of guaiacol in chocolate milk by the psychrotrophic bacterium *Rahnella aquatilis*. *Letters in applied microbiology*, Vol.33, No.5, (November 2001), pp. 339-343, ISBN 0266-8254

Jones, M.E. & Bennett, P.M. (1995). Inducible expression of the chromosomal *cdiA* from *Citrobacter diversus* NF85, encoding an ambler class A beta-lactamase, is under similar genetic control to the chromosomal *ampC*, encoding an Ambler class C enzyme, from *Citrobacter freundii* OS60. *Microbial drug resistance*, Vol.1, No.4, (Winter 1995), pp. 285-291, ISBN 1076-6294

Kati, C.; Bibashi, E.; Kokolina, E. & Sofianou, D. (1999). Case of peritonitis caused by *Ewingella americana* in a patient undergoing continuous ambulatory peritoneal dialysis. *Journal of clinical microbiology*, Vol.37, No.11, (November 1999), pp. 3733-3734, ISBN 0095-1137

Kim, H.; Park, H.-E.; Kim, M.-J.; Lee, H.G.; Yang, J.-Y. & Cha, J. (2003). Enzymatic characterization of a recombinant levansucrase from *Rahnella aquatilis* ATCC 15552.

Journal of microbiology and biotechnology, Vol.13, No.2, (February 2003), pp. ISBN 1738-8872

Kim, K.Y.; Jordan, D. & Krishnan, H.B. (1997). *Rahnella aquatilis*, a bacterium isolated from soybean rhizosphere, can solubilize hydroxyapatite. *FEMS microbiology letters*, Vol.153, No.2, (August 1997), pp. 273-277, ISBN 0378-1097

Labia, R.; Fabre, C.; Masson, J.M.; Barthelemy, M.; Heitz, M. & Pitton, J.S. (1979). *Klebsiella pneumonia* strains moderately resistant to ampicillin and carbenicillin: characterization of a new beta-lactamase. *The Journal of antimicrobial chemotherapy*, Vol.5, No.4, (July 1979), pp. 375-382, ISBN 0305-7453

Laux, P.; Baysal, Ö. & Zeller, W. (2002). Biological control of fire blight by using *Rahnella aquatilis* Ra39 and *Pseudomonas spec.* R1. *Acta Hortiulturae*, Vol.590, (November 2002), pp. 225-229, ISBN 978-90-66058-06-4

Le Gall, S.; Pellissier, L.; Delmas, P.; Esterni, J.P. & Roblin, X. (2000). Septicémie à *Ewingella americana* chez un patient toxicomane, au stade sida. *Médecine et maladies infectieuses*, Vol.30, No.7, (July 2000), pp. 484, ISBN 0399-077X

Liberto, M.C.; Matera, G.; Puccio, R.; Lo Russo, T.; Colosimo, E. & Foca, E. (2009). Six cases of sepsis caused by *Pantoea agglomerans* in a teaching hospital. *The new microbiologica*, Vol.32, No.1, (January 2009), pp. 119-123, ISBN 1121-7138

Lindberg, A.M.; Ljungh, A.; Ahrne, S.; Lofdahl, S. & Molin, G. (1998). Enterobacteriaceae found in high numbers in fish, minced meat and pasteurised milk or cream and the presence of toxin encoding genes. *International journal of food microbiology*, Vol.39, No.1-2, (January 1998), pp. 11-17, ISBN 0168-1605

Lindow, S.E.; Desurmont, C.; Elkins, R.; McGourty, G.; Clark, E. & Brandl, M.T. (1998). Occurrence of indole-3-acetic acid-producing bacteria on pear trees and their association with fruit russet. *Phytopathology*, Vol.88, No.11, (November 1998), pp. 1149-1157, ISBN 0031-949X

Maertens, J.; Delforge, M.; Vandenberghe, P.; Boogaerts, M. & Verhaegen, J. (2001). Catheter-related bacteremia due to *Ewingella americana*. *Clin Microbiol Infect*, Vol.7, No.2, (Febuary 2001), pp. 103-104, ISBN 1198-743X

Maraki, S.; Samonis, G.; Marnelakis, E. & Tselentis, Y. (1994). Surgical wound infection caused by *Rahnella aquatilis*. *Journal of clinical microbiology*, Vol.32, No.11, (November 1994), pp. 2706-2708, ISBN 0095-1137

Martinez, R.J.; Beazley, M.J.; Taillefert, M.; Arakaki, A.K.; Skolnick, J. & Sobecky, P.A. (2007). Aerobic uranium(VI) bioprecipitation by metal-resistant bacteria isolated from radionuclide- and metal-contaminated subsurface soils. *Environmental microbiology*, Vol.9, No.12, (December 2007), pp. 3122-3133, ISBN 1462-2912

Matsukura, H.; Katayama, K.; Kitano, N.; Kobayashi, K.; Kanegane, C.; Higuchi, A. & Kyotani, S. (1996). Infective endocarditis caused by an unusual gram-negative rod, *Rahnella aquatilis*. *Pediatric cardiology*, Vol.17, No.2, (April 1996), pp. 108-111, ISBN 0172-0643

Matsuyama, H.; Sasaki, R.; Kawasaki, K. & Yumoto, I. (1999). Production of a novel exopolysaccharide by *Rahnella aquatilis*. *Journal of bioscience and bioengineering*, Vol.87, No.2, (July 1999), pp. 180-183, ISBN 1389-1723

McGhee, G.C. & Jones, A.L. (2000). Complete nucleotide sequence of ubiquitous plasmid pEA29 from *Erwinia amylovora* strain Ea88: gene organization and intraspecies variation. *Applied and environmental microbiology*, Vol.66, No.11, (November 2000), pp. 4897-4907, ISBN 0099-2240

McNeil, M.M.; Davis, B.J.; Anderson, R.L.; Martone, W.J. & Solomon, S.L. (1985). Mechanism of cross-contamination of blood culture bottles in outbreaks of pseudobacteremia associated with nonsterile blood collection tubes. *Journal of clinical microbiology*, Vol.22, No.1, (July 1985), pp. 23-25, ISBN 0095-1137

McNeil, M.M.; Davis, B.J.; Solomon, S.L.; Anderson, R.L.; Shulman, S.T.; Gardner, S.; Kabat, K. & Martone, W.J. (1987). *Ewingella americana*: recurrent pseudobacteremia from a persistent environmental reservoir. *Journal of clinical microbiology*, Vol.25, No.3, (March 1987), pp. 498-500, ISBN 0095-1137

Müller, H.E.; Fanning, G.R. & Brenner, D.J. (1995). Isolation of *Ewingella americana* from mollusks. *Current microbiology*, Vol.31, No.5, (November 1995), pp. 287-290, ISBN 0343-8651

Naas, T.; Poirel, L. & Nordmann, P. (2008). Minor extended-spectrum beta-lactamases. *Clin Microbiol Infect*, Vol.14, No.1, (January 2008), pp. 42-52, ISBN 1198-743X

Niemi, R.M.; Heikkila, M.P.; Lahti, K.; Kalso, S. & Niemela, S.I. (2001). Comparison of methods for determining the numbers and species distribution of coliform bacteria in well water samples. *Journal of applied microbiology*, Vol.90, No.6, (June 2001), pp. 850-858, ISBN 1364-5072

O'Hara, K.; Chen, J.; Shigenobu, F.; Nakamura, A.; Taniguchi, K.; Shimojima, M.; Ida, H.; Yoshikawa, E.; Tsuboi, I.; Mizuoka, K. & Sawai, T. (1998). Appearance of fosfomycin resistant *Rahnella aquatilis* clinically isolated in Japan. *Microbios*, Vol.95, No.381, (May 1998), pp. 109-115, ISBN 0026-2633

Oh, H.M. & Tay, L. (1995). Bacteraemia caused by *Rahnella aquatilis*: report of two cases and review. *Scandinavian journal of infectious diseases*, Vol.27, No.1, (January 1995), pp. 79-80, ISBN 0036-5548

Olson, A.B.; Silverman, M.; Boyd, D.A.; McGeer, A.; Willey, B.M.; Pong-Porter, V.; Daneman, N. & Mulvey, M.R. (2005). Identification of a progenitor of the CTX-M-9 group of extended-spectrum beta-lactamases from *Kluyvera georgiana* isolated in Guyana. *Antimicrobial agents and chemotherapy*, Vol.49, No.5, (May 2005), pp. 2112-2115, ISBN 0066-4804

Papaefstathiou, C.; Vlassopoulos, D.; Zoumberi, M.; Mangana, P.; Hadjiconstantinou, V. & Kouppari, G. (2004). *Ewingella americana* peritonitis in an adult patient on continuous ambulatory peritoneal dialysis. *Clinical Microbiology Newsletter*, Vol.26, (December 2004), pp. 184-185, ISBN 0196-4399

Peduzzi, J.; Farzaneh, S.; Reynaud, A.; Barthelemy, M. & Labia, R. (1997). Characterization and amino acid sequence analysis of a new oxyimino cephalosporin-hydrolyzing class A beta-lactamase from *Serratia fonticola* CUV. *Biochimica et biophysica acta*, Vol.1341, No.1, (August 1997), pp. 58-70, ISBN 0006-3002

Pien, F.D. & Bruce, A.E. (1986). Nosocomial *Ewingella americana* bacteremia in an intensive care unit. *Archives of internal medicine*, Vol.146, No.1, (January 1986), pp. 111-112, ISBN 0003-9926

Pien, F.D.; Farmer, J.J., 3rd & Weaver, R.E. (1983). Polymicrobial bacteremia caused by *Ewingella americana* (family Enterobacteriaceae) and an unusual *Pseudomonas* species. *Journal of clinical microbiology*, Vol.18, No.3, (Sepember 1983), pp. 727-729, ISBN 0095-1137

Pintado, M.E.; Pintado, I.E. & Malcata, F.X. (1999). Production of polysaccharide by *Rahnella aquatilis* with whey feedstock. *Journal of food science*, Vol.64, No.2, (February 1999), pp. 348-352, ISBN 0022-1147

Pound, M.W.; Tart, S.B. & Okoye, O. (2007). Multidrug-resistant *Ewingella americana*: a case report and review of the literature. *The Annals of pharmacotherapy*, Vol.41, No.12, (December 2007), pp. 2066-2070, ISBN 1542-6270

Raphael, E.; Wong, L.K. & Riley, L.W. (2011). Extended-spectrum beta-lactamase gene sequences in gram-negative saprophytes on retail organic and nonorganic spinach. *Applied and environmental microbiology*, Vol.77, No.5, (March 2011), pp. 1601-1607, ISBN 1098-5336

Reina, J. & Lopez, A. (1996). Clinical and microbiological characteristics of *Rahnella aquatilis* strains isolated from children. *The Journal of infection*, Vol.33, No.2, (September 1996), pp. 135-137, ISBN 0163-4453

Reina, J.; López, A.; Fernández-Baca, V. & Ros, M.J. (1995). Aislamiento de *Ewingella americana* en las heces de un paciente con diarrea scretora. *Revista espanola de pediatria*, Vol.51, No.4, (April 1995), pp. 393-395, ISBN 0034-947X

Reyes, J.E.; Venturini, M.E.; Oria, R. & Blanco, D. (2004). Prevalence of *Ewingella americana* in retail fresh cultivated mushrooms (*Agaricus bisporus*, *Lentinula edodes* and *Pleurotus ostreatus*) in Zaragoza (Spain). *FEMS microbiology ecology*, Vol.47, No.3, (March 2004), pp. 291-296, ISBN 1574-6941

Rhodes, A.N.; Urbance, J.W.; Youga, H.; Corlew-Newman, H.; Reddy, C.A.; Klug, M.J.; Tiedje, J.M. & Fisher, D.C. (1998). Identification of bacterial isolates obtained from intestinal contents associated with 12,000-year-old mastodon remains. *Applied and environmental microbiology*, Vol.64, No.2, (February 1998), pp. 651-658, ISBN 0099-2240

Rodriguez, M.M.; Power, P.; Radice, M.; Vay, C.; Famiglietti, A.; Galleni, M.; Ayala, J.A. & Gutkind, G. (2004). Chromosome-encoded CTX-M-3 from *Kluyvera ascorbata*: a possible origin of plasmid-borne CTX-M-1-derived cefotaximases. *Antimicrobial agents and chemotherapy*, Vol.48, No.12, (December 2004), pp. 4895-4897, ISBN 0066-4804

Rozhon, W.; Khan, M.; Petutschnig, E. & Poppenberger, B. (2011). Identification of *cis*- and *trans*-acting elements in pHW126, a representative of a novel group of rolling circle plasmids. *Plasmid*, Vol.65, No.1, (January 2011), pp. 70-76, ISBN 1095-9890

Rozhon, W.; Petutschnig, E.; Khan, M.; Summers, D.K. & Poppenberger, B. (2010). Frequency and diversity of small cryptic plasmids in the genus *Rahnella*. *BMC microbiology*, Vol.10, (February 2010), pp. 56, ISBN 1471-2180

Rozhon, W.M.; Petutschnig, E.K. & Jonak, C. (2006). Isolation and characterization of pHW15, a small cryptic plasmid from *Rahnella* genomospecies 2. *Plasmid*, Vol.56, No.3, (November 2006), pp. 202-215, ISBN 0147-619X

Ruimy, R.; Brisabois, A.; Bernede, C.; Skurnik, D.; Barnat, S.; Arlet, G.; Momcilovic, S.; Elbaz, S.; Moury, F.; Vibet, M.A.; Courvalin, P.; Guillemot, D. & Andremont, A. (2010a). Organic and conventional fruits and vegetables contain equivalent counts of Gram-negative bacteria expressing resistance to antibacterial agents. *Environmental microbiology*, Vol.12, No.3, (March 2010), pp. 608-615, ISBN 1462-2920

Ruimy, R.; Meziane-Cherif, D.; Momcilovic, S.; Arlet, G.; Andremont, A. & Courvalin, P. (2010b). RAHN-2, a chromosomal extended-spectrum class A beta-lactamase from *Rahnella aquatilis*. *The Journal of antimicrobial chemotherapy*, Vol.65, No.8, (August 2010), pp. 1619-1623, ISBN 1460-2091

Ryoo, N.H.; Ha, J.S.; Jeon, D.S.; Kim, J.R. & Kim, H.C. (2005). A case of pneumonia caused by *Ewingella americana* in a patient with chronic renal failure. *Journal of Korean medical science*, Vol.20, No.1, (Febuary 2005), pp. 143-145, ISBN 1011-8934

Sanmartin Jimenez, O.; Botella Estrada, R.; Roig Rubino, P.; Febrer Bosch, I.; Nieto Hernandez, A. & Navarro Ibanez, V. (1991). Balanitis por *Ewingella americana* en un paciente inmunodeprimido. *Actas dermo-sifiliograficas*, Vol.82, No.3, (March 1991), pp. 125-126, ISBN 1138-8196

Seo, J.W.; Jang, K.H.; Kang, S.A.; Song, K.B.; Jang, E.K.; Park, B.S.; Kim, C.H. & Rhee, S.K. (2002). Molecular characterization of the growth phase-dependent expression of the *lsrA* gene, encoding levansucrase of *Rahnella aquatilis*. *Journal of bacteriology*, Vol.184, No.21, (November 2002), pp. 5862-5870, ISBN 0021-9193

Stock, I.; Gruger, T. & Wiedemann, B. (2000). Natural antibiotic susceptibility of *Rahnella aquatilis* and *R. aquatilis*-related strains. *Journal of chemotherapy (Florence, Italy)*, Vol.12, No.1, (Feburay 2000), pp. 30-39, ISBN 1120-009X

Stock, I.; Sherwood, K.J. & Wiedemann, B. (2003). Natural antibiotic susceptibility of *Ewingella americana* strains. *Journal of chemotherapy (Florence, Italy)*, Vol.15, No.5, (October 2003), pp. 428-441, ISBN 1120-009X

Stock, I. & Wiedemann, B. (1999). Natural antibiotic susceptibility of *Escherichia coli*, *Shigella*, *E. vulneris*, and *E. hermannii* strains. *Diagnostic microbiology and infectious disease*, Vol.33, No.3, (March 1999), pp. 187-199, ISBN 0732-8893

Sykes, R.B. & Matthew, M. (1976). The beta-lactamases of gram-negative bacteria and their role in resistance to beta-lactam antibiotics. *The Journal of antimicrobial chemotherapy*, Vol.2, No.2, (June 1976), pp. 115-157, ISBN 0305-7453

Tamura, K.; Dudley, J.; Nei, M. & Kumar, S. (2007). MEGA4: Molecular Evolutionary Genetics Analysis (MEGA) software version 4.0. *Molecular biology and evolution*, Vol.24, No.8, (August 2007), pp. 1596-1599, ISBN 0737-4038

Tash, K. (2005). *Rahnella aquatilis* bacteremia from a suspected urinary source. *Journal of clinical microbiology*, Vol.43, No.5, (May 2005), pp. 2526-2528, ISBN 0095-1137

Tsokos, M. (2003). Fatal Waterhouse-Friderichsen syndrome due to *Ewingella americana* infection. *The American journal of forensic medicine and pathology*, Vol.24, No.1, (March 2003), pp. 41-44, ISBN 0195-7910

Winder, R.S.; Macey, D.E. & Cortese, J. (2010). Dominant bacteria associated with broods of mountain pine beetle, *Dendroctonus ponderosae* (Colepotera: Curculionidae, Scolytinae). *Journal of the entomological society of Britisch Columbia*, Vol.107, (December 2010), pp. ISBN 0071-0733

Yu, H.; Wang, Z.; Liu, L.; Xia, Y.; Cao, Y. & Yin, Y. (2008). Analysis of the intestinal microflora in *Hepialus gonggaensis* larvae using *16S rRNA* sequences. *Current microbiology*, Vol.56, No.4, (April 2008), pp. 391-396, ISBN 0343-8651

4

Trends of Antibiotic Resistance (AR) in Mesophilic and Psychrotrophic Bacterial Populations During Cold Storage of Raw Milk, Produced by Organic and Conventional Farming Systems

Patricia Munsch-Alatossava[1], Vilma Ikonen[1],
Tapani Alatossava[1] and Jean-Pierre Gauchi[2]
*[1]Department of Food and Environmental Sciences,
Division of Food Technology, University of Helsinki,
[2]Unité de Mathématiques et Informatique Appliquées (UR 341),
Institut National de la Recherche Agronomique, Centre de Jouy en Josas,
[1]Finland
[2]France*

1. Introduction

Antibiotic resistant bacteria continually arise and their increasing prevalence constitutes one of the major public health threat. The problem, earlier mainly confined to hospitals, nowadays encircles the globe (Davies & Davies, 2010; Levy, 2002; Marshall et al., 2009). Perceived once as a consequence of use, overuse and misuse of antibiotics to prevent or treat diseases, as growth promotants for food animals, or as pesticides for agriculture, more explanations for high AR levels in bacteria were recently brought. The picture became darker when came evidences that environmental microbiota present in antibiotic free environments showed to possess an as enormous and diverse number of AR genes as present in pathogenic microbiota (Aminov, 2009). Further evidences point to micro-organisms associated with food, animals, and water as the main sources for resistance genes; commensals among them food commensals are also considered as a reservoir of AR (Knezevic & Petrovic, 2008; Straley et al., 2006), in fact according to Marshall et al. (2009) a rather underappreciated reservoir of AR. In developed countries, several parameters define a raw milk of "good quality" when it is absent of drug or antibiotics residues, when the legal limit of somatic cells per millilitre of milk is below $4x10^5$ /mL (excessive values may be indicating the presence of mastitis in the cow herd), when the bacteriological acceptance level is satisfied. In the later, the sanitation of raw milk is ensured by the determination of the standard plate count (Chambers, 2002) that aims to enumerate aerobic "total bacteria" present in milk; grade A or 1 (acceptable for industrial use) is attributed to milk that contains less than $1x10^5$ CFU/ml, determined on agar plates after 2 days incubation at 32°C, or 3 days at 30°C. After milking, numerous contamination sources raise the bacterial load along the cold chain of raw milk storage and transportation (Chambers, 2002; Cousin, 1982). The cold storage that aims to preserve food or milk from excessive bacterial development, however also selects bacterial types which have perfectly adapted to low temperatures : psychrotrophic bacteria, able to grow below 7°C, present in raw milk are well known for their spoilage features (production of various heat-stable exoenzymes) which affect raw or processed dairy products with significant economic impact. Mainly, out of some exceptions like the human pathogens (toxin producer of *B. cereus* species, or *Listeria* spp: Gray et al., 2006; Schoeni & Lee Wong, 2005), most psychrotrophic bacteria associated to raw milk of which many are Gram-negative, are generally considered as benign.

Foodstuffs are produced by either conventional (CP) or organic (OP) systems. Consumer demands for organic products generally perceived as more safe, is growing in Europe and the United States, offering increased business opportunities and wealth for rural regions (European Commission, 2008; Jacob et al., 2008). The organic food chain supply is guaranteed at the base first by producers which must adhere to strict rules: organic milk is defined by the European Commission as "milk that comes from cows, sheep and goats living in a welfare-oriented animal husbandry: outdoors in summer with access to pasture and indoors in winter when the climate is rough, with organic forage and enough space for regular exercise" (European Commission, 2008). Several principles are underlying organic production such as minimisation of the use of non-renewable resources and off-farms inputs, recycling of wastes and by-products of plant and animal origin as input in plant and livestock production, the feeding of livestock with organic feed (produced mainly at the farm), synthesized allopathic veterinary medicinal products, like antibiotics may be used with restriction on courses of treatment and withdrawal period (European Council Regulation, 2007); organic dairy cattle are treated for mastitis with the same antimicrobials as dairy cows from conventional systems. In Finland, at least 50% of the feed has to be produced by the farm; each cow can only be treated 3 times a year for independent diseases and the time for milk delivery acceptance to dairies is twice as long as for normal systems (Finnish Food Safety Authority, 2008); on a total of 2.2×10^9 L of milk delivered to dairies about 1.3% was produced by organic farming systems (Information Centre of the Ministry of Agriculture and Forestry, 2009). The use of ABs in Finland for cattle was surveyed by Thompson et al. (2008): for acute mastitis, parenteral treatments are based on benzyl penicillins (83%) and fluoroquinolones (11%); ampicillin combined with cloxacillin (36%), or cephalexin combined with streptomycin (26%) were intramammarily administered. Finland, together with Norway and Sweden, have lower ABs usage practices compared to seven other European countries (Grave et al., 2010). Considering the bacteriological quality of the milk, as well as the level of antimicrobial residues (Finnish association for milk hygiene, 2008), altogether the quality of Finnish raw milk is excellent.

While characterizing some raw milk gram-negative psychrotrophs, it was observed that besides having spoilage features (Munsch-Alatossava & Alatossava 2006), these bacteria also carried antibiotic multiresistant features: moreover, the study suggested that the AR load was higher for isolates that apparently spent a longer time in cold storage (Munsch-Alatossava & Alatossava 2007); another study, that considered bacterial raw milk psychrotrophs selected for their spoilage features, compared the AR levels of 79 bacterial isolates originating from CP (6) or OP (9) milk samples. With exception of gentamicin for which similar percentages of AR were recorded for CP and OP samples, we observed a lower prevalence of AR for OP samples; resistance levels to trimethoprim-sulfamethoxazole were 25 and 14% for CP and OP samples respectively, and resistance percentages were higher for ceftazidim and ciprofloxacin (a quinolone) for CP-originating isolates (Munsch-Alatossava, Xheng, Alatossava, unpublished data). To further answer to the question on whether AR levels may be different/lower for isolates retrieved from OP compared to CP milk samples, to follow the respective trends for mesophilic and psychrotrophic populations over time during cold storage (4 days at 4°C), the present study was undertaken: the AR to four ABs (gentamicin, ceftazidim, levofloxacin, and trimethoprim-sulfamethoxazole, representatives of 4 different classes) was evaluated for mesophilic and psychrotrophic bacteria for 12 raw milk samples (6 for each farming system); changes at the bacterial communities level during cold storage were investigated by DGGE.

2. Materials and methods

2.1 Cold storage of raw milk samples

Representative bovine raw milk samples of lorry tanks were collected into sterile bottles; samples were kept on ice until arrival at Helsinki University, at which time 100 ml were added to sterile 250 ml-bottles. Six bottles were placed on a multi-place magnetic stirrer (Variomag) and partially immersed in a refrigerated water bath (MGW Lauda MS/2) which allowed, with help of an immersion thermostat, a constant temperature to be maintained (modified from Munsch-Alatossava et al., 2010). The raw milk samples were continuously mixed at 220 rpm and kept at 4± 0.1 °C for 4 days.

2.2 Antibiotic resistance

The experimental procedures followed the EUCAST guidelines (2000). The microbiological analyses were performed immediately after milk samples arrived; all bacterial counts were determined from duplicate or triplicate agar cultures at day 0 (shortly after reception of the samples) and day 4 (after cold storage); 500 µl or raw milk were serially diluted in saline solution (0.85 % NaCl); 50µl of the diluted samples were spread on Mueller-Hinton (Lab M) agar plates. Four antimicrobial agents [gentamicin (Aminoglycosides), ceftazidim (β-lactams, Cephems), levofloxacin (Quinolones) and trimethoprim-sulfamethoxazole (at a ratio of 1/19, a Folate pathway inhibitor) (Sigma)] were added to agar, according to the EUCAST guidelines (EUCAST, 2000). The ABs solutions were freshly prepared by dissolving the powders in following solvents: water for G (gentamicin), 0.1M phosphate buffer (pH7) for C (ceftazidim), 0.1M NaOH for L (levofloxacin), 0.1M lactic acid for T (trimethoprim), and 95% ethanol for S (sulfamethoxazole) (EUCAST, 2000). With exception of S, all AB solutions were filter sterilized prior to the addition to adequately cooled agar. The AB concentrations were 16 mg/L for GI, 4 mg/L for GII, 32 mg/L for CI, 8 mg/L for CII, 8 mg/L for LI, 2 mg/L for LII, 8 mg/L trimethoprim with 152 mg/L sulfamethoxazole for TSI, and 4 mg/L trimethoprim with 76 mg/L sulfamethoxazole for TSII, which correspond to the MICs (GII, CII, LII and TSII) to 4-fold the MIC (GI, CI, LI), or to 2-fold the MIC (TSI) as indicated by EUCAST for pseudomonads. Agar plates were stored overnight at 4°C, and protected from light. Following the analyses, the plates were incubated for 2-3 days at 30°C, or for 10 days at 7°C to enumerate the "total" bacteria (mesophiles) and psychrotrophs, respectively.

2.3 Statistical analysis

2.3.1 Judicious remarks about ANOVA (ANalysis Of VAriance)

Usual analysis of variance is well known in the field of research and laboratories as an efficient statistical method enabling to analyse results following experimental designs, and to test for significant differences between means. Concerning milk and its microflora, also ANOVA was used (Freitas et al. 2009; Ma et al. 2003). Thanks to the Fisher-Snedecor and Student tests, ANOVA enables to detect factors, to highlight interactions of the considered factors, which both significantly impact on the response (continuous) of the studied phenomenon. However, ANOVA is not considered as robust as it is susceptible to variations of the assumptions on which this method is grounded; more precisely, the statistical tests´ validity of ANOVA are "sensitive" to these variations. The validity is relying on three fundamental restrictive assumptions: A) Distribution of the residuals is normal; B) Variance of errors is constant; C) The data does not contain outliers. If one of these hypotheses is strongly violated, conclusions about significant level of the effects of the factors may be questionable or erroneous. In practice for a particular study, the hypothesis A is very difficult to be proved due to usual low amount of repetitions for a certain treatment (a combination of factors set at a certain level); in addition, if this assumption is not respected the impact on the Student test result is rather low, contrarily to the Fisher Snedecor test; however, this hypothesis has been so often checked by numerous experimental studies, that one may assume it is approximately often respected.

The hypothesis B is easily checked on the graphical analyses of "residuals"; if the hypothesis B is not respected, one common way to proceed even though not optimal consists in stabilizing variation by considering the logarithmic values of the results of the response. Also from the observation of the usual ANOVA graphics (given by standard statistics software) the hypothesis C can be checked. Mathematically it can be demonstrated that statistical tests are hampered by the presence of many outliers which may lead to erroneous conclusions. Moreover in the presence of orthogonal or almost orthogonal experimental designs, the outliers promote high levels (for example triple) of interactions of no meaning; typically one interaction AxBxC between three factors A, B, C may be declared significant, even though in the ANOVA model none of the three main effects of the three factors appears. How to overcome the harmful impact of the outliers on the significance of the ANOVA model? The elimination of extreme results due to outliers constitutes one solution, however in the presence of a limited amount of repetitions in practice this option is not applicable. Consequently it is difficult to validate the hypothesis C. To overcome this problem, no ideal method exists. Nevertheless, to compare several samples one alternative consists in the use of non parametric statistical tests like the Kruskal-Wallis test (Conover 1980) for example, which considers the ranks of the results of the response. For example, for the 6 following results of bacterial counts (expressed as CFU/ml) 0, 1.9×10^4, 1.5×10^5, 2.0×10^5, 2.4×10^5 and $1{,}5 \times 10^9$, the extreme values 0 and $1{,}5 \times 10^9$ may be badly estimated by the ANOVA model, and will generate excessive residuals. With a non parametric statistical approach, the values will be substituted for ranks, here 6, 5, 4, 3, 2, and 1.

2.3.2 RAPD definition

The data analysed in this study are bacterial counts enumerated on Petri dishes, characterized by a rather high variability, which impacted on hypothesis C, and which did not permit the straightforward use of a reliable ANOVA model. Consequently, bacterial counts were transformed into ratios, which were replaced then by ranks according to the prerequisite of the Kruskal-Wallis test, before performing the classical ANOVA. What is meant by ratio? Due to the natural microbiological variability, we considered the CFU (colony forming units) on a Petri dish (in the presence of one AB) not as an absolute value but as a relative value compared to a control plate, which implicated the introduction of a ratio. The ratio here referred to as RAPD was defined for a particular treatment X. RAPD corresponds to the ratio of the amount of bacterial colonies (as CFU/ml) enumerated under this treatment X divided by the number of bacteria enumerated on the corresponding control plates (in the absence of the AB). The treatment X was characterized itself by a combination of factors, like the sample type (milk from CP or OP systems), the population type whether psychrotrophs (P) or mesophiles (M), a sampling day D (D= 0 or 4, that will lead to RAP0 and RAP4 respectively), an AB type, and an AB concentration.

Thus RAPD constitues another way to quantify AR prevalence, while the classical quantification of AR prevalence is generally defined as the percentage of resistant bacteria considering the corresponding "total" bacteria enumerated.

2.3.3 Experimental design

The experimental design was based on the following four fixed factors: the antibiotic (AB) type (whether G, C, L or TS, as detailed above), the concentration of the AB (Dose) which corresponded to a higher level (I) or a lower level (II), the storage time of the milk (day) whether 0 (initial counts) or 4 (after 4 days cold storage), and finally the milk sample noted (ECH) which accounted for the six distinct lorry tanks samples (whether from CP or OP systems). The factor ECH was also introduced as a fixed factor in order to identify an eventual "milk collecting effect". Each treatment corresponded to a defined condition resultant from one modality of every factor (AB, Dose, ECH).

2.3.4 Refinement of ANOVA

Once the ANOVA model has been established, significant factors are identified. If one significant factor presents only 2 modalities, the interpretation is clear: a change of the modality impacts significantly on the level of the response. But if the significant factor presents more than two modalities, the interpretation is not straightforward. Further analyses of the microbiological data are requested, which are not often performed according to the microbiological literature. After the ANOVA table is established, for factors with more than two modalities, pairwise or multiple comparisons of the means of the response associated to the modalities of the factors are requested. On a statistical point of view, as this latter is the most rigorous approach, it was employed in this study. Among the available methods for multiple comparisons of means was chosen the REGW test (Einot & Gabriel, 1975; Ryan, 1959, 1960; Welsch, 1977) that is powerful and particularly adapted for our type of data. The method is available on the SAT/STAT version 8.1 software (SAS Institute, NC, USA).

2.3.5 Use of a non parametric statistical test

One major aim of this study was to compare the trend of RAPD between the two sampling days (Day 0 and Day 4), for a certain treatment. Considering the non normal distribution of the 12 values of RAP0 and RAP4, the mean comparison with a Student test was not possible. Therefore, the analyses were pursued with the use of the non parametric Wilcoxon test (as detailed in page 215 by Conover 1980), implemented in the NPAR1WAY procedure of the SAS/STAT statistical software. This test is also based on ranks: eight treatments (AB=G at dose I, AB=G at dose II.....AB=TS at dose II) were examined for each bacterial type; for both conventional and organic milk types, altogether 32 conditions were considered.

2.4 DGGE (Denaturing Gradient Gel Electrophoresis) analyses

Bacterial DNA was extracted with PathoProof™ mastitis PCR assay kit (Finnzymes, Finland). 16S rDNA sequences were amplified by nested-PCR. Firstly, a 700-bp fragment that comprises the V3 region of bacterial 16S rDNA was amplified, and served as template for the 2nd PCR reaction which yielded PCR products of about 200 bp, as described by Ogier et al. (2002). These primers flank the V3 region (that corresponds for *E.coli* to positions 436-499) which shows variability between different species. DGGE analyses were performed with the BioRad DCode ™ Universal Mutation Detection System (BioRad, USA). The samples were electrophoresed with a denaturing gradient of 35-70% urea and formamide at 70V for 21h. Gels were stained with SYBR Gold (Invitrogen, USA) and photographed on a UV transillumination table (UVItec Ltd, UK). The images were analysed with Gel Compar®II (version 5.1, Applied Maths, Belgium). The similarity between samples was calculated with Pearson´s correlation coefficient and UPGMA (Unweighted pair-group method using arithmetic averages) was used as a clustering method. The maximum parsimony cluster analyses were performed with the boostrap value of 1000. The data is presented as a dendrogram of DGGE profiles from conventional (C1 to C6) and organic (O1 to O6) raw milk samples at days 0 and 4.

3. Results

3.1 Bacterial counts and percentage of psychrotrophs

Initial "total" bacterial counts, determined for the raw milk samples (C1 to C6, O1, O2, O3 and O6), were comprised between 3.4 and 4.12 log-units, indicating that the raw milks were of excellent quality (Fig. 1).

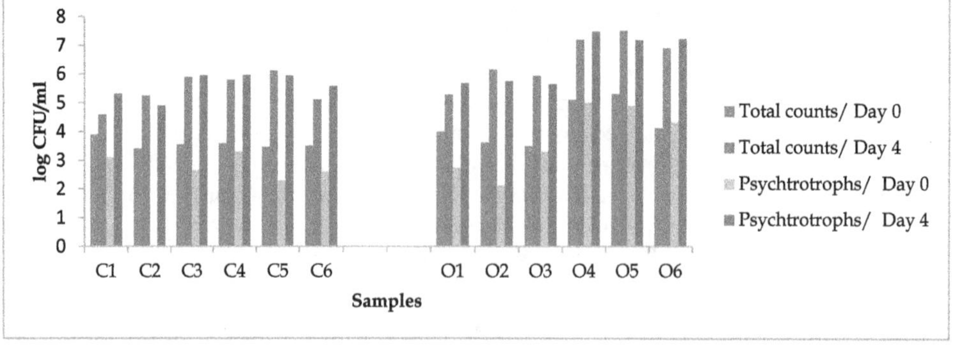

Fig. 1. Bacterial counts on Mueller Hinton agar plates expressed in log CFU/ml, determined for conventional (C1 to C6) and organic (O1 and O6) raw milk samples.

For samples O4 and O5, the mesophilic bacterial counts were 5.1 and 5.3 log-units respectively, suggesting that these milks were longer cold stored prior to the analyses of these samples. At day 4, total counts exceeded 10^5 CFU/ml for all considered samples, to the exception of C1 for which the growth was only of 0.7 log-unit. With exceptions of C4, O3, O4, O5 and O6, psychrotrophic were lower than mesophilic counts for all other samples. The proportion of psychrotrophs (ratio of psychrotrophs/total bacterial counts) increased notably between the two sampling days /day 0 and day 4) for most samples: whereas, the initial proportion of psychrotrophs in samples C1, C2, C3, C5, C6, O1 and O2 was below 20%, considerable higher proportions were determined from C4 (50%), O3 (60%), O4 (80%), O5 (40%) and O6 (100%) at day 0. After 4 days storage at 4°C, psychrotrophic bacteria largely dominated in samples C1, C3, C4, C6, O1, 04, and 06 (100%), whereas the proportions ranged between 40 and 70% for C2, C5, O2, O3 and O5.

3.2 AR load evaluated by RAPD mean values

When combining all results from the different investigated ABs, following observations were made considering RAPD: for CP milk samples, the RAP0 mean values were similar for mesophilic (M) and psychrotrophic (P) populations, whereas for OP samples the RAP0 was slightly lower for mesophiles, contrarily to psychrotrophs for which it was highest (0.245) (Fig.2).

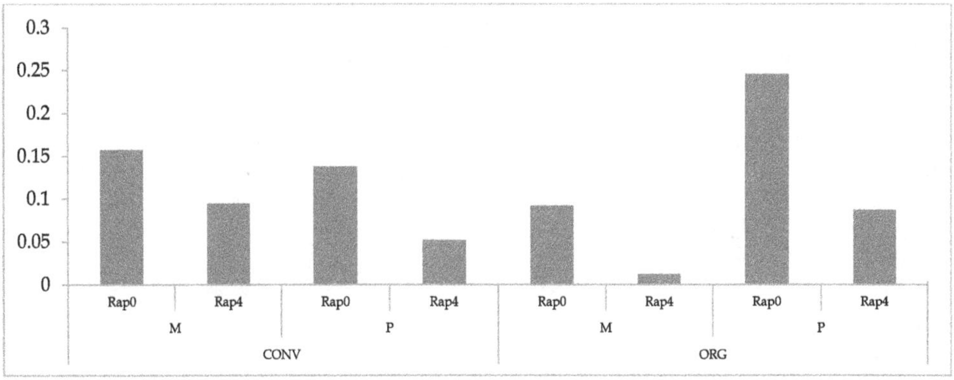

Fig. 2. Mean RAPD values from CP and OP raw milk samples at sampling days 0 or 4, determined for mesophiles (M) and psychrotrophs (P).

All RAP4 mean values were lower than the corresponding RAP0 values, irrespective of the origin of the samples or the bacterial population types. The major drop was observed for psychrotrophic populations retrieved from OP milk samples. For the mesophiles, the AR evaluated through RAPD clearly indicated a decrease for both types of samples, even though more important for bacteria retrieved from OP samples.

3.3 Comparison of RAPD mean values to evaluate the impact of cold storage

The trend of RAPDs were obtained by the results of the NPAR1WAY/REGW procedure (introduced in section 2.3.5). A typical example of the SAS-output where RAP4 was compared to RAP0 is detailed in Table 1.

Wilcoxon Scores (Rank Sums) for Variable rep
Classified by Variable day

Day	N	Sum of Scores	Expected Under H0	Std Dev Under H0	Mean Score
0	12	127.0	150.0	15.060747	10.583333
4	12	173.0	150.0	15.060747	14.416667

Average scores were used for ties.

Wilcoxon Two-Sample Test

Statistic	127.0000
Normal Approximation	
Z	-1.4939
One-Sided Pr < Z	**0.0676**
Two-Sided Pr > |Z|	0.1352
t Approximation	
One-Sided Pr < Z	**0.0744**
Two-Sided Pr > |Z|	0.1488

Z includes a continuity correction of 0.5.

Table 1. Output obtained with the Wilcoxon test applied to mesophiles present in CP raw milk samples, for one AB (G) at concentration I. In this example, RAP0 = 10.58 and RAP4= 14.42, however the t approximation value of 0.1488 indicated that RAP0 and RAP4 were statistically equivalent.

The conclusions from each comparison are summarised in Table 2 a,b. The mean RAP4 values only exceeded the mean RAP0 values for TS (red colour), at both concentrations, for psychrotrophic (P) populations retrieved from CP samples (Table 2a); with the exception of mesophiles (M) enumerated on C-containing plates, for which the RAP4 were lower than the RAP0 values (green colour), in all other conditions (yellow colour), the relative AR levels were equivalent. On the side of the populations retrieved from OP raw milk samples, for half of the conditions, RAP4 values were lower (green colour) or equal (yellow colour) to RAP0; but RAP4 widely exceeded RAP0 for 8 conditions (red colour), mostly for psychrotrophs (Table 2b).

3.4 Mean RAP4 from OP compared to mean RAP4 from CP raw milk samples

The comparison of the mean RAP4 values indicated that for 10 cases out of 16, the AR levels were similar after 4 days storage (yellow colour), irrespective of the milk type; mesophilic populations retrieved on C-containing plates, as well as mesophiles and psychrotrophs enumerated on G-plates (lower concentration, II) from OP samples carried less AR features (green colour)(Table 3); but, psychrotrophs from OP samples, enumerated on L (II) and TS-plates (I), exhibited much superior levels of AR as compared to CP raw milk samples (red colour).

3.5 Ranking of the four considered ABs

For both CP or OP samples, the ranking of the ABs was obtained with REGW based analyses that followed ANOVA. An example is given in Table 4 (a,b).

a)

G	I	M	=
		P	=
	II	M	=
		P	=
C	I	M	<
		P	=
	II	M	<<
		P	=
L	I	M	=
		P	=
	II	M	=
		P	=
TS	I	M	=
		P	>
	II	M	=
		P	>

b)

G	I	M	>
		P	>>
	II	M	=
		P	=
C	I	M	<<
		P	=
	II	M	<<
		P	=
L	I	M	>>
		P	>
	II	M	=
		P	>>
TS	I	M	>>
		P	>>
	II	M	=
		P	>>

Table 2. Mean RAP4 values compared to the mean RAP0 values from CP (a) and OP (b) raw milk samples, for the four ABs tested at concentrations I and II (I>II) for mesophiles (M) or psychrotrophs (P). The symbols =, <, and > are meaning RAP4 equalled, or was significantly below or superior to RAP0, respectively.

G	I	M	=
		P	=
	II	M	<<
		P	<<
C	I	M	<<
		P	=
	II	M	<<
		P	=
L	I	M	=
		P	=
	II	M	=
		P	>>
TS	I	M	=
		P	>>
	II	M	=
		P	=

Table 3. Mean RAP4 values from OP compared to mean RAP4 values from CP raw milk samples, determined for each AB at concentrations I and II (I>II), for mesophiles (M) or psychrotrophs (P). The symbols =, <<, and >> are meaning that RAP4 from OP samples were significantly and respectively equal, much inferior or superior to RAP4 determined for the CP raw milk samples.

Source	DF	Sum of Squares	Mean Square	F Value	Pr > F
Model	32	61772.45833	1930.38932	**10.78**	**<.0001**
Error	63	11279.54167	179.04034		
Corrected Total	95	73052.00000			

R-Square	Coeff Var	Root MSE	RAP4 Mean
0.845596	27.58886	13.38060	48.50000

Source	DF	Type I SS	Mean Square	F Value	Pr > F
AB	3	30643.27083	10214.42361	57.05	<.0001
dose	1	7315.04167	7315.04167	40.86	<.0001
ech	5	8529.00000	1705.80000	9.53	<.0001
AB*dose	3	3033.89583	1011.29861	5.65	0.0017
AB*ech	15	9065.47917	604.36528	3.38	0.0004
dose*ech	5	3185.77083	637.15417	3.56	0.0067

a)

Alpha	0.05		
Error Degrees of Freedom	63		
Error Mean Square	179.0403		
Number of Means	2	3	4
Critical Range	8.8494249	9.2716373	10.19334

Means with the same letter are not significantly different.

	Mean	N	AB
A	**65.125**	**24**	**4**
A	**62.354**	**24**	**2**
B	**46.375**	**24**	**1**
C	**20.146**	**24**	**3**

b)

a) Dependent Variable: RAP4 ; Values of RAP4 were replaced by ranks
b) Ryan-Einot-Gabriel-Welsch Multiple Range Test for RAP4
NOTE: This test controls the Type I experiment wise error rate.

Table 4. a) Analysis of variance of RAP4 ranks from mesophiles present in CP samples. The R-square value was equal to 0.85 and the F p-value was < 0.0001, which was indicative of a good ANOVA model. All three effects (AB, dose, sample /ech) and their interactions were influential with a predominant and significant effect of the AB. b) Output from the REGW test. For the same samples, AB4 (TS) and AB2(C) had equivalent effects, higher to AB1(G) and to AB3 (L); AB1 and AB3 were not equivalent.

No important differences distinguished CP and OP raw milk samples when considering the ranking of the four ABs according to their respective prevalence for mesophiles (M) or psychrotrophs (P) (Fig. 3a, b).

The same ranking, with a preponderant C-resistance was characteristic of day 0 and was observed for all populations types retrieved whether from CP or OP raw milk samples; a slightly higher AR for TS was observed for mesophiles from CP samples, whereas for G and L a similar ranking was noticeable for both sample types. Higher AR was recorded for psychrotrophs from OP samples compared to CP samples for C, TS and L, with the exception of G for which similar levels were observed (Fig. 3a, b). At day 4, the same

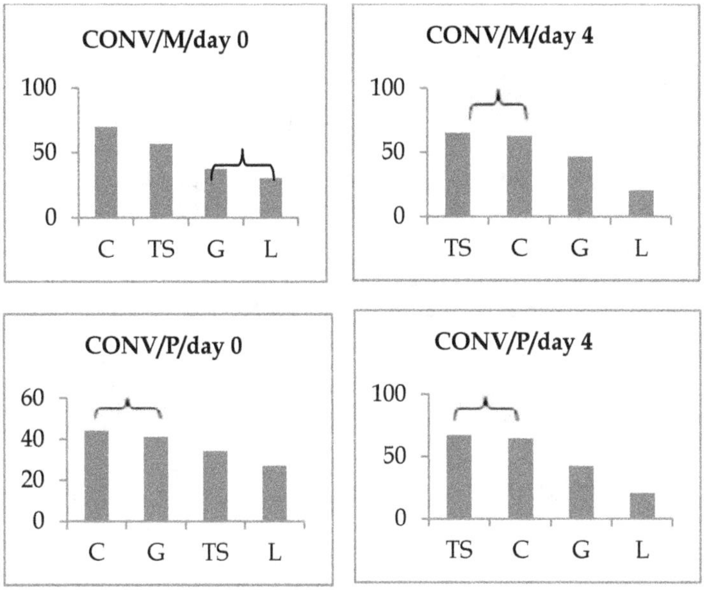

a)

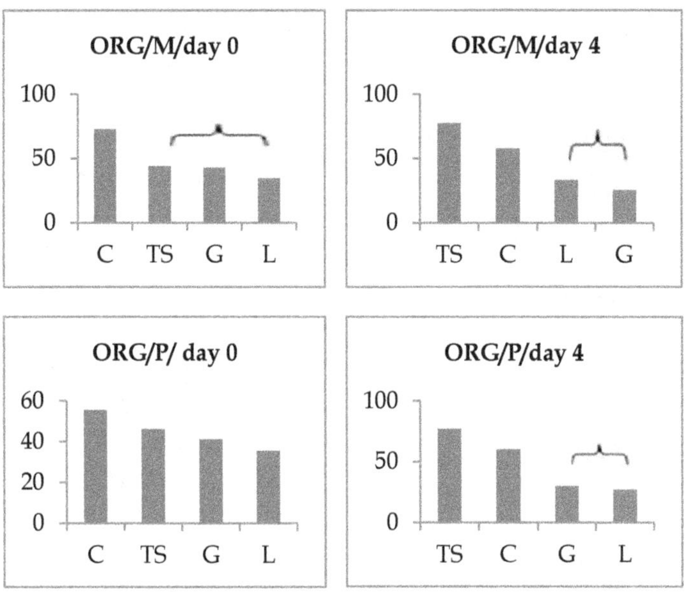

b)

Fig. 3. AR prevalence, estimated by multiple comparison of means from CP (a) and OP (b) raw milk samples over time, determined from combined results with both concentrations (I and II) of each AB. The mean values were obtained with the REGW multiple range test for RAP0 and RAP4. [Noteworthy, ABs that were similarly ranked are grouped in a bracket].

ranking of the ABs was observed for TS and C; the levels were equivalent for psychrotrophs and mesophiles from CP samples (Fig. 3a) whereas TS supplanted C for both mesophiles and psychrotrophs from OP samples (Fig. 3b). For G, similar levels of AR were recorded from CP samples for both psychrotrophs and mesophiles at days 0 and 4, in contrast to OP samples in which the AR dropped over time by about half for both types of bacterial populations (Fig. 3a,b). L-resistance was least prevalent at day 0, mostly also at day 4; a decrease of AR was recorded over time for mesophiles from CP samples and psychrotrophs from CP and OP raw milk samples.

3.6. Ranking of the milk samples according to their total AR load

At day 0, the AR levels (as means determined with the Ryan-Einot-Gabriel-Welsch multiple range test) were comprised between 38-60 and 28-50 for mesophiles and psychrotrophs from CP samples, respectively (Fig. 4a).

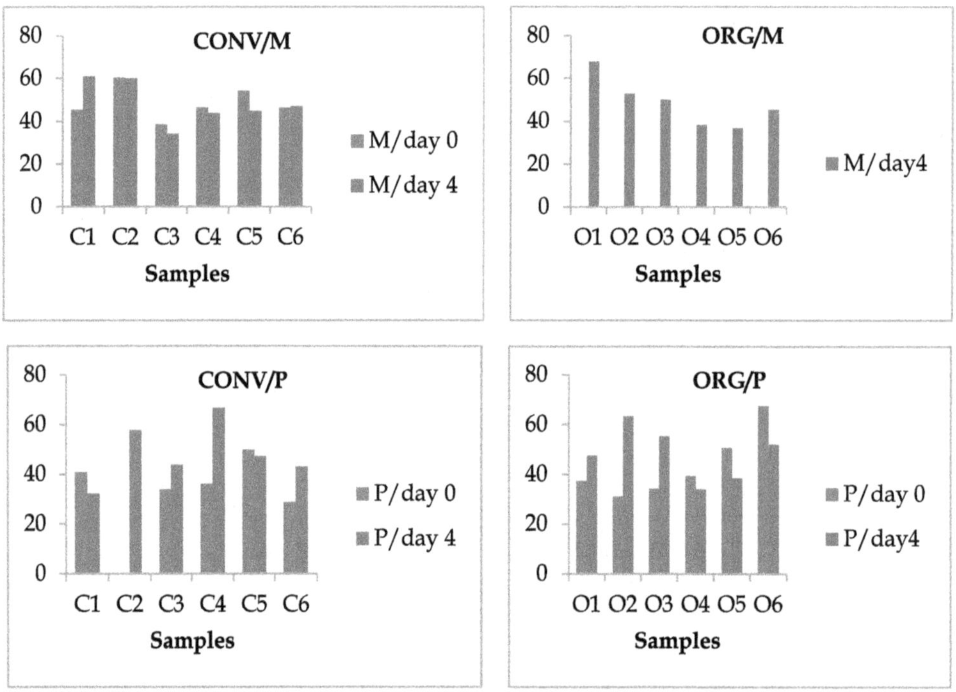

(a) (b)

Fig. 4. AR load from multiple comparison of sample means for CP (a) and OP (b) raw milk samples at days 0 and 4 determined for mesophiles (M) and psychrotrophs (P).

At day 4, the mean values ranged between 32-60 and 32-67 for the mesophiles and psychrotrophs respectively (Fig. 4a). Mesophiles from samples C3, C4, C5 showed moderate decrease of the AR between days 0 and 4, contrarily to the psychrotrophic populations recovered from the same samples, which increased by 10 and 30 for samples C3, C4 respectively, or slightly decreased for C5 (Fig. 4a). Mesophiles from sample C2 were the highest AR carriers at days 0 and 4 whereas sample C3 was the lowest at both sampling days; sample C1 was the second lowest at day 0, and second highest at day 4. No model enabled to rank the six OP samples at day 0; however at day 4, the comparison between mesophiles and psychrotrophs showed that samples may be similarly ranked over time (like O3, O5) or not (sample O1), (Fig. 4b).

3.7 DGGE profile analyses of CP and OP raw milk samples at sampling days 0 and 4.

At day 0, the primer set yielded relatively complex fingerprints for C1, C2, C3, C4, C5, C6, O1, O2, and O3 as the PCR amplicons migrated along the whole length of the denaturing gradient gel (Fig. 5), indicative of a high variability in GC%, hence a high species diversity, irrespective of the milk type.

Based on Gel Compar ™ analyses, some samples displayed profiles with as many as 27 or 26 bands for C6 and O1 respectively, whereas C4, O4, O5 displayed simpler profiles comprising only 10-11 bands. Profiles from CP samples (C1, C5, C6) that yielded the highest amount of bands clustered as well as O1, O2 and O3 from OP raw milk samples (Fig. 5), and showed similar community structure. The 4 days-cold storage implicated for most samples a simpler profile, as less bands were detected; with exception of C1, all CP raw milk samples clustered while the profiles of C5 and C6 still formed a sub-cluster. Cold storage affected O1, O2 and O3 differently: the samples O1 and O2 remained clustered despite a drop of the similarity values (77.2% to 52.3 %) between both sampling days (Fig. 5).

Samples O4, O5 and O6 were least affected by cold storage, as all three samples formed almost exact pairs at days 0 and 4 with similarity values of 75%, 88.5%, and 87.5% for O6, O5 and O4 respectively, indicative of small changes in the bacterial community between the sampling days. For most of the samples, following the cold storage (4°C for 4 days), the banding patterns were more located on the top of the gel, indicative of less bacterial diversity among communities, and domination of species with higher AT%. To some extent, CP and OP samples were distinguished by DGGE analyses.

4. Discussion

The statistical analyses of RAPD means and RAPD trends during cold storage revealed 1) a higher AR level for psychrotrophic populations present in OP compared to CP milk samples at day 0 (Fig. 2); 2) a similar drop of C-resistant mesophilic, and raise of TS-resistant psychrotrophic bacteria over time for both types of samples (Table 2a,b); 3) an increase of L-resistant (at both concentrations) and partial increase (at one concentration) of G-resistant psychrotrophs for OP samples (Table 2a,b); 4) RAP4 from OP was lower to RAP4 from CP in 4 cases of 16, was similar to RAP4 from CP in 10 other tested conditions, but exceeded RAP4 from CP in 2 cases (Table 3). All preceding observations indicate that the AR load on bacterial populations from OP samples may be as high if not higher than for CP samples. When considering the farming type practices, small or no differences in AR levels were reported by Sato et al. (2004) for *Campylobacter* spp. isolates from organic and conventional dairy herds, by Roesch et al. (2006) when the AR of udder pathogens was investigated in dairy cows, by Ray et al. (2006) for *Salmonella,* or by Garmo et al. (2010) for coagulase-negative staphylococci: the frequency of AR in organic farms was not so different from

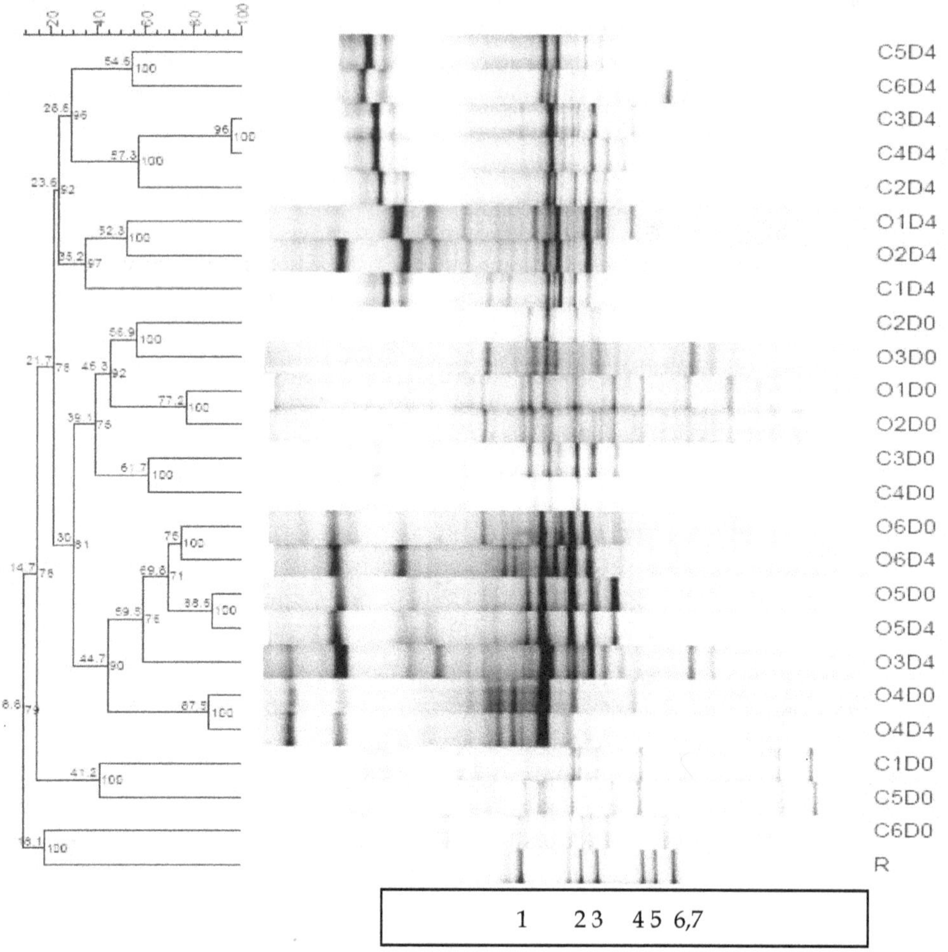

Fig. 5. Dendrogram of DGGE profiles from CP (C1 to C6) and OP (O1 to O6) raw milk samples determined at day 0 (D0) and after 4 days storage at 4°C (D4). The reference standards include the following species: 1, *Listeria innocua* CCUG 15531^{T} (ATCC 33090) ; 2, *Acinetobacter johnsonii* HAMBI 1969 (ATCC 17909) ; 3, *Pseudomonas tolaasii* LMG 2342^{T} (ATCC 33618); 4, *Bacillus cereus* HAMBI 250 (ATCC 10987) ; 5, *Escherichia coli* HAMBI 99 (ATCC 11775) ; 6, *Stenotrophomonas maltophilia* HAMBI 2659 (ATCC 13637) ; 7, *Burkholderia cepacia* HAMBI 1976 (ATCC 25416). [ATTC, American Type Culture Collection; CCUG, Culture Collection University of Göteborg; HAMBI, Culture Collection of the University of Helsinki; LMG, Belgian Collection of Microorganisms].

conventional farms. Also Ruimy et al. (2010) recorded similar levels of resistant Gram-negative bacteria for both organic and conventional produced fruits and vegetables. However, other studies report still higher susceptibilies to antibiotics for samples originating from organic production systems.

Compared to RAP0 values obtained for 18 CP samples (analysed in a previous study), which ranged between 0.0788 and 0.1576, it appeared that the mesophylic populations from organic raw milk samples analysed here had a rather low AR load (0.092), contrarily to the psychrotrophs for which the mean RAP0 value 0.2456 was the highest so far observed for all milk samples investigated and for which the mean values ranged between (0.1378-0.158). The RAP4 value from OP samples (0.0869) was still the highest encountered for psychrotrophs among all so far investigated raw milk samples for which the RAP4 values were comprised between 0.030 and 0.051 (Fig. 2, and Munsch-Alatossava et al. 2012).

In this study, irrespective of the milk type or the investigated bacterial population types (psychrotrophs or mesophiles), C-resistance was most prevalent at day 0 (rather fresh milk) whereas TS-resistance was equivalent to C-resistance (for CP samples) or higher (for OP samples) at day 4 (after the milk underwent a longer cold storage) (Fig. 3a, b). Similar observations were made in the previous study that considered 18 raw milk samples from conventional production systems (Munsch-Alatossava et al. 2012) for which TS-resistance supplanted C-resistance in prevalence following the cold storage. To some extent, AR prevalence at day 0 does mirror AB usage: Kools et al. (2008) in an overview of published data around ABs usage in Europe, indicated the following relative proportions of total AB use for Finland: β-lactams and cephalosporins (62%), Sulfonamides and trimethoprim (16%), Aminoglycosides (2%) and fluoroquinolones/quinolones (0.6%).

By summing up the values obtained from the ranking of the four ABs according to their prevalence at each sampling day and for each population type (Fig. 3a,b), the total of the means (from the REGW test) from each AB reached 194 for mesophiles from both CP and OP raw milk samples at days 0 and 4. Also, psychrotrophs from OP samples exhibited the same level of total AR at day 4 (194), against 178 at day 0. For psychrotrophs from CP samples, the total of the means from each AB was 146 and 184 at days 0 and 4, respectively. From the analysed samples, it appeared that the multiresistant trait was as common among mesophilic bacteria whether they originated from CP or OP samples. Compared to mesophiles, multiresistance seemed to be less common among psychrotrophs at day 0; however, the cold storage permitted a significant raise of the number of multiresistant isolates (more important for CP samples), but the total AR reached a superior value for psychrotrophs from OP samples at day 4. The AB ranking revealed a notable different impact of the cold storage on the AR trend considering the investigated bacterial population types (Fig. 3a, b):

- since the total AR loads were around 194 for both milk types over time, changes at the level of mesophiles appeared to be mainly qualitative (for example, replacement of bacterial species rather resistant to C by species rather resistant to TS)
- changes at the level of psychrotrophs were both qualitative (TS resistance was more frequent than C resistance at day 4 for OP samples), but also quantitative as suggested from the increase of the AR load by respectively 38 and 16 units for psychrotrophs from CP and OP systems during cold storage; the increase may be lower in the later case due to the particular features of samples O4, O5 and O6.

Interestingly, the statistical analyses of RAPD, which enabled a sample ranking according to the "AR loads" revealed that samples may be or not similarly ranked over time following the cold storage, depending on the considered populations (whether mesophiles or psychrotrophs)(Fig. 4a,b). Noteworthy, samples O5 and O6 were ranked as highest AR carriers on the side of the psychrotrophs at day 0 whereas, at day 4, a partition into two classes considered O3, O1 and O2 as high AR carriers, and O6, O5 and O4 as lower ones. Clearly, the cold storage affected differently OP samples while for samples O1, O2 and O3 the AR, estimated as relative amounts, increased, the AR decreased for O4, O5 and O6.

The high RAP0 and RAP4 values of the six considered OP samples (Fig. 2) bring up the question on whether the AR load is the consequence of different milk production practices or may be sample dependant. Part of the answer is given by the RAP0 and RAP4 values, together with their respective variation ranges: the RAP0 and RAP4 variation ranges were comprised between 0-12 (mean 0.2456) and 0-0.996 (mean 0.0869) respectively, for psychrotrophs enumerated from OP samples. In a previous study where the AR was followed over time (at days 0, 2 and 4 of cold storage) from CP raw milk samples it was noticed that RAP2 (determined after 2 days cold storage) and the corresponding variation range largely supplanted RAP0 and RAP4 values and their corresponding variation ranges (Munsch-Alatossava et al. 2012). Moreover ANOVA performed on RAP0 and RAP4 ranks revealed significant main effect (F values from the Fischer-Snedecor test, $p<0.0001$ were highest) of the "AB type" for all analysed conditions (day0/day4; mesophiles/psychrotrophs; conventional/organic production systems) to the exception of psychrotrophs from organic milk samples for which the "sample" was the most important factor.

Consequently, we hypothesize that since total counts for O4 and O5 were highest at day 0 (around and slightly above 10^5 CFU/ml, Fig. 1), lower for O6 which however exhibited the highest percentage of psychrotrophs at day 0 (100%), the excessively high value of Rap0 may be due to the samples O4, O5 and O6, which were most probably longer cold stored prior to the initial analyses as compared to O1, O2 and O3. This point is reinforced by the DGGE based analyses of OP samples, as for the samples O4, O5 and O6 the profiles at day 4 were quite similar as the ones of day 0, indicative of little changes in the bacterial community over time (Fig. 5). Like for other studies, DGGE based data confirmed the potential of this approach to investigate changes in raw milk at population levels. Clearly, the cold storage (4 days at 4°C) promoted a reduction of dominant bacterial species: similar observations were made with DGGE based analyses for raw milk stored at 4°C for 24h by Lafarge et al. (2004), but also for meat (Li et al., 2006).

To some extent, results from DGGE analyses were coherent with plating results: the samples C1, C5, C6, O1 and O2 showed the highest bacterial diversity at day 0 as visible from the most complex banding patterns (Fig. 5). The same samples presented the lowest percentages of psychrotrophs in the initial microflora at day 0 (data not shown), suggesting that these samples were more fresh, and had the lowest storage history. Conversely C4 and O4, for which high percentages of psychrotrophs were recorded at day 0, yielded electrophoretic patterns with fewest bands amounts (Fig. 5).

What could explain such high if not higher AR levels in bacteria from organic compared to conventional production systems? Even though any use of antimicrobials may create the potential for AR development, at day 0, the usage patterns of ABs could somehow constitute one part of the explanation (Kools et al., 2008; Thomson et al., 2008). Manure contains substantial amounts of both antimicrobials and antimicrobial-resistant microorganisms; agricultural practices that prevail in organic production systems where chemical fertilizers are prohibited, and are replaced by antibiotic-polluted manure applications, and where at least 50% of the feed is produced on the farm may also partially explain rather high AR levels in OP compared to CP samples. As milk is the target of numerous sources of contaminations (soil, environment…), it may be not that surprising if AR levels are at least as high for OP as for CP samples .

In 2008, the European Commission launched the European Union ´s new organic farming campaign under the slogan "Organic farming, Good for nature, Good for you". At the same time, the European Food Safety Authority (2008) attempted to evaluate to which extent food serves as a source for the acquisition by human of antimicrobial-resistant bacteria and whether foodborne antimicrobial resistance constitutes a biological hazard.

The statistics applied for data treatment on ranks of RAPD which compared the AR load in milk over time as quantified through RAPD (indicative of relative amounts) suggested that the AR level, the AR trend over time may be less "milk production type" than "sample" dependant; the main determinant may be the initial microflora. Whether cold storage of raw milk promotes the raise of AR, of multiresistant traits among bacteria and whether it affects differently conventionally or organic produced milk needs still to be further investigated. The image of safer and healthier food is most often associated to organic food by consumers. Whether initial good intentions based on a more rare use of ABs (typical for organic production systems), contrarily to conventional systems with more frequent use of ABs, are diverted by microbial activity needs further clarifications.

5. Conclusion

In this study, AR was highest at day 0 for psychrotrophs present in OP samples. Even though the cold storage globally promoted a drop of RAP values (as relative amount of AR) over time, in detail the trends were more contrasted as the AR load increased for psychrotrophs from OP samples for both L and TS at both tested concentrations, during the 4 days storage at 4°C. The AR only dropped for mesophiles, from both sample types, for C at both concentrations. For OP samples, if C-resistance was most frequent at day 0 (which corresponds to rather fresh milk), TS-resistance was more common at day 4 (when the milk already underwent a certain cold storage). Based on DGGE pattern analyses, the bacterial communities fingerprints appeared to be at both sampling days ¨milk age¨ and ¨milk type¨ dependant as the clustering distinguished CP and OP raw milk samples, with different freshness e.g. more or less cold stored. Moreover the changes in bacterial populations structure, following cold storage, indicated a shift in banding patterns towards AT-rich regions, suggesting that the cold storage of raw milk promotes the dominance of AT-rich species over time, irrespective of the milk type.

6. Acknowledgments

We thank J. Rekonen for providing the raw milk samples from conventional dairy farming systems and Juva Organic Ltd for the organic raw milk samples. We are very grateful to Applied Maths (Belgium) for the 2 weeks free access to GelCompar®II.

7. References

Aminov, R.I. (2009). The role of antibiotics and antibiotic resistance in nature. *Environmental Microbiology*, Vol.11, pp. 2970-88.

Chambers, J.V. (2002). The microbiology of raw milk, In: *Dairy Microbiology Handbook, 3rd edition*. Edited by R. K. Robinson, New York: Wiley-Interscience, pp. 39-89.

Conover, W.J. (1980). *Practical Non Parametrics Statistics*, 2nd edition, John Wiley & Sons; New York.

Cousin, M.A. (1982). Presence and activity of psychrotrophic microorganisms in milk and dairy products: a review. *Journal of Food Protection,* Vol. 45, pp. 172-207.

Davies, J.& Davies, D. (2010). Origins and evolution of antibiotic resistance. *Microbiology and Molecular Biology Reviews*, Vol. 74, pp. 417-433.

Einot, I. & Gabriel, K.R. (1975). A study of the power of several methods of multiple comparisons. *Journal of the American Statistical Association*, Vol. 70 (351), pp. 574-583.

European Commission (2008). Organic Farming-What makes milk organic? www.organic-.farming.europa.eu.

European Committee for antimicrobial susceptibility testing (EUCAST), (2000). Determination of minimum inhibitory concentrations (MICs) of antibacterial agents by agar dilution. *CMI* Vol.6, pp.509-515.

European Council Regulation (EC) No834/2007 of June 2007 on organic production and labelling of organic products and repealing regulation (EEC) No2092/91.

European Food Safety Authority (2008). Foodborne antimicrobial resistance as a biological hazard (Question No EFSA-Q-2007-089) by the Biohaz panel (Andreoletti et al.)

Finnish association for milk hygiene. (2008) http://www.maitohygienialiitto.fi

Finnish Food safety authority (2008) http://www.evira.fi

Freitas, R.; Nero, L.A. & Carvalho, A.F. (2009). Technical note: Enumeration of mesophilic aerobes in milk: Evaluation of standard official protocols and Petrifilm aerobic count plates. *Journal of Dairy Science*, Vol. 92, pp. 3069-3073.

Garmo, R.T.; Waage, S.; Sviland, S.; Henriksen, B.F.; Østerås, O. & Reksen, O. (2010). Reproductive performance, udder health, and antibiotic health, and antibiotic resistance in mastitis bacteria isolated from Norwegian red cows in conventional and organic farming. *Acta Veterinaria Scandinavica,* Vol. 52, pp. 1-13.

Gray, M.J.; Freitag, N.E. & Boor, K.J. (2006). How the bacterial pathogen *Listeria monocytogenes* mediates the switch from environmental Dr. Jekyll to pathogenic Mr. Hyde. *Infect ion and Immunity,* Vol. 74, pp. 2505-2512.

Grave, K.; Torren-Edo, J. & Mackay, D. (2010). Comparison of the sales of veterinary antibacterial agents between 10 European countries. *Journal of Antimicrobial Chemotherapy*, Vol. 65, pp. 2037-2040.

Information Centre of the Ministry of Agriculture and Forestry (2009). Matilda tietopalvelu. Maito and kananmunat. http://www.matilda.fi.

Jacob, M.E.; Fox, J.T.; Reinstein, S.L. & Nagaraja, T.G. (2008). Antimicrobial susceptibility of foodborne pathogens in organic and natural production systems: an overview. *Foodborne Pathogens and Disease,* Vol. 5, pp. 721-730.

Knezevic, P. & Petrovic, O. (2008). Antibiotic resistance of commensal *Escherichia coli* of food-producing animals from three Vojvodinian farms, Serbia. *International Journal of Antimicrobial Agents,* Vol. 31, pp. 360-363.

Kools, S.A.E., Moltmann, J.F. & Knacker, T. (2008). Estimating the use of veterinary medicines in the European union. *Regulatory Toxicology and Pharmacology*, Vol. 50, pp. 59-65.

Lafarge, V. ; Ogier, J.-C.; Girard, V.; Maladen, V.; Leveau, J.-Y.; Gruss, A. & Delacroix-Buchet, A. (2004). Raw cow milk bacterial population shifts attributable to refrigeration. *Applied and Environmental Microbiology,* Vol. 70, pp. 5644- 5650.

Levy, S.B. (2002). Factors impacting on the problem of antibiotic resistance. *Journal of Antimicrobial Chemotherapy*, Vol. 49, pp. 25-30.

Li, M.Y; Zhou, G.H.; Xu, X.L. ; Li, C.B. & Zhu,W.Y.(2006). Changes of bacterial diversity and main flora in chilled pork during storage using PCR-DGGE. *Food Microbiology*, Vol.23, pp. 607-611.

Ma, Y.; Barbano, D.M. & Santos, M. (2003). Effect of CO_2 addition to raw milk on proteolysis and lipolysis at 4 °C. *Journal of Dairy Science,* Vol. 86, pp. 1616-1631.

Marshall, B.M.; Ochiend, D.J. & Levy, S.B. (2009). Commensals: Underappreciated reservoir of antibiotic resistance. *Microbe,* Vol. 4, pp. 231-238.

Munsch-Alatossava, P. & Alatossava, T. (2006). Phenotypic characterization of raw milk-associated psychrotrophic bacteria. *Microbiological Research*, Vol. 161, pp. 334-346.

Munsch-Alatossava, P. & Alatossava, T.(2007). Antibiotic resistance of raw-milk associated psychrotrophic bacteria. *Microbiological Research,* Vol. 162, pp. 115-123.

Munsch-Alatossava, P.; Gursoy, O. & Alatossava, T. (2010). Potential of nitrogen gas (N_2) to control psychrotrophs and mesophiles in raw milk. *Microbiological Research*, Vol. 165, pp. 122-132.

Munsch-Alatossava, P.; Gauchi, J.-P.; Chamlagain, B. & Alatossava, T. (2012). Trends of antibiotic resistance in mesophilic and psychrotrophic bacterial populations during cold storage of raw milk, ISRN Microbiology, In Press.

Ogier, J.C.; Son, O. ; Gruss, A.; Tailliez, P. & Delacroix-Buchet, A. (2002). Identification of the bacterial microflora in dairy products by temporal temperature gradient gel electrophoresis. *Applied and Environmental Microbiology*, Vol. 68, pp. 3691-3701.

Ray, K.A.; Warnick, L.D.; Mitchell, R.M.; Kaneene, J.B.; Ruegg, P.L.; Wells, S.J.; Fossier, C.P.; Halbert, L.W. & May, K. (2006). Antimicrobial susceptibility of *Salmonella* from organic and conventional dairy farms. Journal of Dairy Science, Vol. 89, pp. 2038-2050.

Roesch, M.; Perreten, V.; Doherr, M.G.; Schaeren, W.; Schällibaum, S. & Blum, J.W. (2006). Comparison of antibiotic resistance of udder pathogens in dairy cows kept on organic and on conventional farms. *Journal of Dairy Science*, Vol. 89, pp. 989-997.

Ruimy, R.; Brisabois, A.; Bernede, C.; Skurnik, D.; Barnat, S.; Arlet, G.; Momcilovic, S.; Elbaz, S.; Moury, F.; Vibet, M.-A.; Courvalin, P.; Guillemot, D. & Andremont, A. (2010). Organic and conventional fruits and vegetables contain equivalent counts of Gram-negative bacteria expressing resistance to antibacterial agents. *Environmental Microbiology*, Vol. 12, No.3, pp. 608-615.

Ryan, T.A. (1959). Multiple comparisons in psychological research. *Psychological Bulletin*, Vol. 56, pp. 26-47.

Ryan, T.A. (1960). Significant tests for multiple comparisons of proportions, variances and other statistics. *Psychological Bulletin*, Vol. 57, pp. 318-328.

Sato, K.; Bartlett, P.C.; Kaneene, J.B. & Downes, F.P. (2004). Comparison of prevalence and antimicrobial susceptibilities of *Campylobacter* spp. isolates from organic and conventional dairy herds in Wisconsin. *Applied and Environmental Microbiology*, Vol. 70, pp. 1442-1447.

Schoeni, J.L.& Lee Wong, A.C. (2005). *Bacillus cereus* food poisoning and its toxins (Review). *Journal of Food Protection*, Vol. 68, pp. 636-648.

Straley, B.A.; Donaldson, S.C.; Hedge, N.V.; Sawant, A.A.; Srinivasan, V.; Oliver, S.P. & Jayarao, B.M.(2006). Public health significance of antimicrobial- resistant gram-negative bacteria in raw bulk tank milk. *Foodborne Pathogens and Disease*, Vol. 3, pp. 222-233.

Thompson, K.; Rantala, M.; Hautala, M.; Pyörälä, S. & Kaartinen, L. (2008). Cross-sectional prospective survey to study indication-based usage of antimicrobials in animals: Results of use in cattle. *BMC Veterinary Research*, Vol. 4, pp. 15-21.

Welsch, R.E. (1977). Stepwise multiple comparison procedures. *Journal of the American Statistical Association*, Vol. 72 (359), pp. 566-575.

5

Stability of Antibiotic Resistance Patterns in Agricultural Pastures: Lessons from Kentucky, USA

Sloane Ritchey, Siva Gandhapudi and Mark Coyne
University of Kentucky, USA

1. Introduction

Animal and human wastes contain fecal bacteria, including pathogens that can contaminate groundwater, streams, lakes, and reservoirs through runoff and infiltration. Bacterial nonpoint sources of pollution continually impair water quality (Hartel et al., 2002). These pollution sources may come from failed septic systems, large animal operations, land application of wastes, sewage treatment facilities, and wildlife. Fecal pollution of rivers and streams is of great concern due to the direct potential threat to human health, and the increased costs associated with water treatment.

Groundwater contamination from these wastes can be a serious environmental concern in well-drained soils and soils with shallow water tables. Karst topography in Kentucky, for example, constitutes 55% of the land area (KGS, 2002), much of which is in pasture where land application of animal waste is commonly practiced. Of the 4,521 total km (2,810 total mi) of rivers and streams assessed in Kentucky in 2000, 73% were impaired for primary contact (>200 fecal coliforms/100 mL; USEPA, 2000). Similar reports regarding impaired watersheds can be found throughout the United States. Dombek et al. (2000) reported that 47% of assessed river miles in Minnesota were impaired for primary contact due to high levels of fecal coliform bacteria. Graves et al. (2002) reported that approximately 13% of monitored streams and 1% of estuaries in Virginia were impaired, with >60% of the impairments due to fecal contamination. The recurrence of such reports is evidence that tools are needed to identify such pollution sources and facilitate restoration efforts such as implementing total maximum daily loads (TMDLs) or best management practices (BMPs).

The reliance of pollution remediation efforts on TMDLs has been one of the driving forces behind developing techniques to distinguish between human and non-human fecal pollution sources (Johnson et al., 2004). A standard method of assessing water quality impairment based on the potential for pathogenic microbes of intestinal origin is to enumerate commensal bacteria such as coliforms. While total and fecal coliform counts produce an estimate of pollution levels, specific sources of the microbial pollution cannot be determined. Microbial source tracking (MST) techniques offer unique approaches to differentiate nonpoint source pollution. By tracking a pollution source to its origin, resources and management tools may be better allocated to improve water quality. Some issues that affect the usefulness of these MST techniques include the appropriate database portability, size, and temporal characteristics to yield adequate power of prediction given the diversity of antibiotic resistance patterns in a watershed.

The answers to these issues are as yet undetermined. Several reports agree that MST techniques are most applicable to limited geographical areas such as specific watersheds rather than larger geographic regions (Guan et al., 2002; Johnson et al., 2004; Lu et al., 2005; McClellan et al., 2003). There is also no consensus on whether using *Escherichia coli* (EC) or fecal streptococci (FS) is preferred for use as indicator bacteria. Because of the labor-intensive and time-consuming nature of database building, the characteristics of a useful database are critical in the future applicability of MST methodologies.

There is little research that has concluded with any certainty on temporal variability effects on the ability of a host source database to classify nonpoint sources of pollution. There are research papers that have reported on lack of temporal stability due to among-species variation (Caugant et al., 1981; Gordon, 2001). One assumption made for the use of microbial source tracking is temporal stability or the ability to collect samples from the same source over time with little to no change in the outcome. Gordon (2001) reported on the minimal population differentiation in *E. coli* with only 5% of observed diversity derived from among-species variation, and this was considered inadequate. However, with a representative and adequately sized database, is 5% temporal variation significant?

Gordon (2001) continued to report on the most significant problem using *E. coli* in an MST database in which substantial changes in community occur from host to external environment. Caugant et al. (1981) reported that transient and resident strains of *E. coli* are present in the same host and they pose many questions as to the ramifications this may have to the usefulness of MST techniques. Jenkins et al. (2003) reported on the clonal diversity of *E. coli* among the same Black Angus steers sampled four times through one year. They evaluated ribotypes from two herds and discovered that a high clonal diversity index necessitated a large number of isolates (>900) for a database to be independent of temporal variations; however, they were uncertain whether their 20:1 resident to transient ratio could be overcome. Although Wiggins et al. (2003) studied fecal streptococci, they established that separate geographical databases, i.e., several watersheds, could be merged together to create a large, more representative database. Further, they concluded that the profiles were temporally stable for at least one year using antibiotic resistance analysis.

Phenotypic MST techniques such as antibiotic resistance analysis (ARA) have had moderate levels of success in small and relatively simple aquatic systems to differentiate human and nonhuman sources of pollution, or two-way level of classification (Carson et al., 2001; Guan et al., 2002; Graves et al., 2002; Hagedorn et al., 1999; Hartel et al., 2002; Harwood et al., 2000; Ritchey and Coyne, unpublished data; Ritchey and Coyne, 2009; Wiggins et al., 1999). Correct classification rates of ≥50% including five or more sources are considered useful by resource managers and rates of 60-70% are very useful (Harwood et al., 2000). Guan et al. (2002) conducted a study evaluating profiles using 14 antibiotics with a database consisting of 319 EC isolates collected from nine host sources. The database correctly classified 46% of the domestic, 95% of the wildlife, and 55% of the human sources. When the researchers pooled the nonhuman sources and compared the isolates to human sources, the RCC was 86% for human and 92% for nonhuman isolates. Harwood et al. (2000) constructed a database of 6144 fecal coliforms FC and 4619 FS isolates from profiles using 9 antibiotics. For the larger database, when the isolates from the animal sources were analyzed separately, the RCC was 54% for the FC human isolates and 61% for the FS isolates. Pooling the animal sources together increased the human RCCs to 69% for the FC isolates and to 76% for the FS isolates. Reducing the number of sources and pooling the animal sources together, greatly increased RCC values (Carson et al., 2001; Guan et al., 2002; Harwood et al., 2000).

Generally, the primary concern of water resource managers and public health officials is discriminating human and nonhuman sources of contamination followed by secondary information to determine the source of the animal contamination (Harwood et al., 2000). Ritchey and Coyne (unpublished data) reported rates of correct classification of 66% for human and 67% for nonhuman sources at the two-way level of classification. However, caution must be exercised when testing the portability or spatial variability of the database by applying it on a large geographic-scale and in more complex systems. Many researchers (Guan et al., 2002; Johnson et al., 2004; Lu et al., 2005; McLellan et al., 2003) have concluded that because of the importance for an MST database to represent an area, yet exhibit limited temporal variability despite the genetic diversity of bacteria, MST techniques may be more useful when applied to limited geographical areas such as specific watersheds. Work presented by Harwood et al. (2000) with a database of 6144 isolates produced acceptable RCCs. Those RCCs were lower than the RCCs obtained by Wiggins (1996) when using limited geographic areas, but similar to Wiggins et al. (1999) when the geographical area of their study was increased.

Regardless if one is evaluating an aquatic or terrestrial system, the same unresolved issues remain that affect the ability of MST techniques to ascertain the source of contamination from fecal sources to an adequate level of predictability. These issues predominantly lie in the intrinsic resistance and stability, which can vary considerably based on antibiotic profiles chosen, source and type of fecal bacteria, portability, temporal characteristics, and soil and/or water conditions. Based on past and current research, complex environmental systems still require considerable research to adequately evaluate the application of MST.

2. Terrestrial systems and a Kentucky study

Numerous studies show that pollutant concentrations from manure-amended agriculture lands often exceed water quality standards (Howell et al., 1995; Reddy et al., 1981). Bacteria survival also influences bacterial contamination from manure-amended agriculture lands through runoff and infiltration. Some important factors influencing bacteria survival in soil are soil type, moisture, temperature, sunlight, pH, antibiotics, competitive organisms, available nutrients, organic matter, and clay content (Ellis and McCalla, 1978). Few studies have evaluated sod management practices on fecal bacteria survival, but Entry et al. (2000) showed that vegetation type in riparian filter strips had no effect on fecal coliform survival in soils.

Various studies have investigated the correlation behind surface derived fecal sources and elevated fecal levels in groundwater, via infiltration, and surface water, via overland flow or erosion. Several studies have reported that moisture levels play a primary role in determining bacterial growth and duration, while temperature was a secondary factor (Berry and Miller, 2005; Collins, 2004; Sinton et al., 2007; Stoddard et al., 1998; Unc and Goss,

2003). Soil physicochemical characteristics including soil type, structure, depth to water tables, and bedrock, i.e. karstic, should be considered when investigating non point sources of contamination. Stoddard et al. (1998) studied leachate of manure treated and untreated shallow karst tilled and no-tilled soils from central Kentucky (the Bluegrass region). Neither timing of manure application nor tillage method significantly affected leachate concentration of fecal coliforms. Movement of fresh fecal bacteria, within 60 days of application, moved below the root zone upon sufficient rainfall events.

Based on past and current research, complex environmental systems still require considerable research to adequately evaluate the application of MST techniques. Mowing is a common sod management practice that could affect fecal bacteria survival and antibiotic resistance patterns in poultry manure-amended pasture lands because it subjects fecal bacteria to environmental stress. In the Kentucky study Ritchey and Coyne (unpublished data), fecal bacteria survival was examined in frequently mowed, poultry manure-amended sod on Maury silt loam soil for 70 days. Simultaneously evaluated was the efficacy of antibiotic resistance analysis across time for this known animal waste source.

3. Study conditions

The soil consisted of Maury silt loam (fine, mixed, mesic, Typic Paleudalf) in undisturbed sod-covered plots with mixed grass vegetation dominated by fescue. There were 14 experimental units measuring 2.4 m wide by 6 m long, spaced 2.5 m apart. The treatments were undisturbed (n=3), disturbed every week (n=4), and disturbed biweekly (n=4). Disturbance was simulated by using a push mower. Each treatment had one unmanured plot as a control. All treatments received poultry manure at a rate of 20 kg per plot (14 Mg ha^{-1}) in a completely randomized design. Sampling was conducted on day 0, 7, 14, 21, 28, 49, and 70. Because source was known, monitoring the environmental conditions to determine how these sources reacted with the respective condition changes on pasture areas was possible. In this way, behavior of these fecal coliforms with measurable environmental conditions could better be predicted.

Two soil cores, 5 cm deep, were extracted from random locations in each plot, before mowing, at each interval during the experiment. The soil cores were bagged separately and stored at 4 ^{0}C until analysis within 24 h of collection. Each core was separated into vegetative cover and soil for analysis. Fecal coliforms and fecal streptococci from vegetation and soil were enumerated separately. Composite samples of vegetative cover along with the surface residue were prepared from the two cores in each plot and 3 g of composite sample was added to 90 ml of 2 mM phosphate buffer (pH 7.2). The surface 5 cm of soil from each core in each plot was thoroughly mixed and 10 g of field moist soil was added to 90 ml of phosphate buffer. The buffer and samples were agitated on a reciprocating shaker at approximately 160 rpm for 30 min to extract the bacteria. Oven dry weights of vegetative and soil samples were determined and all fecal bacteria concentrations were expressed on a dry weight basis. Samples were analyzed for fecal coliforms and fecal streptococci within 24 h using a spiral plater (Autoplate ® 4000 spiral plater, Spiral Biotech, Inc., Bethesda, MD). Fecal coliforms were incubated on mFC agar (Difco™ mFC Agar, Detroit, MI) at 44.5 °C for 22 h, and fecal streptococci were incubated on KFS agar (Difco ™ KFS Agar, Detroit, MI) at 35 °C for 48 h.

After EC and FS colonies were counted, at least five isolates from each plot were selected at random. To verify the presence of EC and FS, the isolates were grown on EC-MUG broth and mEnterococcus agar, respectively. The positively identified isolates were spiral plated in duplicate onto Mueller Hinton agar. Immediately after plating the *E. coli* isolates, antibiotic diffusion discs (BBL™ Sensi-Disc, Sparks, MD) were placed onto the agar surface using an 8-place dispenser (BBL® Sensi-Disc 8-place dispenser, Cockeysville, MD). Seven antibiotics were evaluated at the following concentrations: ampicillin (10 μg), cephalothin (30 μg), erythromycin (15 μg), rifampin (5 μg), streptomycin (10 μg), tetracycline (30 μg), and trimethoprim (5 μg). The cultures were incubated at 35 °C for 24 h and zones of inhibition for each antibiotic disc were measured at the end of the incubation period. The same procedure was followed for the fecal streptococci isolates except the positively identified isolates were grown in Tryptic Soy Broth (Difco ™ Tryptic Soy Broth, Detroit, MI) at 35 °C for 48 h and then spiral plated onto Mueller Hinton agar that was incubated at 35 °C for 48 h.

Statistical analysis for fecal coliform and fecal streptococci concentrations in sod and soil was performed separately using the PROC MIXED procedure in SAS ® (SAS version 8.2, SAS Institute Inc., Cary, NC) for the analysis of variance and means separation among the treatments were determined by difference in least square means. A linear regression model using a first order decay model (log CFU g^{-1} = K Days + Constant; K= mortality rate) was used to estimate the fecal coliform and fecal streptococci mortality rates in sod and soil. Statistical analysis for *E. coli* and fecal streptococci antibiotic resistance patterns was performed using the PROC GLM procedure in SAS. Repeated measures were used for analysis of variance to detect differences in treatments, collection dates, and interaction of treatments by collection dates. The LSD procedure was used to detect significant pairwise differences. Principle components analysis was performed using the PROC PRINCOMP procedure in SAS. Discriminant analysis was used to evaluate correct rates of classification and was performed using the PROC DISCRIM procedure in SAS.

4. Results and discussion

4.1 Population and survival

The background fecal coliform and fecal streptococci concentrations in the plots were not significantly different from one another prior to manure application. The fecal coliform concentrations in background ranged from non detectable (<1) to 100 CFU g^{-1} in sod and non detectable to 50 CFU g^{-1} in soil. The fecal streptococci concentrations in the background ranged from 1,000 to 16,000 CFU g^{-1} in sod and 100 to 800 CFU g^{-1} in soil. The poultry manure contained approximately 7.9 x 10^8 CFU g^{-1} fecal coliforms, and 2.5 x 10^9 CFU g^{-1} fecal streptococci.

Manure application significantly increased the fecal coliform and fecal streptococci concentrations in sod and soil compared to the respective unmanured controls and remained so for the duration of the experiment. The fecal coliform and fecal streptococci concentrations exceeded 10^6 CFU g^{-1} sod and 10^5 CFU g^{-1} soil seven days after manure application (Tables 1 and 2). Fecal coliform and fecal streptococci concentrations in unmanured control plots also increased after manure application, but this was most likely due to cross contamination resulting from mowing and sample collection. Mowing frequency neither increased nor decreased the fecal coliform and fecal streptococci concentration in either sod or soil in the

Treatment	Day 7	Day 14	Day 21	Day 28	Day 49
			Sod		
Never Mowed	6.9a* †	7.9a*	6.4a*	6.0a*	5.1a*
Never Mowed control	4.1	4.0	4.1	4.0	BD
Mowed Biweekly	6.8a*	7.2ab*	6.3a*	6.4a*	4.6a*
Mowed Biweekly control	4.4	3.9	4.2	3.6	1.9
Mowed Weekly	6.6a*	6.9b*	5.7a*	6.1a*	4.5a*
Mowed Weekly control	5.1	4.9	4.4	4.1	3.2
			Soil		
Never Mowed	5.5a*	4.1a*	4.4a*	4.0b*	2.6a*
Never Mowed control	2.9	2.4	ND	1.2	BD
Mowed Biweekly	5.1a*	5.1a*	5.1a*	3.8b*	2.6a*
Mowed Biweekly control	3.1	2.4	1.9	BD	BD
Mowed Weekly	5.1a*	4.5a*	4.3a*	4.3a*	3.0a
Mowed Weekly control	3.6	3.3	3.1	3.3	3.6

† Values at each interval and sample type sharing the same letter are not significantly different ($p \geq 0.05$). None of the controls were significantly different from one another. * Significantly different ($p \leq 0.05$) from unmanured controls. ND- Not determined. BD - Below detection levels.

Table 1. Average fecal coliform concentration (log CFU g^{-1}) from sod/soil in mowed and poultry manure-amended sod plots.

Treatment	Day 7	Day 14	Day 21	Day 28	Day 49	Day 70
			Sod			
Never Mowed	6.5a*†	6.2a*	6.3a*	6.3a*	6.4a*	4.9a
Never Mowed control	4.8	4.7	4.3	5.1	3.8	4.6
Mowed Biweekly	6.3a*	6.1a*	6.2a*	5.9a*	3.9a*	5.4a
Mowed Biweekly control	4.0	4.8	4.3	4.3	5.1	BD
Mowed Weekly	6.6a*	6.3a*	6.3a*	6.6a*	5.9a*	4.9a
Mowed Weekly control	4.6	4.9	3.9	4.4	4.4	BD
			Soil			
Never Mowed	5.0a*	5.0a*	5.0ab*	4.5a*	4.0a*	3.3a
Never Mowed control	4.1	3.8	3.3	3.1	3.1	3.2
Mowed Biweekly	5.1a*	5.3a*	5.1a*	4.5a*	3.7a	3.6a
Mowed Biweekly control	3.9	2.8	3.7	2.7	3.0	3.7
Mowed weekly	5.2a*	5.2a*	4.6b	4.5a*	4.0a*	3.3a
Mowed weekly control	4.0	4.0	3.9	3.6	3.1	3.5

† Values at each interval and sample type sharing the same letter are not significantly different ($p \geq 0.05$). None of the controls were significantly different from one another. * Significantly different ($p \leq 0.05$) from unmanured controls. ND- Not determined. BD - Below detection levels.

Table 2. Average fecal streptococci concentration (log CFU g^{-1}) from sod/soil in mowed and poultry manure-amended sod plots.

manure-amended plots. These results were consistent with previous rain simulation studies on bacterial survival and infiltration in frequently mowed sod plots (Gandhapudi, 2004) in which mowing did not significantly affect the fecal bacteria concentrations recovered in lysimeters pans.

Because mowing had no effect on bacteria survival, different treatments were used in the study as replicates to study fecal coliform and fecal streptococci survival in sod and soil. The fecal coliform concentration in sod increased from 7 to 14 days after manure application, suggesting net growth, and thereafter decreased slowly for the rest of the study period. In contrast, the fecal coliform concentrations in soil slowly but continuously declined after manure application, without any evidence of net growth during the first 14 days. The fecal coliforms in sod and soil had only an approximate 25-fold decrease in 49 days. However, fecal coliform concentration in sod and soil declined below the detection limits (1000 CFU g^{-1} in sod and 100 CFU g^{-1} in soil) 70 days after manure application. The difference in detection limits was due to the difference in initial dilution.

The fecal streptococci concentration in sod and soil declined very slowly after manure application for the duration of experiment (70 days). There was only an approximate 15-fold decrease in fecal streptococci concentration observed in 70 days and the fecal streptococci concentration exceeded 4×10^4 CFU g^{-1} in sod and 2.0×10^3 CFU g^{-1} in soil even 70 days after manure application. However, fecal streptococci concentrations at 70 days were not different from unmanured control plots.

4.1.1 Mortality rates

A first order die-off model was used to describe fecal coliform and fecal streptococci mortality in this study because the first order die-off model has been widely and successfully used to describe fecal bacteria mortality in bacteria survival studies (Edwards and Daniel, 1992; Reddy et al., 1981; Stoddard et al., 1998). A 35-day model (between Day 14 and Day 49), excluding the periods with net growth, was used to describe the fecal coliform mortality in sod and a 49-day model (between Day 7 and Day 49) was used to describe the fecal coliform mortality in soil. The linear regression model (log CFU g^{-1} = k Days + constant) describing mortality rates indicated that there was no difference between mortality rates in sod and soil, and that the average fecal coliform mortality rate (k) was 0.06 log cells day^{-1} (R^2= 0.57 in sod; R^2 = 0.53 in soil). Redistribution of fecal bacteria in manure during mowing can presumably have facilitated growth, but attempts were not made to calculate growth rates for individual treatments. Lack of significant differences in net mortality rates was likely due to confounding effects of growth and mortality.

A 70-day linear regression model (log CFU g^{-1} = k Days + constant) was used to describe fecal streptococci mortality in sod and soil. The average fecal streptococci mortality rates in this model were 0.02 log cells day^{-1} (R^2= 0.53) in sod and 0.03 log cells day^{-1} (R^2 = 0.69) in soil. We assume that very low fecal streptococci mortality rates in sod and soil might have been influenced by the background fecal streptococci populations. The fecal streptococci mortality rate in the control plots did not correlate with the fecal streptococci mortality rates in the manure-amended population. In unmanured controls, the fecal streptococci concentrations did not change significantly throughout the study.

Studies that used poultry litter as a soil amendment have reported mortality rates ranging from 0.06–0.29 day^{-1} for fecal coliforms and 0.06-0.357 day^{-1} for fecal streptococci (Crane et al., 1980; Zhai et al., 1995). Our mortality rates were comparable to the mortality rates reported elsewhere, although the simple first order die-off model used in this study to describe the mortality of fecal coliform and fecal streptococci in sod and soil showed a poor R^2, indicating that the model was not a good fit for the data.

Moisture, temperature, and nutrient availability are important factors that influence fecal coliform and fecal streptococci mortality in soil. Entry et al. (2000), for example, reported that decreasing soil moisture and increasing soil temperature substantially increased the mortality of total coliforms and fecal coliforms in soil. Our results suggest that fecal coliform and fecal streptococci mortality rates were also influenced by soil moisture and temperature. During the study period almost every sampling period was preceded by a rain event that substantially increased the gravimetric moisture content in the soil to 29-40% (Fig. 1). Weekly rainfall exceeded 5-year averages in 6 of 10 sample periods (Fig. 2). The average 70-day temperature during the study was 17–27 °C in sod and 22–25 °C in soil.

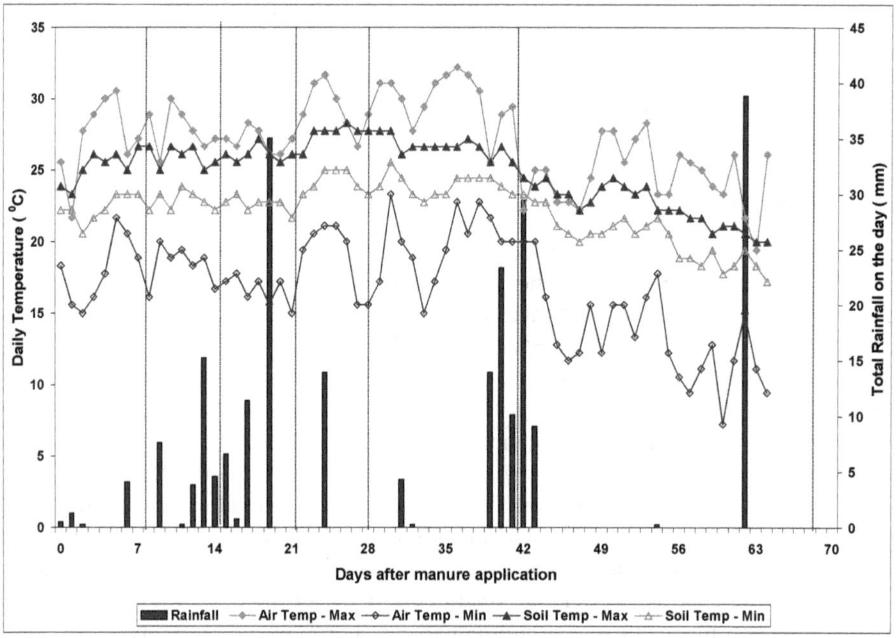

Fig. 1. Daily maximum and minimum air and soil temperatures, and total precipitation during the study period (July 2003 - October 2003) (weather data from Maine Chance Research Farm, Lexington KY). Dotted lines in the graph indicate the sampling periods during the study.

4.2 Antibiotic resistance patterns

Antibiotic resistance patterns of *E. coli* (EC) and fecal streptococci (FS) changed with time. The *E. coli* in sod and soil generally lost resistance followed by a return to initial patterns of resistance; whereas, the fecal streptococci in sod and soil generally had periods of increased resistance followed by a return to initial patterns. A summary of the significant differences of means by antibiotic and date from sod and soil for EC are shown in Table 3. A summary of the significant differences of means by antibiotic and date from sod and soil for FS are shown in Table 4.

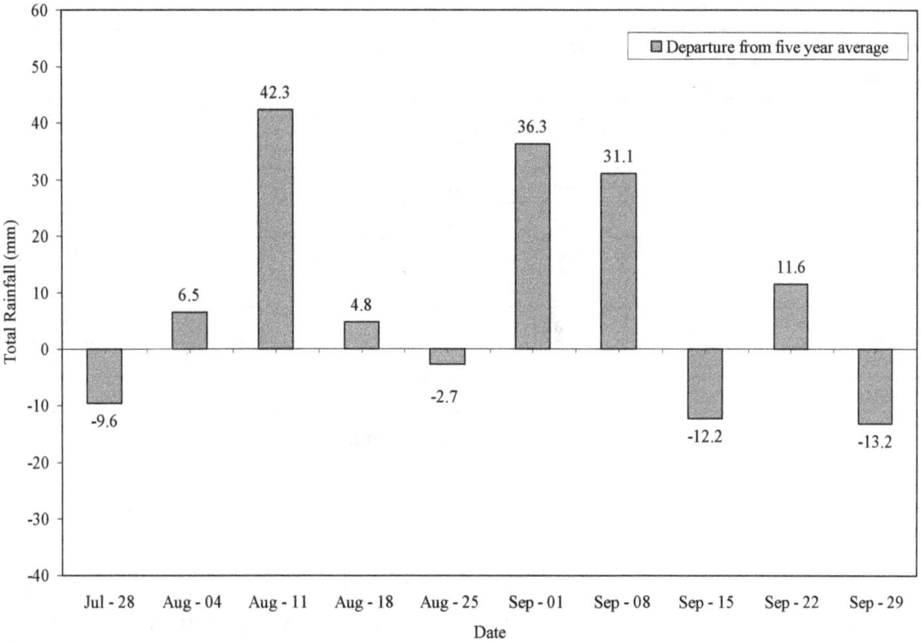

Fig. 2. Weekly rainfall departure during the study period (July - September 2003) from the past five year average (1998-2002). (Data obtained from Spindletop Research Farm Weather Station, Lexington KY).

Escherichia coli (EC) Isolates - Sod. There were five sampling dates for the sod EC isolates. The samples were collected at days 0, 7, 14, 28, and 49 after poultry application. The choice of antibiotic(s) for the study played a large role in the detection of bacterial changes with time. This was evident based on different resistance patterns among the seven antibiotics, thus providing more unique 'signatures' for each isolate. Statistical analysis of the sod data indicated that there was no significant treatment or sampling date main effect or interaction for ampicillin and cephalothin. The remaining antibiotics (i.e., erythromycin, rifampin, streptomycin, tetracycline, and trimethoprim) all produced significantly different antibiotic resistance patterns (ARPs) with sampling date. There were no significantly different date by treatment interactions or treatment main effects.

As the area surrounding the antibiotic or zone of inhibition increases, the resistance of the bacteria to the antibiotic decreases, and vice versa. The resistance of EC to erythromycin, rifampin, streptomycin, tetracycline, and trimethoprim significantly decreased with time. Generally, the bacteria showed initial changes in resistance at day 14 for all of the antibiotics that had significant date effects.

Antibiotic	Day 0	Day 7	Day 14	Day 21	Day 28	Day 49
Sod						
Ampicillin	17a†	16a	17a	ns‡	18a	18a
Cephalothin	18a	15a	17a	ns	17a	18a
Erythromycin	9a	8a	13b	ns	16c	17c
Rifampin	9a	8a	10a	ns	13b	13b
Streptomycin	14a	15a	17b	ns	19c	18bc
Tetracycline	21a	20a	23b	ns	24b	24b
Trimethoprim	18a	23b	26b	ns	29c	28c
Soil						
Ampicillin	18a	19a	ns	18a	19a	17a
Cephalothin	17a	16a	ns	17a	19a	17a
Erythromycin	11a	8a	ns	10a	18b	17b
Rifampin	9a	8a	ns	9a	13b	12c
Streptomycin	16a	17a	ns	17a	20b	18c
Tetracycline	20a	22ac	ns	19a	25b	24bc
Trimethoprim	23a	25ab	ns	26b	28c	28c

† Values at each interval and sample type sharing the same letter are not significantly different ($p \geq 0.05$). ‡ ns = not sampled

Table 3. Date and mean values of antibiotic inhibition zones (mm) for *E. coli* isolates from sod and soil.

E. coli (EC) Isolates - Soil. There were five sampling dates for the soil EC isolates. The samples were collected at days 0, 7, 21, 28, and 49 after poultry application. Similar to the sod data, there was no significant treatment or date main effect or interactions with ampicillin and cephalothin. The sampling dates were significantly different from each other using erythromycin, rifampin, streptomycin, tetracycline, and trimethoprim. The EC from the soil also had decreased resistance to all of the antibiotics with time. However, the initial changes in resistance occurred at day 21 which was approximately one week later than the sod. This would suggest that migration of fecal bacteria from the sod to the soil may have occurred with time.

The treatment by sampling date interactions were significantly different for erythromycin and tetracycline. The resistance of EC decreased with time in the 'Mowed Every Week' and 'Mowed Biweekly' treatments for erythromycin, including the control plots. In the mowed treatments, the significant decrease in antibiotic resistance occurred between day 0 and day 21. However, the 'Never Mowed' treatments receiving poultry manure had increased resistance of bacteria at day 21 followed by a decrease to initial levels of resistance. The resistance of EC to trimethoprim decreased by day 28 and remained at that suppressed level until the last sampling date on day 49 for both the 'Never Mowed' and 'Mowed Every Week' treatments. Similar to the 'Never Mowed' treatment for erythromycin, the 'Mowed Biweekly' treatment for trimethoprim resulted in an increased level of resistance by day 28 and returned to initial levels for the remaining sampling dates. There were no significant changes with time in the control treatment.

Antibiotic	Day 0	Day 7	Day 14	Day21	Day 28	Day 49	Day 70
Sod							
Ampicillin	22a†	23a	22a	ns‡	24a	21a	23a
Cephalothin	15b	10a	9a	ns	17b	14b	18b
Erythromycin	17a	11b	9b	ns	19a	20a	20a
Rifampin	16a	14ab	10b	ns	17a	18a	16a
Streptomycin	6a	7a	6a	ns	9b	10b	7a
Tetracycline	21b	11a	11a	ns	16ab	21b	23b
Trimethoprim	26a	25a	23a	ns	27a	21a	25a
Soil							
Ampicillin	23ab	25a	24a	22ab	23ab	20b	16c
Cephalothin	16ab	9c	10c	16ab	19a	13bc	12bc
Erythromycin	18a	10b	12b	18a	17a	16a	16a
Rifampin	21a	12cd	10d	18ab	15bcd	14bcd	16abc
Streptomycin	8abc	6c	6c	9ab	10a	7bc	7bc
Tetracycline	21a	9c	13bc	17ab	16ab	20a	19a
Trimethoprim	25ab	29a	22b	24ab	20bc	23b	16c

† Values at each interval and sample type sharing the same letter are not significantly different ($p \geq 0.05$). ‡ ns = not sampled

Table 4. Date and mean values of antibiotic inhibition zones (mm) for fecal streptococci isolates from sod and soil.

Fecal Streptococci (FS) Isolates - Sod. There were six collection dates for the sod FS isolates. The samples were collected at days 0, 7, 14, 28, 49, and 70 after poultry application. Trimethoprim produced no statistically significant main effects or interactions. Cephalothin, erythromycin, rifampin, streptomycin, and tetracycline produced significant date main effects. There were no significant treatment main effects for any antibiotic used in this study. The statistical analysis indicated that ampicillin and streptomycin produced significant treatment by date interactions. All of the antibiotics that had significant date effects except for streptomycin went through a phase of increased resistance at approximately day 7 with a subsequent phase at day 28 that was generally not significantly different from day 0. Streptomycin showed an opposite trend, whereby the bacterial response was a slight decrease in resistance at day 28 followed by an increase back to initial patterns of resistance at day 70. This may be an artifact of significant treatment by date interactions for streptomycin.

The most significant differences for treatment by date interactions of ampicillin occurred in the 'Mowed Biweekly' treatment when compared to the other treatments. There was a two phase cycle that was marked by increased resistance of FS to ampicillin followed by a return to initial (day 0) patterns of resistance patterns. There were two of these cycles that were documented over the 70-day sampling period. The first cycle began at day 7 and ended at day 28. The second cycle began at day 49 and ended at day 70. The 'Mowed Weekly' treatment for treatment by date interactions of streptomycin contained ARPs that indicated decreased periods of resistance occurring at day 49 and returning to day 0 patterns at day

70. The treatment by date interactions for the control treatments of ampicillin and streptomycin were also statistically significant. There were decreases in resistance to both antibiotics at day 28.

Fecal Streptococcus (FS) Isolates - Soil. There were seven collection dates for the soil FS isolates. The samples were collected at days 0, 7, 14, 21, 28, 49, and 70 days after poultry application. All seven of the antibiotics used in this study produced significant date main effects, but there were no significant treatment effects or treatment by date interactions. The results for FS in soil were the most ambiguous for this study. The results for FS in sod and EC in sod and soil had definitive resistance patterns that changed similarly with time across antibiotics within each organism and medium. However, upon evaluation of FS in soil, the data suggested an increased resistance at day 7 through day 14. This was more pronounced with cephalothin, erythromycin, rifampin, streptomycin, and tetracycline. Ampicillin and trimethoprim produced ARPs that showed progressively increasing resistance of FS throughout the sampling dates. These results, as those for EC, may be explained by a gradual migration of the organisms from sod to soil.

4.2.1 Rates of correct classification based on antibiotic resistance

The rate of correct classification or RCC for sod and soil by date was analyzed for EC and FS. The six total distinct dates used for EC were divided into two date groups, early and late, and the initial background (day 0) was excluded. The early date included 7, 14, and 21 days after poultry application. The late date included 28 and 49 days after application. The seven total distinct dates for FS were also divided into two groups, early and late, with exclusion of the initial background. The early date for FS included 7, 14, and 21 days after poultry application. The late date included 28, 49, and 70 days after application.

The RCC for EC using resubstitution analysis showed that the database correctly classified 92% of the sod isolates and 70% of the soil isolates for the early collection dates. The database correctly classified 70% of the sod isolates and 85% of the soil isolates for the late collection dates. These results coincided with the analysis of the significant differences of means by antibiotic and date from sod and soil as discussed previously. That is, the data support the idea that migration of fecal bacteria from the sod to the soil may occur with time. The correct classification of bacteria is highest for the early dates of sod while the majority of the bacteria resides in the surface or sod portion of the profile. Over time, the bacteria migrate to the lower area or the soil portion of the profile. For these dates, the RCC becomes lower for sod and higher for soil.

The RCC for FS using resubstitution analysis showed that the database correctly classified 85% of the sod isolates and 59% of the soil isolates for the early collection dates. The database correctly classified 69% of the sod isolates and 58% of the soil isolates for the late collection dates. The results for FS are more ambiguous than those reported for EC. While the RCC for sod also decrease over time, the RCC for soil remain relatively unchanged. It is worth noting that host source origin is typically classified. In this case, the medium, i.e., sod and soil, is effectively being classified with moderate success. Rates of correct classification of 60% or higher are considered useful by resource managers (Harwood et al., 2000), which makes the rates reported here of significant value.

Principle Component Analysis (PCA) was a useful tool when applied to the EC database. The variables used to compute the PCA were the seven antibiotics used for the profiles. The cumulative percent of variability accounted for by the first two axes was 72% which described most of the variability among the seven antibiotics. Axis one, which accounted for 55% of the variability, appeared to be associated with the antibiotics erythromycin, rifampin, and streptomycin. The second axis appeared to have large loadings for ampicillin and cephalothin. The graph of the PCA output for EC is shown in Figure 3 where period 1 = 0 days (background), period 2 = 7, 14, and 21 days, and period 3 = 28 and 49 days after poultry litter application. The dates were combined into early (background, period 1 = 0 days), intermediate (one to three weeks after application, period 2 = 7, 14, and 21 days), and late (anything after three weeks, period 3 = 28 and 49 days). Graphing the two axes based on period reveals grouping in the data. Period 1 data are not structured and agrees with previous findings for these are background data collected prior to poultry application. The data for period 2 resolve as two groups suggesting that a transitional period occurs between one and three weeks after poultry application as bacterial populations migrate from sod to soil. The data for period 3 are grouped together with no further changes up to 7 weeks after poultry application. The groups change relative to axis 1 which suggests that date primarily affects erythromycin, rifampin, and streptomycin antibiotic resistance patterns.

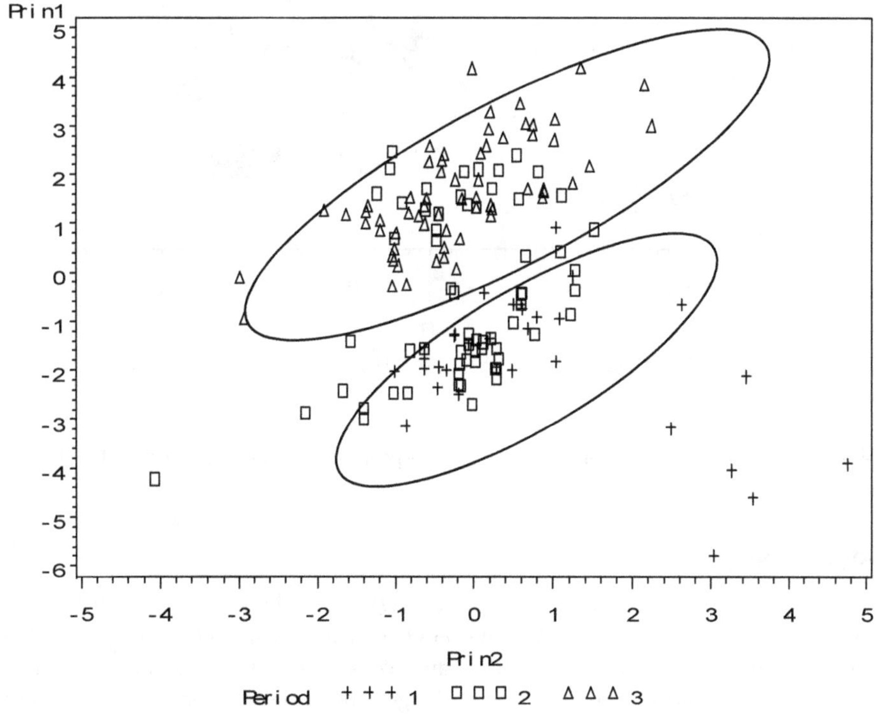

Fig. 3. Principle components analysis for *Escherichia coli* by date. Sod and soil isolates were combined in this analysis.

The graph of the PCA output for FS is shown in Figure 4. The PCA for the FS dataset showed that the cumulative percent of variability accounted for by the first two axes is 64%, which described most of the variability among the seven antibiotics. Axis one, which accounted for 43% of the variability, appeared to be associated with the antibiotics cephalothin, erythromycin, and rifampin. Axis two had large loadings for ampicillin and trimethoprim. The dates are the same as those described for EC with an addition of 70 day data added to period 3. There appeared to be no structure to the data presented in the plot, and no distinct grouping patterns.

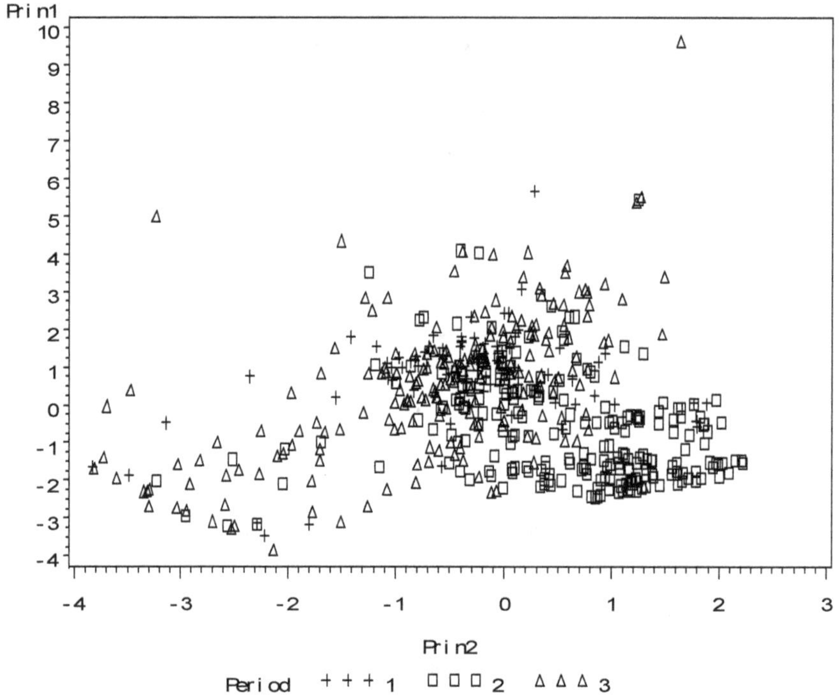

Fig. 4. Principle components analysis for fecal streptococci by date. Sod and soil isolates were combined in this analysis.

5. Conclusions

This study showed that disturbance (e.g. mowing) had little or no effect on EC and FS mortality in sod or soil in our study environment. It was suspected that the selection of mowing height, preservation of residue, and consistently wet weather combined to minimize treatment effects. The relatively prolonged survival of the fecal bacteria promoted the potential for runoff during the study, as well as potential for phenotypic variability as revealed by the MST profiles. The fecal bacteria appeared to persist in the environment for extended periods. Mowing frequency did not appear to affect the resistance profiles of *E. coli* and fecal streptococci for seven antibiotics. However, characterization of the same fecal bacterial population by means of MST was not consistent for that same time period; thereby suggesting that MST by this method was a time-dependent technique. Sampling time after our initial poultry manure application did appear to significantly affect the profiles recovered. Ampicillin and cephalothin were considered good indicators of antibiotic resistance over time for *E. coli* in sod or soil as there were no significant differences between sampling dates.

The selection of antibiotic to identify changes in microbial populations over time appears to play an important role in the effective use of MST. Based on the results from this study (Ritchey and Coyne, unpublished), ampicillin and cephalothin may be good choices to determine sources of EC in soil or sod and trimethoprim may provide useful information when studying FS in sod because there were no significant differences with time which indicates temporal stability when using these antibiotics.

6. Acknowledgement

Funding for this project was provided, in part, by a grant from the General Assembly of the Commonwealth of Kentucky - Senate Bill 271.

7. References

Berry, E.D. & Miller, D.N. (2005) Cattle feedlot soil moisture and manure content: II. Impact on *Escherichia coli* O157. *J. Environ. Qual.*, Vol. 34, No. 2, (March), pp. 656-663, ISSN 0047-2425

Carson, C.A., Shear, B.L., Ellersieck, M.R. & Asfaw, A. (2001) Identification of fecal *Escherichia coli* from humans and animal by ribotyping. *Appl. Environ. Microbiol.*, Vol. 67, No. 4, (April), pp. 1503-1507, ISSN 0099-2240

Caugant, D.A., Levin, B.R. & Selander, R.K. (1981). Genetic diversity and temporal variation in the *E. coli* population of a human host. *Genetics*, Vol. 98, No. 3, (July), pp. 467-490, ISSN 0016-6731

Collins, R. (2004) Fecal contamination of pastoral wetlands. *J. Environ. Qual.*, Vol. 33, No. 5, (September), pp. 1912-1918, ISSN 0047-2425

Crane, S.R., Westerman, P.W. & Overcash, M.R. (1980) Die-off of fecal indicator organisms following land applications of poultry manure. *J. Environ. Qual.*, Vol. 9, No. 1, (January-March), pp. 531-537, ISSN 0047-2425

Dombek, P.E., Johnson, L.K., Zimmerley, S.T. & Sadowsky, M.J. (2000) Use of repetitive DNA sequences and the PCR to differentiate *Escherichia coli* isolates from human and animal sources. *Appl. Environ. Microbiol.*, Vol. 66, No. 6, (June), pp. 2572-2577, ISSN 0099-2240

Edwards, D. R. & Daniel, T.C. (1992) Environmental impacts of on-farm poultry waste disposal - a review. *Bioresource Technology*, Vol. 41, No. 1, pp. 9-33, ISSN 0960-8524

Ellis, J.R. & McCalla, T.M. (1978) Fate of pathogens in soils receiving animal wastes - A review. *Trans. ASAE*, Vol. 21, No. 2, pp. 309-313, ISSN 0309-0313

Entry, J.A., Hubbard, R.K., Thies, J. E. & Furhmann, J.J. (2000). The influence of vegetation in riparian filterstrips on coliform bacteria: II. Survival in soils. *J. Environ. Qual.*, Vol. 29, No. 4, (July-August), pp. 1206-1214, ISSN 0047-2425

Gandhapudi, S.K. (2004) Managing fecal bacteria and nutrient contamination in poultry manure-amended sod by mowing and alum addition. M.S. Thesis, University of Kentucky, Lexington, KY.

Gordon, D.M. (2001). Geographical structure and host specificity in bacteria and the implications for tracing the source of coliform contamination. *Microbiol.*, Vol. 147, No. 5, (May), pp. 1079-1085, ISSN 1350-0872

Graves, A.K., Hagedorn, C., Teetor, A., Mahal, M., Booth, A.M. & Reneau, R.B. (2002) Antibiotic resistance profiles to determine sources of fecal contamination in a rural Virginia watershed. *J. Environ. Qual.*, Vol. 31, No. 4, (July), pp. 1300-1308, ISSN 0047-2425

Guan, S., Xu, R., Chen, S., Odumeru, J., & Gyles, C.. (2002). Development of a procedure for discriminating among *Escherichia coli* isolates from animal and human sources. *Appl. Environ. Technology*, Vol. 68, pp. 2690-2698, ISSN 1994-7887

Hagedorn, C., Robinson, S.L., Filtz, J.R., Grubbs, S.M., Angier, T.A. & Reneau, R.B. (1999). Determining sources of fecal pollution in a rural Virginia watershed with antibiotic resistance patterns in fecal streptococci. *Appl. Environ. Microbiol.*, Vol. 65, No. 12, (December), pp. 5522-5531, ISSN 0099-2240

Hartel, P.G, Summer, J.D., Hill, J.L., Collins, J.V., Entry, J.A. & Segars, W.I. (2002) Geographic variability of *Escherichia coli* ribotypes from animals in Idaho and Georgia. *J. Environ. Qual.*, Vol. 31, No. 4, (July), pp. 1273-1278, ISSN 0047-2425

Harwood, V.J., Whitlock, J. & Withington, V. (2000). Classification of antibiotic resistance patterns of indicator bacteria by discriminant analysis: Use in predicting the source of fecal contamination in subtropical waters. *Appl. Environ. Microbiol.*, Vol. 66, No. 9, (September), pp. 3698-3704, ISSN 0099-2240

Howell, J.M., Coyne, M.S. & Cornelius, P. (1995). Fecal bacteria in agricultural waters of the bluegrass region of Kentucky. *J. Environ. Qual.*, Vol. 24, No. 3, (May-June), pp. 411-419, ISSN 0047-2425

Jenkins, M.B., Hartel, P.G., Olexa, T.J. & Stuedemann, J.A. (2003). Putative temporal variability of *Escherichia coli* ribotypes from yearling steers. *J. Environ. Qual.*, Vol. 32, No. 1, (January), pp. 305-309, ISSN 0047-2425

Johnson, L.K., Brown, M.B., Carruthers, E.A., Ferguson, J.A., Dombek, P.E. & Sadowsky, M.J. (2004) Sample size, library composition, and genotype diversity among natural populations of *Escherichia coli* from different animals influence accuracy of determining sources of fecal pollution. *Appl. Environ. Microbiol.*, Vol. 70, No. 8, (August), pp. 4478-4485, ISSN 0099-2240

Kentucky Geological Survey. (2002). Kentucky landscape-astonishing beauty and hidden hazards. Available from
http://www.uky.edu/KGS/pubs/infocus.htm

Lu, Z., Lapen, D., Scott, A., Dang, A. & Topp, E. (2005) Identifying host sources of fecal pollution: Diversity of *Escherichia coli* in confined dairy and swine production systems. *Appl. Environ. Microbiol.*, Vol. 71, No. 10, (October), pp. 5992-5998, ISSN 0099-2240

McClellan, S.L., Daniels, A.D. & Salmore, A.K. (2003) Genetic characterization of *Escherichia coli* populations from host sources of fecal pollution by using DNA fingerprinting. *Appl. Environ. Microbiol.*, Vol. 69, No. 5, (May), pp. 2587-2594, ISSN 0099-2240

Reddy, K.R., Khaleel, R. & Overcash, M.R. (1981). Behavior and transport of microbial pathogens and indicator organisms in soils treated with organic wastes. *J. Environ. Qual.* Vol. 10, No. 3, (July-Sept), pp. 255-264, ISSN 0047-2425

Ritchey, S.A. and Coyne, M.S. (2009). Applying MAR analysis to identify human and non-human fecal sources in small Kentucky watersheds. *Water Air Soil Pollut* , Vol. 196, No. 1-4, (June), pp. 115-125, ISSN 0049-6979

SAS Institute. (1999). SAS/STAT user's guide version 8. Available from http://v8doc.sas.com/sashtml/

Sinton, L.W., Braithwaite, R.R., Hall, C.H. & Mackenzie, M.L. (2007) Survival of indicator and pathogenic bacteria in bovine feces on pasture. *Appl. Environ. Microbiol.*, Vol. 73, No. 24, (December), pp. 7917-7925, ISSN 0099-2240

Stoddard, C.S., Coyne, M.S. & Grove, J.H. (1998). Fecal bacteria survival and infiltration through a shallow agricultural soil: Timing and tillage effects. *J. Environ. Qual.*, Vol. 27, No. 6, (November-December), pp. 1516-1523, ISSN 0047-2425

Unc, A. & Goss, M.J. (2003) Movement of fecal bacteria through the vadose zone. *Water Air Soil Pollut.*, Vol. 149, No. 1-4, (October), pp. 327-337, ISSN 0049-6979

United States Environmental Protection Agency. (2000) National water quality inventory: 2000 report. Available from http://www.epa.gov/305b/2000report/

Wiggins, B.A., Cash, P.W., Creamer, W.S., Dart, S.E., Garcia, P.C., Gerecke, T.M., Han, J., Henry, B.L., Hoover, K.B., Johnson, E.L., Jones, K.C., McCarthy, J.G., McDonough, J.A., Mercer, S.A., Noto, M.J., Park, Phillips, M.S., Purner, S.M., Smith, B.M., Stevens, E.N. & Varner, A.K. (2003). Use of antibiotic resistance analysis for representativeness testing of multiwatershed libraries. *Appl. Environ. Microbiol.*, Vol. 69, No. 6, (June), pp. 3399-3405, ISSN 0099-2240

Wiggins, B.A., Andrews, R.W., Conway, R.A., Corr, C.L., Dobratz, E.J., Dougherty, D.P., Eppard, J.R., Knupp, S.R., Limjoco, M.C., Mettenburg, J.M., Rinehardt, J.M., Sonsino, J., Torrijos, R.L. & Zimmerman, M.E. (1999) Use of antibiotic resistance analysis to identify nonpoint sources of fecal pollution. *Appl. Environ. Microbiol.*, Vol. 65, No. 8, (August), pp. 3483-3486, ISSN 0099-2240

Wiggins, B.A. (1996) Discriminant analysis of antibiotic resistance patterns in fecal streptococci, a method to differentiate human and animal sources of fecal pollution in natural waters. *Appl. Environ. Microbiol.*, Vol. 62, No. 11, (November), pp. 3997-4002, ISSN 0099-2240

Zhai, Q., Coyne, M.S. & Barnhisel, R. I. (1995) Mortality rates of fecal bacteria in subsoil amended with poultry manure. *Bioresource Technology*, Vol. 54, No. 2, pp. 165-169, ISSN 0960-8524

6

Emergence of Antibiotic Resistant Bacteria from Coastal Environment – A Review

K.C.A. Jalal[1], B. Akbar John[1], B.Y. Kamaruzzaman[1] and K. Kathiresan[2]
[1]*Department of Biotechnology, Kulliyyah of Science, International Islamic University Malaysia,*
[2]*Centre of Advanced Studies in Marine Biology, Annamalai University,*
[1]*Malaysia*
[2]*India*

1. Introduction

Antibiotic resistance in microbes is a growing issue of human health. The extraordinary ability of microbes to develop resistance to various antibiotics attracted evolutionary scientists and environmental biologists in recent years. Historically, the use of antimicrobial agents started in 1904 with the discovery of Tripan red by Ehrlich and Shiga (Browning & Gulbransen, 1936). In 1929, penicillin was discovered by Alexander Fleming when his group found that the fungus *Penicilium notatum* produces a very selective inhibitor for *Staphylococcus* sp. Fleming's discovery showed that not only synthetic agents like Ehrlich's "Magic Bullet" but also a microbial product can be an effective antimicrobial drug (Hare, 1970). In 1943, Waksman started to use the word "antibiotics" when he discovered streptomycin (Wainwright, 1988). After the initial age of discovery and since the 1970s many antimicrobial agents have been developed together with the discoveries of new antibiotics. It is well documented that the evolution of antibiotic resistance in bacterial strains is a direct consequence of natural selection applied by widespread use of antibiotic drugs (Benveniste & Davies, 1973). The providential experiment by Fleming demonstrated the production of antibiotics (Penicillin) which eventually led to its large-scale production from mold *Penicillium notatum* in the 1940s. As early as the late 1940s resistant strains of bacteria began to appear due to their extraordinary ability in gaining resistance towards any particular antibiotics with elapsing generation (Shoemaker et al., 2001; Chopra & Roberts et al., 2001; Doern et al., 2001). In 1980 it was estimated that 3–5% of *S. pneumoniae* were penicillin-resistant and by 1998, 34% of the *S. pneumoniae* sampled were resistant to penicillin. Currently, it is estimated that more than 70% of the bacteria that cause hospital-acquired infections are resistant to at least one of the antibiotics used to treat them (NIAID, 2006).

Antibiotics are defined as a chemical substance derived from microorganisms, which have the capacity to inhibit growth, and even destroying other microorganisms in a dilute solution (ICON, 2003). Antibiotics are low-molecular-mass (<1500 kDa), products of secondary metabolism and nonessential for the growth of producing organisms, but are very important for human health. They have unusual structures and are most often formed during the late growth phase of the producing microorganisms. These secondary metabolites have exerted a major impact on the control of infectious diseases and other medical conditions, and the development of pharmaceutical industry. Their use has contributed to an increase in the average life expectancy in the USA, which increased from 47 years in 1900 to 74 years (in men) and 80 years (in women) in 2000 (Reynolds, 2010). Probably, the most important use of secondary metabolites has been as anti-infective drugs. In 2000, the market for such anti-infectives was US$55 billion and in 2007 it was US$66 billion, with the estimated global antibiotic consumption of between 100,000 and 200,000 tonnes per year (Demain & Sanchez, 2009).

Coastal environment plays a very important role as habitat to a number of plants and animals. They serve as breeding and nursery grounds, shelters, sources of food for various marine lives. In the recent times, pollution of coastal areas represents one of the most important environmental problems because it causes economic and tourism damages as well as affects health quality. It was noted that antibiotics released into the aquatic environment are of great concern for the three important reasons: (1) Contamination of water used for drinking, irrigation and recreation, (2) Widespread occurrence of bacterial resistance to antibiotics, and (3) Negative effect on microbes which play vital role in nutrient cycling (e.g. nitrogen cycle) and regeneration of nutrients in aquatic ecosystems (Costanzo et al., 2005). The use of antibiotics is the main treatment applied to control bacterial illness in fish farms (Castro et al., 2008). Due to the use of a wide variety of antibiotics, aquaculture has been implicated as potential environment to the development and selection of resistant bacteria and a source of these pathogens to other animals and humans (Hatha et al., 2005; Serrano, 2005). It has also been noted that sediment samples containing microorganisms with antibiotic resistance alter the production of β-lactamase in the human defence system (Lu, et al., 2010). The issue of antibiotic resistance was extensively addressed in the scientific literature describing the presence of antibiotics in the environment (e.g. Nygaard et al., 1992; Samuelsen et al., 1992). But, a comprehensive review on the emergence of antibiotic resistance strains from the aquatic habitat is still scanty.

3. Antibiotic resistance an ecological perspective

Although antibiotics have been used in large quantities for some decades, until recently the existence of these substances in the environment has received little attention. It is only in recent years that a more complex investigation of antibiotic substances has been undertaken in order to permit an assessment of the environmental risks (Kümmerer, 2009a & b). Within the last decade, an increasing number of studies covering antibiotic input, occurrence, fate and effects have been published (Kümmerer, 2009 b; Björkman et al., 2000; Alanis, 2005). Antibiotic resistance is one of the major challenges for human medicine and veterinary medicine. However, there is still a lack of understanding and knowledge about sources, presence and significance of resistance of bacteria against antibiotics in the aquatic environment despite the numerous studies performed (Kümmerer, 2009b).

Antibiotic resistance can reach the environment with the potential of adversely affecting aquatic and terrestrial organisms which eventually might reach humans through drinking water and food chain (Edquist & Pedersen, 2001; Prior, 2008; Aarestrup et al., 2008). The history of resistance due to the use of antibiotics has only recently been described in more detail (Edquist & Pedersen, 2001; Prior, 2008). In general, the emergence of resistance is a highly complex process which is not yet fully understood with respect to the significance of the interaction of bacterial populations and antibiotics, even in a medicinal environment (Björkman et al., 2000; Martinez & Baquero, 2000; Alanis, 2005). The transfer of resistant bacteria to humans could occur via water or food if plants are watered with surface water or sewage sludge, if manure is used as a fertilizer, or if resistant bacteria are present in meat (Perreten et al., 1997; Khachatourians, 1998; Dolliver & Gupta, 2008). The significance of the transfer of antibiotic resistance from animals to humans is not clearly understood. However, to minimize this route and the unwanted intake of antibiotics, the antibiotic content of fishery products is monitored by authorities in many countries (WHO, 2003; IM, 1989; FAAIR, 2002).

Many bacterial species multiply rapidly enough to double their numbers every 20–30 minutes, therefore, their ability to adapt to changes in the environment and survive unfavorable conditions often results in the development of mutations that enable the species to survive in changing external conditions (Ferenci, 2008). Research on the use of antibiotics in aquaculture shows similar results with the medical use of antibiotics (Weston, 1996). The important research findings in this regard are: (1) The use of one antibacterial agent can increase levels of resistance not only to that specific drug but also to many others, even those using very different modes of antibacterial action (cross-resistance). (2) Antibacterial resistance does not always respond in a predictable fashion correlating with the amount of drugs used or with the concentrations of residues in the environment (Hernando et al., 2006).

3.1 Coastal environment

Coastal Environment plays a very important role as habitat to a number of microbes, plants and animals. They serve as breeding grounds, shelters, sources of food for marine life, and are home to a number of endangered species (Kuijper, 2003). Over half of the current global population lives within 200 km of the coastline. For the future, the Centre for Climate Systems Research (CCSR) of the Earth Institute at Columbia University estimates a strong growth of coastal population by 2025. The coastal zone contains natural systems that provide more than half of the global ecosystem goods (e.g., fish, oil, minerals) and services (e.g., natural protection from storms and tidal waves, recreation). In addition, 14 of the world's 17 largest megacities are located along coasts and most of them are located in Asia's fastest growing economies (www.loicz.org). The overcrowding of beaches has led to large-scale destruction of some of these habitats and has reduced their ability to adapt to drastic environmental changes. Development, climate change, and commercialization have all contributed a major part in increasing the pressure on beach ecosystems. Besides this fact, anthropogenic input of various pollutants especially antibiotics into the aquatic environment has increased the resistant capacity of the bacterial strains. In general, bacterial load is higher in the sediments compared to the overlying water body. Hence, more investigations were carried out on surface soil samples (Jensen et al., 2001; Tolls, 2001; Marengo et al., 1997. It has been noted that persistence of antibiotics in soil depends on many factors including soil type, climate, and class of antibiotics (Bonaventura, 2004). Most antibiotics are recycled in soils through natural cycles but some of them have a long half-life (Kumar et al., 2005; Kümmerer, 2009a). According to Marengo et al. (1997), less than 1% of sarafloxacin, an antibiotic used widely in poultry production, degrades in the soil after 80 days of incubation. These antibiotics may leach to ground water or move to surface waters via surface runoff. Olapade et al., (2006) have reported that these antibiotics find their way to the coastal and marine environment.

Antibiotics have both quantitative and qualitative effects on the native microbial communities in soil environment (Nygaard et al., 1992). Although antibiotic concentrations in most soils are not at therapeutic levels to cause inhibitory effects on bacterial population, it may still influence the selection of antibiotic resistant bacteria in the niche (USEPA, 2002). Jensen et al. (2001) have recorded an increased antibiotic resistance among *Pseudomonas* sp. and *Bacillus cereus* after exposure to soil sediments. Many antibiotics have a strong tendency to bind with soil particles (Tolls, 2001; Kummerer et al., 2003). Distribution coefficients ($K_{d,solid}$) as high as 2300, 6310, and 128 L kg^{-1} have been reported for tetracycline, enrofloxacin, and tylosin, respectively (Kummerer et al., 2003). Our research team has earlier shown that the bacterial isolates from the tropical mangrove sediments are 100% resistant against β - lactam antibiotics (ampicillin, amoxicillin and penicillin). Bacterial isolated from mangrove sediment soil have exhibited 66.7 and 77.8% resistance against chloramphenicol and streptomycin, respectively, suggesting that the lipid composition may play a key role in preventing the entrance or binding of antibiotics to the cell (Jalal et al., 2010). Interestingly, All the isolates are susceptible to ciprofloxacin since it inhibits the enzyme topoisomerase II that causes the negative super-coil in DNA strands and thus permits transcription or replication. All the bacterial isolates display Multi Antibiotic Resistance (MAR) index higher than 0.2 indicating the high-risk sources of contamination in the environment (Jalal et al., 2010).

3.2 Aquaculture

In aquaculture fields, high loads of antibiotics in sediments at concentrations potent enough to inhibit the growth of bacteria have been reported (Costanzo et al., 2005; Hatha et al., 2005; Hirsch et al., 1999; Holmström et al., 2003; Kümmerer, 2009a &b). Resistant bacteria may be present in sediments because of the application of antibiotics in fish farming or because of selection through the antibiotics present in the sediments. The fact that the exposure is highly concentrated must also be considered to be critical. The substances used in fish farming can enter sediments directly from water without undergoing any kind of purification process. Some investigations have demonstrated the presence and persistence of antibiotics applied extensively in fish farming in sediments beneath fish farms (Kümmerer, 2003). Fluoroquinolones, sulphonamides and tetracyclines are strongly adsorbed (Kümmerer, 2009b) and therefore, they can readily accumulate in the sediments. It is not clearly known as to what degree and under what circumstances the compounds are effective after sorption or whether they are released to contribute to resistance. Antimicrobials can have qualitative and quantitative effects upon the resident microbial community in sediments. In the fish farming sector (aquaculture, mariculture, etc.), the widespread use of antibiotics for treating bacterial diseases is associated with the development of antibiotic resistance in *Aeromonas hydrophila, Aeromonas salmonicida, Edwardsiella tarda, Edwardsiella icttaluri, Vibrio anguillarum, Vibrio salmonicida, Pasteurella piscida* and *Yersinia ruckeri* (Serrano, 2005). Bacteria resistant against these compounds have been detected in sediments. Increased antibacterial resistance in sedimentary bacteria is often the most sensitive environmental indicator of past antibacterial use (Kümmerer, 2003). Various patterns of resistance among strains were isolated from very close geographical areas during the same year, suggesting diverse patterns of drug resistance in environmental bacteria within this area. In addition, the cross-resistance patterns have suggested that the resistance determinants among *Vibrio* spp. are acquired differently within sediment and seawater environments (Neela et al., 2007).

As far as intensive shrimp culture goes, a large amount of shrimp food and antibiotics have been used to increase production and to protect shrimp from diseases (EJF, 2003). Consequently, a large portion of feeds and antibiotics enters the water as wastes, causing water pollution (Le et al., 2003). Several studies have demonstrated the presence of antibacterial residues in fish farms (Weston, 1996; Capone et al., 1996; Herwig et al., 1997). Recent studies have shown that many antibiotics persist in the sediment and in the aquatic environment for several months following administration (Bjorklund et al., 1991; Lai et al., 1995; Pouliquen & Le, 1996; Hirsch et al., 1999; Miranda & Zemelman, 2002).The residues of antibacterial agents may affect the sedimentary microbial community and introduce antibiotic resistance in the bacteria (Hektoen et al., 1995; Tendencia & Dela Pena, 2002). Mc Phearson et al. (1991) have observed that individual and multiple antibiotic resistances are associated with antimicrobial use. A study in Thailand has indicated that the pattern of antibiotic use among the farms can cause the risk of the development of resistant bacteria strains (Holmostro¨m et al., 2003). Little is known about the occurrence of antibiotic resistant bacteria in marine sediments near fish farms (Schmidt et al., 2000; Tendencia & DelaPena, 2001).

4. Antibiotic resistance in sea food

Sea foods are often susceptible to spoilage by putrefactive microorganisms. Sea foods usually spoil much more rapidly than meats obtained from warm blooded animals when stored at ordinary refrigerator temperatures, and the reason for this is almost certainly because of the marine products that are invariably contaminated with psychrophilic bacteria (Witter, 1961). These organisms not only multiply quite rapidly at refrigerator temperatures, but spoil fish about twice as fast at 37^0 F as at 30^0 F (Bluhm et al., 1956). Though proper vessel and fish plant sanitation are obviously highly desirable for production of high quality fish, it is quite possible to prepare fish of excellent bacteriological quality in quite primitive premises. In other words, the maintenance of high sanitary standards on fishing vessels and at shore plants does not necessarily insure good quality fish, though from an aesthetic stand point alone such conditions are highly desirable. It is the actual handling and treatment of the fish themselves which is of prime importance in determining their quality.

Reviews and original articles dealing with antibiotics in fish or shellfish preservation have been published from other laboratories (Tomiyama et al., 1955; Ingram et al., 1956). Antibiotics have been commonly used to preserve the fish from bacterial contamination. In 1943 penicillic acid was prepared and tested as a possible preservative for fish with poor success (Tarr, 1944). Later penicillin and streptomycin were examined with similar disappointing results (Tarr, 1948). In the spring of 1950, a number of the newer antibiotics were studied and the findings were much more encouraging since Aureomycin, Terramycin and Chloromycetin all gave quite significant preservation in comparatively low concentration (Boyd & Tarr, 1956). Further experiments proved that of 14 antibiotics examined, Aureomycin (chlortetracycline, CTC) was found most effective (Tarr et al., 1954) and it is with this antibiotic that all applied studies have been conducted (Gillespie et al., 1955; Steiner and Tarr, 1955; antibiotics as food preservatives; Tarr et al., 1954).

Effect of several new antibiotics and furan derivatives on growth of bacteria in fish products have been studied and they are: (1) Antibiotics: Aureomycin (Lederle Laboratories), Amphomycin, Etamycin, Bryamycin (Bristol Laboratories, Inc.); and (2) Furan derivatives: Furoxone, Furadantin, Nitrofurazone (Furacin), and N. F. 56 (N-5-nitro-2 furfurylidene-l-aminoguanidine sulphate) (Eaton Laboratories, Inc.) (**Table 1**). The technique is similar to that employed in previous studies with ground flesh (Tarr et al., 1950).

Compound	concentration (μg/g)	Bacterial counts (colony forming units × 10^6/g) at temperature			
		1^0C		5^0C	
		6	8	6	6
None		27	>600	600	130
Aureomycin (CTC)	2.5	1.3	0.5	7	19
Amphomycin	5			450	
Bryamycin	5				98
	10	92	340		
	20	19	470		
Etamycin	5		910		
	10		380		
Furoxone	2.5				32
Furadantin	2.5				85
Nitrofurazone	2.5				114
	10	37	>900		
	25	57	310		
	50	19	900		
NF-56	2.5				63
	25	157	837		
	50	76	367		
CTC+ Bryamycin	5				
	10	2.7	8		
CTC+ Bryamycin	2.5				
	5	4	1		
NF-56+ Bryamycin	25		>900		
	10				
Nitrofurazone+ Bryamycin	25				
	10	18	400		

Table 1. Effect of various antibiotics and Furan derivatives on growth of bacteria in Minced Lingod muscle at 0^0 and 4^0C (Boyd et al., 1955).

The search for antibiotics or other substances which could prove valuable in preventing microbiological spoilage of fish or fish waste products is continuing, and the results of trials with several new antibiotics and furan derivatives are presented. It has been argued that suppression of natural bacterial flora of fish by introduction of CTC might create favorable conditions for the growth of food poisoning microorganisms.

5. Antimicrobial resistance in drug development

5.1 Mechanism of antibiotic resistance in bacteria

A key factor in the development of antibiotic resistance is the ability of infectious organisms to adapt quickly to new environmental conditions. Bacteria are single-celled organisms that, compared with higher life forms, have small numbers of genes. Therefore, even a single random genetic mutation can greatly affect their ability to cause disease. And because most microbes reproduce by dividing every few hours, bacteria can evolve rapidly. A mutation that helps a microbe surviving to an antibiotic exposure will quickly become dominant throughout the microbial population. Microbes also often acquire resistance genes from each other through horizontal gene transfer mechanism which might enable them to be a multiple antibiotic resistant strain. It is also noted that the specificity of the interactions between antibiotics and various protein sequences within a bacterium resultse in significantly high ratio of mutations in its genome which leads to antibiotic resistance. There is also a relatively high possibility that a particular mutation in a certain target sequence will result in antibiotic resistance.

Antibiotics generally target a variety of essential bacterial functions. For instance, the β-lactam antibiotics and vancomycin interrupte cell wall synthesis of pathogens, whereas macrolides and tetracyclines disrupt the protein synthesis at ribosomal level. Bacteria may develop their antibiotic properties by a variety of mechanisms. According to a study by Nicolaou (2001), one mechanism of resistance is by degrading the antibiotic in a step by step process. This degradation starts when bacterial β-lactamases hydrolyzes the β-lactam ring thus rendering these antibiotics ineffective. A secondary resistance mechanism is then triggered when the antibiotic target is altered. As the next step, bacteria may block the entry of antibiotic to the site of action, resulting in decreased absorption, which in turn results in bacteria with decreased sensitivity to vancomycin due to thicker cell walls. Finally, bacteria may develop efflux pumps that actively pump antibiotics out of the cell so that they do not reach their target. Nicolaou also tested the findings experimentally with macrolides and has found that if the ribosomal binding site for macrolides changes so that these antibiotics bind with decreased affinity, then protein synthesis will not be disrupted.

5.2 Drug discovery

When bacteria contact with chemical substances, they show a positive or negative chemotaxis. If the substrates are acceptable for bacteria or can support bacterial growth, they show a positive chemotaxis and utilize the substrate as an organic source. If toxic, they respond by escaping from the chemical(s). Antibiotics selectively inhibit bacteria based on targeting a specific structure or function of bacteria, which means antibiotics act as toxins to bacteria. Mostly the targets of antibiotics are prokaryote-specific mechanisms and structures, which are not present in eukaryotes or they have different characteristics from those of eukaryotic cells. However, bacteria inherently have potential drug resistance mechanisms or they can acquire exogenous genes conferring drug resistance. Drug resistance therefore, occurs by such mechanisms. At present, four main categories of drug resistance mechanisms are known (Li & Nikadio, 2009). They are: (1) Drug inactivation or modification: for example, enzymatic deactivation of *Penicillin* G in some penicillin-resistant bacteria through the production of β-lactamases, (2) Alteration of target site: for example, alteration of PBP—the binding target site of penicillins—in MRSA and other penicillin-resistant bacteria, (3) Alteration of metabolic pathway: for example, some sulfonamide-resistant bacteria do not require para-aminobenzoic acid (PABA), an important precursor for the synthesis of folic acid and nucleic acids in bacteria inhibited by sulfonamides. Instead, like mammalian cells, they turn to utilizing preformed folic acid, and (4) Reduced drug accumulation: by decreasing drug permeability and/or increasing active efflux (pumping out) of the drugs across the cell surface (Li & Nikadio, 2009) .Some of these mechanisms have been well studied at the molecular level (Walsh, 2003).

The integrated approaches for maximizing the diversity of microbes in drug discovery programs have been reviewed recently, with selective isolation of novel microorganisms (Knight et al., 2003; Zhang et al., 2005; Bian et al., 2008; Wagner-Dobler et al., 2002). Recently Cubist Pharmaceuticals has constructed a multi-drug resistant *E. coli* strain, which carries resistance markers for 17 of the most frequently produced antibiotics. Thus, a comparison of extract activities against sensitive and resistant *E. coli* strains will allow researchers to rapidly discovering novel and specific active compounds that can be used as effective drugs against pathogenic strains (Baltz, 2008). From these studies, it is strongly anticipated that metagenomic libraries of the drug resistant microbial strains will drive drug discovery process now and in the future. Hence, undoubtedly, metagenome analysis technology combined with high throughput screening will bring innovation to the drug discovery.

6. Impact of antibiotic resistance on human health

It has been widely understood that the bacteria and other microorganisms that often cause infections are known to be remarkably resilient and have the ability to develop ways for surviving drugs that are meant to kill or weaken them. Recent scientific evidence suggests that during the last decade, antibiotic resistance by various mechanisms has increased worldwide in bacterial pathogens leading to treatment failures in human and animal infections (Singer et al., 2003). However, the resistance against different types of biocides (including disinfectants, antiseptics, preservatives, sterilants) has been studied and characterized (Russell, 1990 & 1995). Only limited sound scientific evidence to correctly assess the risks of antibiotic resistance induced by resistance to biocides is available (SCENIHR, 2009). Furthermore, research indicates that biocides and antibiotics may share some common behaviour and properties in their respective activity and in the resistance mechanisms developed by bacteria (Russell, 2003, Sheldon 2005).

Although antibiotic usage has clearly benefited the animal industry and helped providing affordable animal protein to the growing human population, the use of antibiotics in food production has also contributed to the emergence and spread of antibiotic multiple resistance (AMR). Along with antibiotics used for human medicine, the use of antibiotics for animal treatment, prophylaxis and growth promotion exerts an inestimable amount of selective pressure toward the emergence and propagation of resistant bacterial strains.

Animals can serve as mediators, reservoirs and disseminators of resistant bacterial strains and/or AMR genes. Consequently, imprudent use of antimicrobials in animals may eventually result in increased human morbidity, increased human mortality, reduced efficacy of related antibiotics used for human medicine, increased healthcare costs, increased potential for carriage and dissemination of pathogens within human populations and facilitated emergence of resistant human pathogens (**Figure 1**).

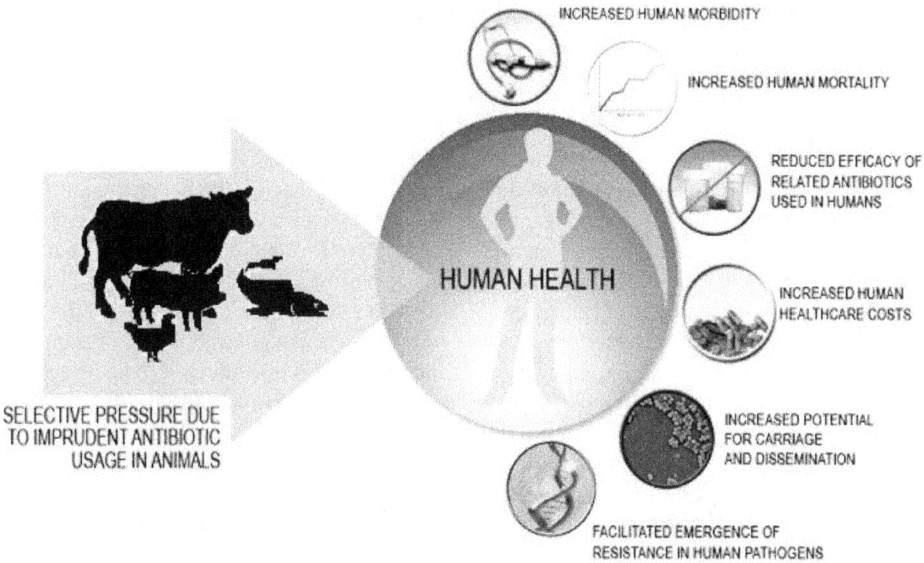

Fig. 1. The Human Health Impact of Antimicrobial Resistance in Animal Populations

According to Helms et al., (2002), the patients infected with pansusceptible *Sal*monella typhimurium are 2.3 times more likely to die within 2 years after infection than persons in the general Danish population, and that patient infected with strains resistant to amplicillin, chloramphenicol, streptomycin, suldonamide and tetracycline are 4.8 times (95% CI 2.2 to 10.2) more likely to die within 2 years. Furthermore, they have established that quinolone resistance in this organism is associated with a mortality rate 10.3 times higher than the general population.

It has been well documented that antimicrobial resistance due to a particular antibiotic used in food animals may result in reduced efficacy of most or all members of that same antibiotic class, some of which may be extremely important for human medicine (McDonald et al., 2001). The current pharmaceutical era faces multi resistant infectious disease organisms that are difficult and, sometimes, impossible to treat successfully. When there is an increase in numbers of bacteria that are resistant to antibiotics, it will be more difficult and more expensive to treat human bacterial infections. According to a study published by the Centers for Disease Control and Prevention (CDC), up to date, there are more than 100 antibiotics approved by the US Food and Drug Administration for human use. As antibiotics fail to treat recurring infections, the consequences include frequent visits to the doctor, hospitalization or even a need for a more expensive medication as a replacement for the existing ineffective ones (Levy, 2002). Increased healthcare costs are another important consequence of antimicrobial resistance. Increased costs are due to the need for additional antibiotic treatments, longer hospitalization, more diagnostic tests, higher professional costs and more pain management. In 1998, the Institute of Medicine estimated the annual cost of infections caused by antibiotic-resistant bacteria at US$ 4 to 5 million per year (McGowan, 2001). This occurrence of antibiotic resistance is found all over the world and has become a very serious problem in the treatment of diseases. The US Office of Technology Assessment report has attributed a cost of $1.3 billion per year for antibiotic-resistant infections in US hospitals. The fiscal cost of treating antibiotic resistant infections worldwide has been estimated to be many billions of dollars per year.

7. Conclusion

At present, there is insufficient information available to reach a final conclusion on the significance and impact of the presence of resistant bacteria in the environment which would allow the assessment of the potential risks related, for instance, to human health and ecosystem functions. Currently, it is thought that the input of antibiotics in general as well as from hospitals seems to be of minor importance, at least in terms of resistance. Up to now, antibiotics have not been detected in drinking water. The impact of antibiotics present in the aquatic environment on the frequency of resistance transfer is questionable. The information available to date suggests that the input of resistant bacteria into the environment from different sources seems to be the most important source of resistance in the environment. Therefore, the prudent use of antibiotics and disinfectants will significantly reduce the risk for the general public and for the environment. This not only means limiting the duration of selective pressure by reducing the treatment period and the continuous use of sub-therapeutical concentrations, but also includes controlling the dissemination of antibiotics being used, as well as prudent monitoring of resistance. However, a full environmental risk assessment cannot be performed on the basis of the data available; the availability of such data is a prerequisite if proper risk assessment and risk management programs for both humans and the environment are to be undertaken. Therefore, the careful use of antibiotics and the restriction of their input into the aquatic environment are the matters of necessity.

8. References

Aarestrup, F.M.,. Wegener, H.C., & Collignon, P. 2008. Resistance in bacteria of the food chain: epidemiology and control strategies. Expert Review of Anti-Infective Therapy. 6(5): p. 733-50.

Alanis, A.J. 2005. Resistance to Antibiotics: Are We in the Post-Antibiotic Era? Archives of Medical Research 36, 697-705.

Baltz, R. H. 2008. Renaissance in antibacterial discovery from actinomycetes. Current Opinion in Pharmacology. 8, 557–563.

Benveniste R, & Davies J. 1973. Mechanisms of antibiotic resistance in bacteria. Annual Review of Biochemistry. 42:471-506.

Bian, J., Song, F. & Zhang, L. 2008. Strategies on the construction of high-quality microbial natural product library. A review. Wei Sheng Wu Xue Bao 48, 1132–1137.

Bjorklund, H, Bergh, R.B., CMI, & Bylund, G. 1991. Residues of oxolinicacid and oxytetracycline in fish and sediments from fish farms. Thesis, Bjdrklund, H.

Oxytetracycline and oxolinic acid as antibacterials in aquaculture analysis, pharmacokinetics and environmental impacts. Department of Biology, Abe Akademi University, Finland.

Björkman, J., Nagaev, I., Berg, O.G., Hughes, D., & Andersson, D.I. 2000. Effects of Environment on Compensatory Mutations to Ameliorate Costs of Antibiotic Resistance. Science 287, 1479-1482.

Bluhm, H.M., Boyd, J.W., Muirhead, C.R., Tarr, H.L. 1956. Use of antibiotics for the preservation of fish and sea foods. American Journal of Public Health Nations Health. 46(12):1531-9.

Bonaventura, C., & Johnson, F.M. 2004. Healthy Environments for Healthy People. EHPS. Vol 1/105. Environmental Health Perspectives.

Boyd, J.W., & Tarr, H.L.A., 1956. Effect of chlortetracycline and storage temperatures on quality of shucked oysters. fishery research. Bd. Canada, Prog. Rep. Pacific coast stas., No. 105: 12-13.

Boyd, J.W., Bissett, H.M., & Tarr, H.L.A., 1955. Further observations on the distribution of chlortetracycline throughout ice blocks. Ibid. No. 102-14-15.

Browning, C.H., & Gulbransen, R., 1936. Immunity following cure of experimental Trypanosoma brucei infection by a chemotherapeutic agent. The Journal of Pathology and Bacteriology 43, 479-486.

Capone, D.G., Weston, D.P., Miller, V., & Shoemaker, C., 1996. Antibacterial residues in marine sediments and invertebrates following chemotherapy in aquaculture. Aquaculture 145, 55-75.

Castro, S.B.R., Leal, C.A.G., Freire, F.R., Carvalho, D.A., Oliveira, D.F., & Figueiredo, H.C.P. 2008. Antibacterial activity of plant extracts from Brazil against fish pathogenic bacteria. Brazilian Journal of Microbiology.39. No. 4. doi: 10.1590/S1517-83822008000400030

Chopra, I., & Roberts, M., 2001. Tetracycline Antibiotics: Mode of Action, Applications, Molecular Biology, and Epidemiology of Bacterial Resistance. Microbiology and Molecular Biology Reviews. 65, 232-260.

Costanzo, S.D., Murby, J., & Bates, J. 2005. Ecosystem response to antibiotics entering the aquatic environment. Marine Pollution Bulletin 51, 218-223.

Demain, A.L., & Sanchez, S., 2009. Microbial drug discovery: 80 years of progress. Journal of Antibiotics. 62, 5-16.

Doern, G.V., Heilmann, K.P., Huynh, H.K., Rhomberg, P.R., Coffman, S.L., & Brueggemann, A.B., 2001. Antimicrobial Resistance among Clinical Isolates of Streptococcus pneumoniae in the United States during 1999-2000, Including a Comparison of Resistance Rates since 1994-1995. Antimicrobial Agents Chemotheraphy. 45, 1721-1729.

Dolliver, H.A., & Gupta, S.C., 2008. Antibiotic losses from unprotected manure stockpiles. Journal of Environmental Quality. 37, 1238–1244.

Edquist, L.E., & Pedersen, K.B. 2001. Antimicrobials as growth promoters: resistance to common sense. In: Harremoës, P. (Chairman), Gee, D. (EEA Ed.), MacGarvin, M. (Executive Ed.), Stirling, A., Keys, J., Wynne, B., Guedes Vas, S. (Eds.), Late lesson From Early Warnings: The Precautionary Principle 1896–2000. Environmental Issue Report No. 22, European Environment Agency, Copenhagen, pp. 93–109.

EJF. 2003. Risky Business: Vietnamese Shrimp Aquaculture – Impacts and Improvements. London, UK7 Environmental Justice Foundation. pp. 44.

FAAIR, Policy recommendations. Clinical Infectious Diseases, 2002. 34 Suppl 3: p. 76-87.

Ferenci T. 2008. Bacterial physiology, regulation and mutational adaptation in a chemostat environment. Advances in Microbial Physiology. 53:169-229.

Gillespie, D.C., Boyd, J.W., Bissett, H.M., & Tarr, H.L.A., 1955. Ices containing chlortetracycline in experimental fish preservation. Ibid. 9:296-300.

Hare, R. 1970. The Birth of Penicillin, Allen & Unwin, London.

Hatha, M., Vivekanandhan, A.A., Julie Joice, G., & Christol, 2005. Antibiotic resistance pattern of motile aeromonads from farm raised fresh water fish. International Journal of Food Microbiology 98, 131-134.

Hektoen, H., Berge, J.A., Hormazabal, V., & Yndestad, M., 1995. Persistence of antibacterial agents in marine sediments. Aquaculture 133, 175-184.

Helms, M., Vastrup, P., Gerner-Smidt, P., & Molbak, K. 2002. Excess Mortality Associated with Antimicrobial Drug-Resistant *Salmonella*Typhimurium. Emerging Infectious Diseases. 8(5):490-495.

Hernando, M.D., Mezcua, M., Fernández-Alba, A.R., & Barceló, D., 2006. Environmental risk assessment of pharmaceutical residues in wastewater effluents, surface waters and sediments. Talanta 69, 334-342.

Herwig, R.P., Gray, J.P., & Weston, D.P., 1997. Antibacterial resistant bacteria in surficial sediments near salmon net-cage farms in Puget Sound, Washington. Aquaculture 149, 263-283.

Hirsch, R., Ternes, T., Haberer, K., & Kratz, K.L., 1999. Occurrence of antibiotics in the aquatic environment. The Science of The Total Environment 225, 109-118.

Holmström, K., Gräslund, S., Wahlström, A., Poungshompoo, S., Bengtsson, B.E., & Kautsky, N., 2003. Antibiotic use in shrimp farming and implications for environmental impacts and human health. International Journal of Food Science & Technology 38, 255-266.

ICON, 2003. Antibiotics: A Medical Dictionary, Bibliography, and Annotated Research Guide to Internet References. San Diego, CA: ICON Health Publications, 2003. http://www.answers.com/topic/antibiotic#ixzz1SzZAoJuz

IM, 1989. Institute of Medicine. Human health risks with the subtherapeutic use of penicillin or tetracyclines in animal feed. 1989. Washington, D.C.: National Academy Press.

Ingram, M., Barnes,E., & Shewan, J.M., 1956. Problems in the use of antibiotics for preserving meat and fish. Food science abstracts 28: 121-136.

Jalal, K.C.A., Fatin, Mardiana, Akbar John, B., Kamaruzzaman, Y.B., & Mohd. Nor. 2010. Antibiotic Resistance Microbes in Tropical Mangrove Sediments, East Coast Peninsular Malaysia. African Journal of Microbiology Research Vol. 4 (8), pp. 640-645

Jensen, L.B., Baloda, S., Boye, M., & Aarestrup, F.M., 2001. Antimicrobial resistance among Pseudomonas spp. and the Bacillus cereus group isolated from Danish agricultural soil. Environment International 26, 581-587.

Khachatourians, G.G., 1998. Agricultural use of antibiotics and the evolution and transfer of antibiotic-resistant bacteria. Canadian Medical Association Journal 159, 1129-1136.

Knight, V., Sanglier, J.J., DiTullio, D., Braccili, S., Bonner, P., Waters, J., Hughes, D., & Zhang, L., 2003. Diversifying microbial natural products for drug discovery. Applied Microbiology and Biotechnology 62, 446-458.

Kuijper, M.W.M., 2003. Marine and coastal environmental awareness building within the context of UNESCO's activities in Asia and the Pacific. Marine Pollution Bulletin 47, 265-272.

Kumar, K., Gupta, S., Chander, Y., Singh, A.K., 2005. Antibiotic Use in Agriculture and Its Impact on the Terrestrial Environment, in: Donald, L.S. (Ed.), Advances in Agronomy. Academic Press, pp. 1-54.

Kümmerer, K., 2003. Significance of antibiotics in the environment. Journal of Antimicrobial Chemotherapy 52, 5-7.

Kümmerer, K., 2009a. Antibiotics in the aquatic environment - A review - Part I. Chemosphere 75, 417-434.

Kümmerer, K., 2009b. Antibiotics in the aquatic environment - A review - Part II. Chemosphere 75, 435-441.

Lai, H.T., Liu, S.M. & Chieln, Y.H. 1995. Transformation of chloramphenicol and oxytetracycline in aquaculture pond sediments. Journal of Environmental Science and Health, Part A. Toxic / Hazardous Substances and Environmental Engineering. A30:1987–1993.

Le Tuan Xuan, Munekage Yukihiro, Phan Dao Anh Thi, Quan Dao & Quynh Thi. 2003. The environmental quality of shrimp ponds in mangrove areas. Proceedings of the Thirteenth (2003) International Offshore and Polar Engineering Conference Honolulu, HI, USA, May25 – 30; ISSN: 1098-6189 (set) 1-880653-60-5 (set). p. 255–262.

Levy, S. B. 2002. The antibiotic paradox: How the misuse of antibiotics destroys their curative powers. Cambridge: Perseus Publishing.

Li, X, & Nikadio H. 2009. Efflux-mediated drug resistance in bacteria: an update. Drug 69 (12): 1555–623.

Lu, S.Y., Zhang, Y.L., Geng, S.N., Li, T.Y., Ye, Z. M., Zhang, D.S., Zou, F., & Zhou, H.W., 2010. High Diversity of Extended-Spectrum Beta-Lactamase-Producing Bacteria in an Urban River Sediment Habitat. Applied Environmental Microbiology. 76, 5972-5976.

Marengo, J.R., Kok, R.A., O'Brien, K., Velagaleti, R.R., & Stamm, J.M., 1997. Aerobic biodegradation of (14C)-sarafloxacin hydrochloride in soil. Environmental Toxicology and Chemistry 16, 462-471.

Martinez, J.L., & Baquero, F., 2000. Mutation Frequencies and Antibiotic Resistance. Antimicrobial Agents Chemotheraphy. 44, 1771-1777.

McDonald, L.C., Rossiter, S., Mackinson, C., Wang, Y.Y., Johnson, S., Sullivan, M., Sokolow, R., DeBess, E., Gilbert, L., Benson, J.A., Hill, B. & Angulo, F.J. 2001. Quinupristin-Dalfopristin resistant *Enterococcus faecium* on chicken and in human stool specimens. New England Journal of Medicine. 345(16):1155-60.

McGowan Jr, J.E. 2001. Economic Impact of Antimicrobial Resistance. Emerging Infectious Diseases. 7(2):286-292.

McPhearson, R.M., DePaola, A., Zywno, S.R., Motes Jr, M.L., & Guarino, A.M., 1991. Antibiotic resistance in Gram-negative bacteria from cultured catfish and aquaculture ponds. Aquaculture 99, 203-211.

Miranda, C.D., & Zemelman, R., 2002. Bacterial resistance to oxytetracycline in Chilean salmon farming. Aquaculture 212, 31-47.

Neela, F., Nonaka, L., Rahman, M., & Suzuki, S., 2009. Transfer of the chromosomally encoded tetracycline resistance gene *tet* (M) from marine bacteria to; *Escherichia coli* and; *Enterococcus faecalis*. World Journal of Microbiology and Biotechnology 25, 1095-1101.

NIAID, 2006. The problem of antimicrobial resistance. National Institute of Allergy and Infectious Diseases, Division of Microbiology and Infectious Diseases, www.niaid.nih.gov/dmid/antimicrob

Nicolaou, K.C. 2001. A close look at the inner workings of microbes in the era of escalating antibiotic resistance is offering new strategies for designing drugs. Scientific American 2001; Vol 284: p 54-61.

Nygaard, K., Lunestad, B.T., Hektoen, H., Berge, J.A., & Hormazabal, V., 1992. Resistance to oxytetracycline, oxolinic acid and furazolidone in bacteria from marine sediments. Aquaculture 104, 31-36.

Olapade, O.A., Depas, M.M., Jensen, E.T., & McLellan, S.L., 2006. Microbial Communities and Fecal Indicator Bacteria Associated with Cladophora Mats on Beach Sites along Lake Michigan Shores. Applied Environmental Microbiology. 72, 1932-1938.

Perreten, V., Schwarz, F., Cresta, L., Boeglin, M., Dasen, G., & Teuber, M., 1997. Antibiotic resistance spread in food. Nature. 389, 801-802.

Pouliquen, H., & Le Bris, H., 1996. Sorption of oxolinic acid and oxytetracycline to marine sediments. Chemosphere 33, 801-815.

Prior, L.S.O.S., 2008. The 2008 Garrod Lecture: Antimicrobial resistance—animals and the environment. Journal of Antimicrobial Chemotherapy 62, 229-233.

Reynolds, D., 2010. Modern Medicine and The Overuse Of Antibiotics. http://www.healthytheory.com/modern-medicine-and-the-overuse-of-antibiotics

Russell, A.D. 2003. Biocide use and antibiotic resistance: the relevance of laboratory findings to clinical environmental situations. Lancet Infectious Disease. 3:794-803.

Russell, A.D., 1990. Mechanisms of bacterial resistance to biocides. International Biodeterioration 26, 101-110.

Russell, A.D., 1995. Mechanisms of bacterial resistance to biocides. International Biodeterioration & Biodegradation 36, 247-265.

Samuelsen, O.B., Torsvik, V., & Ervik, A., 1992. Long-range changes in oxytetracycline concentration and bacterial resistance towards oxytetracycline in a fish farm sediment after medication. Science of The Total Environment 114, 25-36.

SCENIHR, 2009. Scientific Committee on Emerging and Newly Identified Health Risks. Assessment of the Antibiotic Resistance Effects of Biocides. European Commission. pp.1-87.

Schmidt, A.S., Bruun, M.S., Dalsgaard, I., Pedersen, K., & Larsen, J.L., 2000. Occurrence of Antimicrobial Resistance in Fish-Pathogenic and Environmental Bacteria Associated with Four Danish Rainbow Trout Farms. Applied Environmental Microbiology. 66, 4908-4915.

Serrano, P.H. 2005.. Responsible use of antibiotics in aquaculture. In: Food and Agriculture Organization (FAO) Fisheries Technical Paper, 469, Roma, 97 p.

Sheldon, A.T. Jr. 2005.Antiseptic "resistance": real or perceived threat? Clinical Infectious Diseases. 40:1650-6.

Shoemaker, N.B., Vlamakis, H., Hayes, K., & Salyers, A.A., 2001. Evidence for Extensive Resistance Gene Transfer among Bacteroides spp. and among Bacteroides and Other Genera in the Human Colon. Applied Environmental Microbiology. 67, 561-568.

Singer, R.S., Finch, R., Wegener, H.C., Bywater, R., Walters, J., Lipsitch, M., 2003. Antibiotic resistance--the interplay between antibiotic use in animals and human beings. The Lancet Infectious Diseases 3, 47-51.

Steiner, G., & Tarr, H.L.A., 1955. Transport and storage of fish in refrigerated sea water: II. Bacterial spoilage of blue black salmon in refrigerated sea water and in ice, with and without assed chlortetracycline. Fish research Bd. Canada, Prog. Rep. pacific coast sras, No: 104: 7-8.

Tarr, H.L.A., & Deas, C.P., 1948. Action of sulpha compounds, antibiotics and nitrite on growth of bacteria in fish and flesh. Journal of fishery research. Bd. Canada. 7: 221-223.

Tarr, H.L.A., 1944. Chemical Inhibition of Growth of Fish Spoilage Bacteria. Journal of the Fisheries Research Board of Canada 6c, 257-266.

Tarr, H.L.A., Boyd, J.W., & Bissett, H.M., 1954. Antibiotics in food processing. Experimental preservation of fish and beef with antibiotiocs. Journal of Agriculture Food chemistry. 2: 372-375.

Tarr, H.L.A., Southcott, B.A., & Bissett, H.M., 1950. Effect of several antibiotics and food preservatives in retarding bacterial spoilage of fish. Fish. Res. Bd, Canada, Prog. Rep. pacific coast stas. No. 83:35-38.

Tendencia, E.A., & Dela Peña, L.D., 2002. Level and percentage recovery of resistance to oxytetracycline and oxolinic acid of bacteria from shrimp ponds. Aquaculture 213, 1-13.

Tolls, J., 2001. Sorption of Veterinary Pharmaceuticals in Soils: A Review. Environmental Science & Technology 35, 3397-3406.

Tomiyama, T., Nomura, M., & Kuroki,S. 1955. Effectiveness of aureomycin on keeping quality of sardine. Bulletin of Japanese society of scientific fisheries. 21: 262-266.

USEPA, 2002. Environmental and Economic Benefit Analysis of Final Revisions to the National Pollutant Discharge Elimination System Regulation and the Effluent Guidelines for Concentrated Animal Feeding Operations. EPA 821-R-03-003. USEPA Office of Water, Washington, DC.

Wagner-Döbler, I., Beil, W., Lang, S., Meiners, M., Laatsch, H., 2002. Integrated Approach To Explore the Potential of Marine Microorganisms for the Production of Bioactive Metabolites, in: Schügerl, K., Zeng, A.P., Aunins, J., Bader, A., Bell, W., Biebl, H., Biselli, M., Carrondo, M., Castilho, L., Chang, H., Cruz, P., Fuchs, C., Han, S., Han, M.R., Heinzle, E., Hitzmann, B., Köster, D., Jasmund, I., Jelinek, N., Lang, S., Laatsch, H., Lee, J., Miirkl, H., Maranga, L., Medronho, R., Meiners, M., Nath, S., Noll, T., Scheper, T., Schmidt, S., Schüigerl, K., Stäirk, E., Tholey, A., Wagner-Döbler, I., Wandrey, C., Wittmann, C., & Yim, S.C. (Eds.), Tools and Applications of Biochemical Engineering Science. Springer Berlin / Heidelberg, pp. 207-238.

Wainwright, M. 1988. Selman A.Waksman and the streptomycin controversy. Soc.gen. Microbial. Quarterly, 15: 90-92

Walsh, C. 2003. Antibiotics—Action, Origin, Resistance. ASM Press, Washington, D.C.

Weston, D.P. 1996. Environmental considerations in the use of antibacterial drugs in aquaculture. In: Baird D, Beveridge M, Kelly L,Muir J, editors. Aquaculture and Water Resources Management. Black-well Science; 140–65.

Witter, L.D., 1961. Psychrophilic Bacteria--A Review. Journal of Dairy Science 44, 983-1015.

World Health Organization 2003. Dept. of Communicable Disease Prevention Control and Eradication., Danish Veterinary Institute., and Danmarks jordbrugs forskning, Impacts of antimicrobial growth promoter termination in Denmark : the WHO international review panel' s evaluation of the termination of the use of antimicrobial growth promoters in Denmark : Foulum, Denmark 6-9, Geneva: World Health Organization. 57 p.

Zhang, L., An, R., Wang, J., Sun, N., Zhang, S., Hu, J., & Kuai, J., 2005. Exploring novel bioactive compounds from marine microbes. Current Opinion in Microbiology 8, 276-281.

7

Biofilms: A Survival and Resistance Mechanism of Microorganisms

Castrillón Rivera Laura Estela and Palma Ramos Alejandro
Universidad Autónoma Metropolitana, Departamento de Sistemas Biológicos, México

1. Introduction

Biofilms are microbial monoespecie or multispecie (consortium) communities that are the most successful colonization among microorganisms, are ubiquitous in nature and responsible for many diseases. They are considered growing communities of microorganisms embedded in a self-produced exopolysaccharide matrix and are attached to an inert surface or living tissue (Castrillón et al., 2010).

It is believed that this organization represents the mode of cell growth that allows cells to survive in hostile environments, disperse to form new niches and gives them significant advantages in protection against environmental fluctuations such as humidity, temperature, pH, the concentration of nutrients and waste removal (Costerton et al., 1987, Hall-Stoodley et al., 2004).

There is an association between the presence of biofilm-grown microorganisms with delayed wound healing and various diseases such as endocarditis, otitis media, chronic prostatitis, cystic fibrosis, periodontitis, and related infections medical devices and implants responsible for nosocomial infections (Castrillón et al., 2011, Donlan & Costerton, 2002). The latter share common features, although the causative organism and the site of infection are very different, they all evade host defenses and resist treatment with antimicrobials. In general, bacteria in biofilms tolerate high levels of antibiotics compared with planktonic cells (free). The ability of biofilm formation is not restricted to any specific group of bacteria or fungus and is now considered that under ideal conditions all microorganisms can form biofilms (Lasa et al., 2005).

2. Stages of development of biofilms

The main experimental models for studying bacterial biofilms are four: *Escherichia coli, Psedomonas aeruginosa, Bacillus subtilis and Staphylococcus aureus* (Lopez et al., 2010) and fungi *Candida albicans* and *Aspergillus fumigatus* (Kumamoto, 2002, Müller et al. 2011). In these works describes the development of a biofilm which begins with planktonic bacteria (free) that bind irreversibly to a surface in a continuous process in accordance with various stages of development are:, b) adhesion, c) synthesis of extracellular matrix, d) maturation and e) dispersion, which leads to the formation of a uniform structure of deposits and accumulations of viscous and homogeneous material surrounding the cells by a polymer matrix with open channels for water movement (Figure 1).

Any natural or synthetic surface is covered by the constituents of the local environment, electrolytes, water and organic materials form a film before the arrival of the organism which neutralize the charge over the surface (conditioning) that prevents the aproximation between bacterial cells fungi and so begins adherence, these organic compounds can serve as nutrients for these microorganisms.

Free (or planktonic) cells form a layer that is adsorbed to the surface for short periods by electrostatic attraction forces and released from it by reversible adsorption (Bos et al., 1999). In this phase the microorganisms are still susceptible to action of antibiotics.

The microorganisms in suspension are aggregated and cell adhesion occurs with same or different cells (co-aggregation) to the surface conditioned, this process is favored by several bacterial components involved in this process by overcoming the repulsive forces such as pili or flagella, and surface polymers such as lipopolysaccharide in Gram-negative bacteria and mycolic acid in Gram-positive. The expression of these microbial structures may change depending on the environment in which they are and thus change the phase of biofilm formation. Mutants no-mobile fail to form monolayers and their union as microcolonies therefore mobility structures play an important role in the initiation of biofilm (Stickler, 1999).

The physicochemical properties of the surface can exert a strong influence on the degree and extention of adherence, the germs adhere more readily to hydrophobic surfaces, non-polarized and plastics such as Teflon, compared to hydrophilic metals such as glass or metal.

Once irreversible adhesion is achieved, the cells divide and colonize the surface and when the local concentration of chemical signals produced by microbial metabolism reaches a threshold level, suggesting that the microbial population density has reached a minimum, this determines the start of phenotypic changes in the community.

The process in which a microbial cell senses the proximity of other cells reaching a critical number in a limited space in the environment, chemical signals are generated corresponding to secondary metabolites, known as *quorum sensing*, this fact results in the autoinduction in the synthesis of the extracellular matrix or exopolysaccharide (composed of polysaccharides, proteins, nucleic acids and lipids), and thus gets to the maturation of biofilm formation with subsequent three-dimensional structure, generated by water channels that serve as the microcirculation in colonies. When the message is large enough, the organism responds like a mass and behaves as a group (Keller & Surette, 2006). The composition of the exopolysaccharide or glycocalyx is different for each bacteria and fungus, and varies depending on culture conditions, medium and substrates which are: alginate in *P. aeruginosa*, cellulose in *S. typhimurium*, rich in galactose in V. *cholerae* and poly-N-acetylglucosamine in *S. aureus* (Whitehead et al., 2001, Sutherland 1997). This matrix allows the interconnection of immobilized cells and acts as a digestive system that keeps external extracellular enzymes close to the cells and enables them to metabolize biopolymers and colloidal solids (Sauer et al., 2002, Flemming & Wingender, 2010).

The detachment may be seen as another stage of the life cycle of the biofilm, which can be reached or not depending on environmental conditions such as nutrient availability, oxygenation, pH and specific compounds because at some point the high density cell can result in severe, dynamic gradients of nutrients and toxic metabolic sub-products, then some cells are released from the matrix to colonize other surfaces closing the process of formation and development of biofilms, this process may be the result of several factors such as are: mechanical forces as the flow of blood vessel, cessation of production of exopolysaccharides and detachment factors such as enzymes that destroy the matrix or surfactants.

Fragments of biofilm with viable cells can be dispersed in liquids or aerosols. The scattering process is of interest for their potential to promote the spread of bacteria or fungi in the ambient or their ability to exploit these processes to combat infections (Hall-Stoodley & Stoodley, 2005).

For the development cycle of *Candida albicans* biofilms has shown that scattered cells show a distinct phenotype associated with increased virulence (Uppuluri et al., 2010). When the extracellular medium accumulates enough of these molecules activate specific receptors that alter gene expression and affect different phenotypes that produce virulence factors such as enzymes and toxins or rhamnolipid of *P. aeruginosa* cell that are protective of fagocytosis, the *quorum sensing* determines tolerance to antibiotics and innate inflammatory response dependent on polymorphonuclear cells.

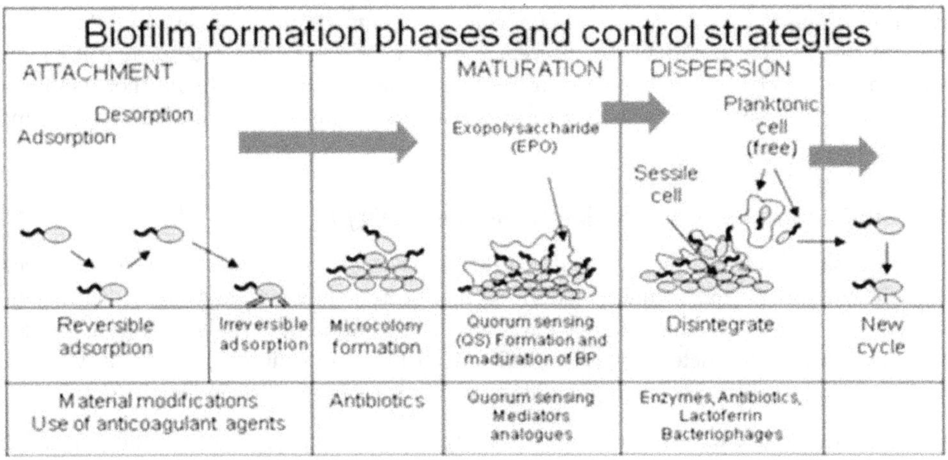

Biofilm formation occurs as a series of sequential events that depend on the interaction of microorganisms on inert surfaces or living, by overcoming the repulsive forces to achieve irreversible adsorption followed by the formation of a microcolony. Upon reaching a certain population density, induce the synthesis of secondary metabolites (*quorum sensing*) that produces an exopolysaccharide formation until maturation of the biofilm. Disintegration allows the formation of a new colony or elimination. It shows the treatment options for different stages of biofilm development.

Fig. 1. Phases of biofilm formation and dispersal strategies.

The main characteristic that best distinguishes chronic infections associated with biofilm to acute infections is their response to treatment with antibiotics, in general biofilm microorganisms tolerate high levels of antibiotics compared to planktonic cells and cause recurrent episodes. In the case of acute infections these are eliminated after a short treatment. In addition, acute infections are more aggressive than those associated with chronic infections or implants as the latter persist for months or years and progress through periods of rest alternating with exacerbations.

3. Host resistance to biofilm

Biofilms cause chronic infections characterized by persistent inflammation and tissue damage despite treatment with antibiotics and innate and adaptive immune responses of the host.

Planktonic cells that are released directly from the biofilm was removed by the action of antibiotics and phagocytic cells activated, but the organization as a biofilm is considered as a very efficient defensive strategy adopted since these microorganisms grow slowly and are protected mechanisms of host resistance through various strategies among which are a) inability of antibodies, complement and lysozyme to penetrate these organizations multicellular b) production of catalase bacteria that prevents the action of hydrogen peroxide produced by oxidative mechanisms of phagocytic cells c) inhibition of host immune function such as chemotaxis, opsonization and bactericidal potential exopolysaccharide (Lasa et al., 2005).

A study has demonstrated inability of the immune system clearance sessile cells that persist for weeks and months was observed when the peritoneal cavity of rabbits were inoculated mature biofilms of *P. aeruginosa* in immunocompetent animals, the penetration of phagocytic cells in the biofilm was detected, however, these cells were unable to phagocytose the bacteria (Ward et al., 1992). A similar response was described with the inoculation of fragments of the same biofilm bacteria trapped in agar beads and introduced into the lung (Woods et al., 1980).

4. Identification tests and antibiotic susceptibility in biofilms

In clinical samples, a biofilm is difficult to detect in routine diagnosis but may be recognized by light microscopy and accurate identification of bacteria in a biofilm can only be done by techniques of hybridization, fluorescein staining, the molecular probe 16SRNA domain eubacteria (EUB 338), determining live cell / dead BacLight staining or by identifying the matrix components by specialized staining techniques (Veeh et al., 2003).

Routine microbial cultures provide misleading results because they do not reflect the increasing resistance of bacteria growing in biofilms. The minimum inhibitory concentration (MIC) of bacteria grown as biofilm is 100 to 1000 times higher compared to planktonic cells despite antibiotic susceptibility in the laboratory (Costerton et al., 1999).

There are no standardized methods to date used routinely to determine the antibiotic sensitivity of bacteria grown as biofilms. When sampling swab and plating growth obtained in cultures performed standardized susceptibility testing, these same antibiotics fail to solve conventional bacterial infections This is because bacteria grow attached and the surface as a biofilm. However, in many cases it is not possible to recover the bacteria by traditional culture methods. This has been reported in infections where *Staphyococcus* biofilms emerging vascular grafts stimulate the production of antibodies against biofilms initiated within 10 days of colonization, however, cells were never recovered by conventional techniques of microbial culture (Costerton al ., 2003), another case is related to infections in medical devices where antibiograms shown susceptibility against some microorganisms but the infection fails to be eliminated by these antibiotics (Fux et al., 2005).

It is very important to point out that the systems sensitivity to antibiotics were traditionally performed on cells in suspension, which is equivalent to the population of planktonic cells, for this reason, is necessary to design new laboratory techniques that reveal the sensitivity of these substances directly on biofilms, this idea has been reported that antibiotics active against stationary phase bacteria *in vitro* are successful in removing biofilms *in vitro* infections (Zimmerli et al., 1998).

This information is important to consider that when it is mentioned that biofilm infection has hematogenous dissemination must specify if they are planktonic cells or biofilm fragments because there are differences in their ability to resist antibiotics, adherence and host response resistance.

5. Horizontal gene transfer

Mobile elements such as plasmids and transposons, have proven important in the transfer of antibiotic resistance is enhanced when the cell density increases and competition genetic, hence that biofilms are an ideal state to promote the horizontal transfer of genes (Ghigo, 2001). However, there is evidence that when bacteria of a biofilm is dispersed is rapidly becoming susceptible so their resistance is not the result of mutations and mobile elements (Stewart & Costerton, 2001, Stewart, 2002).

Increasing resistance to beta-lactams, aminoglycosides and fluoroquinolones has been correlated to the frequency of mutations in bacteria that grow as biofilms (Hoiby et al., 2010). These facts lead to rapid and global spread of genes in natural environments and in hospitals favoring nosocomial infections associated with biofilms.

6. Mechanisms of resistance associated with biofilms

The conventional mechanisms of resistance to antibiotics and biocides fall into four categories: direct inactivation of the active molecule, altering the body's sensitivity by changing its target of action, reducing the concentration of the drug reaches its target unchanged its chemical composition and efflux systems (Hogan & Kolter, 2002, Poole 2002). However, most information comes from studies that were performed in suspension cultures and in general, bacteria in biofilms tolerate high levels of antibiotics compared to what their planktonic cells. In different settings, the level of antibiotic resistance may vary and the factors causing this increase may differ.

The primary evidence indicates that conventional mechanisms do not explain the high resistance to antimicrobial agents associated with biofilms, although this evidence does not exclude the possibility of resistance in the growth of adherent cells. This suggests that the development of resistance in bacteria that are aggregated on surfaces or biofilm has its own intrinsic mechanisms are different and are responsible for those conventional antibiotic resistance, and although currently no single accepted mechanism, we have explored several potential candidates as responsible for this high resistance characteristic of biofilms among which are: Diffusion limited, neutralizing enzymatic, functional heterogeneity, slow growth, persistent cells and biofilm phenotype corresponding to adaptive mechanisms to stress such as efflux pumps and alterations in membrane. (Figure 2).

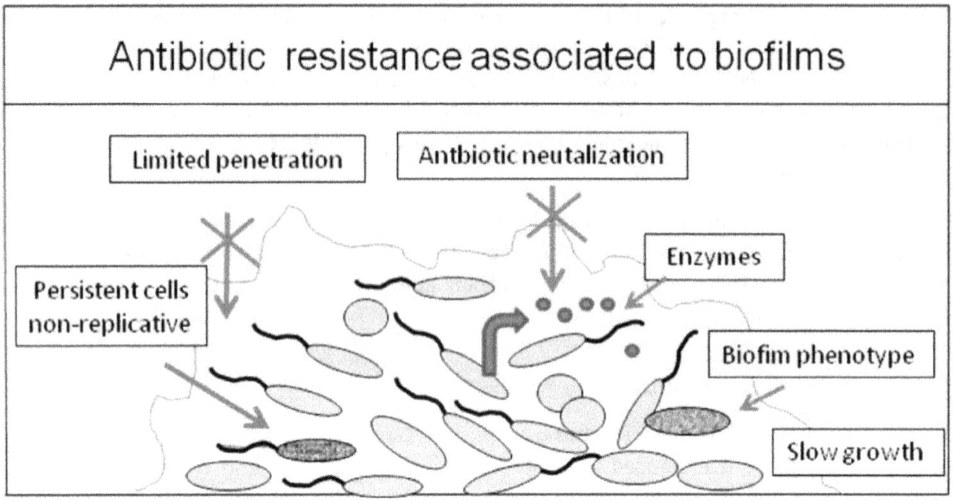

The antibiotic may be retained by interactions with the extracellular matrix or be neutralized by the production of enzymes that modify it. The metabolic heterogeneity may alter the growth preventing antibiotic action if its molecular target requires active metabolic pathways, or the oxygenation or pH gradients inhibit the action of the antimicrobial. The appearance of persistent or phenotype within biofilm makes it insensitive to the antibiotic

Fig. 2. Antibiotic resistance associate to biofilms.

6.1 Low penetration

Antibiotics can diffuse through the biofilm matrix, to inactivate the cells trapped, but this exopolysaccharide behaves as a physical barrier affecting its spread to deeper layers by direct interaction of these molecules to modify their transport to the interior, causes resistance to these antimicrobials, as well as high molecular weight molecules with cytotoxic properties as lysozyme and complement. So, while planktonic cells are quickly exposed to high concentrations of antibiotics, the microorganisms in deep layers are gradually exposed to increasing the concentration of antibiotics.

Bacteria that are deficient in polysaccharide synthesis and therefore of produce biofilm, escape from the biofilm and are susceptible to attack by immunocompetent cells. An antibiotic may be inactivated or sequestered by binding to the extracellular matrix as in the case of the alginate exopolysaccharide of *P. aeruginosa* which is anionic nature. Which explains why the fluoroquinolones and aminoglycosides penetrate slowly rapidly since the latter positively charged bind to the matrix has a negative charge, but this mechanism can be saturated if repeated doses are administrated (Lewis, 2001, Gordon et al. , 1988, Mah & O'Toole, 2001).

The penetration of chlorine does not reach concentrations greater than 20% in mixed cultures of *K. pneumoniae* and *P. aeruginosa* biofilms. In case of biofilms of *S. epidermidis* vancomycin reaches deep layers but not rifampin (Mah & O'Toole, 2001).

Has also been observed that the thickness of the biofilm is important for the penetration of hydrogen peroxide was allowed in layers with 3.5 log CFU *P. aeuroginosa* and not diffusion when the layer was 7.6 log CFU, however, the absence of catalase gene (kata) makes it easy access even if the biofilm is thick (Stewart et al., 2000).

The dissemination and death from alkaline hypochlorite (pH 11) and chlorosulphamate (pH 5.5) was evaluated on biofilms of *P. aeruginosa.* The chlorosulfamate transport was not affected unlike hypochlorite delaying their penetration, however both biocides enter to the biofilm and fail to kill cells suggesting an alternative mechanism to explain the resistance to these substances (Stewart et al., 2001).

Other explanations for the failure to altering the penetration of antimicrobial agents in biofilms *K. pneumoniae* are that the cells are stacked or is the result of problems of bioavailability of the drug (Smith, 2005).

Reduced mobility of an antibiotic is not an impenetrable barrier and is not sufficient to explain the resistance, it is assumed that other mechanisms must be involved. Recently it has been suggested that the delay in permeability through the biofilm allows the bacteria have enough time to implement adaptive responses to stress.

6.2 Neutralization

If an antibiotic penetrates the biofilm enzyme production by microorganisms can degrade or modify are synthesized by enzymes that selectively destroy the activity of antibiotics. These enzymes are a series of proteins that use multiple adaptive strategies to confer resistance such as hydrolysis (β-lactams, macrolide esterases epoxidase) and modification of antibiotics by acyltransferases, phosphorylation, glycosylation, nucleotidilación, ribosylation and transfer of thiol groups (Wright, 2005, Castrillón et al., 2003, Gallant et al., 2005, Martinez-Suarez et al., 1985). These enzymes accumulate in the glycocalyx as a result of its secretion or cell lysis (by action of the antibiotic on the microorganisms from the biofilm surface or planktonic).

Neutralization acts synergistically with delayed diffusion and degradation of the antimicrobial into the biofilm. An important mechanism of resistance in cystic fibrosis by *P. aeruginosa* is due to the overproduction of cephalosporinase AmpC enzymes which is its main mechanism of resistance to beta lactam in the presence of high levels of carbapenems such as imipenem which is a strong inducer in contrast with ceftazidime is weak probably due to its inactivation in the biofilm (Del Valle, 2009, Giwercman, 1991).

The filters impregnated with antibiotics and its direct action on biofilms *K. pneumoniae* has shown that the antibiotic diffuses only in the presence of mutant cells β-lactamases but growth is observed, suggesting that another mechanism of resistance must be considered (Anderl et al., 2000).

6.3 Heterogeneity

To determine the rate of microbial growth within a biofilm microelectrodes were used with probes for direct measurement of oxygen in different areas of the biofilm, and the use of acridine orange to identify fast-growing cells (stained orange) or slow (stained yellow/ green) according to their relative concentration of RNA / DNA. (Mah & O'Toole 2001). These studies demonstrate that biofilms are structurally and metabolically heterogeneous in which aerobic and anaerobic processes occur simultaneously and display areas so that metabolically inactive antimicrobial response may vary depending on the location of an individual cell within the community and that the high level of activity on the surface and limited or absent growth inside reduces the susceptibility to antibiotics.

These studies have shown that biofilms are heterogeneous structures with three chemical patterns that correspond to differences in concentration gradients from outside to inside the biofilm. The pattern of metabolic substrate induces a higher concentration on the outside and less inside, the metabolic product pattern is reversed to the previous and the pattern of metabolic intermediates shows a greater concentration between the boundary of the biofilm in the aqueous phase (Stewart & Franklin , 2008). These patterns bring the result that within these structures are established differences in pH gradients and oxygenation as it has been shown that the penetration of oxygen as high as 25% in the depth of the biofilm (Borriello et al., 2004). These facts are installed microbial populations aerobic or facultative anaerobes within the different layers of the biofilm, allowing us to understand the differences in susceptibility to treatment with antibiotics, which is different from the response to the free forms (plankton) that the attached (sessile).

Deprivation of oxygen and anaerobic growth of microorganisms affects the action of aminoglycosides which is modulated by the availability of oxygen and pH gradients (Wimpenny, 2000).

6.4 Slow growth

When an organism is limited nutrients, slow growing and may cause resistance to antibiotics. Cells within biofilms are under a gradient of nutrients resulting in metabolically active cells with access to these nutrients in the surface layer or on the periphery of the biofilm, in contrast, metabolically inactive cells are found within its interior. These different areas of metabolic activity correspond to different areas of antimicrobial susceptibility

The decrease in growth rate and low metabolic activities decrease the cell permeability and therefore the access of antimicrobial substances, metabolic inactivity can also reach a level where the bacteria are viable but have lost their ability to be cultivated this state of non-culturable viable cells is the main reason for the low detection of biofilm infections by standardized culture methods.

The cytotoxic action of many antibiotics is dependent on the growth of microorganisms such as penicillins that are active are active only in growing cells, many antibiotics are targeting some kind of molecular synthesis and have no effect on bacteria where this synthesis has stopped, and cells in the interior might be protected from the cytotoxic action of these substances (Brown and Allison, 1988). Penicillin and ampicillin do not attack cells that are not growing and its action is proportional to its activity, other antibiotics such as β-lactams, cephalosporins, aminoglycosides and fluoroquinolones attack stationary phase cells, but are more active in dividing cells (Costerton et al., 1999). It has been determined resistance to cetrimide on *E. coli*, ciprofloxacin on *S. epidermidis*, tobramycin and piperacillin in *P. aeruginosa*, this effect is associated with decrease in growth rate (Donlan & Costerton, 2002).

Antimicrobial peptides are natural products produced as part of the arsenal of protection in the host innate responses and target microbial membrane (Castrillón et al., 2007). Colestine peptide (polymyxin E) has been used in the treatment of multidrug-resistant cancer patients and cystic fibrosis by *P. aeruginosa* (Hachem et al., 2007), this antibiotic is the only antimicrobial activity against the central part of biofilms *in vitro,* while the metabolically active at the surface become tolerant due to the regulation system *pmr* operon genes and the MexAB-OprM. Ciprofloxacin and tetracycline are able to clear metabolically active cells so it is suggested that combination therapy with these antibiotics colistin for early eradication of *P. aeruginosa* in patients with cystic fibrosis (Pamp et al., 2008).

6.5 Persistent cells

A small percentage of the cell population remains viable after prolonged exposure (or overdoses) to antibiotics known as persistent, and gives (or not) their resistance to progeny once the selective pressure is removed. This susceptibility to the threshold of growth varies depending on the mode of action of antibiotic used.

Persistent cells are cells that temporarily quit the replication for the survival of the community and their strategy is different from the stress-related adaptive responses in which the population expresses resistance proteins in response to potential environmental damage. Persistent cells survive doses of antibiotics that kill normal cells and increase in number when there is a high cell density reached the highest number in the stationary phase suggesting that their main role is to ensure the survival of cells that are not growing (Lewis 2008).

These cells are different from the antibiotic-resistant mutants do not produce offspring resistant to the antibiotic in his absence and can grow in the presence of the antibiotic while maintaining the same minimum inhibitory concentration (MIC) in contrast to the mutants.

The main evidence of the existence of persistent cells in biofilms are: a) there is a biphasic dimension in biofilms wich means that much of the population is attacked fast and another is not affected even with a prolonged course of antibiotics, b) description of gene of persistence (*hip*) that act as regulatory circuits that allow them to enter and leave this state as a protective response, c) bacteriostatic antibiotics inhibit the growth of sensitive cells are those that contribute to persistent cell growth and preservation of biofilm d) when therapy is withdrawn biofilm again reshape (Herrera 2004).

The production of persistent cells in biofilms in bacteria is highest during the stationary phase in planktonic culture of the biofilm, however, in the case of *Candida albicans* their formation occurs only when growth occurs as a biofilm (Spoering & Lewis, 2001).

Although the date is unknown the basics of the physiology of these persistent cells, several genes involved has been described for their generation, including locus have identified three hip (high-level-persistence): A, B and AB control the frequency of this phenotype. The identification of genes and their products may be targets for developing new therapies (Keren et al., 2004).

All *hip* mutant cells produce a thousand times more cells persistent than the wild variant (Moyed & Broderick 1986). The importance of the appearance of these cells determines the success of treatment with antimicrobial use as the minimum bactericidal concentration would kill 99.9% of cells in biofilms, and the remaining would be eliminated by the immune system, without however, the presence of persistent cells limits the removal of the population of microbial cells or in the case of a dysfunction in the patient's immune response may be the cause of recurrent infections.

6.6 Biofilm phenotype

Nutritional starvation and high cell density in a limited space are important features in in the physiology of planktonic cultures reaching stationary phase. Hence the formation of a biofilm represents this natural phase of bacterial growth by increasing production of secondary metabolites such as antibiotics, pigments and other molecules, which act as signaling molecules to form (or inhibition of growth of other microorganisms) of biofilms (Lopez et al., 2010).

The response to environmental stresses such as heat shock, pH changes, oxygen and chemicals among others, cause physiological changes that act as protective antagonizing the harmful effects by inducing protective mechanisms such as efflux pumps of antibiotics, changes membrane level or phase variation.

In biofilms in response to treatment with antibiotics, appear subpopulations with different phenotypes that vary in their gene expression but not in their genetic material (Fux et al, 2005). This was confirmed when performing subcultures in fresh medium in which not only provide nutrients but also dilutes the cell-cell signaling, the cells regain susceptibility to the antibiotic, demonstrating the absence of mutations.

The gene expression patterns in biofilms of *P. aeruginosa* produce different phenotypes that differ from their planktonic counterparts (Sauer et al., 2002) and a small proportion of cells develop a protective phenotype that coexists with the cells sensitive to antibiotics and has been suggested by some authors that corresponds to that expressed by a spore (Stewart & Costerton, 2001).

A biofilm community that shows resistance to treatment by antibiotics and develops a characteristic phenotype such as biofilm growth has been called "biofilm phenotype" and have come to propose the existence of specific genes and reference to their therapeutic targets, however , DNA microarrays and gene expression in *Bacillus subtilis* biofilms differ only 6% compared to their planktonic cells and only 1% in *Pseudomonas aeruginosa*. At present, the differential expression of these genes has not proven useful for this purpose (Fux et al., 2005).

6.6.1 Efflux pumps

Accumulation of antibiotics in the periplasmic space inside the bacteria is antagonized by efflux pumps that are resistant to several classes of antibiotics including tetracyclines, macrolides, fluoroquinolones, β-lactam and reducing their concentration at sub-toxic level (Van Bambeke et al ., 2003).

Efflux pumps are protein structures that are able to expel from the bacterial cytoplasm and periplasm for bacteria toxic compounds such as antibiotics. The expression of these pumps can be permanent (constitutive expression) or intermittent (expression can be induced). These pumps may be specific to a substrate or similar compounds can be transported and may be associated with multidrug resistance (MDR). (Sánchez-Suarez et al., 2006, Grkovic et al., 2002).

In prokaryotes there are five families of efflux transporters: MF (major facilitator), MATE (multidrug and toxic efflux), RND (resistance-nodulation-division), SMR (small multidrug resistance) and ABC (ATP binding cassette). All of them require proton motive power and power supply.

The main systems reported in bacteria of interest in the clinic are: *Campylobacter jejuni* (CmeABC), *E. coli* (AcrAB-TolC, TolC-AcrEF, EmrB, EmrD), *Pseudomonas aeruginosa* (MexXY-OprM, MexCD-OprJ, and OprN MexEF Mex-XY-OprM), *Streptococcus pneumoniae* (PmrA), *Salmonella typhimurium* (AcrB) and *Staphylococcus aureus* (NorA) and *Candida albicans* (MRD1, CDR1 and CDR2) (Webber & Piddock, 2003).

It has been speculated the possibility of antibiotic resistance in biofilms of *P. aeruginosa* by the expression (or overexpression) of these pumps, however, none of the four efflux pumps in the genome of this bacterium contributes to the resistance (De Kievit et al., 2001). In contrast to these results, resistance to azithromycin is associated pumps MexAB-OprM and MexCD-OprJ to biofilm resistance mechanisms in *P. aeruginosa* (Gillis et al., 2005) and PA1874-1887 pump that is expressed at high level in both biofilms and planktonic cells (Zhang & Mah, 2008). Although the results are still inconclusive, have proposed the use of anti-inhibitor drugs efflux pumps (EPI) as potential anti-biofilm treatment have been well tolerated in humans (Kvist et al., 2008).

When cells bind to a surface, expressed a different phenotype to the planktonic cells and may be expressed as a resistance mechanism multidrug efflux pump as reported in *Escherichia coli* (AcrAB operon *mar)*. When *mar* expression was evaluated in a bioreactor and as growth in biofilm, the results support the idea that *mar* operon was expressed in biofilms where the lowest level was detected compared with the equivalent in stationary phase fermenter cultures (Maira Litrán et al., 2000a). The loss of acrAB *mar* did not affect the growth as biofilms of *E. coli* and resistance to ciprofloxacin is not dependent on the regulation of *mar* operons or acrAB (Maira Litrán et al., 2000b).

In the case of *Candida albicans* pumps for azoles was noted that in mutants *cdr* planktonic cells and *mdr* were hypersusceptible to fluconazole in contrast to cells that were resistant biofilm showing that resistance is a complex phenomenon that can not be explained by a single mechanism (Ramage et al., 2002).

6.6.2 Alterations in membrane proteins

The diffusion of any antibiotic depends on the permeability of its outer membrane that allows its diffusion of different routes to the periplasmic space. Porins are channel proteins of the outer membrane of Gram-negative bacteria involved in the transport of hydrophilic molecules from the external environment to the periplasmic space.

The genes encoding porins can mutate and produce nonfunctional or altered proteins can decrease their expression. Both processes give rise to mutant bacteria deficient in porins, which have low permeability to hydrophobic molecules pass (Hancock, 1997).

A quick change of balance in the expression of porins in response to antibiotic therapy confers an advantage to the pathogen compared with the commensal microflora that is susceptible to β–lactams (Pagés et al., 2008). In the case of *P. aeruginosa porin* OprD is used for the dissemination of imipenem and resistance is associated with its three-dimensional disturbance.

Porins in *E. coli* are OmpF and OmpC operated in response to changes in osmolarity. Mutations in ompB (regulator of OmpF and OmpC) increase resistance to β-lactam antibiotics, the mutants lacking OmpF are resistant to chloramphenicol and tetracycline.

The genes encoding porins are differentially expressed in biofilms and may contribute to antibiotic resistance. The expression of ompC and three other osmotically regulated genes are increased when the bacteria grow as biofilms in the environment a protective mechanism (Mah & O'Toole 2001).

6.6.3 Phase variation

In biofilm there is capacity development of subpopulations of bacteria or fungi to switch to the dormant metabolic state as small-colony known variants (SCVs) in which they are less susceptible to growth-dependent antibiotic killing, have a defective catalase activity interfere with oxidative metabolism and uptake of aminoglycoside modifying its minimum inhibitory concentration of 8 to 16 times compared with large colonies and normal as in the case of *Enterobacter aerogenes* (Neut et al., 2007, Rusthoven al., 1979).

The phase variation plays an integral role in the formation of diverse phenotypes within biofilms and is largely responsible for the recalcitrance of infections caused by biofilms, the increase in the reversal phase coincides with the antibiotic treatment. This phenomenon has been reported for several genera and species, including *Staphylococcus* and *Pseudomonas* genus, and certain species of Enterobacteriaceae and fungi. (Costerton et al., 1999).

The phase variation causes detectable changes in colonial morphology, the small colony variants of phase variant (SCVs) in biofilms develop properties hyperadherence, autoaggregation, increased hydrophobicity and reduced motility, it has been suggested that tolerate a wide variety of aggressive environmental conditions so that this process is considered a survival mechanism.

It was considered that the phase variation is a process of cellular internal rearrangement, however recently it has been considered to occur by interactions with genetic elements outside the cell as an internal bacteriophage genetic rearrangement by suggesting a model where mobile genetic elements generate the phase variation through a collective mechanism (Chia et al., 2008).

In *Pseudomonas aeruginosa* has shown that under different environmental pressures will favor the appearance of morphological variants that relate to the phenotype of biofilm among which are the small-colony variants (SCVs), rough small-colony variant (RSCVs), wrinkled variants, and rugose colonies autoaggregating cells. The phenotypes RSCVs and SCVs play a critical role in the colonization in cystic fibrosis and mutations in the *psl* locus in variants RSCVs lose their hyperadherence and autoaggregation abilities (β Häubler et al, 2003, Kirisits et al., 2005).

The SCVs of *S. aureus* differ from normal phenotype in size as they are ten times smaller than the wild colonies and are deficient in electron transport by auxotrophism to hemin / menadione, thiamine or thymidine. Their colonies are non-pigmented on agar plates and reduced coagulase production increases resistance to aminoglycosides and cell-wall active antibiotics. The specific role of the SCVs of *S. aureus* resistance to antibiotics in biofilms is still unknown (Proctor & Peters, 1998) although its presence in mixed biofilms with *Pseudomonas* has proven to be a survival mechanism against the attack of the exotoxins of *Pseudomonas* for which its wild form is sensitive (Biswas et al., 2009).

In staphylococcal biofilm formation requires intercellular adhesin (PIA) is a polymer whose main component is N-acetylglucosamine and is synthesized by several enzymes encoded by intercellular adhesion cluster (*ica*), the presence of these genes correlated with the morphology colonial and the ability to form biofilms, so the net growth in Congo red agar form black colonies when the adhesin is present and red in its absence (Ziebuhr et al., 1997). The *ica* operon is constituted by a group of four structural genes icaA, icaB, icaC and a regulatory component icaR (Diemond & Miranda, 2007). Adhesin negative mutants do not produce biofilms due to an IS256 transposon in the gene icaC (Cho et al., 2002).

It has recently been reported in strains of methicillin resistant *Staphylococcus aureus* (MRSA) that the presence of *ica* locus does not guarantee that its expression and does not directly reflect the ability of biofilm formation. Has been evaluated the participation of three regulatory genes *agr* and *sar*A and as well as the alternative transcription sigma factor *sig*B latter being responsible for the variation of biofilm (Jong-Hyun et al., 2008, Eftekhar & Dadaei T, 2011).

In *S. pneumoniae* have described two variants of colonial morphology between colonies spontaneously switched between transparent and opaque, the latter capable of forming two to six times the capsule, with limited bonding capacity and the possibility of evasion of host immune system, this variation observed both in planktonic growth conditions and in biofilm. Other variants described in aged biofilms are small and not mucoid without capsule (SCVs) with capacity to form hyperadherent biofilms, in contrast to the large and mucoid variants that appear late in the biofilm adhere poorly to surfaces forming flat structures unable to form biofilms. The SCVs of *S. pneumoniae* correlated with reduced capsule production and an increase in initial attachment instead to the opaque and transparent colonies, the SCV non capsule cells are not reversible due to a deletion in the capsule operon cps3DSU (Allegrucci & Sauer, 2007).

In *Candida parapsilosis* was previously thought that it was not able to form true filaments and biofilms, we now know they are not as large as those of *Candida albicans* and concentric phenotype forms quantitatively more biofilm in contrast to the smooth phenotype as it does in lesser extent and does not invade the agar (Laffey & Butler, 2005).

The coexistence of microorganisms in biofilms may lead to the emergence of phenotypic variants as in the case of *Pseudomonas putida* and *Acinetobacter* strain C6 where the excretion of benzoate by *Acinetobacter* as a result of the metabolism of benzyl alcohol, induces phase variation in *Pseudomonas* as rough colony (Kirkelund et al., 2007).

The importance of knowledge and isolation of these slow-growing variants (SCVs) are often misdiagnosed by routine microbiological analysis due to its unusual morphology and biochemical reactions which complicates eradication by failures in the antibiotic treatment

7. Biofilm control

Biofilms can be reformed if: a) there is growth of fragments, followed by debridement and cleaning, b) planktonic bacteria is spread, released from the biofilm residual, c) there is new growth of microorganisms in the biofilm (Cooper & Okhiria, 2010) .

Antibiofilms actions can be divided in two: 1) Prevention of formation. and 2) removal or destruction of biofilms. Among the prevention strategies for catheter-related infections that have developed protocols aqre aseptic filtered air in operating rooms which has reduced the incidence of these infections and are based on the correct implementation of the measures of asepsis during insertion and maintenance of vascular pathways. The formation and training of staff on the recommendations of the indication, insertion and maintenance of intravascular devices are the backbone of the prevention of catheter-associated infections.

The methods for controlling biofilms are basically: prevent adhesion (material handling, use of antibiotics or anticoagulants) to prevent bacterial differentiation and congregation (quorum sensing antagonists or use of lactoferrin), matrix elimination (enzymes) and recently the administration of specific bacteriophages (Figure 1).

Many of catheter-related infections due to microorganisms present in the skin are acquired when the catheters are inserted so that alternative strategies anti-colonization are being explored. Other alternatives would be to coat catheters or medical devices with antimicrobial agents (antibiotics, antiseptics and silver) incorporated into the implant material, with limited success. This is due to several reasons among which are the fact that biofilm infections are chronic and the half-life of these substances is shorter on the other hand the incorporation of these drugs can damage the implanted material or incompatibility with the host.

The coating of catheters with antibiotics or biocides such as rifampin and minocycline or cefazolin, chlorex, silver sulfadiazine and silver impregnation decreases the possibility of colonization, has also proved successful when the catheter is used for short periods and as a prophylactic measure, but counterproductive in the long term the huge problem of resistance (Lewis, 2001, Raad & Hanna, 1999).

The coating material with enzymes may be another option to prevent infections resulting from medical devices, recently reported peroxidase titanium coating which can generate antimicrobial hypothiocyanite hypoiodite or to form hydrogen peroxide or thiocyanate. This coated material and a liquid environment with substrates of the enzyme has been shown to limit the formation of biofilms of *Candida albicans* (Ahariz & Courtois, 2010).

Recently have proposed new alternatives for delivery of antibiotics into the biofilm with the use of liposomes or biodegradable complexes that allow the drug concentration at the interfaces of the biofilm (Smith, 2005).

The discovery of bacterial communication systems (*quorum sensing*) as a temporary facility during the infectious process has given an opportunity to decrease the bacterial infection by means other than growth inhibition. Because many bacteria use this communication system and control of virulence, *quorum sensing* mediators are the new targets for drug design (Hentzer & Givskov, 2003). These substances are known as quorum sensing inhibitors (QSI), which have been identified in nature and analogs have been synthesized by modifying its structure and assessed its activity in experimental systems *in vivo* and *in vitro*. QSI resistance occurs only in bacterial mutations.

In the case of gram-negative bacteria depends on the communication mechanism of the synthesis of N-acyl homoserinlactones (AHL), so they have developed analogs of this substance that are aimed at inhibiting biofilm formation by several mechanisms: a) inhibition of AHL signal generation, b) inhibiting the spread of the intracellular signal and c) inhibiting the reception of AHL. In Gram-positive bacteria that use peptides as signaling molecules of *quorum sensing*. A synthetic peptide called RIP interferes with the reception of these signals in *Staphylococcus aureus*, is active in its ability to inhibit biofilm formation in animal models (Balaban et al., 2007).

Substances that interfere in the formation of exopolysaccharide as xylitol and gallium have been used in formulations of oral biofilms management and iron chelating agents such as lactoferrin, deferoxamine and EDTA are candidates for use in controlling biofilms. Recently it was shown that lactoferrin, a ubiquitous and abundant substance in secretions, stimulates the disintegration of biofilms depends on its ability chelator of iron, essential for bacterial growth, and stability of the links necessary for the extracellular matrix biofilms. Their use encourages the release of planktonic cells rather than their aggregation and biofilm (Castrillón 2010, Rodríguez-Franco et al., 2005).

Endogenous production of enzymes allows degradation of exopolysaccharides of the biofilm to achieve dispersion of microorganisms for the generation of a new colony once the biofilm is mature and begin a new cycle of development, this allows us to propose the use of different enzymes for removal, however, due to the heterogeneity of extracellular polysaccharide, it is necessary to use a mixture enzymes for degradation. Among the most commonly used are dispersin D alginase, phage depolimerase, proteases, glycosidases: pectinase arabanase, cellulase, hemicellulase, beta-glucanase, xylanase, glucose oxidase and lactoperoxidase (Johansen et al., 1997, White, 2006, Kaplan et al., 2004).

A different approach for the treatment of biofilms is the use of bacteriophages, viruses that are specific for the bacteria to replicate inside and kill them. It has been demonstrating its effectiveness with the use of bacteriophage T4, which can infect and replicate in *Escherichia coli* breaking up the morphology of the biofilm and killing the bacteria, or in the case of phage 456 on *S. epidermidis*. (Curtin & Donlan, 2006). A bacteriophage expressing enzymes that degrade the biofilm matrix has been designed and simultaneously attack the bacterial cells of *Escherichia coli*. This design eliminates the need to express, purify and deliver large doses of enzymes to specific sites of infection that impede access by the presence of the extracellular matrix (Lu & Collins, 2007).

Pretreatment of catheters with hydrogel with a hydrolyzate of bacteriophage *P. aeruginosa* M4 reached lower cell density in biofilms after bacterial inoculation suggesting its potential use to prevent biofilm formation (Fu et al., 2010).

8. Conclusions and perspectives

The organization of the microorganisms to grow as a biofilm has been shown to have their own intrinsic mechanisms of resistance differ from those described stop the growth of microorganisms in free form. Therefore, these strategies should be considered resistance to explain therapeutic failure in the treatment of patients for whom laboratory results provide suitable sensitivity patterns.

Growth as a biofilm is a risk factor for the spread of resistance to antibiotics and biocides as a long-term treatment with a microorganism determines their survival by developing a biofilm phenotype.

Therapy in the future against biofilm-related infections should be considered as a priority to have standardized methods of diagnosis (still non-existent at the routine level) to determine differential management strategies of these infections.

As biofilms are heterogeneous in nature, antibiotics are useful to control those who are active in cells with low metabolic activity or non-actively growing cells so requires the search for new antibiotics that fit this profile.

The main strategy for controlling these infections is the use of agents that prevent biofilm formation as (*quorum sensing* inhibitors, inhibitors of synthesis of exopolysaccharides or material handling to prevent sticking) and its growth has been kept as planktonic cells to be susceptible to the action of antibiotics and host immune system. Other possible control strategies for mature biofilm consisting of dispersal of the organism by specific enzymes responsible or bacteriophage that allow differential lysis.

In conclusion, biofilm growth as a major advantage for microorganisms because of the variety of strategies developed by them not only to ensure their survival in hostile environments but to evade the antibiotics, so knowledge of the process and the mediators involved will allow us to direct them to our benefit.

9. References

Ahariz M, Courtois P. (2010). *Candida albicans* biofilm on titanium: effect of perodxidase precoating. *Medical devices: evidence and research*.Vol.3 pp. 33-40.

Allegrucci M & Sauer K (2007) Characterization of colony morphology variants isolated from *Streptococcus pneumoniae* biofilms. *J Bacteriol.* Vol. 189 pp. 2030-2038.

Anderl JN, Franlin JM, Stewart SP. (2000). Role of antibiotic penetration limitation in *Klebsiella pneumoniae* biofilm resistance to ampicillin and ciprofloxacin. *Antimicrob Agents Chemother.* Vol. 44 pp. 1818-1824.

Balaban N, Cirioni O, Giacometti A, Ghiselli R, Braunstein BJ, Silvestri C, Mocchegiani F, Saba V, Scalise G. (2007) Treatment of *Staphylococcus aureus* biofilm infection by the Quorum-sensing inhibitor RIP. *Antimicrob Agents Chemother.* Vol. 51 pp. 2226- 2229.

Biswas L, Biswas R, Schlag M, Bertram R, Götz F. (2009). Small-colony variant selection as a survival strategy for *Staphylococcus aureus* in the presence of *Pseudomonas aeruginosa. Appl Environ Microbiol.* Vol. 75 pp. 6910-6912.

Borriello G, Werner E, Roe F, Kim AM, Ehrlich GD, Stewart PS. (2004). Oxygen limitation contributes to antibiotic tolerance of *Psedomonas aeruginosa* biofilms. *Antimicrob Agents Chemother.* Vol.4 pp. 2659-2666.

Brown MR Allison DG, Gilbert P .(1988). Resistance of bacterial biofilms to antibiotics: a growth-rate related effect? *J Antimicrob Chemother.* Vol. 22 pp. 777-780.

Bos R, van der Mei CH, Busscher JH. (1999). Physico-chemistry of initial microbial adhesive interactions. Its mechanisms and methods for study. *FEMS Microbiol Rev.* Vol. 23 pp. 179-230.

Castrillon RLE, Palma RA, Desgarennes PC. (2003) Aminoglucósidos: una revisión reciente. *Dermatología Rev Mex.* Vol. 47 pp. 178-193.

Castrillón RLE, Palma RA, Desgarennes PC. (2007). Péptidos antimicrobianos: antibióticos naturales de la piel. *Dermatología Rev Mex.* Vol. 51 pp. 57-67.

Castrillón RLE, Palma RA, Desgarennes PMC.(2010). Importancia de las biopelículas en la práctica médica. *Dermatología Rev Mex* Vol. 54 pp. 14-24

Castrillón RLE, Palma RA, Padilla DMC. (2011) Interferencia de las biopelículas en el proceso de curación de heridas. *Dermatología Rev Mex.* Vol. 55 pp. 127-139.

Chia N, Woese CR, Goldenfeld N (2008) A collective mechanism for phase variation in biofilms. *PNAS* Vol 105 pp. 14597-14602.

Cho SH, Naber K, Hacker J, Zibuhr W. (2002) Detection of the *ica*ADBC gene cluster and biofilm formation in *Staphylococcus epidermidis* isolates from catheter-related urinary tract infections. *Int J Antimicrob Agents.* Vol. 19 pp. 570-575.

Cooper R., Okhiria O. (2010) Biofilms, wound infection and the issue control. *Wounds UK.* Vol. 6 pp. 84-90

Costerton JW, Cheng KJ, Geesey GG, Ladd TI,, Nickel JC, Dasgupta M, Marrie TJ. (1987). Bacterial biofilms in nature and disease. *Ann Rev Microbiol.* Vol. 987 pp. 435-464.

Costerton JW, Stewart PS, Greenberg EP. (1999) Bacterial biofilms: a common cause of persistent infections. *Science.* Vol. 284 pp. 1318-1322.

Costerton W, Veeh R, Shirfliff M, Pasmore M, Post Ch, Ehrlich G. (2003). The applications of biofilm science to the study and control of chronic bacterial infections. *J Clin Invest.* Vol. 112 pp. 1466-1477.

Curtin JJ, Donlan RM.(2006). Using bacteriophages to reduce formation of catheter-associated biofilms by *Staphylococcus epidermidis. Antimicrob Agents Chemother.* Vol.50 pp. 1268-1275.

De Kievit TR, Parkins MD, Gillis RJ, Srikumar H, Ceri H, Poole BH, Iglewski DG, Storey DG. (2001). Multidrug efflux pumps: expression patterns and contribution to antibiotic resistance in *Pseudomonas aeruginosa* biofilms, *Amtimicrob Agents Chemother.* Vol. 45 pp. 1761-1770.

Del Valle Martínez Rojas D. (2009) Betalactamasas tipo AmpC: generalidades y métodos para su detección fenotípica. *Rev Soc Venezolana Microbiol.* Vol. 29 pp. 78-83.

Diemond HJB, Miranda NG. (2007) Biofilm: ¿amenaza latente o factor de protección? Estado del arte. *Enf Inf Microbiol.* Vol. 27 pp. 22-28.

Donlan MR, Costerton W. (2002). Biofilms: survival mechanisms of clinically relevant microorganisms. *Clin Microb Rev.* Vol.15 pp. 167-193.

Eftekhar F, Dadaei T. (2011). Biofilm formation of *Ica*AB genes in clinical isolates of methicillin resistant *Staphylococcus aureus. Iranian J Basic Med Sci.* Vol. 14 pp. 132-136.

Flemming HC, Wingender J. (2010). The biofilm matrix. *Nature Rev Microbiol.* Vol. 8 pp. 623-633.

Fu W, Forster T, Mayer O, Curtin JJ, Lehman MS, Donlan MR (2010) Bacteriophage cocktail for the prevention of biofilm formation by *Pseudomonas aeruginosa* on catheters *in vitro* model. *Antimicrob Agents Chemother.* Vol 54 pp. 397-404

Fux CA, Costerton JW, Stewart PS, Stoodley P.(2005). Survival strategies of infectious biofilms. *Trends Microbiol.* Vol. 13 pp. 34-40.

Gallant VC, Daniels C, Leung MJ, Ghosh SA, Young DK, Kotra LP, Burrows LL.(2005). Common beta-lactamases inhibit bacterial biofilm formation. *Mol Microbiol.* Vol.58 pp. 1012-1024.

Ghigo JM. (2001). Natural conjugative plasmids induce biofilm development. *Nature.* Vol. 412 pp. 442-445.

Gillis, R., K. White, K. Choi, V. Wagner, H. Schweizer, and B. Iglewski. (2005) Molecular basis of azithromycin-resistant *Pseudomonas aeruginosa* biofilms. *Antimicrob. Agents Chemother.* Vol. 49 pp. 3858–3867.

Giwercman B, Jensen ETT, Hoiby N.. (1991) Induction of β–lactamase production in *Pseudomonas aeruginosa* biofilm. *Antimicrob Agents Chemother.* Vol.35 pp. 1008-1010.

Grkovi S, Brown MH,m Skurray RA. (2002). Regulation of bacterial drug export systems. *Microbiol Mol Biol Rev.* Vol. 66 pp. 671-701.

Gordon CA, Hodges NA, Marriott C. (1988). Antibiotic interaction and diffusion through alginate and exopolysaccharide of cystic fibrosis-derived *Pseudomonas aeruginosa. J Antimicrob Chemother* Vol. 22 pp. 667-674.

Hachem YR, Chemaly FR, Ahmar AC, Jiang Y, Boktour RM, Rjaili AG, Bodey PG, Raad II. (2007). Colistin is effective in treatment of infectious caused by multidrug-resistant *Pseudomonas aeuroginosa* in cancer patients. *Antimicrob Agents Chemother.* Vol. 51 pp. 1905-1911.

Hall-Stoodley L, Costerton WJ, Stoodley P. (2004). Bacterial biofilms: from the natural environment to infectious diseases. *Nat Rev Microbiol* Vol. 2 pp. 95-108.

Hall-Stoodley, L. & Stoodley, P. (2005). Biofilm formation and dispersal and the transmission of human pathogens. *Trends Microbiol.* Vol. 13. pp. 7-10.

Hancock RE. (1997). The bacterial outer membrane as a drug barrier. *Trends Microbiol.* Vol. 5 pp. 37-42.

Häubler S, Ziegler I, Löttel A, Götz F Rhode M, Wehmhöhner D, Saravanamuthu S, Tümmler B, Steinmetz I. (2003). Highly adherent small-colony variants of *Pseudomonas aeruginosa* in cystic fibrosis lung infection. *J Med Microbiol.* Vol. 52 pp. 295-301.

Hentzer M, Givskov M. (2003). Pharmacological inhibition of quorum sensing for the treatment of chronic bacterial infections. *J Clin Invest.* Vol 112. pp 1300-1307.

Herrera Mendoza MT. (2004). El papel del biofilm e el proceso infeccioso y la resistencia. *Nova Publicación científica.* Vol. 2 pp. 71-80.

Hogan D, Kolter R. (2002). Why are bacteria refractory to antimicrobials? *Curr Opin Microbiol.* Vol. 5 pp. 472-477.

Hoiby N, Bjarnsholt T, Givskov M, Molin S, Ciofu O. (2010). Antibiotic resistance of bacterial biofilms. *Int J Antimicrob Agents* Vol. 35 pp. 322-332.

Johansen Ch, Falholt P, Gram L.(1997). Enzymatic removal and disinfection of bacterial biofilms. *Appl Environ Microbiol,* Vol. 63 pp. 3724-3728.

Jong-Hyum K, Kim Ch, Hacker J, Ziebuhr W, Lee KB, Cho SH. (2008). Molecular characterization of regulatory genes associated with biofilm variation in a *Staphylococcus aureus* strain. *J Microbiol Biotechnol.* Vol. 18 pp. 28-34.

Kaplan BJ, Ragunath C, Velliyagounder K, Fine HD, Ramasubbu N. (2004). Enzymatic detachment of *Staphylococcus epidermidis* biofilms. *Antimicrob Agents Chemother.* Vol. 48 pp. 2633-2636.

Keller L, Surette GM. (2006). Communication in bacteria: an ecological and evolutionary perspective. *Nat Rev Microbiol.* Vol. 4 pp. 249-258.

Keren I, Shah D, Spoering A, Wang Y, Lewis I. (2004). Specialized persister cells and the mechanism of multidrug tolerance in *Escherichia coli. J Bacteriol.* Vol. 186 pp. 8172-8180.

Kirisits MJ, Prost L, Starkey M, Parsek RM (2005) Characterization of colony morphology variants isolated from *Pseudomonas aeruginosa* biofilms *Appl Environ Microbiol.* Vol 71 pp. 4809-4821.

Kikerlund HS, Haagensen AJJ, Gjrmansen M, Jorgensen MT, Tolker-Nielsen T, Molin S. (2007). Characterization of *Pseudomonas putida* rough variant evolved in a mixed-species biofim with *Acinetobacter* sp. Strain C6. *J Bacteriol.* Vol. 189 pp. 4932-4943.

Kumamoto AC. (2002). Candida biofilms. *Curr Opin Microbiol.* Vol. 5 pp. 608-611.

Kvist M, Hancock V, Klemm P. (2008). Inactivation of efflux pumps abolishes bacterial biofilm formation. *App Environ Microbiol.* Vol. 74 pp. 7376-7382.

Laffey S, Butler G (2005) Phenotype switching affects biofilm formation by *Candida parapsilosis. Microbiology* Vol 151 pp. 1073-1081.

Lasa I, del Pozo JL, Penadés JR, Leiva J. (2005). Biofilms bacterianos e infección. *An Sist Sanit Navar.* Vol. 28 pp. 163-175.

Lewis K. (2001). Riddle of biofilm resistance. *Antimicrob Agents Chemother.* Vol. 45 pp. 999-1007.

Lewis K. (2008). Multidrug tolerance of biofilms and persister cells. *Curr Topics Microbiol Immunol.* Vol. 322 pp. 107-131.

López D, Vlamakis H, Kolter R. (2010). Biofilms. *Cold Spring Harb Perspect Biol.* Vol. 2 pp. 1-11.

Lu TK, Collins JJ. (2007). Dispersing biofilms with engineered enzymatic bacteriophage. *PNAS* Vol.104 pp. 11197-11202.

Mah TFC, O'Toole GA. (2001). Mechanisms of biofilm resistance to antimicrobial agents. *Trends Microbiol.* Vol. 9. pp. 4-39.

Maira-Litrán T, Allison DG, Gilbert P. (2000a). Expression of the multiple antibiotic resistance operon (*mar*) during growth of *Escherichia coli* as a biofilm. *J Appl Microbiol.* Vol. 88 pp. 243-247.

Maira-Litrán T, Allison GD, Gilbert P. (2000b). An evaluation of the potential of the multiple antibiotic resistance operon (mar) and the multidrug efflux pump acrAB to moderate resistance towards ciprofloxacin en *Escherichia coli* biofilms. *J Antimicrob Chemother.* Vol. 45 pp. 789-795.

Martínez-Suárez VJ, Baquero F, Reig M, Pérez-Díaz JC. (1985). Transferable plasmid-linked chloramphenicol acetytransferase conferring high-lvel resistance in Bacteroides uniformis. *Antimicrob Agents Chemother.* Vol. 28 pp. 113-117.

Moyed HS, Broderick SH. (1986). Molecular cloning and expression of *hip* A, gene of *Escherichia coli* K-12 that affects frequency of persistence after inhibition of murein synthesis. *J Bacteriol.* Vol. 166 pp. 399-403.

Müller CFM, Seider M, Beauvais A. (2011). *Aspergillus fumigatus* biofilms in the clinical setting. *Medical Micology* Vol. 49(Suppl. 1)pp S96-S100.

Neut D, van der Mei H, Bulstra KS, Busscher JH. (2007). The role of small-colony variants in failure to diagnose and treat biofilm infections in orthopedics. *Acta Orthopaedica* Vol. 78 pp. 299-308.

Pagés JM, James ECh. Winterhalter M. (2008). The porin and the permeating antibiotic: a selective diffusion barrier in Gram-negative bacteria. *Nat Rev Microbiol.* Vol. 6 pp. 893-903.

Pamp JS, Gjermansen M, Johansen KH, Tolker-Nielsen T. (2008). Tolerance to the antimicrobial peptide colistin in *Pseudomonas aeruginosa* biofilms in linked to metabolically active cells, and depends on the pmr and mexAB-oprM genes. *Mol Microbiol.* Vol. 68 pp. 223-240.

Poole K. (2002). Mechanisms of bacterial biocide and antibiotic resistance. *J Appl Microbiol.* Vol. 92 pp. 55S-64S.

Proctor RA, Peters G. (1998). Small colony variants in staphylococcal infections: diagnostic and therapeutic implications. *Clin Infect Dis.* Vol. 27 pp. 419-423.

Raad I, Hanna H.(1999). Intravascular catheters impregnated with antimicrobial agents: a milestone in the prevention of bloodstream infections. *Support Care Cancer.* Vol. 7 pp. 386-390.

Ramage G, Bachmann S, Patterson FT, Wickes LB, López-Ribot JL. (2002). Investigation of multidrug efflux pumps in relation to fluconazole resistance in *Candida albicans* biofilms. *J Antimicrob Chemother.* Vol. 49 pp. 973-980.

Rodríguez-Franco DA, Vázquez-Moreno L, Ramos-Clamont, Monfort G. (2005). Actividad antimicrobiana de la lactoferrina: Mecanismos y aplicaciones clínicas potenciales. *Rev Latinoam Microbiol.* Vol. 47 pp. 102-111.

Rusthoven JJ, Davis TA, Lerner SA. (1979). Clinical isolation and characterization of aminoglucoside-resistant small colony variants of *Enterobacter aerogenes. Am J Med.* Vol. 67 pp. 702-706.

Sánchez-Suárez P, Bentiez-Bibriesca L. (2006) Procesos biomoleculares de la Resistencia a drogas. *Cancerología* Vol 1 pp. 187-199.

Sauer K, Camper AK, Ehrlich GD, Costerton JW, Davies DG. (2002). *Pseudomonas aeruginosa* displays multiple phenotypes during development as a biofilm. *J Bacteriol.* Vol. 184 pp. 1140-1154.

Smith WA. (2005). Biofilms and antibiotic therqapy: Is there a role for combating bacterial resistance by the use of novel drug delivery system? *Adv Drug Delivery Rev.* Vol. 57 pp. 1539-1550.

Stewart SP, Roe F, Rayner J, Eldins GJ, Lewandowski Z, Oschsner AU, Hassett JD. (2000). Effect of catalase on hydrogen peroxide penetration into *Pseudomonas aeruginosa* biofilms. *Appl Environ Microbiol.* Vol. 66 pp. 836-838.

Stewart SP, Costerton WJ. (2001) Antibiotic resistance of bacterial biofilms. *Lancet* Vol. 358 pp. 135-138.

Stewart SP. (2002). Mechanism of antibiotic resistance in bacterial biofilms. *Int J Med Microbiol.* Vol. 292 pp. 107-113.

Stewart SP, Franklin JM. (2008). Physiological heterogeneity in biofilms. *Nat Rev Microbiol.* Vol.6 pp. 199-210.

Stickler D., (1999). Biofilms. *Curr Opin Microbiol.* Vol. 2 pp. 270-275.

Spoering AL, Lewis K. (2001). Biofilms and planktonic cells of *Pseudomonas aeruginosa* have similar resistance to killing by antimicrobials. *J Bacteriol.* Vol. 183 pp. 6746-6751.

Sutherland WI. (1997). Microbial exopolysaccharides-structural subtleties and their consequences. *Pure & Appl Chem.* Vol. 69 pp. 1911-1917.

Uppuluri P., Ashok K. Chaturvedi KA, Srinivasan A, Banerjee M, Ramasubramaniam KA, Köhler RJ, David Kadosh D, Lopez-Ribot J. (2010). Dispersion as an important step in the *Candida albicans* biofilm developmental cycle. *PLoSPatog.* Vol. 6 pp. 1-13.

Van Bambeke F., Glupczynski Y., P. Plésiat P., J. C. Pechère JC., P. M. Tulkens PM. (2003). Antibiotic efflux pumps in prokaryotic cells: occurrence, impact on resistance and strategies for the future of antimicrobial therapy. *J Antimicrob. Chemother.* Vol. 51 pp. 1055-1065.

Veeh RH, Shirtliff EM, Petik RJ, Flood AJ, Davis CC, Seymor LJ, Hansmann AM, Kerr MK, Pasmore EM, Costerton WJ. (2003). Detection of *Staphylococcus aureus* biofilm on tampons and menses components. *J Infect Dis.* Vol. 188 pp. 519-530.

Ward KH, Olson ME, Lam K, Costerton JW. (1992). Mechanism of persistent infection with peritoneal implants. *J Med Micro.* Vol. 36 pp. 406-413.

Webber MA, Piddock LJV. (2003) The importance of efflux pumps in bacterial antibiotic resistance. *J Antimicrob Chemother.* Vol 51 pp.9-11.

White R. (2006). Flaminal®: a novel approach to wound bioburden control. *Wounds.* Vol. 2 pp. 64-77.

Whitehead AN, Barnard MLA, Slater H, Simpson JLN, Salmond PCG. (2001). Quorum-sensing in Gram-negative bacteria. *FEMS Microbiol Rev.* Vol. 25 pp. 365-404.

Wimpenny J, Manz W, Szewzyk U. (2000). Heterogeneity in biofilms. *FEMS Microbiol Rev.* Vol. 24 pp. 661-671.

Woods DE, Bass JA, Johanson WG. (1980). Role of adherence in the pathogenesis of *Pseudomonas aeruginosa* lung infection in cystic fibrosis patients. *Infect Immun.* Vol. 30 pp. 784-790.

Wright DG. (2005). Bacterial resistance to antibiotics: Enzymatic degradation and modification. *Adv Drug Deliv.* Vol. 57 pp. 1451-1450.

Zhang, L., & T.-F. Mah.. (2008). Involvement of a novel efflux system in biofilm-specific resistance to antibiotics. *J Bacteriol.* Vol. 190 pp. 4447–4452.

Ziebuhr W, Heilmann Ch, Götz F, Meyer P, Wils K, Straube E, Hacker J. (1997). Detection of the intercellular adhesion gene cluster (ica) and phase variation in *Staphylococcus epidermidis* blood culture strains and mucosal isolates. *Infect Immun.* Vol. 65 pp. 890-896.

Zimmerli W, Widmer FA, Blatter M, Frei R, Ochnsner EP. (1998). Role of rifampin for treatment of orthopedic implant-related stapylococcal infections: a randomized controlled trial. Foreign-body infection (FBI) Study Group. *JAMA.* Vol. 279 pp. 1537-1541.

8

Antibiotic Resistance, Biofilms and Quorum Sensing in *Acinetobacter* Species

K. Prashanth*, T. Vasanth, R. Saranathan,
Abhijith R. Makki and Sudhakar Pagal
Laboratory No. 6, Department of Biotechnology, Pondicherry University, India

1. Introduction

Acinetobacter is a Gram-negative coccobacillus that is strictly aerobic, nonmotile, catalase positive and oxidase negative. It is ubiquitous in nature, being found in soil and water. Members of the genus *Acinetobacter* have now clearly emerged as opportunistic nosocomial pathogens (Forster et al., 1998). Bacteremia, pneumonia, meningitis, urinary tract and surgical wound infections are the most common infections caused by this organism (Cisneros et al., 2002; Dijkshoorn et al., 2007). The taxonomy of the genus *Acinetobacter* has undergone extensive revision during the last two decades, and at least 31 named and unnamed species have now been described (Dijkshoorn et al., 2007). Of these, *Acinetobacter baumannii* and the closely related unnamed genomic species 3 and 13 sensu Tjernberg and Ursing (13TU) species were the most clinically relevant. In recent years, multidrug-resistant (MDR) *A. baumannii* are increasingly held responsible for nosocomial infections and MDR *A. baumannii* clones are spreading into new geographic areas with increasing number of strains acquiring many resistance genes (Navon venezia et al., 2005). Unfortunately, newer extended-spectrum β-lactamases and different carbapenemases are emerging fast, leading to pan-resistant strains of *A. baumannii*.

A. baumannii appears to have the propensity for developing multiple antimicrobial resistances extremely rapidly. This bacterium has shown a remarkable tendency to develop resistance to virtually every antibiotic class (Henwood et al., 2002). The emergence and quick dissemination of multiple drug resistant (MDR) *A. baumannii* and its genetic potential to carry and transfer diverse antibiotic resistance determinants pose a major threat in hospitals world-wide. The complex interplay of MDR clones, its rapid spread, their persistence through biofilm formation, their regulation by quorum sensing (QS), transfer of resistance elements and other interactions are contributing to the increasing woes and creating additional difficulties in treating infections caused by these organisms. This review article mainly focus on antibiotic resistance in *Acinetobacter*, the current understanding of biofilm production and its correlation with antibiotic resistance as well the quorum sensing mechanisms in *Acinetobacter* species.

---

* Corresponding Author

2. Antibiotic resistance in *Acinetobacter* spp.

A. baumannii is considered the paradigm of multi-resistant bacteria as the organism has an ever-increasing list of resistance determinants that can rapidly nullify most of the therapeutic armamentarium. Both acquired and intrinsic resistance mechanisms can contribute this multi-resistance. The ability to acquire such resistance for multiple drugs may be due to either the acquisition of genetic elements carrying multiple resistant determinants or mutations affecting the expression of porins and/or efflux pump(s), which can minimize the activity of unrelated antimicrobial agents (Vila, 2007). It is also indicated that the outer membrane of *Acinetobacter* spp. acts as a substantial barrier against the penetration of these antibiotics. The results of one of the earliest studies suggest that one of the causes for the high antibiotic resistance of *Acinetobacter* is attributable to the presence of a small number of small-sized porins (Sato et al., 1991). Apart from this, it was also shown earlier that the amount of *Acinetobacter* porin was less than 5% of the Total outer membrane proteins (OMP), while that of *E. coli* it was reported to be about 60% (Rosenbusch, 1974) that contributes to reduced permeability. The most widespread β-lactamases with carbapenemase activity in *A. baumannii* are carbapenem hydrolysing class D β-lactamases mediated by OXA genes that are most specific for this species. In addition, metallo-β-lactamases have now been reported worldwide that confer resistance to all β-lactams except aztreonam (Dijkshoorn et al., 2007). Resistance to aminoglycosides in *A. baumannii* is mediated principally by aminoglycoside-modifying enzymes (AME's). Further, multidrug efflux pump such as AdeABC may have a role in aminoglycoside resistance (Wieczorek et al., 2008). Quinolone resistance is often caused by modifications in the structure of DNA gyrase secondary to mutations in the quinolone resistance determining regions of the *gyrA* and *parC* genes.

The main underlying resistance mechanisms to multiple antibiotics in *Acinetobacter* sp. can be summarily outlined as follows (i) production of hydrolysing enzymes for e.g. β-lactam hydrolysis by different kinds of β-lactamases (Class A to D β-lactamases), (ii) changes in penicillin-binding proteins (PBPs) that prevent action of β-lactams, (iii) alterations in the structure and number of porin proteins that result in decreased permeability to antibiotics through the outer membrane of the bacterial cell and (iv) the activity of efflux pumps that further decrease the concentration of antibiotics within the bacterial cell. But, among these β-lactamases, OXA- and metallo-carbapenemases seem to be more significant with their increasing incidence when compared to other β-lactamases (Livermore et al., 2006).

2.1 Resistance to β-lactam antibiotics

Resistance for β-lactams in *Acinetobacter* is been associated with the production of β-lactamases.

2.1.1 β-lactamases

Resistance due to the expression of hydrolysing enzymes such as cephalophorinases and amber class A-D β-lactamases remains as one of the extensively studied and skilful resistance mechanism among the species of *Acinetobacter*. These enzymes to some extent hydrolyze carbapenems along with other β-lactams. The most common carbapenemases detected in *A. baumannii* were either Class B β- lactamases such as metallo β- lactamases

(MBL) or class D β- lactamases (also referred as carbapenem hydrolyzing oxicillinases (CHDLs)) (Livermore, 2007). While class A carbapenemases have been frequently detected in bacteria belonging to *Enterobacteraceae* family, they were not usually found in *Acinetobacter* spp. However, *A. baumannii* producing extended-spectrum β-lactamases (ESBLs) have been reported, though it is not a common phenomenon (Livermore & Woodford, 2006). As there are emerging reports of arrival of newer broad spectrum β- lactamases such as New Delhi metallo-beta lactamase -1 (NDM-1) (Karthikeyan et al., 2010) among Gram-negative pathogens including *Acinetobacter* and their progressing hydrolysing abilities makes this group of Gram-negative bacterial pathogens as superbugs by assisting them to survive in extreme conditions. The genes that code for multiple resistances are reported to be plasmid as well as chromosomally encoded.

2.1.2 A- Class

A. baumannii, like *Pseudomonas aeruginosa,* produces a naturally occurring AmpC β-lactamase, together with a naturally occurring oxacillinase with carbapenemase properties. ESBLs are plasmid-mediated β-lactamases of predominant class A. ESBLs are capable of efficiently hydrolyzing penicillin, cephalosporin, the oxyimino group containing cephalosporins (cefotaxime, ceftazidime) and monobactams (aztreonam). β-lactamase inhibitors (clavulanic acid, sulbactam and tazobactam) generally inhibit ESBL producing strains. A wide range of class A ESBLs have been reported in *Acinetobacter* sp. such as TEM, SHV, CTX-M, GES, SCO, PER and VEB. However, these resistant determinants are not universally present in *Acinetobacter,* as there are only isolated reports of them. Some of the documented ESBLs world-wide are PER-1 from Turkey, Korea, Russia, Romania, Belgium and France; VEB-1 from France and Belgium; TEM-116 and SHV-12 from China and The Netherlands; CTX-M-2 from Korea; *bla* Shv-5 -EBSL, TEM -92 from Italy and VEB -1 from Northern France and Belgium (Naiemi et al., 2005; Nass et al., 2006, 2007; Endimiani et al., 2007). Nevertheless, they were not as common as MBL and CHDL in *Acinetobacter* species.

2.1.3 B- Class

Carbapenemases are the most versatile of all β-lactamases and many of them recognize almost all hydrolysable β-lactams. The most common hydrolyzing enzyme carbapenemases found in *A. baumannii* belong to either the class B family of beta-lactamases such as MBLs (IMP/VIM) or the OXA class D family of serine β-lactamases (Poirel, 2006). Class B β-lactamases are also referred as MBLs has the highest level of carbapenem-hydrolyzing activity among the three classes of carbapenemases. MBLs have been identified in many Gram-negative bacteria including *Acinetobacter* genomic species 13 TU and *A. baumannii* and are resistant to the commercially available β-lactamase inhibitors but susceptible to inhibition by metal ion chelators. Potent class B metallo-carbapenemases of the IMP, VIM, SIM and NDM type have been found in *A. baumannii.*

There are numerous existing reports on IMP type of MBL in *Acinetobacter* spp (Lee et al., 2003; Livermore, 2007). In *A. baumannii,* six IMP variants belonging to three different phylogroups have been identified and reported namely IMP-1 in Italy, Japan and South Korea; IMP-2 in Italy and Japan; IMP-4 in Hong Kong; IMP-5 in Portugal; IMP-6 in Brazil and IMP-11 in Japan (Poirel and Nordmann, 2006). In addition, IMP-4 has been identified in clinical isolates of *Acinetobacter junii* in Australia (Peleg et al., 2006). On the contrary, there are only few studies that have documented MBL VIM type in *Acinetobacter*. In fact more than 100 clinical isolates screened by our group showed non-existence of VIM in this part of world. Surprisingly, *P. aeruginosa* isolates collected from the same hospital in our region showed the presence of VIM type of MBL and there was no cross transmission observed (Unpublished data). VIM-2-producing *Acinetobacter* spp. have been isolated in the Far East (Lee, et al., 2003) and in Germany (Toleman, 2004), while the VIM-1 determinant has been reported only in Greece (Tsakris 2006). One study recently identified VIM-4, which is nothing but a point mutant of VIM-1 and that has been previously identified only in *Enterobacteriaceae* (Luzzaro et al., 2008) and *Pseudomonas* spp. (Pournaras et al., 2003). This report on MBL VIM-4 determinant in *Acinetobacter* spp., emphasizes the fact that CHDLs are not the solitary factor for emergence of resistance to carbapenems in this genus. Interestingly, *bla*VIM-4 was identified in a non-*A. baumannii* isolate, thereby indicating that clinically insignificant Gram-negative bacterial species may also be reservoirs for MBL-encoding genes. It is also noteworthy that the occurrence of VIM-4 in *Acinetobacter* in a country that has reported VIM-4 in *P. aeruginosa* previously (Pournaras et al., 2003). Concurrently, it was also observed in Greece that *bla*VIM-1 which is widespread in *P. aeruginosa* had apparently crossed the species barrier to reach *Acinetobacter* spp. Such examples might be yet another example of resistance genes crossing genus barrier (Tsakris et al., 2006).

A small number of reports are available on other MBL types such as SIM-1, NDM-1 encountered in *Acinetobacter* spp (Lee et al., 2005, Karthikeyan et al., 2010). Recently, a novel acquired MBL gene namely *bla*SIM-1 was detected in clinical isolates of *A. baumannii* from Korea (Lee et al., 2005). This SIM-1 is encoded by a class 1 integron-borne gene cassette and is more closely related to IMP-type enzymes than to other MBLs. Very recently new β-lactamase such as NDM-1 has been reported in *A. baumannii* (Karthikeyan et al., 2010). Interestingly, in this report NDM-1–positive isolate was also positive for both OXA-23 and IMP. The *bla*NDM-1– positive strain was more resistant to antibiotics than the strains that were harbouring both OXA-23 and IMP. Fortunately, it was found that this *bla*NDM-1–positive *A. baumannii* strain was susceptible to several fluoroquinolone antibiotics and to polymyxin B (Chen et al., 2011).

2.1.4 D- Class

The most common carbapenemases detected in *Acinetobacter* are CHDLs that are also referred as Class-D oxacillinases. Among the nine clusters of carbapenem hydrolysing oxacillinases, four have been identified to date in *A. baumannii*. These included members of OXA-23, -24, -51, and -58 families. In addition, recently a novel class D enzyme named OXA-143 has been reported from Germany. OXA-58 oxacillinase was the first enzyme to be identified in an *A. baumannii* isolate in France and subsequently this has been reported among *A. baumannii* isolates in several countries (Coelo et al., 2006). Contrary to many workers, one investigation opined that the carriage of OXA-58 but not of OXA-51 β-lactamase gene correlates with carbapenem resistance in *A. baumannii* (Tsakris, 2007). In one of the studies, epidemiologically unrelated *Acinetobacter* isolates that were positive for the presence *bla*OXA-51- and *bla*OXA-58-like carbapenemase genes was also shown to carry the *bla*VIM-1 in a class 1 integron, which is of much concern (Tsakris, 2008).

Recently, a new OXA class D β–lactamase Oxa-97 has been reported in Tunisia which belongs to Oxa58-like (subgroup) in Africa (Poirel et al., 2008). In one instance, a novel Oxa-

143- CHDL in *A. baumannii* (Higgins et al., 2009) which is not associated with insertion sequence (IS) elements or integron features has been reported, which is bracketed by 2 replicase genes and its incorporation was shown to be by homologous recombination. Oxa-143 is a class D carbapenemase is similar to OXA-66/OXA-51-like enzyme that contributes to imipenem resistance, which was first reported from Taiwan. Off late, OXA-72 oxacillinase has been also reported in several carbapenem resistant *A. baumannii* isolates in Taiwan (Lu et al., 2009).

It has also been discovered that *bla*OXA-51-like genes may be associated with carbapenem resistance in isolates with an adjacent copy of insertion sequence (IS) ISAbA1 (Turton et al., 2006). IS elements presumed to enhance β-lactamase gene expression by providing additional promoters. Repeated observations such as ISAba1, ISAba2, ISAba3, ISAba4 IS elements being often found upstream of the different β- lactamases genes in *A. baumannii* can be taken as evidence for such assumption (Chen et al., 2008; Poirel 2006a. 2006b & 2008). In addition, one recent work demonstrated that a plasmid-borne CHDL with appropriate upstream ISs was enough to confer a high level of carbapenem resistance in *A. baumannii*. Moreover, a *bla*OXA-58 gene with an upstream insertion of a truncated ISAba3 and IS1008 was detected on a plasmid obtained from a clinical carbapenem resistant isolate in one of the studies (Chen et al., 2008). Acquisition of a plasmid-borne *bla*OXA-58 gene with an upstream IS1008 insertion is also shown to confer a high level of carbapenem resistance to *A. baumannii* (Chen et al., 2008). Therefore, as observed for the natural *bla*AmpC gene of *A. baumannii*, ISAba1 might provide promoter sequences that enhance expression of associated genes. These promoter sequences are probably extremely efficient in *A. baumannii*, so that insertion of ISAba1 upstream of *bla*OXA-51-like genes might represent a true mechanism of carbapenem resistance, or at least decreased susceptibility. Hence, it is sensible to believe that the association of *bla*OXA -51 like genes with IS elements may have a role in increasing carbapenem resistance. At least in one instance, it was conclusively shown that the reduced susceptibility to carbapenems was related to selection of the ISAba1-related overexpression of *bla*OXA-66 that belongs to *bla*OXA-51 subgroup (Figueiredo et al., 2009).

2.2 Modifications in target proteins

2.2.1 Penicillin binding protein

Carbapenem resistance in *A. baumannii* may be because of penicillin binding proteins (PBP) or porin modifications. The penicillin-binding domains of PBPs are transpeptidases or carboxypeptidases involved in peptidoglycan metabolism. Reduced expression level of PBP was observed in multidrug resistant strains in order to resist the activity of antibiotics. Some of the strategies adopted by *A. baumannii*, which have been uncovered, are the acquisition of an additional low-affinity PBP, overexpression of an endogenous low-affinity PBP and alterations in endogenous PBPs by point mutations or homologous recombination.

One recent study strongly indicated an association between down-regulation of PBPs and/or alteration in PBPs for β-lactam resistance in *A. baumannii* (Vashist et al., 2011). In this study, it was shown that one of the PBP designated PBP-7/8 is critical for the survival of *A. baumannii* strain AB307-0294 in the rat soft tissue infection and pneumonia models. Furthermore, it was shown PBP-7/8 either directly or indirectly contributes to the resistance of this strain to complement-mediated bactericidal activity (Russo, 2009).

2.2.2 *gyr*A and *par*C

Quinolone resistance is often caused by modifications in the structure of DNA gyrase secondary to mutations in the quinolone resistance determining regions (QRDR) of the *gyr*A and *par*C genes. DNA gyrase and DNA topoisomerase IV encoded by *gyr*A and *par*C genes respectively, are among the housekeeping genes involved in DNA replication and processing are the targets for ciprofloxacin and other fluoroquinones. A point mutation on the *gyr*A gene (Ser-83 to leu) was observed in MDR strains of *A. baumannii* which is consistent with fluoroquinolone resistant phenotype. Sequencing of the *par*C gene also indicated mutations in the *par*C gene that caused an amino acid change at either Ser-80 or Glu-84 (Deccache et al., 2011)

2.3 Alternations in permeability

2.3.1 Changes in OMPs & porins

Reducing the transport of β-lactam into the periplasmic space via changes in porins or OMPs reduces the access to PBPs. The outer membrane in MDR *A. baumannii* is less permeable to antimicrobial agents than that in other susceptible ones. Alternations in permeability characteristics disturbs the β-lactam assimilation into the periplasmic space, resulting in the weak activity of antibiotics. Several porins, including the 33-kDa CarO protein, that constitute a pore channel for influx of carbapenems, might be involved in such resistance. Sometimes disruption of OMP genes by ISAba10 element may lead to the inactivation of the OMPs like CarO thereby reducing the extent of which the antibiotic enters the cell. When the chromosomal locus containing the *car*O gene was cloned from clinical isolates and characterised, it was shown that only a single copy of *car*O, present in a single transcriptional unit, was present in the *A. baumannii* genome. The *car*O gene encodes a polypeptide of 247 aminoacid residues, with a typical N-terminal signal sequence and a predicted trans-membrane β-barrel topology (Siroy et al., 2006). Remarkably, many recent studies have revealed that disruption of the *car*O gene by the IS elements such as ISAba1, ISAba125, or ISAba825 results in loss of activity of CarO OMP leading to carbapenem resistance in *A. baumannii* (Mussi et al., 2005; Poirel et al., 2006). Many recent reports of outbreaks caused by carbapenem resistant phenotypes and their characterization having revealed the loss or reduction of porins such as OMPs of 22-29 kDa, 47, 44, and 37kDa and one of 31 to 36 kDa substantiates the findings of many previous investigations on OMPs. Additional gene expression studies, along with phenotypic characterization, of these membrane proteins will conclusively clarify the role of membrane permeability in β-lactam resistance.

2.4 Efflux pumps

Efflux pumps are the ones among the well studied mechanisms of resistance in *A. baumannii*, by which the bacterial cells overcome the action of antibiotics by expelling them out. For example the 3.9-Mb genome of *A. baumannii* AYE is reported to harbour 46 open reading frames (ORFs) encoding putative efflux pumps of different families (Fournier et al., 2006). The over expression of efflux pump genes have been reported in the antibiotic resistant strains which provides the evidence for the role of efflux pumps in making the bacteria multi-drug resistant. To date, five classes of efflux pumps have been reported to be present in *A. baumannii* such as ATP binding cassette (ABC), major facilitator superfamily (MFS), multidrug and toxic compound extrusion (MATE), resistance-nodulation-cell division (RND) and small multidrug resistance (SMR).

The efflux systems in *A. baumannii* that are completely characterized functionally so far include AdeABC, AdeFGH and AdeIJK (RND type), AbeM (MATE type), and CraA (MFS type) (Peleg, 2008; Roca, 2009; Damier-Piolle, 2009). We have only partial knowledge on the functionality of ABC and SMR efflux pumps (Iacono et al., 2008; Srinivasan et al., 2009)

2.4.1 RND type efflux pump

The RND class efflux pumps that are commonly found in Gram-negative bacteria are usually tripartite in nature, i. e. they comprise of three protein components such as cytoplasmic, inter-membrane or membrane fusion protein (MFP) and peripalsmic or outer membrane protein which are encoded by three different genes present in a single operon. The cytoplasmic protein is otherwise termed as transporter protein which is involved in the export of substrates such as drugs or antibiotics from the cell, MFP and OMP help in export mechanisms. Different classes of RND family efflux pumps have been reported till date in *Acinetobacter* sp. Among these *ade*ABC, *ade*FGH and *ade*IJK functions and specificities have been studied extensively and overexpression of all these efflux pumps is controlled by two-component regulatory systems such as sensor and regulator kinase cascade.

In *A. baumannii*, AdeABC is one of the common types of efflux pumps which are involved in posing resistance to antibiotics such as aminoglycosides, β-lactams, chloramphenicol, tetracyclin, trimethoprim, erythromycin and drugs such as ethidium bromide (Magnet et al., 2001; Peleg et al., 2008). However, many studies seemed to indicate that the presence of *ade*ABC and *ade*DE is species specific, wherein *ade*ABC is being restricted to *A. baumannii* and adeDE to *Acinetobacter* genomespecies 3 (Chau et al., 2004). Contrastingly, one recent study for the first time showed the involvement of AdeABC pump in a non-*A. baumannii* strain and this study also described it in detail and characterized this pump. This investigation had also revealed that all three types of RND pumps coexist in non-*A. baumannii* strains (Roca et al., 2011). In AdeABC pump, AdeB is the multidrug transporter protein, AdeA is the membrane fusion protein and AdeC is the OMP. The efflux transporter AdeB captures the substrates either from within the phospholipid bilayer or the cytoplasm and then transports them out via OMP (AdeC). The periplasmic protein AdeA acts as an intermediate component which acts as an overpass between AdeB and AdeC components. AdeR-S two-component system is likely to control the expression of AdeABC type pumps. Further, point mutations in components of AdeABC and its regulatory proteins have been associated with overexpression of AdeABC leading to multidrug resistance (Marchand et al., 2004).

One study supports the hypothesis that the increased expression of *ade*B is associated with increased MICs of tigecycline. However, in the absence of an *ade*B gene knockout experiments, it is difficult to ascertain the overall contribution of the AdeABC efflux pump to tigecycline nonsusceptibility (Peleg et al., 2007; Hornsey et al., 2010). But, one recent study demonstrated that overexpression of the *ade*ABC efflux pump resulted in tigecycline nonsusceptibility by quantizing transcripts of the *ade*B gene and demonstrating conversion of the tigecycline resistance pattern in the presence of an efflux pump inhibitor without any previously known mutation (Sun et al., 2010). When the isolates were analysed separately, there was an association between a higher MIC and elevated *ade*ABC expression, although more isolates would need to be investigated to confirm this observation.

AdeIJK is the second RND type efflux pump reported in *A. baumannii*, in which *ade*I, *ade*J, and *ade*K genes encode the MFP, transporter and outer membrane components of the pump, respectively. This type of pumps are found to be involved in exporting β-lactams, chloramphenicol, tetracycline, erythromycin, lincosamides, fluoroquinolones, fusidic acid, novobiocin, rifampin, trimethoprim, acridine, safranin, pyronine and sodium dodecyl sulphate (Piolle et al., 2008).

The third RND type efflux pump is AdeFGH, which was found to be functional in the mutant in which AdeABC and AdeIJK were non-functional. In one clinically relevant study, it was shown that the increased expression of AdeFGH in *A. baumannii* is an additional mechanism for high-level resistance to fluoroquinolones and decreased susceptibility to tigecycline. The efficiency of AdeFGH pump is less when compared to the other type of efflux pumps because its overexpression was not reported during antibiotic stress and is found be constitutively expressed in the cells. AdeL, a LysR type regulator controls the expression of AdeFGH operon. The presence of the *ade*FGH operon in 90% of the strains was shown in one study (Coyne et al., 2010). This work also revealed that overexpression of *ade*FGH is likely due to point mutation in *ade*L, suggesting that this event may possibly occur in all clinical strains under selection pressure. More molecular and biochemical studies on the transcriptional regulator AdeL should allow better understanding of the mechanism of AdeFGH expression in *A. baumannii* (Coyne et al., 2010)

2.4.2 MFS type efflux pump

Major facilitator superfamily (MFS) acts as efflux pumps to decrease the intracellular concentrations of multiple toxic substrates and confer multidrug resistance. TetA and TetB efflux pumps from the MFS, involved in the tetracycline and minocycline resistance in *A. baumannii*. Many believe that MFS efflux pump is also responsible for the intrinsic chloramphenicol resistance described in *A. baumannii* strains, and therefore it was suggested that it can be named CraA, for **c**hloramphenicol **r**esistance ***A**cinetobacter* (Magnet et al., 2001; Peleg et al., 2008). Recently, a novel efflux pump AmvA (Methyl Viologen resistance) that mediates antimicrobial and disinfectant resistance in *A. baumannii* has been characterized (Rajamohan et al., 2010). AmvA is known to be responsible for the transport of toxic substances such as acridine orange, acriflavine, benzalkonium chloride, DAPI, deoxycholate, ethidium bromide, methyl viologen, SDS and tetraphenylphosphonium chloride(TPPCl). In yet another study, two different MFS type efflux pumps such as CmlA and CraA that are specific for chloramphenicol resistance have been reported (Roca et al., 2009).

2.4.3 MATE type efflux pump

The MATE (Multidrug and Toxic Compound Extrusion) family is the most recently categorized, one among the five multidrug efflux transporter families. There are almost twenty different types of MATE type transporters reported in bacteria. A proton driven

MATE family of efflux pump AbeM is reported in *Acinetobacter* which was characterized to be responsible for exerting resistance to kanamycin, erythromycin, chloramphenicol, tetraphenylphosphonium chloride (TPPCl), norfloxacin, ciprofloxacin and trimethoprim (Su et al., 2005)

2.4.4 SMR type efflux pump

One most recent study for the first time described the role of the SMR efflux pump in *Acinetobacter* spp (Srinivasan et al., 2009). The regulatory protein of this pump AbeS mediates resistance to various antibiotics, hydrophobic compounds, detergents, and disinfectants in *A. baumannii* strain AC0037 (Srinivasan et al., 2009). The SMR type pump is composed of four transmembrane α-helices of approximately 100–140 amino acids in length driven by H+ gradient. A related study concluded that the coupling ion in the AbeM pump is H+ and not Na+. It is worthwhile to note that some H^+ - norfloxacin antiport activity is seen earlier in vesicles of *E. coli* KAM32/pUC18 (Su et al., 2005).

2.4.5 ABC transporters

ATP Binding Cassette (ABC) transporters form a special family of membrane proteins, characterized by homologous ATP-binding and large, multispanning transmembrane domains. Several members of this family are primary active transporters. Whole cell proteome analysis of *Acinetobacter* has revealed the presence ABC transporters which are proposed to be responsible for the transport of ferric ion and drug resistance (Iacono et al., 2008).

2.5 Aminoglycoside-modifying enzymes (AMEs)

Resistance to aminoglycosides by AMEs is also a major threatening feature which leads to resistant phenotypes which shows resistance to aminoglycoside antibiotics such as gentamycin, kanamycin and streptomycin in *Acinetobacter* spp. All three classes of aminoglycoside-modifying enzymes reported have been found in *Acinetobacter.* These enzymes are the O-nucleotidyltransferases (ANT) and O-phosphotransferases (APH) that catalyse the nucleotidylation (adenylation) and phosphorylation of the hydroxyl groups and finally the N-acetyltransferases (AAC) that catalyse acetylation of amino groups thereby rendering the antibiotics inactive. Studies have shown that the genes encoding all these enzymes to be present on plasmids, transposons or within integron-type structures.

In summary, emergence of MDR *A. baumannii* isolates that are resistant to almost all available antibiotics are a serious problem in clinical settings. More ominously, pan drug-resistant (PDR) and extremely drug-resistant (XDR) *A. baumannii* isolates that have been recently emerged (Park et al., 2009). As a consequence, colistin is now considered as a therapy of last resort against MDR *Acinetobacter* infections (Nation & Li, 2009). Unfortunately, colistin resistance has also been reported now (Adams et al., 2009). The overexpression of components of PmrAB two-component system such as *pmr*B and/or *pmr*A appear to be only partially responsible for colistin resistance as shown by Park et al (Park et al., 2011). All kinds of mechanisms of antimicrobial resistance in *Acinetobacter* species have been clearly illustrated in Figure - 1.

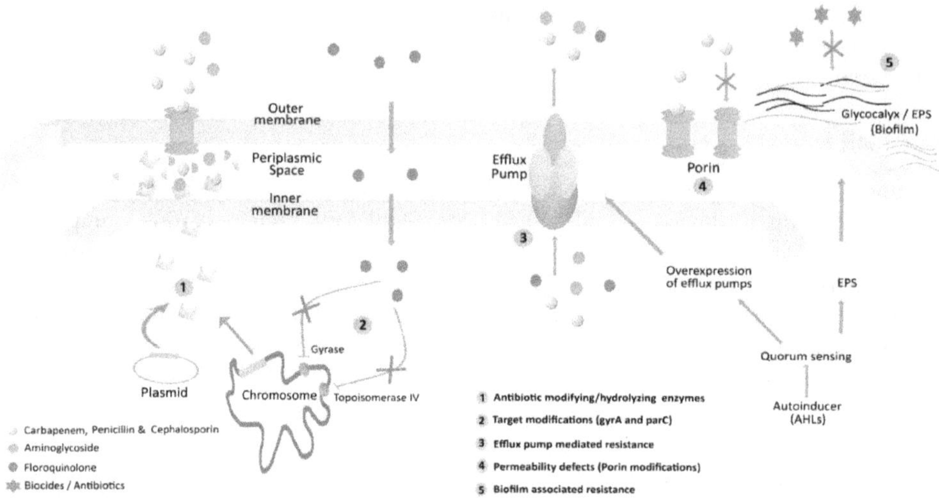

Fig. 1 Potential mechanisms of antimicrobial resistance in *Acinetobacter* species. General depiction of different kinds of antimicrobial resistance mechanisms operating in *Acinetobacter* spp. Five types resistance mechanisms are illustrated in the figure, which is of self explanatory

Finally, more experiments are in need that elucidates the performance of gene knockout studies particularly, knockout of the genes for β-lactamases and efflux systems and restoration of the genetic support for deficient mechanisms (e.g., porins) will further define their roles in *Acinetobacter* clinical isolates.

3. Biofilms and antibiotic resistance

The ability of *A. baumannii* to adhere to and form biofilms on biotic and abiotic surfaces (inanimate objects) may explain its success in the hospital environment. Biofilms might contribute to the environmental persistence of *Acinetobacter* leading to host infection and colonization

3.1 Bacterial biofilms

The bacterial biofilm have been in nature since very long but, it was not until 1970s that science could decipher and appreciate the biofilm lifestyle of bacteria. Biofilm is a complex aggregation of microorganisms, wherein the cells are embedded in a self-produced matrix of extracellular polymeric substance (EPS). The new definition of a biofilm is a microbially derived sessile community characterized by cells that are irreversibly attached to a substratum or interface or to each other, are embedded in a matrix of extracellular polymeric substances that they have produced, and exhibit an altered phenotype with respect to growth rate and gene transcription (Donlan & Costerton, 2002). It is now becoming clear that aggregation of bacterial cells are natural assemblages of bacteria within the biofilm matrix and it functions as a cooperative consortium, in a relatively complex and coordinated manner. Biofilm phenotype of a pathogen promotes increased colonization and persistence and therefore is the leading cause for device-related infections. The ability of these pathogens to adhere to human tissues and medical devices and produce biofilms is a major virulence factor that correlates with increase in antibiotic resistance, reduced phagocytosis, and overall persistence of the bacterial population. Moreover, these biofilms are notoriously difficult to eradicate and are a source of many recalcitrant infections. The medical importance of the scientific studies of biofilms and its architecture resides more in our ability to explain the characteristics of device-related infections and other chronic infections and to design strategies to counter their refractory nature.

3.1.1 Biofilms and resistance

The mechanisms by which biofilms contribute to reduced susceptibility still remain unclear, but a number of different explanations have been proposed. Biofilms are inherently resistant to the antimicrobial agents, reasons being failure of an agent to penetrate full depth to cells of biofilm or cells slow growing state due to the organism's slow metabolism. For chemically reactive disinfectants such as chlorine, iodine and peroxygens, and for highly charged antibiotics, such as the glycopeptides, the glycocalyx does indeed greatly affect the ability of the antimicrobial agent to reach those cells that are deep within the biofilm. On the other hand, for relatively unreactive, uncharged agents, such as the β-lactams, such reaction-diffusion limitation is unlikely to occur. The glycocalyx may however, contribute to reduced susceptibility to β-lactams, if the antibiotic is susceptible to inactivation by β–lactamases and if the β-lactamase is derepressed while the bacterium is in the biofilm mode of growth. In such cases, the enzyme is concentrated within the extracellular polymer matrix and hydrolyses the drug as it penetrates (Gilbert & Brown, 1998). Reduced susceptibility to β-lactams amongst biofilm bacteria is more likely to be a function of a diminished growth rate within the deeper recesses of the biofilm which causes the expression of penicillin-binding proteins that are unrepresentative of those normally targeted by these antibiotics (Gilbert & Brown, 1998). Retarded growth also affects the bactericidal action of the β-lactams because transpeptidase inhibition, which induces cellular injury, is directly related to growth rate. One investigation revealed that gene transfer in biofilms occurs far more frequently than previously noticed (Hausner & Wuertz, 1999) and horizontal gene transfer inside a biofilm matrix offers a great advantage in terms of both frequency and stability (Hausner & Wuertz, 1999). The knowledge that attached cells of the same species differ in their ability to maintain incoming plasmids hints at specific physiological conditions in biofilms which lead to individual cells experiencing different environmental pressures.

3.1.2 Biofilm cycle – a multistep process

Attachment to abiotic surface is mainly dependent on cell surface hydrophobicity, whereas surface proteins mediate adhesion to host matrix-covered implants. After adhesion to the surface, exopolysaccharide, specific proteins and accessory macromolecules aid in intercellular aggregation (Otto, 2009). At critical cell density, cells co-ordinate through a communication pathway involving signalling molecules, termed quorum sensing (QS), resulting in biofilm formation (Costerton et al., 1999). Further, at a later stage, due to physical forces or intercellular signalling, the cells detach and disperse to colonize new areas (Costerton et al., 1999).

3.1.3 Biofilm and disease

While many biofilm infections are "stealthy," in that they develop slowly and initially produce few symptoms, they may be very damaging because they promote immune complex sequelae and act as reservoirs for acute exacerbations in hosts. Many a times host immune response products of oxidative bursts rarely penetrate the biofilm matrix accounting for the inability of phagocytes to destroy the pathogen (Costerton et al., 1999). The exact processes by which biofilm associated organisms elicit disease in the human host are poorly understood. However, suggested mechanisms include: (i) detachment of cells or cell aggregates from indwelling medical device biofilms, resulting in bloodstream or urinary tract infections, (ii) production of endotoxins and (iii) resistance to the host immune system (Peleg et al., 2008). One should begin to examine any infection that is refractory to antibiotic therapy and to host defences in terms of the genes that are expressed to produce the refractory bacterial phenotype. Furthermore, one must begin to use the biofilm phenotype of each chronic pathogen in the development of new vaccines and antibiotics aimed at biofilm-specific targets that can be the means of controlling burgeoning group of diseases caused by biofilm phenotype.

3.2 Biofilm development mechanisms in *A. baumannii*

There are three important factors which contribute to the persistence of *A. baumannii* in the hospital environment, namely: resistance to major antimicrobial drugs, resistance to desiccation and resistance to disinfectants. This survival property is most likely to play a significant role in the outbreaks caused by this pathogen (Tomaras et al., 2003). The potential ability of *Acinetobacter* to form biofilms may explain its outstanding antibiotic resistance against a wide range of antibiotics (Rao et al., 2008; Dijkshoorn et al., 2007; Donlan & Costerton, 2002). *A. baumannii* has the ability to colonize both abiotic and medical devices (Tomoras et al., 2003) and form biofilms that display decreased susceptibility to multiple antibiotics (Uma Karthika et al., 2008). Adherence of *A. baumannii* to human bronchial epithelial cells and erythrocytes has already been demonstrated, with pilus like structures appear to be important for adherence (Gospodarek et al., 1998, Lee et al., 2006). This process is considered to be a first step in the colonization process of *A. baumannii.* Survival and growth on host skin and mucosal surfaces requires the clones that can resist inhibitory agents and the conditions that are exerted by these surfaces. Outgrowth on mucosal surfaces and medical devices, such as intravascular catheters and endotracheal tubes can result in *A. baumannii* biofilm formation, which enhances the risk of infection of the bloodstream and airways (Tomoras et al., 2003). One of the studies had showed that the common source of *Acinetobacter* bacteremia is intravascular catheters and the colonization of respiratory tract (Cisneros et al., 2002). Interestingly, it has also been demonstrated that biofilm formation in *Acinetobacter* is phenotypically associated with exopolysaccharide (EPS) production and pilus formation (Tomoras et al., 2004). The protein equivalent to CsuE of *Vibrio parahaemolyticus,* a chaperone has been identified as a key factor in pilus and biofilm formation in a pioneer study (Tomoras et al., 2004). Surprisingly, considerable variation in quantitative adherence was observed among different strains of *A. baumannii* isolated from the same geographical region (Lee et al., 2006). This observation of varying degree of adherence among the strains is in concordance with our studies (unpublished data). Our earlier investigation also demonstrated a high propensity among the clinical isolates of *A.*

baumannii to form biofilm and a significant association of biofilms with multiple drug resistance (Rao et al., 2008). Thus, biofilm production by *A. baumannii* promotes increased colonization and persistence leading to higher rates of device related infections. Identification of new genes involved in biofilm formation is required for better understanding of molecular basis of strain variation and various pathogenic mechanisms implicated in chronic *Acinetobacter* infections.

3.2.1 Factors associated with *A. baumannii* biofilm formation

3.2.2 Poly-β-(1, 6)-N-acetlyglucosamine (PNAG)

One of the important polysaccharides is poly-β-(1, 6)-N-acetlyglucosamine (PNAG), which has been now portrayed as a major component of biofilms of bacteria was first described in the genus *Staphylococci* (Maira-Litran et al., 2002). PNAG seems to be having profound effects on host-microbe interactions. PNAG affects colonization, virulence, and immune evasion in infections caused by both Gram-positive and Gram-negative species (Itoh et al., 2008). Apart from its role in surface and cell-to-cell adherence (Cramton et al., 1999), PNAG is described as an important virulence factor (Kropec et al., 2005) and provides protection against the antibiotics and shown to protect *Staphylococci* against innate host defences (Lewis 2001 and Voung et al., 2004). Pga locus encodes for the proteins involved in the synthesis and translocation of PNAG on to the bacterial surface (Kropec et al., 2005; Shiro et al., 1995; Vuong et al., 2004). In *S. aureus*, PNAG confers resistance to killing mediated by innate host immune mediators. Overall, PNAG production by *S. aureus* appears to be a critical virulence factor as assessed in murine models of systemic infection (Kropec et al., 2005). PgaB and IcaB (from *Staphylococci*) contain polysaccharide N-deacetylase domains belonging to carbohydrate esterase family 4. PNAG is also shown to be essential for the formation of the nonrandom or periodic cellular architecture in *E. coli* biofilm microstructure and for conversion from temporary polar cell surface attachment to permanent lateral attachment during the initial stages of biofilm development (Itoh et al., 2008). PgaB of *pga*ABCD peron of *E. coli* is predicted to be an outer membrane lipoprotein. The *hms* locus in *Yersinia pestis,* which is equivalent to PNAG operon apparently promotes the transmission of the plague bacillus *Y. pestis* from the flea vector to the mammalian host (Jarrett et al., 2004). PgaB ortholog in *Y. pestis* designated as HmsF, co-purifies with the outer membrane fraction in this bacterium.

PNAG, the most important EPS secreted by the bacterial population also forms the major component of the biofilms in *Acinetobacter* spp. (Choi et al., 2009). Recent study on *pga*ABCD of Gram-negative bacteria with the typical reference strain of *A. baumannii* showed that the four gene loci share a high degree of similarity with *E. coli* and *Y. pestis* (Choi et al., 2009). *A. baumannii pga*A encodes for a predicted 812-amino-acid OMP and it contains a porin domain suggesting that it facilitates PNAG translocation across the outer membrane and a superhelical periplasmic domain that is thought to play a role in protein-protein interaction (Itoh et al., 2008). PgaB is made up of 510 amino acids with a putative polysaccharide deacetylase domain. PgaB is an outer membrane lipoprotein that along with PgaA, is necessary for PNAG export (Itoh et al., 2008). *pga*C encodes for a 392-amino-acid N-glycosyltransferase that belongs to the glycosyltransferase 2 family. Gene *pga*D encodes for a 150 amino acid protein which localizes in the cytoplasm and assists PgaC in the synthesis of PNAG (Itoh et al., 2008). One recent investigation speculated that in a more dynamic environment with higher shear forces, PNAG is more essential for maintaining the integrity of *A. baumannii* biofilms (Choi et al., 2009).

3.2.3 Biofilm-associated protein (Bap)

Biofilm-associated proteins (Bap) were first characterized in *S. aureus* (Cucarella et al 2001) and recent research findings indicated that *Acinetobacter* has a homologue of Bap protein of *Staphylococcus.* Bap family members are high-molecular weight proteins present on the bacterial surface, contain a core domain of tandem repeats, and play a critical role in cell-cell interactions and biofilm maturation (Loehfelm et al., 2008; Lasa & Penades, 2006). Bap is made up of 8620 amino acids, arranged in tandemly repeated modules A-E (Rahbar et al 2010). It has a higher proportion of negatively charged amino acids in the tandem repeats compared to non-tandem repeat parts (Loehfelm et al., 2008). As it has no transmembrane anchoring domain, its interaction with the cell wall is unclear and yet to be investigated.

The mechanism by which the Bap contributes to biofilm development is unknown, though their large size and the presence of a high number of repeats suggest that these proteins could mediate homophilic or heterophilic intercellular interactions (Lasa & Penades, 2006). Structural studies suggest that the main target for Bap is carbohydrates, for maintenance of biofilm complex (Rahbar et al., 2010). Time course confocal laser scanning microscopy and three-dimensional image analysis of actively growing biofilms demonstrate that Bap mutant is unable to sustain biofilm thickness and volume, suggesting a role for Bap in supporting the development of the mature biofilm structure. In *A. baumannii,* Bap is identified as a specific cell surface protein and is involved in intercellular adhesion within the mature biofilm. Future studies in *A. baumannii* must explore Bap-mediated interactions like direct mediation of intercellular adhesion from one bacterium to a surface receptor on a neighboring bacterium, autoadhesion between Bap molecules on adjacent bacteria and/or whether cells may be linked indirectly via shared interactions with some extracellular biofilm matrix component. However, one can hope that Bap can be a potential target to develop a novel vaccine that can abolish biofilm development (Rahbar et al., 2010).

3.2.4 Chaperone-usher secretion system

A. baumannii require chaperone-usher pili assembly for the production of biofilm on inanimate surfaces as revealed from the study of Tomaras et al (2003). This secretion system encodes for a putative pili-like structure/adhesion protein essential for the initiation of biofilm formation. The *csu* operon expressing chaperone-usher pili assembly comprised of a gene cluster that encompasses six ORFs: *csu*AB-A-B-C-D-E and is polycistronic in nature (Tomaras et al., 2003). The translational products of the *csu*D and *csu*E are highly related to chaperone and usher bacterial proteins, respectively, the four remaining ORFs encode hypothetical proteins potentially involved in pili assembly (Tomaras et al., 2003). The *csu* operon is regulated by a two-component system, *bfm*RS. BfmS is a sensor kinase, which senses environmental conditions and activates a response regulator encoded by *bfm*R. Over-expression of the *csu*AB operon is caused by higher BfmR intracellular concentration (Tomaras et al., 2003). Current models on biofilm formation clearly implicate the participation of bacterial surface related flagella and pili (O' Toole & Kolter, 1998) and cellular appendages (Tolker-Nielson et al., 2000). Bacterial cells in the biofilm community are linked to each other through extracellular appendages that resemble pili structures (Tomaras et al., 2003).

All the above data suggest that there may be an overlap in factors required for the initiation and maturation of biofilms on abiotic and biotic surfaces, bacterial attachment and pathogenesis *in vivo.* Though one can articulate that quorum sensing may be a central mechanism for autoinduction of multiple virulence factors such as genes those involved in the cell envelope, EPS production, pilus biogenesis, iron uptake and metabolism (Smith, 2007) and type IV virulence/secretion systems.

4. Quorum sensing in bacteria

Many bacteria use cell to cell communication to monitor their population density, synchronize their behavior and socially interact. Such communication used by the bacteria is chemical in nature and generally designated as quorum sensing (QS) which is nothing but a coordinated gene regulation and is generally termed as QS. Small diffusible molecules produced by bacteria are 'signals' which can reach other cells and elicit 'answers'. This phenomenon relies mainly on cell density and with the increase in cell density, a critical concentration of signaling molecule will be reached that allows sensing of the signalling molecule and enables the other bacteria to respond. QS is a type of community behaviour prevalent among a diverse group of bacteria to switch between planktonic phenotype to high cell density biofilm phenotype. Irrespective of either Gram-negative or Gram-positive bacteria, the process of QS is analogous in both the groups. The stepwise process involving intracellular synthesis of low molecular weight molecules and secrete them to the extracellular milieu. When the number of cells in a population increases, the concentration of QS molecules also increases and once the minimal threshold level crosses, the molecules are recognised by the receptors that trigger signal transduction cascades that result in a population wide change in gene expression. Such molecular cascades enable the population to function in harmony to survive and proliferate. Depending upon the bacterial species, the physiological processes regulated by QS are extremely diverse, ranging from maintaining the biofilms to regulating the antibiotic resistance. A flurry of research over the past decade has led to significant understanding of many aspects of QS molecules including their synthesis, the receptors that recognize the signal and transduce this information to the level of gene expression and the interaction of these receptors with the transcriptional machinery. Recent studies have begun to integrate QS into global regulatory networks and establish its role in developing and maintaining the structure of bacterial communities.

QS network in Gram-negative bacteria regulate the expression of specific sets of genes in a cell density-dependent fashion (Ng & Bassler, 2009). Pathogenic bacteria typically use QS in the regulation of genes encoding extracellular virulence factors. Gram-positive bacteria like *S. aureus* secrete small peptides for cell to cell communication. On the other hand Gram-negatives like *A. baumannii* predominantly produce small molecules like acylated homoserine lactones (Acyl-HSL) as QS entities. Sometimes other signalling molecules such as 2-heptyl-3-hydroxy-4-quinolone and diketopiperazines are also produced by Gram-negative bacteria (Holden et al., 2000)

4.1 Quorum sensing molecules

Acyl homoserine lactones (AHLs) are a major class of autoinducer signals used by Gram-negative proteobacteria for intraspecies communication that are best characterised till date. AHLs of QS signalling system seem to control diverse physiological functions such as biofilm formation, Ti plasmid conjugation, production of antibiotics, and competence in certain bacteria (Fuqua et al., 2001; Antunes et al., 2010). AHLs are composed of HSL rings carrying acyl chains of C4 to C18 in length. These side chains harbour occasional modification, notably at the C3 position or unsaturated double bonds. The first AHL autoinducer and its cognate regulatory circuit has been first discovered in the bioluminescent marine bacterium *Vibrio fischeri*. Two proteins, LuxI and LuxR, are essential for QS control of bioluminescence in *V. fischeri*. The LuxI/LuxR regulatory system of *V. fischeri* is considered the paradigm for the control of gene expression by QS in Gram-negative bacteria. Homologs of *lux*I and *lux*R have been identified in a large number of bacterial genomes and these other LuxIR-type QS systems control global cell density dependent gene expression. In *V. fischeri*, LuxI is the synthase of the QS autoinducer N-3-(oxo-hexanoyl)-homoserine lactone (3OC6HSL). LuxI catalyzes acylation and lactonization reactions between the substrates S-adenosylmethionine (SAM) and hexanoyl-ACP. Following synthesis, 3OC6HSL diffuses freely in and out of the cell and its concentration increases as the cell density of the population increases (Stevens et al., 1994). LuxR is the cytoplasmic receptor for 3OC6HSL as well as the transcriptional activator of the luciferase operon. Without the 3OC6HSL ligand, the LuxR protein is unstable and is rapidly degraded. When 3OC6HSL accumulates, it is bound by LuxR and the LuxR-AHL complex recognizes a consensus binding sequence (*lux* box) upstream of the luciferase operon and activates its expression. Because expression of luxI is also activated by 3OC6HSL-bound LuxR, when the QS circuit engages, autoinducer production is induced, and the surrounding environment is flooded with the signal molecule. This autoinduction positive feedback loop is presumed to enforce synchrony as the population of cells switches from low cell density mode to high cell density QS mode (Stevens et al., 1994; Schaefer et al., 1996).

The QS networks are increasingly gaining importance in clinical isolates as they function as global regulators. One of the well studied organisms in clinical context is *P. aeruginosa,* which uses AHL as a QS signaling molecule. In *P. aeruginosa,* the QS network is found to play a major role in maintaining biofilm, this biofilm matrix in turn helps the bacteria to survive hostile conditions by becoming resistance to bactericidal agents, resisting nutrition depleted conditions and thereby helps them to remain persistent in hospital environment that makes complete eradication of this organism a challenging quest.

4.2 Quorum sensing in *A. baumannii*

Quorum sensing (QS) in *A. baumannii* appears to have a regulatory role in biofilm formation (Smith et al., 2007). Environmental survival and growth require attributes such as resistance to desiccation and antibiotics, versatility in growth requirements, biofilm forming capacity and possibly, QS activity (Dijkshoorn et al., 2007; Smith, 2007). QS has been shown to regulate a wide array of virulence mechanisms in many Gram-negative organisms (Antunes et al., 2010) and *Acinetobacter* is no different. The presence of QS has been inferred from the detection of a gene that is involved in autoinducer production (Gaddy et al., 2009) that could control the various metabolic processes, production of virulence factors, including biofilm formation. QS network in *Acinetobacter* is mediated by acyl homoserine lactones (AHL). Up to five different QS signal molecules that are more detectable (produced abundantly) during the stationary phase have been identified in *Acinetobacter*, indicating that this may be a central mechanism for autoinduction of multiple virulence factors (Gonzalez et al., 2001;Joly-Guillou et al., 2005; Niu et al., 2008; Gonzalez et al., 2009). In one most recent study, different species of *Acinetobacter* were analyzed for the production of AHL and it was shown that QS sensors were not homogenously distributed among species, though one particular AHL was specifically present in most of the strains belonging to *A. calcoaceticus-A. baumannii* complex (Gonzalez et al., 2009). Furthermore, it was revealed that no distinction could be made between the QS signals secreted by typical opportunistic strains of the *A. calcoaceticus-A. baumannii* complex isolated from patients and strains belonging to other species of the genus (Gonzalez et al., 2009). In our investigation, we have also identified more than six different QS signal molecules in majority of the *A. baumannii* clinical isolates wherein chromatographic separation (Thin Layer Chromatography) of ethyl acetate extracts followed by β-galactosidase assay for determining QS activity using *A. tumefaciens* reporter strain NT1, containing plasmid pZLR4 carrying traR and a traG::lacZ reporter fusion was used. However, among these only one kind of QS molecule was produced abundantly (Figure - 2).

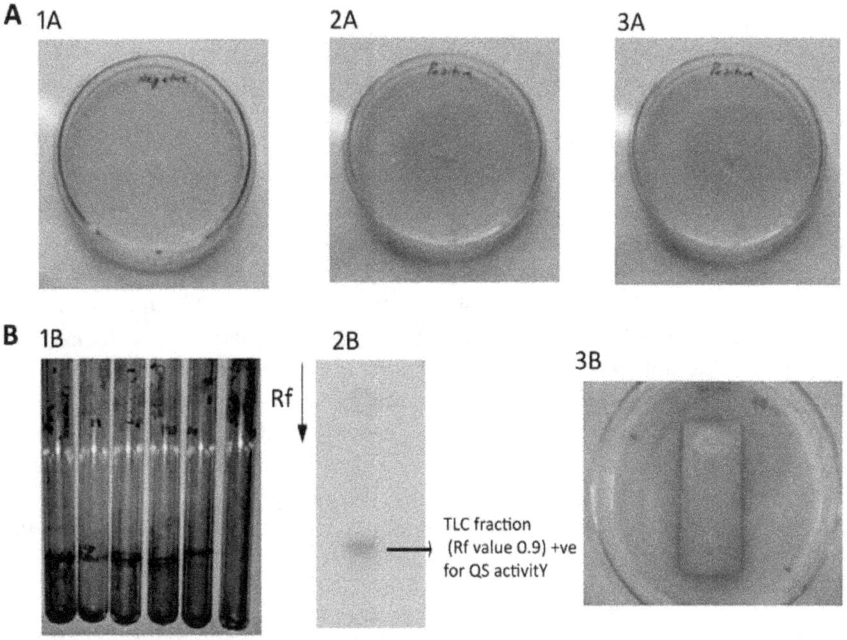

A:- Biosensor overlay test using reporter strain (*Agrobacterium tumefaciens* pZLR4) for detection of quorum sensing (QS) molecules; 1A – Negative control; 2A *A. tumefaciens* Positive control NTL4(pTiC58ΔaccR); 3A - QS activity positive reaction produced ethyl acetate extract of *A. baumannii* clinical isolate confirming the production Acyl Homoserine lactone
B:- 1B- Biofilm production in *A. baumannii* isolates detected through Tube method using 1% crystal violet stain. Thick violet ring was witnessed between liquid air interfaces; 2B - Thin layer chromatography (TLC) of crude ethyl acetate extract of *A. baumannii* culture supernatant; 3B - Ethyl acetate extracts obtained from *A. baumannii* culture supernatants were separated by TLC and over laid with *A. tumefaciens* (pZLR4).

Fig. 2. Quorum sensing activity in *A. baumannii*

Another recent investigation on *A. baumannii* M2 strain characterized an AHL and one AHL synthase gene was identified, which was held responsible for predominant of kind QS molecule produced (Niu et al., 2008). Although additional AHLs were detected in this study, they were not able detect any other gene related to them. Hence, it appears that the auto inducer synthase that was discovered has low specificity and may be capable of synthesizing other QS signals as well. Some interesting questions arising out of above study are: do the diversity of QS signals observed respond only to particular synthase? or is there any existence of more than one AHL synthase?

However, since AHL signals produced by acyltransferases do not have similarity to LuxI or LuxM/AinS, it cannot be ruled out that additional AHL signals are present in *A. baumannii* M2. The AbaI protein was similar to members of the LuxI family of autoinducer synthases and was predicted to be the only autoinducer synthase encoded by *A. baumannii*. The expression of *aba*I at the transcriptional level was activated by ethyl acetate extracts of *A. baumannii* culture supernatants or by synthetic 3-hydroxy-C12-HSL. Further an *aba*I mutant failed to produce any detectable AHL signals and was impaired in biofilm development indicting that there is direct role QS molecules in biofilm development (Niu et al., 2008). QS machinery in *A. baumannii* appear to be mediated by a two component system AbaIR (Niu et al., 2008). This two-component system is homologous to a typical LuxIR family of proteins found in Gram- negative bacteria. This system includes a sensor protein AbaI that functions as an enzyme synthesizing AHLs and AbaR that functions as receptor by recognizing the AHL and induces a cascade of signaling pathway(s). QS was found to play a major role in biofilm maintenance and maturation in *Acinetobacter*. Niu et al (2008) have revealed that in abaI null mutants, there is about 40% reduction of biofilm and this was restored when AHL supplied externally. Consistent with this study, scanning electron microscopy (SEM) analysis data from our laboratory has shown biofilm formation in biofilm-negative clinical isolates when AHL was provided exogenously, as well there was enhanced biofilm formation in weakly adherent clinical isolates after such supplementation (Figure- 3). *A. baumannii* was found to produce more than 5 types of AHLs with varying fatty acid chains (Gonzalez et al., 2001 & 2009; Niu et al., 2008). The *aba*I autoinducer synthase was found to produce N-(3-hydroxydodecanoyl)-L-HSL (3-hydroxy-C12-HSL) when cloned and expressed in *E. coli*. Genomic sequence analysis of *A. baumannii* ATCC 17978 has revealed that *aba*I and acyltransferase may be the core mediator for synthesis of AHLs with varying chemical nature. Such observations as whole underpin a positive correlation between QS and biofilm formation

A comparative study using *in silico* tools have shown that the autoinducer synthase gene *aba*I is more than 45% identical to autoinducer synthase gene from environmental non-pathogenic organisms like *Halothiobacillus neapolitanus, Acidithiobacillus ferrooxidans* ATCC23270 and less identical to RhlI and LasI system of pathogenic *P. aeruginosa* but about 47.3% identical to autoinducer synthase genes of an environmental strain *Pseudomonas* sp RW10S (Bhargava et al., 2010). These similarities and dissimilarities between environmental and clinical isolates clearly demonstrates how *Acinetobacter* as evolved from an environmental form to a pathogenic individual. Further, in-depth analysis has revealed that *A. baumannii* has more similarity with *Burkholderia ambifaria* at organism level and in stark contrast, its *aba*I gene shares similarity with *H. neapolitanus*. Similarly, *aba*R was found to share more similarity to *H. neapolitanus* but it is unrelated to *B. ambifaria*. This can raise another question that *aba*I and *aba*R are two different genes yet they share similarity with homologs of another organism and it is because *aba*R is present just 63 base pairs upstream of *aba*I and it can be easily transferred as a single unit from one organism to the other.

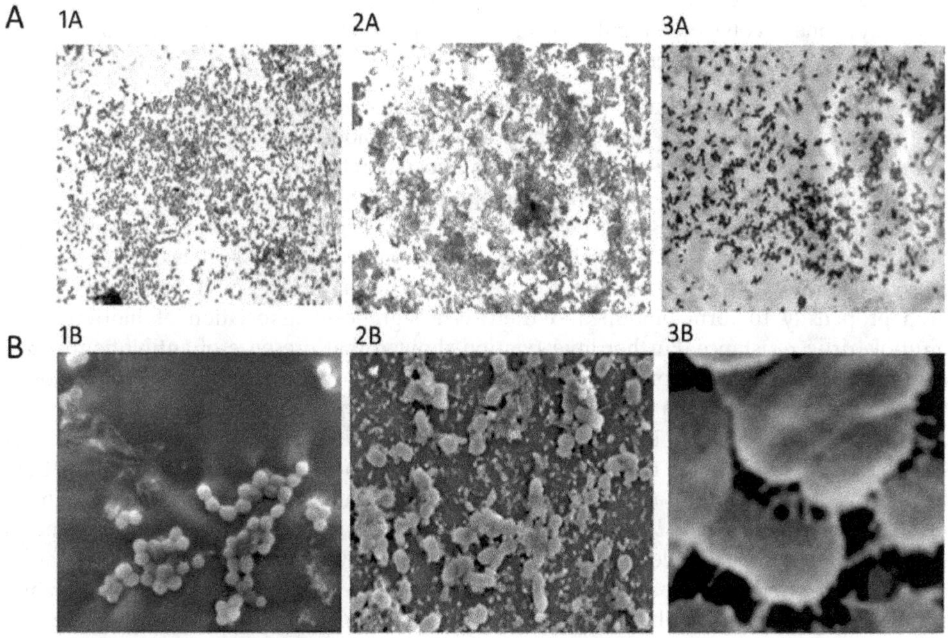

1A- Growth of *A. baumannii* (biofilm-negative) on glass cover slip stained with 0.1% of crystal violet; 2A- Effect of N-AHL (200μM) extracted from *A. baumannii* biofilm phenotype on growth of biofilm non-producer; biofilm development can be observed. 3A - Effect of garlic extract on growth and biofilm formation; inhibition of biofilm was observed.
1B & 2B - SEM images of preparations similar to 1A & 2A respectively (X 5000 magnification); 3B magnified images showing cell to cell adherence through pili-like appendages (X 15000 magnifiction).

Fig. 3. A & B – Microscopic and scanning electron microscopic (SEM) analysis of effect of N-Acyl homoserine lactone (AHL) and garlic extract (Quorum quenching agent) on biofilm-negative strains of *A. baumannii* of clinical origin.

The likely lateral gene transfer between two distinct bacteria can be attributed to the natural competence of *A. baumannii* that has made them to acquire genetic information from other organisms. Interestingly, QS sensing is well known to increase competence in bacteria which further illuminates the importance of these chemical mediators.

A. baumannii being found to be a major threat in many hospitals, recent studies have clearly demonstrated the alarming need for an intense research on QS in *A. baumannii*. Pandrug resistance of *A. baumannii* is attributed to a number of antibiotic resistance mechanisms and biofilm formation. This biofilm formation is in turn regulated by QS networks, which make them to be considered as an important drug target to combat these multidrug resistant superbugs.

4.3 Quorum sensing and Antibiotic resistance

Multiple drug resistance can be attributed to a number of mechanisms, which includes synthesis of enzymes that degrade the drugs, modified targets that does not respond to the drug and presence of efflux pumps that pumps out the bactericidal drugs from the bacterial system to the extracellular milieu. QS was found to be regulating multidrug resistance in two ways, one involves up regulation of biofilm associated EPS matrix and other by up regulation of efflux pump genes.

The production of an EPS matrix is one of the distinguishing characteristics of biofilm and it has been suggested that EPS prevents the access of antibiotics into the bacterial community. Our investigations reveal that there is a strong association between multidrug resistance and biofilms wherein majority of our clinical isolates, which were strong biofilm producers were also exhibiting multidrug resistance (Rao et al., 2008). Compared to non-biofilm producers, biofilm producers showed a significantly higher resistance to cephotaxime, amikacin, ciprofloxacin and aztreonam. Thus, it is clear that clinical isolates of *A. baumannii* have a high propensity to form biofilm and there is a significant association of biofilms with multiple drug resistance. Further investigation showed that presence of antibiotic resistant determinant *bla*PER-1 is more critical for cell adherence, which is the first step in biofilm formation cycle. One of the success stories of *Acinetobacter* is its ability to withstand stress conditions like exposure to high dose of antibiotics. Previous studies on *Pseudomonas* have shown that exposure to the macrolide antibiotics found to enhance biofilm formation. Such responses suggest biofilm as a potential defence mechanism against antibiotics. Similar mechanism is seen in *A. baumannii* in which strong biofilm producers are commonly multidrug resistant. The role of QS molecule as a key player in antibiotic resistance can be understood from their mechanism of enhancing replication and transfer of plasmids, which are the major carriers of antibiotic resistant genes. Thus in a biofilm microstructure there is an increased possibility of gene transfer including genes for antibiotic resistance. Consequently, the biofilm forming capacity of *A. baumannii* combined with its multidrug resistance contributes to the organism's survival and further dissemination in the hospital settings.

Evidences for the role of QS in upregulating efflux pumps arise from studies in *E. coli* in which over expression of *E. coli* luxR homologue SdiA lead to the overexpression of AcrAB efflux pumps and its knockout lead to decrease in AcrAB efflux gene expression. This study clearly demonstrates how QS directly play an indispensable role in regulating efflux pump gene expression. SdiA as well regulates cell division in a cell density-dependent manner. It was also shown that SdiA controls multidrug resistance by positively regulating the MDR pump AcrAB and overproduction of SdiA confers multidrug resistance and increased levels of AcrAB. Conversely, *sdi*A null mutants are hypersensitive to drugs and have decreased levels of AcrB protein. These observations provide a direct link between QS and MDR achieved through efflux pump. Combined with earlier reports, this data support a model in which a role of drug efflux pumps is to mediate cell–cell communication in response to cell density (Rahmati et al., 2002). Now, it is clear that *sdi*A positively regulates the AcrAB efflux pump to mediate multiple drug resistance in *E. coli.*

In *P. aeruginosa,* when the cells are in the logarithmic growth phase, the MexR repressor negatively regulates *mex*AB-*opr*M efflux pump expression by binding at the MexR-MexAB-OprM operator-promoter region. As the cells enter the stationary growth phase, they sense a high population density and turn on a QS switch producing an autoinducer, C4-HSL, which independently induces the expression of *mex*AB-*opr*M operon directly or it inactivates the MexR repressor, as a consequence it enhances the transcription of MexAB-OprM efflux pump (Maseda et al., 2004). This study also revealed that MexAB mutants accumulate 3O-C12-HSL intracellularly, which shows how QS signals form a part of efflux pump networks. In *A. baumannii*, antibiotic resistance is also brought about by a number efflux pump genes and the RND efflux genes which are found to share about 47% similarity with MexAB pumps are the major efflux pumps in *A. baumannii*. *A. baumannii* also produces C12-HSL compounds as QS molecules, which shows that there may be an interconnecting role between efflux pumps and QS that imparts multiple drug resistance.

To overcome stress, cells express various factors and one of them is RpoS which is regulated by the global regulator Hfq. In one of the studies conducted in *P. aeruginosa*, *las*R knockout mutants showed decreased resistance to ofloxacin, whereas the resistance was restored when RpoS was over expressed in *las*R knockouts. This finding suggests the strong role of stress regulators in multiple-drug resistance. As Hfq was found to regulate RpoS which in turn involved in orchestrating QS controlling antibiotic resistance, one can understand the pivotal role of stress regulators in QS and multidrug resistance. *Acinetobacter* genome analyses provide evidences for the presence of both Hfq and RpoS in *A. baumannii* though their interconnecting role is not yet elucidated.

4.4 Biofilm associated gene expression and virulence factors

Many recent investigations have revealed differential gene expression of genes during biofilm formation. Since biofilm helps in persistence of the organism in various stressful environments including survival in human hosts, many stress tolerating factors (can also termed as virulence factors) are produced to overcome a range of stress conditions. In this regard, our investigations have shown a positive correlation between biofilm and virulence factors. Our study which included majority of clinical isolates of *A. baumannii* that are biofilm producers were also found to be positive for production of virulence factors like protease, gelatinase, phospholipase, serum resistance and haemolysis (unpublished data). These factors are highly helpful for the pathogens survival in human hosts. Thus our observation sturdily supports a positive correlation between biofilm and virulence factors. Some cells in biofilm have slow growth rate, which is related to general stress response rather than nutrient limitations. To overcome stress, cells express various factors and one of them is RpoS which is regulated by the global regulator Hfq. As Hfq was found to regulate RpoS which in turn leads to QS controlled expression of virulence factors, one can understand the pivotal role of Hfq during harsh conditions. A general model of QS network with overall role of AHL in signal transduction regulated by AbaR, possible role of AbaI, Hfq, RpoS in *Acinetobacter* spp. is depicted in Figure - 4.

In conclusion, QS sensing works as a global regulator in regulating a diversified network of signalling cascades which helps the organism to resist infinite hostile conditions that are yet to be unveiled. Bacterial virulence being shown as one of the functions regulated by QS may therefore be a right target for designing newer therapeutics. Consequently, interference with QS-based inter-cellular communication might become the basis of new therapeutic schemes. Moreover, understanding QS cascades apart from revealing the communal relationships between the cells may help in designing potential drugs which can tackle multidrug resistant superbug *A. baumannii*.

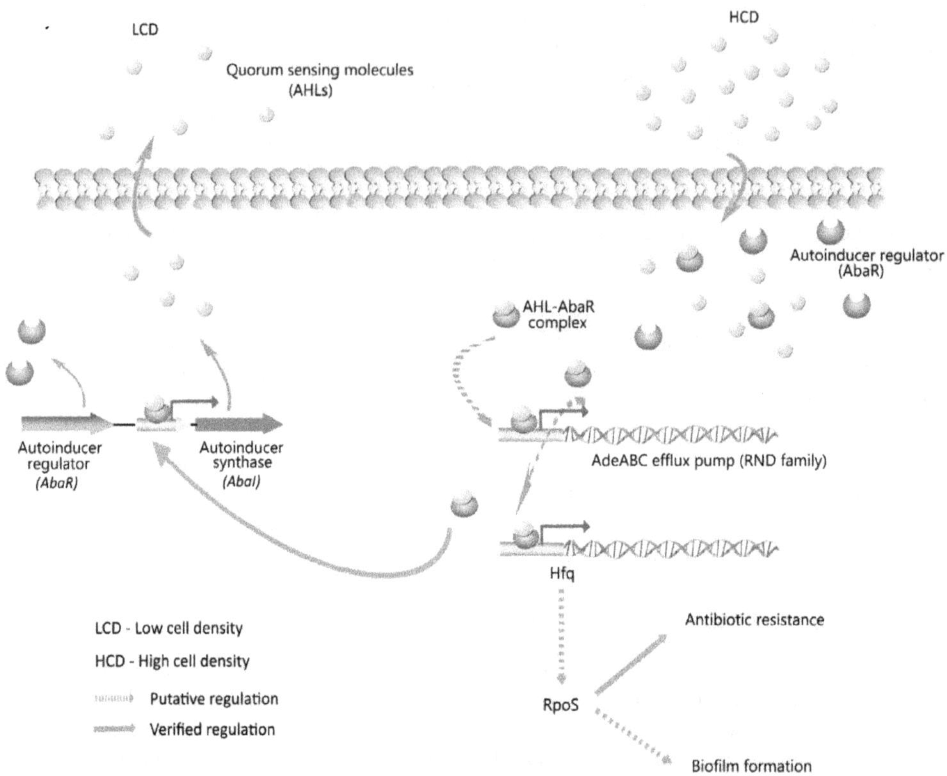

Fig. 4. A General model of acyl-homoserine lactone (AHL) signal transduction in *Acinetobacter* spp. by quorum sensing is shown. Tentative model for AHL synthesis (*left side*) and AHL interaction with AbaR-type regulatory proteins (*right side*) are depicted. Green solid arrows on the outer membrane indicate the potential two-way traffic of AHLs into and out of the cell. Putative regulatory role of AbaR and its interaction with AbaI or AbaI-type protein is shown at left side. Putative activation and overexpression of AdeABC efflux pump by AHL- AbaR complex is depicted by green dotted arrows at the right side. The presumed role of AHL- AbaR complex in up regulation of Hfq expression and putative regulation of RpoS by Hfq are shown. Finally, role of RpoS in antibiotic resistance and its probable role in biofilm development are illustrated.

5. Future prospective

Ironically, many have started believing that we are nearing the post antibiotic era as no new groups of antibiotics have been discovered after 1980s. As such, we are in a desperate need for searching new therapeutic solutions for infections caused pan-drug resistant bacteria. We might achieve this with respect to nosocomial pathogen *A. baumannii* after some careful studies of the genomics and proteome of *Acinetobacter* species looking for possible promising targets. In the following paragraphs, we describe one of the potential targets as an example, where we have tried to relate iron metabolism to biofilm production, which is based entirely on indirect evidences but strong correlation of *A. baumannii* with its other close relatives in a genomic perspective.

The remarkable similarities between the prokaryote and eukaryote iron transport systems underscore the importance of our analysis with respect to the host-bacteria interactions leading to disease. An increased knowledge of the molecular mechanisms of microbial pathogenicity mediated by iron and host resistance will undoubtedly help in finding potential drug targets. The iron-scarce environment of a vertebrate host generates a non-specific defence mechanism as most iron is bound with host proteins such as haemoglobin, or complexed with high affinity ligands such as transferrin and lactoferrin (Neilands et al., 1995). To overcome this, *A. baumannii* and other Gram-negatives secrete high affinity iron chelators, called siderophores that gather this micro- but essential nutrient (Neilands et al., 1995; Crosa, 1989). Siderophores (from the Greek: "iron carriers") are defined as relatively low molecular weight, ferric ion specific chelating agents elaborated by bacteria and fungi growing under low iron stress environment. The role of these compounds is to scavenge iron from the environment and to make the mineral and make it available to the cell. The ability to extract iron from these iron-scarce environments of the host often contributes to the virulence of a successful pathogen.

5.1 Iron metabolism in *Y. pestis* and *A. baumannii*

Indeed, there have been reports that iron deficient media suppress biofilm formation and hence decrease virulence (Weinberg, 2004; Yang et al., 2007). But, this would do nothing to hinder the growth of the pathogen as the siderophores perform superbly, the task of iron acquisition with their extremely high affinity for ferric ion (Neilands et al., 1995; Braun and Hantke, 2011). We certainly have a choice of targeting the iron acquisition system so as to abolish the virulence. Recent studies on human Gram-negative pathogen *Y. pestis* suggest that the HmsHFRS and HmsT operons regulating hemin-binding and storing system are also involved in biofilm formation (Perry et al., 1990; Kirillina et al., 2004). In fact, *Y. pestis* Hms+ phenotype, described by enormous adsorption of hemin or congo red to become red coloured, is a manifestation of biofilm formation during growth at 26–34 °C (Perry et al., 2004). *A. baumannii* has genes homologous to HmsH, HmsF and HmsR that occur end-to-end and (may) constitute an operon having a pair of hypothetical genes and spanning about a 4.7 kb region along the complementary strand of the genome (Figure-5).

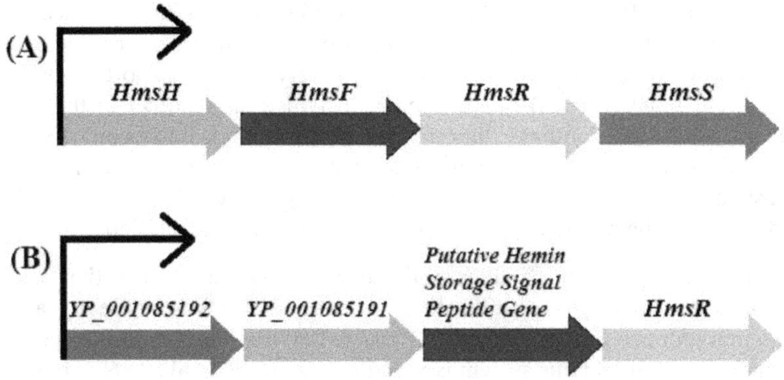

Fig. 5. A comparison between (A) *Y. pestis* Hms operon and (B) a 4.7 kb region of *A. baumannii* genome (see text) having four genes. Matching colours except dark grey colour showing homologues. Dark grey segments do not match. Promotor and intergenic sequences are ignored for the sake of simplicity.

Y. pestis HmsH is an outer membrane protein with a predicted β-barrel domain (Wortham et al., 2010) and has a weak homology to *A. baumannii* poly-beta-1, 6-N-acetyl-D-glucosamine (PGA) synthesis protein. HmsF is also an outer membrane protein with a predicted deacetylase domain. HmsR and HmsS are inner membrane proteins (Wortham et al., 2010). HmsR has a putative glycosyl-transferase domain where as HmsS homologue Ica is linked to the *Y. pestis* biofilm PGA synthesis protein PgaD. *Y. pestis* HmsH, HmsF, HmsR and HmsS have 58.2%, 60.8%, 83% and 50% sequence similarities to *E. coli* PgaA, PgaB, PgaC, PgaD respectively (Forman et al., 2006). But, they have very weak similarities with their (predicted) *A. baumannii* counterparts. Yet, from some recent investigations, it is now becoming obvious that genes from Hms operon have corresponding counterparts in *A. baumannii* (Zhou and Yang, 2001).

The above mentioned 4.7 kb region in genome of *A. baumannii* contains 4 genes in tandem, which consists of a pair of hypothetical proteins, bearing IDs YP_001085192 and YP_001085192 followed by a putative hemin storage signal peptide protein and hemin storage system protein HmsR. Neither the sequence nor the structural topology of YP_001085192 fits into any of the genes of *Y. pestis* HmsHFRS operon. Rather, according to UniProtKB annotations, it is a putative phosphotransferase, containing a nucleotide (possibly ATP) binding motif. There have been some evidences of phosphoenolpyruvate phosphotransferase (PTS) systems being involved in biofilm formation in *Vibrio cholerae, E. coli* and *Streptococcus gordonii* (Houot and Watnick, 2008; Lazazzera, 2010; Houot et al., 2010). YP_001085191, when searched against RefSeq (Pruitt et al., 2000) database, comes to be *A. baumannii* poly-beta-1, 6 N-acetyl-D-glucosamine export porin PgaA, which could be involved in the export of PGA to the cell exterior. The putative hemin storage signal peptide gene, as the name suggests, is involved in hemin storage. Searching results in the Conserved Domain Database (CDD) (Marchler- Bauer et al., 2011) suggested further that it has one each of polysaccharide deacetylase and poly-beta-1,6-N-acetyl-D-glucosamine N-deacetylase PgaB domains. The polysaccharide deacetylase domain is found in polysaccharide deacetylase. This family of polysaccharide deacetylases includes NodB (nodulation protein B from *Rhizobium*), which is a chito-oligosaccharide deacetylase. It also includes chitin deacetylase from yeast and endoxylanases which hydrolyses glucosidic bonds in xylan (Fukushima et al., 2004). Poly-beta-1, 6-N-acetyl-D-glucosamine N-deacetylase PgaB produces polysaccharides based on N-acetyl-D-glucosamine in straight chains with beta-1, 6 linkages. Deacetylation by this protein appears necessary to allow export through the porin PgaA (Itoh et al., 2008). The last one in the order, HmsR, as resulted in the CDD search, belongs to the cellulose synthase superfamily (Roberts and Bushoven, 2007) and also contains a DXD motif which binds to a metal ion that is used to coordinate the phosphates a nucleotide-sugar at the active site. These features suggest that *A. baumannii,* like its near relatives, depends on hemin-adsorption and storage for biofilm formation.

Neither the hemin acquisition (Zimbler et al., 2009) nor the biofilm function has remained uncharacterized in *A. baumannii.* But the above discussion correlates these two and suggests that they are not independent of each other. Even *A. baumannii* is able to survive without the help of iron chelators, if its Hms system is functional (Zimbler et al., 2009). On the contrary, an Hms negative almost does not develop biofilms (Figure-6) (Jarrett et al., 2004). One previous work (James et al., 2006) had revealed that genes coding for hemin and iron acquisition systems in *Porphyromonas gingivalis* are regulated by QS protein LuxS. Again QS is well known for inducing biofilm formation.

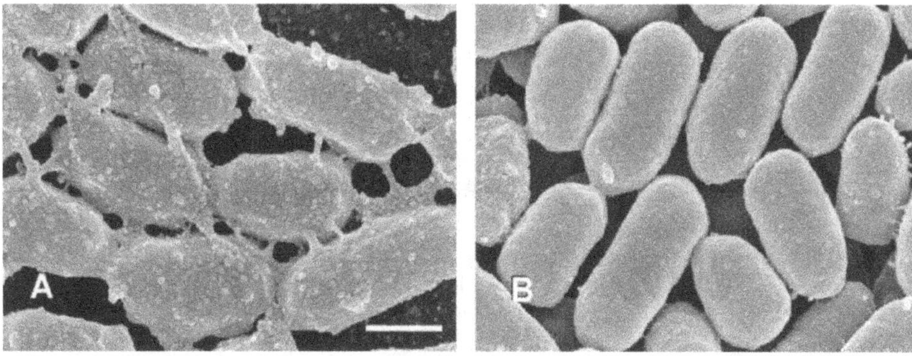

Fig. 6. Scanning electron microscopy of Hms-positive (A) and Hms-negative (B) *Yersinia pestis* grown on agar plates at 21°C. Bar, 0.5 µm. Reproduced with the permission from Jarret et al., 2004.

6. Conclusion

This review attempted to give a glimpses of multiple mechanisms of antimicrobial resistance adopted by various species of *Acinetobacter*, described the current understanding of biofilm development and various factors regulating the biofilm formation in *Acinetobacter*. This write up also explained about the biofilm development and different virulence factors elaborated by *Acinetobacter* and its correlation with antibiotic resistance. Finally, quorum sensing has been elucidated in detail, which works as a global regulator in controlling and regulating diverse physiological functions such as biofilm formation, pilus biogenesis, production of multiple virulence factors, development of antibiotic resistance and increasing the competence of cells that helps in gene transfer. All the information discussed here will definitely help the future research in this area.

In conclusion, all the available evidence implies that *A. baumannii* is very important human pathogen that is gradually gaining more attention as a major global public health problem. It is responsible for a significant proportion of nosocomial infections among patients who are critically-ill receiving intensive care in the ICUs. With this situation together with the fact that certain biofilm phenotypes of *A. baumannii* being highly refractile and recalcitrant that are highly resistant to multiple drugs due to intrinsic resistance properties and those that can acquire resistant determinants with increasing propensity, makes this pathogen one of the most difficult challenges of the present days.

7. Acknowledgment

We are very grateful to **Dr. Stephen K. Farrand**, Departments of Crop Sciences and of Microbiology, University of Illinois at Urbana-Champaign, USA for generously providing *Agrobacterium tumefaciens* NTL4 (pZLR4) indicator strain, *A. tumefaciens* Positive control NTL4(pTiC58ΔaccR) and *A. tumefaciens* NTL4 negative control strains and for helpful discussions.

Authors would also like to thank Indian Council of Medical Research (ICMR), Government of India for funding the Project No.5/3/3/14/2007-ECD and University Grant Commission (UGC), Government of India for funding under Special Assistance Programme (UGC-SAP)

8. References

Adams, M.D. Nickel, G.C. Bajaksouzian, S. Lavender, H. Murthy, A.R. Jacobs, M.R. & Bonomo, R.A. (2009). Resistance to colistin in *Acinetobacter baumannii* associated with mutations in the PmrAB two-component system, *Antimicrob. Agents and Chemother*, Vol. 53, No. 9, (September 2009), pp. 3628-3634, ISSN 0066-4804

Antunes, L.C. Ferreira, R.B. Buckner, M.M. Finlay B.B (2010). Quorum sensing in bacterial virulence. *Microbiology*, Vol. 156, No. 8, (August 2010), pp. 2271-2282, ISSN 1350-0872

Bhargava, N. Sharma,P. Capalash,N. (2010). Quarum sensing in *Acinetobacter*: an emergingPathogen. *Critical Reviews in Microbiology*, Vol.36, No.4, (November 2010), pp.349-360, ISSN 1040-841X

Braun, V. & Hantke, K. (2011). Recent insights into iron import by bacteria. *Current Opinion in Chemical Biology*, Vol.15, No.2, (April 2011), pp. 328–334, ISSN 1367-5931

Chau, S.L. Chu, Y.W. Houang, E.T. (2004). Novel resistance-nodulation-cell division efflux system AdeDE in *Acinetobacter* genomic DNA group 3. *Antimicrob Agents and Chemotherapy* Vol. 48, No. 10, (October 2004) pp. 4054-4055, ISSN 0066-4804

Chen, T. Wu, R. Shaio, M. Fung, C. & Cho, W. (2008). Acquisition of a plasmid-borne blaOXA-58 gene with an upstream IS1008 insertion conferring a high level of carbapenem resistance to *Acinetobacter baumannii*. *Antimicrobial Agents and Chemotherapy* Vol.52, (July 2008) pp.2573–2580, ISSN 0066-4804

Chen, Y. Zhou, Z. Jiang, Y. & Yu, Y. (2011). Emergence of NDM-1-producing *Acinetobacter baumannii* in China. *Journal of Antimicrobial Chemotherapy* Vol. 66, No. 6 (June 2011) pp. 1255-9, ISSN 0305-7453

Choi, AHK; Slamti, L; Avci, FY; Pier, GB; & Maira-Litra´n, T. (2009) The *pga*ABCD locus of *Acinetobacter baumannii* encodes the production of Poly--1-6-N-acetylglucosamine, which is critical for Biofilm formation. *Journal of Bacteriology*. Vol. 191, No. 19, pp. 5953–5963, ISSN 1098-5530

Cisneros, J.M. & Rodríguez-Baño, J. (2002). Nosocomial bacteremia due to *Acinetobacter baumannii*: epidemiology, clinical features and treatment. *Clinical Microbiology Infection*, Vol. 8, No. , pp. 687-693, ISSN 1469-0691

Coelho, J. Woodford, N. Afzal-Shah, M. & Livermore, D. (2006). Occurrence of OXA-58-like carbapenemases in *Acinetobacter* spp. collected over 10 years in three continents. *Antimicrobial Agents and Chemotherapy* Vol. 50, No. 2, (February 2006) pp. 756–758, ISSN 0066-4804

Coelho, J.M. Turton, J.F. Kaufmann, M.E. Glover, J. Woodford, N. Warner, M. Palepou, M.F. Pike, R. Pitt, T.L. Patel, B.C. & Livermore, D.M. (2006). Occurrence of carbapenem-resistant *Acinetobacter baumannii* clones at multiple hospitals in London and Southeast England, *Journal of Clinical Microbiology* Vol.44, No.10 (October 2006) pp.3623–3627, ISSN 0095-1137

Costerton, J.W. Stewart, P. S. & Greenberg, E.P. (1999). Bacterial biofilms: a common cause of persistent infections. *Science* Vol. 284, No. 5418, (May 1999) pp. 1318-1322, ISSN 0036-8075

Coyne, S. Rosenfeld, N. Lambert, T. Courvalin, P. & Perichon, B. (2010). Overexpression of Resistance-Nodulation-Cell Division Pump AdeFGH Confers Multidrug Resistance in *Acinetobacter baumannii*, *Antimicrobial Agents and Chemotherapy* Vol.54, No.10, (October 2010) pp. 4389-4393, ISSN 0066-4804

Crosa J. H. (1989). Genetics and molecular biology of siderophore-mediated iron transport in bacteria. *Microbiological Reviews*, Vol.53, No.4, (December 1989), pp. 517-530, ISSN 1098-5557.

Cucarella, C; Solano, C; Valle, J; Amorena, B; Lasa, I & Penades, JR (2001). Bap, a *Staphylococcus aureus* surface protein involved in biofilm formation. *Journal of Bacteriology* Vol. 183, pp. 2888–2896, ISSN 1098-5530

Deccache, Y. Irenge, L.M. Savov, E. Ariciuc, M. Macovei, A. Trifonova, A. Gergova, I. Ambroise, J. Vanhoof, R. & Gala, J.L. (2011). Development of a pyrosequencing assay for rapid assessment of quinolone resistance in *Acinetobacter baumannii* isolates. *Journal of Microbiol Methods* Vol.86, No. 1, (July 2011), pp. 115-118, ISSN 0167-7012

Donlan, RM & Costerton, JW. (2002) Biofilms: Survival mechanisms of clinically relevant microorganisms. *Clinical Microbiology Reviews*. Vol. 15, No. 2, pp. 167-193, ISSN: 0983-8512.

Dijkshoorn, L. Nemec, A. & Seifert, H. (2007). An increasing threat in hospitals: multidrug resistant *Acinetobacter baumannii. Nature Reviews Microbiology*. Vol. 5, No. pp. 939-950, ISSN 1740-1526

Endimiani, A. Luzzaro, F. Migliavacca, R. Mantengoli, E. Hujer, A.M. Hujer, K.M. Pagani, L. Bonomo, R. A. Rossolini, G. M. & Toniolo, A. (2007). Spread in an Italian Hospital of a Clonal *Acinetobacter baumannii* Strain Producing the TEM-92 Extended-Spectrum β-Lactamase. *Antimicrobial agents and chemotherapy* Vol. 51, No. 6 (June 2007) pp. 2211–2214, ISSN 0066-4804

Figueiredo, S. Poirel, L. Croize, J. Recule, C. & Nordmann, P. (2009). In Vivo Selection of Reduced Susceptibility to Carbapenems in *Acinetobacter baumannii* Related to ISAba1-Mediated Overexpression of the Natural blaOXA-66 Oxacillinase Gene, *Antimicrob. Agents and Chemother*, Vol.53, No.6, (June 2009) pp. 2657-2659, ISSN 0066-4804

Forman, S., Bobrov, A. G., Kirillina, O., Craig, S. K., Abney, J., Fetherston, J. D. & Perry, R. D. (2006). Identification of critical amino acid residues in the plague biofilm Hms proteins. *Microbiology*, Vol.152, No.11, (November 2006), pp. 3399–3410, ISSN 1465-2080.

Forster, D.H. & Daschner, F.D. (1998). *Acinetobacter* Species as Nosocomial Pathogens. *European Journal of Clinical Microbiology Infectious* Disease Vol. 17, No. 2, (February 1998), pp.73–77, ISSN 0934-9723

Fournier, P.E. Vallenet, D. Barbe, V. Audic, S. Ogata, H. Poirel, L. Richet, H. Robert, C. Magnet, S. Abergel, C. Nordmann, P. Weissenbach, J. Raoult, D. & Claverie, J.M. (2006), *PLoS genetics*, Comparative Genomics of Multidrug Resistance in *Acinetobacter baumannii*, Vol.2, No.1 (January 2006) pp. 62-72, ISSN 1553-7390

Fukushima, T., Tanabe, T., Yamamoto, H., Hosoya, S., Sato, T., Yoshikawa, H. & Sekiguchi, J. (2004). Characterization of a polysaccharide deacetylase gene homologue (pdaB) on sporulation of *Bacillus subtilis*. *Journal of Biochemistry*, Vol.136, No.3, (September 2004), pp. 283-291, ISSN 1098-5530.

Fuqua, C. Parsek, M.R. Greenberg, E.P. (2001). Regulation of gene expression by cell-to-cell communication: acyl-homoserine lactone quorum sensing. *Annual Reviews Genetics*, Vol. 35, (December 2009), pp.439–68, ISSN 0066-4197.

Gaddy, J.A. & Actis, L.A. (2009). Regulation of *Acinetobacter baumannii* biofilm formation. *Future Microbiol* Vol. 4, No.3, (Aril 2009), pp.273-278, ISSN 1746-0913

Gilbert, P. & Brown, M. R. W. (1998). Biofilms and β-lactam activity. *Journal of Antimicrobial Chemotherapy* Vol. 41, No. 5 (May 1998), pp 571-572, ISSN 0305-7453

Gonzalez, R.H, Nusblat A. & Nudel B. C. (2001). Detection and characterization of quorum sensing signal molecules in *Acinetobacter* strains. *Microbiology Research* Vol. 155, No. 4, (March 2001), pp. 271–277.

González, R.H. Dijkshoorn, L. Van den Barselaar, M. Nudel, C. (2009). Quorum sensing signal profile of *Acinetobacter* strains from nosocomial and environmental sources. *Revista Argentina de Microbiología,* Vol.41, (March 2009), pp. 73-78, ISSN 0325-757413

Gospodarek E, Grzanka A, Dudziak Z et al. (1998). Electron-microscopic observation of adherence of *Acinetobacter baumannii* to red blood cells. *Acta Microbiol* Pol Vol. 47, No. 2, (February 1998), pp.213–217.

Hausner, M & Wuertz, S. (1999) High rates of conjugation in bacterial biofilms as determined by quantitative in situ analysis. *Applied Environmental Microbiology.* Vol 65, pp. 3710–3713, ISSN 0099-2240

Henwood C. J, Gatward T. & Warner M et al. (2002). Antibiotic resistance among clinical isolates of *Acinetobacter* in the UK and in-vitro evaluation of tigecycline (GAR-936). *Journal of Antimicrobial Chemotherapy* Vol. 49, No. 3, (March 2002), pp. 479–487, ISSN 0305-7453

Higgins, P.G. Poirel, L. Lehmann, M. Nordmann, P. Seifert, H. (2009). OXA-143 a novel carbapenem hydrolyzing class D β-lactamase in *Acinetobacter baumannii. Antimicrobial Agents and Chemotherapy* Vol. 53, No. 12, (December 2009), pp.5035–5038, ISSN 0066-4804

Holden I, Swift I, Williams I. (2000). New signal molecules on the quorum-sensing block. *Trends Microbiology* Vol. 8, No. 3, (March 2000), pp. 101-104. ISSN 0966-842X

Hornsey, M. Ellington, M.J. Doumith, M. Thomas, C.P. Gordon, N.C. Wareham, D.W. Quinn, J. Lolans, K. Livermore, D.M. & Woodford, N. (2010). AdeABC-mediated efflux and tigecycline MICs for epidemic clones of *Acinetobacter baumannii, J Antimicrob Chemother,* Vol. 65, (June 2010), pp. 1589-1593, ISSN 0305-7453

Houot, L. & Watnick, P. I. (2008). A novel role for enzyme I of the *Vibrio cholerae* phosphoenolpyruvate phosphotransferase system in regulation of growth in a biofilm. *Journal of Bacteriology,* Vol.190, No.1, (January 2008), pp. 311–320, ISSN 1098-5530.

Houot, L., Chang, H., Pickering, B. S., Absalon, C. & Watnick, P. I. (2010). The phosphoenolpyruvate phosphotransferase system regulates *Vibrio cholerae* biofilm formation through multiple independent pathways. *Journal of Bacteriology,* Vol.192, No.12, (June 2010), pp. 3055-3067, ISSN 1098-5530.

Itoh, Y., Rice, J. D., Goller, C., Pannuri, A., Taylor, J., Meisner, J., Beveridge, T. J., Preston, J. F. 3rd & Romeo, T. (2008). Roles of *pgaABCD* genes in synthesis, modification, and export of the *Escherichia coli* biofilm adhesin poly-beta-1, 6-N-acetyl-D-glucosamine. *Journal of Bacteriology,* Vol.190, No.10, (May 2008), pp. 3670-3680, ISSN 1098-5530.

James, C. E., Hasegawa, Y., Park, Y., Yeung, V., Tribble, G. D., Kuboniwa, M., Demuth, D. R. & Lamont, R. J. (2006). LuxS involvement in the regulation of genes coding for hemin and iron acquisition systems in *porphyromonas gingivalis. Infection & Immunity,* Vol.74, No.7, (July 2006), pp. 3834–3844, ISSN 1098-5522.

Jarrett, C. O., Deak, E., Isherwood, K. E., Oyston, P. C., Fischer, E. R., Whitney, A. R., Kobayashi, S. D., DeLeo, F. R. & Hinnebusch, B. J. (2004). Transmission of Yersinia pestis from an Infectious Biofilm in the Flea Vector. *The Journal of Infectious Diseases,* Vol.190, No.4, (August 2004), pp. 783–92, ISSN 1537-6613

Joly-Guillou M. L. (2005). Clinical impact & pathogenicity of *Acinetobacter. Clinical Microbiology and Infection* Vol. 11, No. 11, (November 2005), pp.868–873. ISSN 1469-0691

Karthikeyan, K., Thirunarayan, M.A. & Krishnan, P (2010). Coexistence of blaOXA-23 with blaNDM-1 and armA in clinical isolates of *Acinetobacter baumannii* from India, *J Antimicrob Chemother*, Vol.65, (July 2010) pp. 2253-2270, ISSN 0305-7453

Kirillina, O., Fetherston, J. D., Bobrov, A.G., Abney, J. & Perry, R. D. (2004). HmsP, a putative phosphodiesterase, and HmsT, a putative diguanylate cyclase, control Hms dependent biofilm formation in *Yersinia pestis. Molecular Microbiology*, Vol.54, No.1, (October 2004), pp. 75–88, ISSN 1365-2958.

Kropec, A; Maira-Litran, T; Jefferson, KK; Grout, M; Cramton, SE; Gotz, F; Goldmann, DA & Pier, GB. (2005) Poly-N-acetylglucosamine production in *Staphylococcus aureus* is essential for virulence in murine models of systemic infection. *Infection and. Immunity*. Vol 73, pp. 6868–6876, ISSN: 0019-9567.

Lasa, I & Penades, JR. (2006) Bap: A family of surface proteins involved in biofilm formation. *Research in Microbiology* Vol. 157, pp. 99–107. ISSN: 0923-2508.

Lazazzera, B. A. (2010). The phosphoenolpyruvate phosphotransferase system: as important for biofilm formation by *Vibrio cholerae* as it is for metabolism in *Escherichia coli. Journal of Bacteriology*, Vol.192, No.16, (August 2010), pp. 4083-4085, ISSN 1098-5530.

Lee, K. Lee, W. G. Uh, Y. et al. (2003). VIM- and IMP-type metallo-blactamase-producing *Pseudomonas* spp. and *Acinetobacter* spp. in Korean hospitals. *Emerging Infectious Disease* Vol. 9, No. 7, (July 2003) pp. 868–871, ISSN1080-6059

Lee, K. Yum, J.H. Yong, D. Lee, H.M. Kim, H.D. Docquier, J.D. Rossolini, G.M. & Chong, Y. (2005). Novel Acquired Metallo- β -Lactamase Gene, blaSIM-1, in a Class 1 Integron from *Acinetobacter baumannii* Clinical Isolates from Korea, *Antimicrobial Agents and Chemotherapy* Vol. 49, No. 11, (November 2005) pp. 4485-4491, ISSN 0066-4804

Lee JC, Koerten H, van den Broek P, et al. (2006). Adherence of *Acinetobacter baumannii* strains to human bronchial epithelial cells. *Research Microbiology* Vol. 157, No. 4, (May 2006), pp. 360–366. ISSN - 0923-2508

Lewis, K. (2001). Riddle of biofilm resistance. *Antimicrobial Agents and Chemotherapy*. Vol. 45, No. 4, (April 2001), pp. 999-1007, ISSN: 0066-4804.

Loehfelm, T.W. Luke, N. R. & Campagnari, A. A.. (2008). Identification and characterization of an *Acinetobacter baumannii* biofilm-associated protein. *Journal of Bacteriology*. Vol. 190, No. 3, (February 2006), pp. 1036-1044, ISSN: 1098-5530.

Livermore, D.M. & Woodford, N. (2006). The beta-lactamase threat in *Enterobacteriaceae, Pseudomonas* and *Acinetobacter. Trends in Microbiology* Vol. 14, No. 9 (September 2006), pp. 413-420. ISSN 0966-842X

Livermore, D. (2007). The zeitgeist of resistance. *Journal of Antimicrobial Chemotherapy* Vol. 60, No. suppl 1, (August 2007) pp. i59-61. ISSN 0305-7453

Lu, P.L. Doumith, M. Livermore, D.M. Chen, T.P. & Woodford, N. (2009). Diversity of carbapenem resistance mechanisms in *Acinetobacter baumannii* from a Taiwan hospital: spread of plasmid-borne OXA-72 carbapenemase. *Journal of Antimicrobial Chemotherapy* Vol.63 (April 2009), pp.641–647, ISSN 0305-7453

Maglott, D.R., Katz, K. S., Sicotte, H. & Pruitt, K. D. (2000) NCBI's LocusLink and RefSeq. Nucleic Acids Research Vol. 28, No. 1, (January 2000), pp. 126-128, ISSN 0305-1048

Magnet, S. Courvalin, P. & Lambert, T. (2001). Resistance-Nodulation-Cell Division-Type Efflux Pump Involved in Aminoglycoside Resistance in *Acinetobacter baumannii*

Strain BM4454, *Antimicrob. Agents and Chemother,* Vol.45, No.12, (December 2011) pp. 3375-3380, ISSN 0066-4804

Maira-Litrán, T. Kropec, A. Abeygunawardana, C. Joyce, J. Mark, G. Goldmann, D. A. & Pier, G. B. Immunochemical properties of the staphylococcal poly-N-acetylglucosamine surface polysaccharide. (2002). *Infection Immunity* Vol. 70, No. 8 (August 2002) pp. 4433-4440, ISSN 0019-9567

Marchler-Bauer, A., Lu, S., Anderson, J. B., Chitsaz, F., Derbyshire, M. K., Deweese-Scott, C., Fong, J. H., Geer, L. Y., Geer, R. C., Gonzales, N. R., Gwadz, M., Hurwitz, D. I., Jackson, J. D., Ke, Z., Lanczycki, C. J., Lu, F., Marchler, G. H., Mullokandov, M., Omelchenko, M. V., Robertson, C. L., Song, J. S., Thanki, N., Yamashita, R. A., Zhang, D., Zhang, N., Zheng, C. & Bryant, S. H. (2011). CDD: a Conserved Domain Database for the functional annotation of proteins. *Nucleic Acids Research,* Vol.39, Database issue (January 2011), pp. D225-D229, ISSN 1362-4962

Marchand, I. Piolle, L.D. & Courvalin, P. (2004). Expression of the RND-type efflux pump AdeABC in Acinetobacter baumannii is regulated by the AdeRS two-component system. *Antimicrob Agents Chemother,* Vol.48 (September 2004) pp. 3298– 30, ISSN 0066-4804

Maseda, H. Sawada, I. Saito, K. Uchiyama, H. Nakae, T. Nomura, N. (2004). Enhancement of the *mexAB-oprM* efflux pump expression by a quorum-sensing autoinducer and its cancellation by a regulator, MexT, of the*mexEF-oprN* efflux pump operon in *Pseudomonas aeruginosa. Antimicrobial Agents Chemother*apy, Vol.48, No.4, (Apirl 2004), pp. 1320-1328, ISSN 0066-4804

Mussi, M.A. Limansky, A.S. & Viale, A.M. (2005). Acquisition of resistance to carbapenems in multidrug-resistant clinical strains of *Acinetobacter baumannii*: natural insertional inactivation of a gene encoding a member of a novel family of b-barrel outer membrane proteins. *Antimicrob Agents Chemother,* Vol.49 (April 2005), pp.1432-1440, ISSN 0066-4804

Naas, T. Namdari, F. Poupet, H.R. Poyart, C & Nordmann, P. (2007). Panresistant extended-spectrum β-lactamase SHV-5-producing *Acinetobacter baumannii* from New York City. *Journal of Antimicrobial Chemotherapy* Vol. 60, No. 5, (November 2007) pp. 1174–1176, ISSN 0305-7453

Naiemi, N.A. Duim, B. Savelkoul, P.H.M. Spanjaard, L. Jonge, E.D. Bart, A. Grauls, C.M.V. & Jong, M.D. (2005). Widespread Transfer of Resistance Genes between Bacterial Species in an Intensive Care Unit: Implications for Hospital Epidemiology, *J. Clin. Microbiol.* Vol.43, No.9 (September 2005), pp. 4862-4864, ISSN 0095-1137

Nation, R. L. & Li, J. (2009). Colistin in the 21st century. *Current Opinion in Infectious Disease* Vol. 22, No. 6 (December 2009) pp. 535-543. ISSN 0951-7375

Navon-Venezia, S. Ben-Ami, R. Carmeli, Y. (2005). Update on *Pseudomonas aeruginosa* and *Acinetobacter baumannii* infections in the healthcare setting. *Current Opinion in Infectious Disease* Vol. 18, No. 4, (August 2005) pp. 306–313, ISSN 0951-7375

Neilands, J. B. (1995). Siderophores: structure and function of microbial iron transport compounds. *Journal of Biological Chemistry,* Vol.270, No.45, (November 1995), pp. 26723-26726, ISSN 1083-351X.

Ng, W.L., & Bassler, B.L. (2009). Bacterial quorum-sensing network architectures. *Annual Reviews Genetics,* Vol. 43, (August 2009), pp.197–222, ISSN 0066-4197

Niu, C. Clemmer, K.M. Bonomo, R.A. Rather, P.N. (2008). Isolation and characterization of an autoinducer synthase from *Acinetobacter baumannii*. *Journal of Bacteriology*, Vol.190, No.9, (February 2008), pp.3386-3392, ISSN 0021-9193

Otto, M. (2009) *Staphylococcus epidermidis* – the 'accidental' pathogen. *Nature Reviews Microbiology*. Vol. 7, No. 8, (August 2009), pp. 555-567, ISSN: 1740-1526.

O'Toole, GA & Kolter, R. (1998). Flagellar and twitching motility are necessary for *Pseudomonas aeruginosa* biofilm development. *Molecular Microbiology*. Vol. 30, No. 2, (October 1998), pp. 295–304, ISSN: 1365-2958.

Park, Y.K. Jung, S.I. Park, K.W. Cheong, H.S. Peck, K.R. Song, J.H. Ko, K.S. (2009). Independent emergence of colistin-resistant *Acinetobacter spp.* Isolates from Korea, *Diagnostic Microbiology and Infectious Disease*, Vol.64, (January 2009), pp.43-51, ISSN 0732 8893

Park, Y.K. Choi, J.Y. Shin, D. & Ko, K.S. (2011), Correlation between overexpression and amino acid substitution of the PmrAB locus and colistin resistance in *Acinetobacter baumannii*, *International Journal of Antimicrobial Agents*, Vol. 37, (February 2011) pp. 525-530, ISSN 0924-8579

Peleg, A.Y. Franklin, C. Walters, L. J. Bell, J.M. & Spelman, D.W. (2006). OXA-58 and IMP-4 carbapenem-hydrolyzing b-lactamases in an *Acinetobacter junii* blood culture from Australia. *Antimicrobial Agents and Chemotherapy* Vol. 50, No. 1, (January 2006) pp. 399–400, ISSN 0066-4804.

Peleg, A.Y. Adams, J. & Paterson, D.L. (2007). Tigecycline Efflux as a Mechanism for Nonsusceptibility in *Acinetobacter baumannii*, *Antimicrobial Agents and Chemotherapy* Vol. 51, No. 6, (June 2007) pp. 2065-2069, ISSN 0066-4804

Peleg, A.Y. Seifert, H. & Paterson, D.L. (2008). *Acinetobacter baumannii*: Emergence of a Successful Pathogen, *Clin. Microbiol. Rev.* Vol.21, No.3, (July 2008), pp. 538–582, ISSN 0893-8512

Perry, R. D., Pendrak, M. L. & Schuetze, P. (1990). Identification and cloning of a hemin storage locus involved in the pigmentation phenotype of *Yersinia pestis*. *Journal of Bacteriology*, Vol.172, No.10, (October 1990), pp. 5929–5937, ISSN 1098-5530.

Perry, R. D., Bobrov, A. G., Kirillina, O., Jones, H. A., Pedersen, L., Abney, J. & Fetherston, J. D. (2004). Temperature regulation of the hemin storage (*Hms+*) phenotype of *Yersinia pestis* is posttranscriptional. *Journal of Bacteriology*, Vol.186, No.6, (March 2004), pp. 1638–1647, ISSN 1098-5530.

Piolle, L.D. Magnet, S. Bremont, S. Lambert, T. & Courvalin, P. (2008). AdeIJK, a Resistance-Nodulation-Cell Division Pump Effluxing Multiple Antibiotics in *Acinetobacter baumannii*, *Antimicrob. Agents and Chemother*, Vol.52, No.2, (February 2008) pp. 557-562, ISSN 0066-4804

Rahbar, MR; Rasooli, I; Gargavi, SLM; Amani, J & Fattahian, Y. (2010) In silico analysis of antibody triggering biofilm associated protein in *Acinetobacter baumannii*. *Journal of Theoretical Biology*. Vol. 266, pp. 275-290, ISSN: 0022-5193.

Poirel, L. Lebessi, E. Heritier, C. Patsoura, A. Foustoukou, M & Nordmann, P (2006). Nosocomial spread of OXA-58-positive carbapenem-resistant *Acinetobacter baumannii* isolates in a paediatric hospital in Greece, *Clinical Microbiology and Infection*, Vol.12 No.11, (November 2006) pp.1138-1141, ISSN 1198-743X

Poirel, L. & Nordmann, P. (2006). Genetic structures at the origin of acquisition and expression of the carbapenem-hydrolyzing oxacillinase gene blaOXA-58 in *Acinetobacter baumannii*. *Antimicrobial Agents and Chemotherapy* Vol. 50, No. 4, (April 2006) pp. 1442–1448. ISSN 0066-4804.

Poirel, L. Mansour, W. Bouallegue, O & Nordmann, P (2008). Carbapenem-Resistant *Acinetobacter baumannii* isolates from Tunisia Producing the OXA-58-Like Carbapenem-Hydrolyzing Oxacillinase OXA-97, *Antimicrob. Agents and Chemother,* Vol.52, No.5, (May 2008) pp. 1613-1617, ISSN 0066-4804

Pournaras, S. Maniati, M. Petinaki, E. Tzouvelekis, L. S. Tsakris, A. Legakis, N. J. & Maniatis, A.N. (2003). Hospital outbreak of multiple clones of *Pseudomonas aeruginosa* carrying the unrelated metallo-beta-lactamase gene variants blaVIM-2 and blaVIM-4. *Journal of Antimicrobial Chemotherapy* Vol. 51, No. 6 (June 2003) pp. 1409-1414, ISSN 0305-7453

Pruitt, K., Brown, G., Tatusova, T., & Maglott, D., (2002). Chapter 18, The Reference Sequence (RefSeq) Project, *The NCBI Handbook,* http://www.ncbi.nlm.nih.gov/books/NBK21091/

Rahbar, M. R. Rasooli, I. Mousavi Gargari, S. L. Amani, J. & Fattahian, Y. (2010). In silico analysis of antibody triggering biofilm associated protein in *Acinetobacter baumannii. Journal of Theoretical Biology* Vol. 266, No. 2 (September 2010) pp. 275-90, ISSN 0022-5193

Rahmati, S. Yang, S. Davidson, A.L. Zechiedrich, E.L. (2002). Control of the AcrAB multidrug efflux pump by quorum-sensing regulator SdiA. *Molecular Microbiology,* Vol. 43, No.3, (February 2002), pp.677–685, ISSN 0950-382X

Rajamohan, G. Srinivasan, V.B, & Gebreyes, W.A. (2010). Molecular and functional characterization of a novel efflux pump, AmvA, mediating antimicrobial and disinfectant resistance in *Acinetobacter baumannii, J Antimicrob Chemother,* Vol.65, (June 2010), pp.1919-1925, ISSN 0305-7453

Rao, RS; Karthika, RU; Singh, SP; Shashikala, P; Kanungo, R; Jayachandran, S & Prashanth, K. (2008) Correlation between biofilm production and multiple drug resistance in imipenem resistant clinical isolates of *Acinetobacter baumannii. Indian Journal of Medical Microbiology.* Vol. 26, No. 4, pp. 333-337, ISSN: 02550857

Roberts, A. W. & Bushoven, J. T. (2007). The cellulose synthase (CESA) gene superfamily of the moss *Physcomitrella patens. Plant Molecular Biology,* Vol.63, No.2, (January 2007), pp. 207-219, ISSN 1573-5028.

Roca, I. Marti, S. Espinal, P. Martínez, P. Gibert, I. & Vila, J. (2009). CraA, a major facilitator superfamily efflux pump associated with chloramphenicol resistance in *Acinetobacter baumannii. Antimicrobial Agents and Chemotherapy* Vol. 53, No. 9 (September 2009) pp. 4013-4014. ISSN 0066-4804.

Roca, I., Espinal, P. Marti, S. & Vila, J. (2011). First Identification and Characterization of an AdeABC-Like Efflux Pump in *Acinetobacter* Genomospecies 13TU, *Antimicrob. Agents and Chemother,* Vol.55, No.3, (March 2011) pp. 1285-1286, ISSN 0066-4804

Rosenbusch, J. P. (1974). Characterization of the major envelope protein from *Escherichia coli. Journal of Biological Chemistry* Vol. 249, No. 24, (December 1974) pp. 8019-8029, ISSN 0021-9258

Russo, T.A. Donald, U.M. Beanan, J.M. Olson, R., MacDonald, I.J. Sauberan, S.L. Luke, N.R. Schultz, L.W. & Umland, T.C. (2009). Penicillin-Binding Protein 7/8 Contributes to the Survival of *Acinetobacter baumannii* In Vitro and In Vivo, *The Journal of Infectious Diseases,* Vol. 199, (February 2009) pp. 513-21, ISSN 0022-1899

Sato, K. & Nakae T. (1991). Outer membrane permeability of *Acinetobacter calcoaceticus* and its implication in antibiotic resistance. *Journal of Antimicrobial Chemotherapy* Vol. 28, No. 1, (July 1991) pp. 35-45, ISSN 0305-7453

Schaefer, A.L. Hanzelka, B.L. Eberhard, A. Greenberg, E.P. (1996). Quorum sensing in *Vibrio fischeri*: probing autoinducer-LuxR interactions with autoinducer analogs. *J ournal of Bacteriology,* Vol.178, No.10, (May 1996), pp. 2897-2901, ISSN 0021-9193

Shiro, H. Meluleni, G. Groll, A. Muller, E. Tosteson T. D, Goldmann, D.A. Pier, G. B. (1995). The pathogenic role of *Staphylococcus epidermidis* capsular polysaccharide/adhesin in a low-inoculum rabbit model of prosthetic valve endocarditis. *Circulation* Vol. 92, No. 9 (November 1995) pp. 2715-2722, ISSN 0009-7322

Siroy, A. Molle, V. Guillier, C.L. Vallenet, D. Caron, M.P. Cozzone, A.J. Jouenne, T. & De, E. (2006). Channel Formation by CarO, the Carbapenem Resistance-Associated Outer Membrane Protein of *Acinetobacter baumannii, Antimicrobial Agents and Chemotherapy* Vol.49, No.12, (December 2005) pp. 4876-4883, ISSN 0066-4804

Smith MG, Gianoulis TA, Pukatzki S et al. (2007). New insights into *Acinetobacter baumannii* pathogenesis revealed by high-density pyrosequencing and transposon mutagenesis. Genes and Development Vol. 21, No. 5, (March 2007), pp.601-614. ISSN - 0890 9369

Srinivasan, V.B. Rajamohan, G. & Gebreyes, W.A. (2009). Role of AbeS, a Novel Efflux Pump of the SMR Family of Transporters in Resistance to Antimicrobial Agents in *Acinetobacter baumannii. Antimicrobial Agents and Chemotherapy* Vol. 53, No. 12, (December 2009) pp. 5312-5316, ISSN 0066-4804

Stevens, A.M. Dolan, K.M. Greenberg E.P. (1994). Synergistic binding of the *Vibrio fischeri* LuxR transcriptional activator domain and RNA polymerase to the *lux* promoter region. *Proceedings of National Academy of Sciences,* Vol. 91, (December 1994), pp.12619-12623, ISSN 0027-8424

Su, X.Z. Chen, J. Mizushima, T. Kuroda, T. & Tsuchiya.T. (2005). AbeM an H^+ Coupled *Acinetobacter baumannii* Multidrug Efflux Pump Belonging to the MATE Family of Transporters, *Antimicrobial Agents and Chemotherapy* Vol. 49, No. 10, (October 2005) pp. 4362-4364, ISSN 0066-4804

Sun, J.R. Chan, M.C. Chang, T.Y. Wang, W.Y. Chiueh, T. S. (2010). Overexpression of the adeB gene in clinical isolates of tigecycline-nonsusceptible *Acinetobacter baumannii* without insertion mutations in adeRS. *Antimicrobial Agents and Chemotherapy* Vol. 54, No. 11, (November 2010) pp. 4934-4938, ISSN 0066-4804.

Toleman, M.A. Biedenbach, D. Bennett, D.M. Jones, R. N. & Walsh, T.R. (2005). Italian metallo-beta-lactamases: a national problem? Report from the SENTRY Antimicrobial Surveillance Programme. *Journal of Antimicrobial Chemotherapy* Vol. 55, No. 1, (January 2005) pp. 61-70, ISSN 0305-7453

Tolker-Nielsen, T; Brinch, UC; Ragas, PC; Andersen, JB; Jacobsen, CS & Molin, S. (2000). Development and dynamics of Pseudomonas sp. biofilms. *Journal of Bacteriology.* Vol. 182, pp. 6482-6489, ISSN: 1098-5530.

Tomaras, AP; Dorsey, CW; Edelmann, RE & Actis, LA. (2003) Attachment to and biofilm formation on abiotic surfaces by *Acinetobacter baumannii*: involvement of a novel chaperone-usher pili assembly system. *Microbiology.* Vol. 149, pp. 3473-3484, ISSN: 0099-2240.

Tsakris, A. Ikonomidis, A. Pournaras, S. Tzouvelekis, L.S. Sofianou, D. Legakis, N.J. & Maniatis, A.N. (2006). VIM-1 Metallo-β-lactamase in *Acinetobacter baumannii, Emerg Infect Dis.* Vol.12, No. 6, (June 2006) pp. 981-983, ISSN 1080-6059

Tsakris, A. Ikonomidis, A. Spanakis, N. Pournaras, S. & Bethimouti, K. (2007). Identification of a novel blaOXA-51 variant, blaOXA-92, from a clinical isolate of *Acinetobacter baumannii, Clinical Microbiology and Infection,* Vol.13, No.3 (March 2007) pp.347-349, ISSN 1198-743X

Tsakris, A. Ikonomidis, A. Poulou, A. Spanakis, N. Vrizas, D. Diomidous, M. Pournaras, S. & Markou, F. (2008). Clusters of imipenem-resistant *Acinetobacter baumannii* clones producing different carbapenemases in an intensive care unit. *Clinical Microbiology and Infection* Vol. 14, No. 6, (June 2008) pp. 588-594, ISSN 1198-743X

Turton, J.F. Ward, M.E. Woodford, N. Kaufmann, M.E. Pike, R. Livermore, D.M. & Pitt, T.L. (2006). The role of ISAba1in expression of OXA carbapenemase genes in *Acinetobacter baumannii, FEMS Microbiol Lett,* Vol.258 (March 2006) pp.72–77, ISSN 0378-1097

Uma Karthika, R. Srinivasa Rao, R. Sahoo, S. Shashikala, P., Kanungo, R. Jayachandran, S. & Prashanth, K. (2009). Phenotypic and Genotypic assays for detecting the prevalence of Metallo-β- lactamases in clinical isolates of *Acinetobacter baumannii* from a South Indian tertiary care hospital. *Journal of Medical Microbiology,* Vol. 58, No. 4, (April 2009) pp 430-435, ISSN 0022-2615

Vashist, J. Tiwari, V. Das, R. Kapil, A. & Rajeswari, M.R. (2011). Analysis of penicillin-binding proteins (PBPs) in carbapenem resistant *Acinetobacter baumannii, Indian J Med Res,* Vol.133, (March 2011) pp. 332-338, ISSN 0971-5916

Vila, J. Marti, S. & Cespedes, J.S. (2007). Porins, efflux pumps and multidrug resistance in *Acinetobacter baumannii, J Antimicrob Chemother,* Vol.59, (February 2007) pp. 1210-1215, ISSN 0305-7453.

Vuong, C; Voyich, JM; Fischer, ER; Braughton, KR; Whitney, AR; DeLeo, FR & Otto, M. (2004) Polysaccharide intercellular adhesin (PIA) protects *Staphylococcus epidermidis* against major components of the human innate immune system. *Cellular Microbiology.* Vol 6, pp. 269–275, ISSN: 1462-5822.

Weinberg, E. D. (2004). Suppression of bacterial biofilm formation by iron limitation. *Medical Hypotheses,* Vol.63, No.5, (August 2004), pp. 863–865, ISSN 0306-9877.

Wieczorek P, Sacha P, Hauschild T et al. (2008). Multidrug resistant *Acinetobacter baumannii* – the role of AdeABC (RND family) efflux pump in resistance to antibiotics. Folia *Histochemica Et Cytobiologica* Vol. 46, No. 3, (March 2008), pp.257-267, 0239-8508

Wortham, B. W., Oliveira, M, A., Fetherston, J. & Perry, R. D. (2010). Polyamines are required for the expression of key Hms proteins important for *Yersinia pestis* biofilm formation. *Environmental Microbiology,* Vol.12, No.7, (July 2010), pp. 2034–2047, ISSN 1462-2920.

Yang, L., Barken, K. B., Skindersoe, M. E., Christensen, A. B., Givskov, M. & Tolker-Nielsen, T. (2007). Effects of iron on DNA release and biofilm development by *Pseudomonas aeruginosa. Microbiology,* Vol.153, No.5, (May 2007), pp. 1318–1328, ISSN 1465-2080.

Zhou, D. & Yang, R. (2011). Formation and regulation of *Yersinia* biofilms. *Protein & Cell,* Vol.2, No.3, (March 2011), pp. 173-179, ISSN 1674-8018.

Zimbler, D. L., Penwell, W. F., Gaddy, J. A., Menke, S. M., Tomaras, A. P., Connerly, P. L. & Actis, L. A. (2009). Iron acquisition functions expressed by the human pathogen *Acinetobacter baumannii. Biometals,* Vol.22, No.1, (February 2009), pp. 23–32, ISSN 1572-8773.

9

Prevalence of Carbapenemases in *Acinetobacter baumannii*

M.M. Ehlers, J.M. Hughes and M.M. Kock
University of Pretoria/NHLS
South Africa

1. Introduction

Acinetobacter baumannii (A. baumannii) is an important opportunistic pathogen and causes a variety of nosocominal infections especially in Intensive Care Units (ICU's) (Bergogne-Berezin & Towner, 1996; Villegas & Harstein, 2003). These infections include bacteraemia, surgical-site infections, secondary meningitis, urinary tract infections and ventilator associated pneumonia (Bergogne-Berezin & Towner, 1996; Villegas & Harstein, 2003). *Acinetobacter baumannii* has multiresistant phenotypes, including resistance to broad-spectrum β-lactams, fluoroquinolones, aminoglycosides and carbapenems and therefore treatment of this pathogen is complicated (Coelho et al., 2004; Dalla-Costa et al., 2003; Jeon et al., 2005; Landman et al., 2002; Naas et al., 2005; Vahaboglu et al., 2006; Zarrilli et al., 2004). The multiresistant phenotypes of *A. baumannii* also contributed to the emergence of multi drug resistant *Acinetobacter baumannii* (MDRAB), which have become more prevalent within the past decade (Coelho et al., 2004) and has also caused an increase in the number of nosocomial infections in the past decade (Joly-Guillou, 2005).

Over the last 20 years, there has been an increase in the interest of the *Acinetobacter* species (Giamarellou et al., 2008). The increase in interest is due to i) worldwide expansion of ICU's, leading to a change in the types of infections caused by *Acinetobacter spp* and ii) due to the emergence of MDRAB and cases of pan-drug resistant *A. baumannii* (PDRAB) have also been reported (Giamarellou et al., 2008).

The acquired carbapenem resistance in *A. baumannii* is often associated with carbapenemase production; IMP, VIM and SIM-type metallo-β-lactamase production or the OXA-24, OXA-23 and OXA-58 type class D carbapenemases (Brown & Amyes, 2006; Poirel & Nordmann, 2006). Also associated with acquired carbapenem resistance in *A. baumannii* is the over production of natural oxacillinase (OXA-51) (Poirel & Nordmann, 2006).

Carbapenemases are the most versatile of all β-lactamases and many of them recognize almost all hydrolysable β-lactams (Livermore & Woodford, 2006; Nordmann & Poirel 2002; Walther-Rasmussen & Hoiby, 2006). Most carbapenemases are resistant to commercial β-lactamase inhibitors (Livermore & Woodford, 2006; Nordmann & Poirel, 2002; Walther-Rasmussen & Hoiby, 2006). Carbapenemases are divided into three subclasses on the basis of their hydrolysis characteristics (Frere et al., 2005). The first carbapenemases described were from Gram-positive bacilli and were inhibited by EDTA (Frere et al., 2005). These carbapenemases were described as metalloenzymes and have one zinc atom in the active site (Frere et al., 2005). This zinc atom facilitates hydrolysis of a bicyclic β-lactam ring (Frere et al., 2005). The second form of carbapenemases use serine at the active sites and are inactivated by clavulanic acid and tazobactam (β-lactamase inhibitors) (Rasmussen et al., 1996; Yang et al., 1990). Molecular classes A, C and D have serine in the active site and form part of the β-lactamases (Bush, 1988). The molecular class B of the β-lactamases are metalloenzymes and have zinc in the active site (Bush, 1988). The enzymes from the molecular classes A, B and D have the ability to hydrolyse carbapenems, which results in an elevated carbapenem minimum inhibitory concentration (Bush, 1988).

The aim of this study was to optimise and evaluate multiplex polymerase chain reaction (PCR) assays to rapidly differentiate the four subgroups of the oxacillinase (OXA) genes and the five subgroups of the metallo-β-lactamase (MBL) antibiotic resistant genes. The PCR assays results were compared to the phenotypic tests i) Hodge test and ii) Double disk synergy test. Antibiotic resistance testing is important to decrease the spread of antibiotic resistant strains of *A. baumannii* in clinical settings.

2. History of Acinetobacter baumannii

Acinetobacter baumannii (Figure 1) was first isolated in 1911 from a soil sample by MW Beijerink (Kuo et al., 2004). *Acinetobacter spp* were first thought to be non-virulent saprophytes (Bergogne-Berezin & Towner, 1996). In the 1970s the widespread use and misuse of antibiotics started (Kuo et al., 2004). In 1986 *Acinetobacter baumannii* was taxonomically classified (Bouvet et al., 1986). The first carbapenem resistant *A. baumannii* (CRAB) isolates were discovered in 1991 (Kuo et al., 2004). The first carbapenem hydrolyzing oxacillinase (CHDL's) was identified in 1995 (Scaife et al., 1995). It was initially named ARI-1 and was later renamed OXA-23 (Scaife et al., 1995).

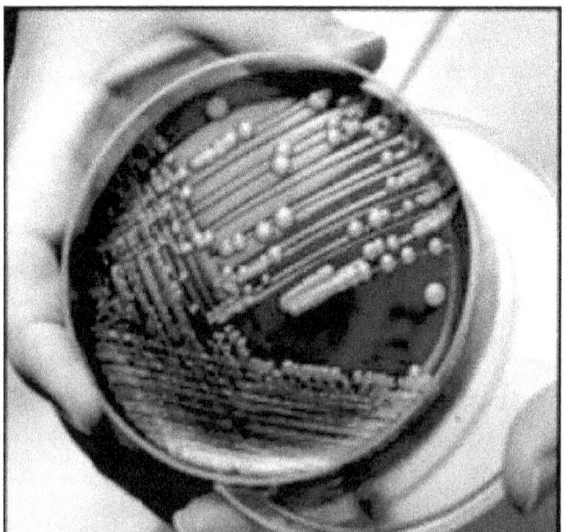

Fig. 1. *Acinetobacter baumannii* isolates (www.acinetobacter.org)

The first reported outbreak of CRAB occurred in the USA in 1991 (Go et al., 1994). Carbapenem Resistant *A. baumannii* isolates were isolated from a leukaemia patient in the oncology ward of a Taiwanese hospital in May 1998 (Hsueh et al., 2002). These isolates were observed to be resistant to almost all antibiotics e.g. cephalosporins, aztreonam, aminoglycosides and ciprofloxacin and were therefore named pan-drug resistant *A. baumannii* (PDRAB) (Hsueh et al., 2002). The rise in the number of multi drug resistant *A. baumannii* (MDRAB) strains has been due to the extensive use of antimicrobial chemotherapy against bacterial infections (Hsueh et al., 2002).

3. Classification of *Acinetobacter baumannii*

In 1986 *Acinetobacter baumannii* was taxonomically classified (Bouvet et al., 1986). *Acinetobacter* are grouped into three main complexes: i) *Acinetobacter calcoaceticus-baumannii* complex, which is glucose oxidizing and non-haemolytic; ii) *Acinetobacter lwoffii,* which are glucose negative and non-haemolytic and iii) *Acinetobacter haemolyticus,* which is haemolytic (Euzeby, 2008). The full classification of *A. baumannii* is listed in Table 1.

Domain	*Bacteria*
Phylum	*Proteobacteria*
Class	*Gammaproteobacteria*
Order	*Pseudomonadales*
Family	*Moraxellaceae*
Genus	*Acinetobacter*
Species	*A. baumannii* *A. baylyi* *A. beijerinckii* *A. bouvetii* *A. calcoaceticus* *A. gerneri* *A. grimontii* *A. gyllenbergii* *A. haemolyticus* *A. johnsonnii* *A. junnii* *A. lwoffii* *A. parvus* *A. radioresistens* *A. schindleri* *A. soli* *A. tandoii* *A. tjernbergiae* *A. towneri* *A. ursingii* *A. venetianus* 14 species are still unnamed

Table 1. Nomenclature of *Acinetobacter baumannii* (Euzeby, 2008)

There are 21 recognized genomic species of the genus *Acinetobacter* and 14 unnamed genomic species (Euzeby, 2008).

4. General characteristics of *Acinetobacter baumannii*

Acinetobacter baumannii are Gram-negative, non-fermentative, non-motile, oxidase-negative, aerobic coccobacilli that are ubiquitous in nature and commonly found within the hospital environment causing a variety of opportunistic nosocomial infections (Bergogne-Berezin et al., 1996). The bacteria can be isolated from water, soil and the environment and from human skin (Bergogne-Berezin et al., 1996). The morphology of *Acinetobacter* spp is variable in Gram-stained human clinical specimens and thus cannot be used to differentiate *Acinetobacter* from other causes of common nosocomial infections (http://microbewiki.kenyon.edu/index.php/Acinetobacter_baumannii). *Acinetobacter baumannii* are non-lactose fermenting bacteria, however they partially ferment lactose on MacConkey agar (http://microbewiki.kenyon.edu/index.php/Acinetobacter_baumannii). All the species of the *Acinetobacter* genus grow well on MacConkey agar (except for *A. lwoffii*), when salt is absent (http://microbewiki.kenyon.edu/index.php/Acinetobacter_baumannii). *Acinetobacter baumannii* are strict aerobes and grow well on nutrient agar (http://microbewiki.kenyon.edu/index.php/Acinetobacter_baumannii). Infection by *A. baumannii* is difficult to combat due to the Gram-negative nature of the cell wall as the outer wall provides a barrier so that the antimicrobial agent is unable to enter the bacterial cell (Projan, 2004).

Acinetobacter baumannii is an opportunistic pathogen that is successful in colonizing and persisting in the hospital environment and is able to resist desiccation (Getchell-White et al., 1989; Jawad et al., 1996). The bacterium is also able to survive on inanimate surfaces for months (Kramer et al., 2006). *Acinetobacter baumannii* is among the most common causes of device related nosocomial infections (Dima et al., 2007; Thongpiyapoom et al., 2004), resulting when the bacterium is able to resist both physical and chemical disinfection, by forming a biofilm (Cappelli et al., 2003; Loukili et al., 2006; Pajkos et al., 2004). Biofilm associated proteins (BAP's) were first characterized in *S. aureus* (Cucarella et al., 2001) and have been found in a number of other Gram-positive and Gram-negative pathogenic bacteria.

4.1 Optimal Growth conditions for *Acinetobacter baumannii*

Acinetobacter baumannii form part of the natural flora of the skin and mucous membranes of humans (Seifert et al., 1997). *Acinetobacter baumannii* are ubiquitous in clinical and natural environments and commonly colonises the skin, oropharynx secretions, respiratory secretions, urine, irrigating and intravenous solutions (Seifert et al., 1997). *Acinetobacter baumannii* can be cultured from sputum or respiratory secretions, wound and urine (Go & Cuhna, 1999). The pathogen colonises the gastro-intestinal tract and is associated with nosocomial meningitis, nosocomial pneumonia and bacteraemia (Go & Cuhna, 1999).

Acinetobacter baumannii grown on trypticase soy agar produce circular, convex, smooth and slightly opaque colonies, which are 1.5 to 2.0 mm in diameter after 24 hours at 30°C or 3.0 to 4.0 mm after 48 hours (Garrity et al., 2005). *Acinetobacter baumannii* do neither haemolyse horse blood nor sheep blood when grown on blood agar plates (Garrity et al., 2005). Seasonal variations have been reported for nosocomial *A. baumannii* infections and bacteraemia, with increased incidences occurring in the summer months (McDonald et al., 1999).

5. Risk factors for *Acinetobacter baumannii* infections

Acinetobacter baumannii can survive on various surfaces within hospitals, including catheters and other medical equipment (http://microbewiki.Kenyon.edu/index.php/Acinetobacter_baumannii). Thus environmental contamination is an important source of infection as pathogens are spread directly from surfaces or through the hands of healthcare workers to patients (Corbella et al., 1996). Infected or colonized patients are important reservoirs of *A. baumannii. Acinetobacter baumannii* is passed from patient to patient via direct and indirect contact (D'Agata et al., 2000). The main risk factors of *Acinetobacter baumannii* bacteraemia are invasive procedures e.g. central venous catheterization, mechanical ventilation and surgery (Seifert et al., 1995b). Another major risk factor for *A. baumannii* infections is the widespread use of broad-spectrum antibiotics (Cisneros & Rodriguez-Bano, 2002). Other risk factors include prolonged hospital stay, ICU stay, enteral feeding, previous administration to another unit and previous use of third generation cephalosporins (Mulin et al., 1995; Scerpella et al., 1995).

The risk factors within the ICU's concern the immunosuppressed patients, patients previously exposed to antimicrobial therapy, patients who underwent high invasive procedures and patients who suffered from previous sepsis (Garcia-Garmendia et al., 2001). Other risk factors include pneumonia as a source of infection, inappropriate empirical treatment and prior treatment with carbapenems (Robenshtok et al., 2006). Surgical procedures performed within the emergency operating theatre is another major risk factor contributing to the spread of epidemic cases of *A. baumannii,* however the main risk factor was the previous use of fluoroquinolones (Villers et al., 1998).

5.1 Pathogenesis of Acinetobacter baumannii

Acinetobacter baumannii infections are associated with systems of high fluid content e.g. lungs, cerebrospinal fluid, peritoneal fluid and the urinary tract and usually only occur in the immunocompromised patients (Cuhna, 2007). Patients with *A. baumannii* bacteraemia usually have signs and symptoms that are related to the organ system involved (Cuhna, 2007). Symptoms include wound infections, outbreaks of nosocomial pneumonia, catheter associated bacteriuria, urethritis and continuous ambulatory peritoneal dialysis (CAPD) associated peritonitis (Cuhna, 2007). Bacteraemia results in septic shock in 25-30% of all cases and disseminated intravascular coagulation frequently occurs (Cisneros et al., 1996: Seifert et al., 1997). Colonisation may occur after an invasive infection (Corbella et al., 1996), especially in burn patients (Wisplinghoff et al., 2004). Problems rarely associated with *A. baumannii* infections include meningitis, endocarditis, urinary tract infections, pneumonia and cholangitis (Cuhna, 2007). Other problems that rarely occur are soft tissue infections and complicated skin, abdominal infections and central nervous system (CNS) infections (Fournier & Richet, 2006). Allen and Green documented the first report of airborne spread of *A. baumannii* in 1987. *Acinetobacter baumannii* survives much better on fingertips or on dry surfaces when tested under stimulated hospital environmental conditions (Jawad et al., 1996). The skin of patients and medical personnel is involved in the transmission of *A. baumannii* strains and in some outbreaks; molecular typing has identified the epidemic strain on the skin of the patients (Gerner-Smidt, 1987; Patterson et al., 1991). Contaminated reusable medical equipment e.g. ventilator tubing, respirometers and arterial pressure monitoring devices are used for the management of severely ill patients serve as another route of transmission to patients (Beck-Sague et al., 1990; Cefai et al., 1990). Fomites e.g. bed mattresses (Sheretz & Sullivan., 1985), pillows (Weernink et al., 1995), a tape recorder, television set and a fan (Jawad et al., 1994) were found to be contaminated with *Acinetobacter* and served as reservoirs during nosocomial outbreaks.

The mortality rate within the hospitals is high, with a 23% mortality recorded for hospitalized patients and a 43% mortality rate among patients in intensive care (Falagas et al., 2006). The Antimicrobial Availability Task Force (AATF) of the Infectious Disease Society of America identified *Acinetobacter baumannii, Aspergillus* spp, extended spectrum β-lactamase producing *Enterobacteriaceae, Pseudomonas aeruginosa, Staphylococcus aureus* as "particularly problematic pathogens" and there is a desperate need for new drug development (Talbot et al., 2006).

It is difficult to distinguish between colonization and infection regarding *A. baumannii* (Joly-Guillou, 2005). There is controversy over whether infections caused by *A. baumannii* result in unfavourable outcomes (Blot et al., 2003; Falagas et al., 2006). The isolation of *A. baumannii* in hospitalized patients is an indicator of severe illness with an associated mortality of approximately 30% (Wilson et al., 2004).

Community acquired *A. baumannii* (CAAB) occurs within an individual with one or more cultures of blood, collected within 48 hours of admission, that is positive for *A. baumannii* complex and is identified by a biochemical method (API 20NE system) (bioMerieux, France) (Schreckenberger & Von Graevenitz, 2000). Patients with CAAB associated pneumonia had an increased mortality rate and presented with a more severe disease than the patients without pneumonia (Wang et al., 2002). The development of CAAB is associated with underlying malignancies e.g. lung cancer, lymphoma and thymic carcinoma (Wang et al., 2002). *Acinetobacter baumannii* genomic species were responsible for CAAB; however there is no evidence of clonal spread of *A. baumannii* in the community (Wang et al., 2002). Carbapenems, cefopirome, cefepime, ceftazidime, aminoglycosides and fluoroquinolones are the antimicrobials of choice for treating CAAB (Wang et al., 2002).

5.2 Virulence factors of *Acinetobacter baumannii* strains

Acinetobacter baumannii have very few virulence factors (Cisneros & Rodriguez-Bano, 2002), however some strains have virulence factors associated with invasiveness, transmissibility or the enhanced ability to colonise immunocompromised patients (Dijkshoorn et al., 1996). Ethanol stimulates the virulence of *A. baumannii* (Smith et al., 2004), which led to the identification of a number of genes, affecting virulence towards *Caenorhabditis elegans* and *Dictyostelium discoideum* (Smith et al., 2007).

A new strain (OXA-23 clone II) was identified in a military hospital and was found to be a particularly virulent strain, which is very difficult to eliminate from medical facilities (promedmail). There are three major European clones of *A. baumannii* (Giamarellou et al., 2008) Clone I, found in South Africa, Czech Republic, Poland, Italy and Spain; Clone II, found in South Africa, Spain, Turkey, Greece and France and clone III is found in the Netherlands, Italy, France and Spain (Van Dessel et al., 2004). Clones I and II are responsible for the outbreaks of

A. baumannii bacteraemia in South Africa and Northern Europe (Van Dessel et al., 2004). *Acinetobacter* can efficiently transfer genes horizontally (only observed and analysed in *A. baylyi*), especially the genes encoding antibiotic resistance (Gerischer, 2008).

A large portion of the *A. baumannii* genome is dedicated to pathogenesis, with a large number of genes occurring within virulence islands (Perez et al., 2007). *Acinetobacter baumannii* together with *Acinetobacter* DNA group13TU is involved in the majority of *Acinetobacter* hospital outbreaks (Bergogne-Berezin & Towner, 1996). Strains of the *Acinetobacter* DNA group 3 and *A. junii* have only occasionally been implicated in outbreaks of nosocomial infections (Bernards et al., 1997). *Acinetobacter baumannii* has environmental resilience and a wide range of resistance determinants, therefore making it a successful nosocomial pathogen (Nordmann, 2004). *Acinetobacter baumannii* has caused numerous global outbreaks and displayed ever increasing rates of resistance (Villegas & Harstein, 2003). In hospital outbreaks the emergence of imipenem-resistant strains has been documented (Brown et al., 1996; Go et al, 1994).

6. Clinical manifestations of *Acinetobacter baumannii* infections

The clinical manifestations of *A. baumannii* are non-specific and present as a trans-maculopapular rash affecting the palms of the hands and the soles of the feet of endocarditis patients, or necrotic lesions of the skin and soft tissue (Seifert et al., 1995). *Acinetobacter baumannii* bacteraemia is polymicrobial, and is often associated with *Klebsiella pneumoniae* (Seifert et al., 1995).

6.1 Treatment of *Acinetobacter baumannii* infections

Acinetobacter baumannii are Gram-negative bacteria and therefore are particularly difficult to treat due to the presence of an outer membrane (Projan, 2004). The recommended treatment therefore is a limited spectrum active β-lactam e.g. ceftazidime or imipenem the most active agent against *A. baumannii* and an aminoglycoside (Cisneros & Rodriguez-Bano, 2002).

There is incomplete current knowledge of the clinical response and bacterial mechanisms of resistance to antimicrobials (Kahlmeter et al., 2006). The reliability and comparability of different methods of susceptibility testing e.g. disc diffusion and broth microdilution have not been consistent for *A. baumannii* (Swenson et al., 2004). The persistence of subtle growth beyond an obvious end point by broth microdilution is of great concern in the case of β-lactams, which therefore explains its poor reaction with the disc diffusion method (Swenson et al., 2004). Doripenem, a novel carbapenem is active against susceptible *A. baumannii* (Fritsche et al., 2005; Jones et al., 2004; Jones et al., 2005; Mushtaq et al., 2004). Doripenem was not effective against *A. baumanni* isolates producing bla_{OXA-23} or bla_{IMP-4} or metallo-β-lactamases (Mushtaq et al., 2004).

6.2 Carbapenems as treatment for *Acinetobacter baumannii* infections

Carbapenems are structurally related to the penicillins ("penams"), differing only by the substitution of carbon ("carba") for the sulfur atom at position 1 and the presence of a double bond between C2 and C3 (Bradley, 1997; Wise, 1986). A hydroxyethyl side chain instead of the acylamino group found in penicillins and cephalosporins is present and provides resistance to most β-lactamases (Bradley, 1997; Wise, 1986).

Carbapenems were introduced into clinical practice in the 1970's and the 1980's marked the emergence of Gram-negative bacterial resistance to carbapenems (Nordmann & Poirel, 2002; Walsh, 2005). Carbapenems were derived from the naturally occurring antibiotic, thienamycin, which is produced by the soil microorganism *Streptomyces cattleya* (Jacobs, 1986). The first carbapenemases described were from Gram-positive bacilli and were inhibited by EDTA (Frere et al., 2005). Carbapenems are recognised as the gold standard for treating infections caused by resistant Gram-negative bacteria (Rahal, 2006).

6.3 Combination therapy as a strategy for the treatment of multiple drug resistant *Acinetobacter baumannii*

Sulbactam is an inhibitor of β-lactamases and has *in vitro* bactericidal activity against *Acinetobacter spp* (Cisneros & Rodriguez-Bano, 2002). The efficacy of sulbactam against susceptible *A. baumannii* is similar to imipenem (Rodriguez-Hernandez, 2000). Sulbactam exhibits bacteriostatic action against *A. baumannii* (Corbella et al., 1998). Sulbactam is also used to treat meningitis caused by multiple drug resistant *Acinetobacter baumannii* (MDRAB) (Cisneros & Rodriguez-Bano, 2002). Combinations of sulbactam with aminoglycosides, rifampin and azithromycin have demonstrated synergy against imipenem susceptible strains (Appleman et al., 2000; Savov et al., 2002). There is little or no advantage to the combination sulbactams with cephalosporins (Appleman et al., 2000; Savov et al., 2002).

Polymyxins (colistimethate and polymyxin B) are the only alternative treatment for sulbactam resistant *A. baumannii* strains (Wood & Reboli, 1993). Colistin was used in the 1960's and the 1970's, but had many adverse side effects, including nephrotoxicity, neuro-muscular blockage (Cisneros & Rodriguez-Bano, 2002). Colistin disrupts the outer cell membranes of many Gram-negative bacilli by changing the permeability of the membrane and causing a bactericidal effect (Cisneros & Rodriguez-Bano, 2002). Colistin is only recommended for patients who have no other treatment alternatives (Cisneros & Rodriguez-Bano, 2002). Rifampicin combined with colistin or sulbactam acts synergistically against MDRAB (Hogg et al., 1998).

7. Mechanisms of antibiotic resistance in *Acinetobacter baumannii*

The general mechanisms of resistance are enzyme-mediated resistance, genetic adaption, efflux pumps and changes in the structure of outer membrane components (Cloete, 2003). Enzyme mediated resistance is the ability of the bacteria to produce enzymes that transform the antibiotics into non-toxic or inactivated forms (Ma et al., 1998). Efflux pumps involve a large number of seemingly unrelated (structurally) compounds, pumped out of the cell, which lowers the concentration of the drug within the cell and therefore prohibits the drug to take proper effect (Nikaido, 1996). Changes in the structure of the outer membrane and its components e.g. porins and alterations in the penicillin binding proteins (PBP's), allows for the cells to develop resistance to antimicrobials on the basis of exclusion because the drugs are no longer able to penetrate the cells and therefore the drugs can't reach their intended site of action in the cell (Cloete, 2003).

Acinetobacter baumannii has become resistant to many classes of antibiotics and is well suited for genetic exchange (Lorenz & Wackernagel, 1994; Metzgar et al., 2004). *Acinetobacter baumannii* are among a unique class of Gram-negative bacteria that are described as "naturally transformable" (Lorenz & Wackernagel, 1994; Metzgar et al., 2004). *Acinetobacter* strains lack the *mut*S gene, which is part of the mismatch repair system that preserves genetic stability and exhibits increased mutation rates (Young & Ornston, 2001). It is unknown whether *A. baumannii* are naturally competent or whether through the alteration of environmental conditions facilitates pathogenicity or antibiotic resistance gene acquisition (Fournier et al., 2006). The key resistance genes identified were those coding for VEB-1, AmpC, and OXA-10 beta-lactamases, various amino glycoside-modifying enzymes (AME) and those genes encoding for the tetracycline efflux pumps (Fournier *et al.*, 2006).

Plasmids, transposons and the bacterial chromosome are involved in antibiotic resistance within *A. baumannii* (Bergogne-Berezin & Towner, 1996). Carbapenemases occurring within *A. baumannii* belong to the class D family of serine-β-lactamases or the imipenemase (IMP)/Verona integrase (VIM) class B family of metallo-β-lactamases (Brown & Amyes, 2006). Imipenem is the most active drug against *A. baumannii* (Cisneros & Rodriguez-Bano, 2002). Resistance to carbapenems is associated with reduced drug uptake due to porin deficiency and reduced affinity for the drug due to modification of the PBP's by mutations (Clark, 1996).

Acinetobacter baumannii's largest virulence island contains genetic elements, which are homologous to the type IV secretion systems of *Legionella* and *Coxiella burnetti* (Goldstein et al., 1983). Over 25 years ago *A. baumannii* was observed to acquire antimicrobial resistance factors through conjugation of plasmids (Goldstein et al., 1983). Transposons are important in the dissemination of genetic determinants of resistance in *Acinetobacter* spp (Devaud et al., 1982; Palmen & Hellingwerf, 1997) and many of the transposons contain integrons, predominantly from class I. Integrons contain an *int* gene and gene cassettes that can be mobilized to other integrons or to secondary sites in the bacterial genome (Poirel et al., 2005).

A multi drug resistant (MDR) phenotype in *A. baumannii* occurs when integron-born resistance determinants acting against different classes of antibiotics co-exist, giving rise to MDR gene cassettes (Seward, 1999; Yum et al., 2002). Insertion sequences (IS), which promote gene expression, have played an important role in explaining the regulation of resistance (Segal et al., 2005). The IS_{Aba1} element found in *A. baumannii* but not in *Enterobacteriaceae* or in *Pseudomonas aeruginosa* (Segal et al., 2005), results in the over expression of Amp C and OXA-51/OXA-69-like beta-lactamases and in decreased levels of susceptibility to ceftazidime and carbapenems (Heritier et al., 2006).

7.1 Oxacillinase (OXA) genes in *Acinetobacter baumannii*

Carbapenemases are classified into four major functional groups (groups 1 to 4) with multiple subgroups of group 2 that are differentiated according to a group specific inhibitor or substrate profiles (Bush et al., 1995). According to this classification scheme carbapenemases are found primarily in group's 2f and 3 (Nordmann et al., 1993; Yang et al., 1990).

Class D carbapenemases are classified into four subgroups (Vahaboglu et al., 2006). Subgroup 1, the OXA-23 group (including OXA-27 and OXA-49), are the plasmid encoded genes (Vahaboglu et al., 2006). The OXA extended spectrum beta-lactamases are able to hydrolyze extended spectrum cephalosporins (Aubert, 2001; Walther-Rasmussen & Hoiby, 2006). The OXA-23 was the first OXA carbapenemase (OXA β-lactamases that inactivate carbapenems) within *A. baumannii* obtained from a clinical isolate (Aubert, 2001; Walther-Rasmussen & Hoiby, 2006). The OXA-23 genes originated in *A. radioresistens* (Turton et al., 2005). This plasmid-encoded enzyme was found in 1985 in Scotland before the introduction of carbapenems (Paton et al., 1993). It was initially named "*Acinetobacter* resistant to imipenem" (ARI-1) and has been discovered in Brazil, England, Polynesia, Singapore, Korea and China (Brown & Amyes, 2006; Jeon et al., 2005). Subgroup 2 is the OXA-24 group (including OXA-25, OXA-26 and OXA-40), which is chromosomally encoded (Vahaboglu et al., 2006). The OXA-24 carbapenemase has a crystal structure and therefore suggests a novel catalytic role for Tyr112 and Met223 side chains (Santillana et al., 2007). Subgroup 1 and 2 share 60% identity (Heritier et al., 2005b).

Subgroup 3 consists of OXA-51 and its variants, which are chromosomally encoded (Vahaboglu et al., 2006). The OXA-51/69 expression varies according to the presence of IS_{Aba1} (Poirel & Nordmann, 2006). The OXA-51 gene was first detected in Argentina in 2005, within genetically distinct *A. baumannii* isolates (Brown & Amyes, 2005). Subgroup 3 has 56% identity with subgroup 1 and 61% to 62% identity with subgroup 2 (Brown et al., 2005). Subgroup 4 contains OXA-58, which is a plasmid-encoded gene (Vahaboglu et al., 2006) and was first detected in Toulouse (France) in 2003 (Heritier et al., 2005a; Poirel et al., 2005). Subgroup 4 shares less than 50% homology with the other three groups (Poirel et al., 2005). The OXA-58 gene is rapidly disseminating and those isolates, which contain both OXA-51-type and OXA-58 genes, are pandrug-resistant *A. baumannii* (PDRAB) (Coelho et al., 2006). The plasmid borne carbapenemase, OXA-58, was found in France, England, Argentina, Spain, Turkey, Romania, Austria, Greece, Scotland and Kuwait (Coelho et al., 2006; Marque et al., 2005; Pournaras et al., 2006). It is uncertain whether these genes are acquired or occur naturally in *A. baumannii* (Brown & Amyes, 2006). In *A. baumannii* isolates with OXA-51 as the sole carbapenemase, carbapenem resistance was associated with an insertion sequence IS_{AbaI} and it is thought that this might be the promoter for the hyper-production of β-lactamase genes (Turton et al., 2006).

Bacteria producing carbapenemase enzymes have a reduced susceptibility to imipenem (Ambler et al., 1991). However, the minimum inhibitory concentration (MIC) of imipenem can range from mildly elevated to fully resistant (Ambler et al., 1991). Therefore, these β-lactamases may not be recognised following routine susceptibility testing (Ambler et al., 1991). Beta-lactamases have the ability to hydrolyse carbapenems, resist commercially available β-lactamase inhibitors and are susceptible to inhibition by metal ion chelators (Lim et al., 1988). The widespread presence of oxacillinases and their division into distinct subgroups, indicates that these enzymes are an essential component of the genetic makeup of *Acinetobacter* spp (Walther-Rasmussen & Hoiby, 2006). The OXA enzymes as emerging carbapenemases are increasingly associated with outbreaks of *A. baumannii containing OXA-40 and OXA-58* in the United States (Hujer et al., 2006; Lolans et al., 2006). The OXA-51/69-like beta-lactamase is a "naturally occurring" chromosomal enzyme in *Acinetobacter baumannii* and has been found in isolates from four continents (Heritier et al., 2005a).

7.2 Metallo-β-lactamase (MBL) genes in Acinetobacter baumannii

Metallo-β-lactamases form part of the class B β-lactamases, capable of hydrolyzing carbapenems and other β-lactam antibiotics except for aztreonam (Walsh et al., 2005; Walsh,

2005). Class B β-lactamases differ from class A and class D carbapenemases by having a metal ion, zinc, in their active site, which participates in catalysis (Walsh et al., 2005; Walsh, 2005). There are five types of metallo-β-lactamases (MBL's) that have been identified in *A. baumannii* (Brown & Amyes, 2006). The most common metallo-β-lactamases include "Verona integron-encoded metallo-β-lactamases" (VIM), "Imipenem hydrolyzing β-lactamase"(IMP), "German Imipenemase" (GIM), Seoul imipenemase (SIM) and Sao Paulo metallo-β-lactamases (SPM-1) enzymes, which are located on a variety of integron structures and are incorporated as gene cassettes (Brown & Amyes, 2006). The integration of the integron on the plasmids or transposons allows for facilitated transfer between bacteria (Watanabe et al., 1991).

Imipenem (IMP) metallo-β-lactamases were first described in a *P. aeruginosa* strain found in Japan in 1988 (Watanabe et al., 1991). Metallo-β-lactamases is not the predominant carbapenemases found within *A. baumannii* however the following carbapenemases have been described: IMP-1, IMP-2, IMP-4, IMP-5, IMP-6, and IMP-11 (Walsh et al., 2005; Walsh, 2005). The IMP type MBL's have stronger carbapenem-hydrolysing activity than the OXA-type-β-lactamases (Laraki et al., 1999). The VIM, IMP, SPM, and GIM genes are found on cassettes in class 1 integrons, although IMP genes have also been found on class 3 integrons (Collis et al., 2002). Watanabe et al. (1991) reported the detection of IMP-1, located on an integron situated on a conjugative plasmid, in *Serratia marcescens* and other *Enterobacteriaceae* in Japan. The imipenem-hydrolyzing β-lactamase has been detected in rare clinical isolates of *Enterobacter cloacae* in Argentina, the USA and France (Nordmann et al., 1993; Pottumarthy et al., 2003; Radice et al., 2004; Rasmussen et al., 1996).

Imipenem hydrolyzing β-lactamase contains the conserved active site motifs S-X-X-K, S-D-N and K-T-G of the class A β-lactamases (Aubron, 2005; Yu et al., 2006). The carbapenemases have conserved cysteine residues at positions 238 and 69 that form a disulfide bridge (Aubron, 2005; Yu et al., 2006). Genes encoding IMP-2 β-lactamases were found on plasmids in *Enterobacter asburiae* isolated from river water in the US and on plasmids from an *E. cloacae* isolated from China (Aubron, 2005; Yu et al., 2006). The disulfide bond is necessary for the hydrolytic activity and is used to stabilize the enzyme structurally (Majiduddin & Palzkill, 2003; Sougakoff et al., 2002). The mechanism of cleavage of the β-lactam ring is different for MBL's as compared to β-lactamases, however, both gene products still share a unique αββα fold in the active sites of the enzymes (Ullah et al., 1998). The bla_{IMP} is a foreign gene that is introduced from another species of bacteria and *A. baumannii* only retain the gene in environments where there is selective pressure in the form of the presence of imipenem (Takhashi et al., 2000).

Pandrug-resistant *A. baumannii* (PDRAB) are resistant to nearly all the commercially available antibiotics including amikacin, aztreonam, cefepime, ceftazidime, ciprofloxacin, gentamycin, imipenem, meropenem, ofloxacin, ticarcillin-clavulanate and piperacillin-tazobactam (Hsueh et al., 2002). Carbapenem-resistant *A. baumannii* are usually susceptible to ciprofloxacin, ofloxacin, gentamycin or amikacin (Hsueh et al., 2002). Increasing the use of carbapenems and ciprofloxacin has contributed to the development and spread of PDRAB strains (Hsueh et al., 2002).

Verona integron-encoded MBL (VIM-1) was first identified in Italy in 1997 in a *P. aeruginosa* isolate (Lauretti et al., 1999). *Acinetobacter baumannii* containing the VIM-2 gene has been reported only in Korea (Yum et al., 2002). *Acinetobacter baumannii* isolates producing metallo-β-lactamases from Korea were reported to be incredibly diverse, containing Seoul imipenemase (SIM-1), which is a novel metallo-β-lactamase (Lee et al., 2005).

7.3 Non-enzymatic mechanisms of antibiotic resistance

In *A. baumannii* isolates from Madrid the loss of the 22-kDa and 33-kDa outer membrane proteins combined with the production of OXA-24, resulted in resistance to carbapenems (Bou et al., 2000). A homologue of OprD, a 43-kDa protein was identified in *A. baumannii* (Dupont et al., 2005). The 43-kDa protein is a well studied porin, which is frequently associated with imipenem resistance in *P. aeruginosa* (Dupont et al., 2005). Confirming resistance to imipenem and meropenem in *A. baumannii* is the channel formation of CarO, a 29-kDa outer membrane protein (Limansky et al., 2002; Mussi et al., 2005; Siroy et al., 2005). Reduced expression of PBP-2 within isolates from Seville, Spain explained the resistance of *A. baumannii* to carbapenems (Fernandez-Cuenca et al., 2003).

7.3.1 Efflux pumps as mechanisms of resistance in *Acinetobacter baumannii*

Efflux pumps cause resistance against several different classes of antibiotics and mediate the efflux of compounds that are toxic to the bacterial cell, including antibiotics, in a coupled exchange with protons (Poole, 2005). The distinct families of efflux pumps the major facilitator superfamily, the small multidrug resistance superfamily, the multidrug and toxic compound extrusion superfamily and the resistance-nodulation-cell division family are found in various species of bacteria (Poole, 2005). Over expression of the AdeABC efflux pump, which forms part of the resistance-nodulation-cell division family, confers high-level resistance to carbapenems, together with carbapenem-hydrolyzing oxacillinase (Marque et al., 2005). The mechanism, which controls the expression of the efflux pump, functions as a two-step regulator (adeR) and sensor (adeS) system (Marchand et al., 2004). A single point mutation within the *ade*R and *ade*S genes results in increased expression and increased efflux (Marchand et al., 2004).

8. Resistance of *Acinetobacter baumannii* to various antibiotics

Resistance to aminoglycosides is mediated by aminoglycoside-modifying enzymes (AME's) (Perez et al., 2007). Examples of such enzymes include aminoglycoside phosphotransferases (aph), aminoglycoside acetyltransferases (acc) and aminoglycoside adenyltransferase (aad) (Perez et al., 2007). *Acinetobacter baumannii* have transposon mediated efflux pumps, which involves tetracycline A (Tet) and TetB (Guardabassi et al., 2000). Tetracycline A allows for the efflux of tetracycline, while TetB allows for the efflux of both tetracycline and minocycline (Huys et al., 2005). The other mechanism of resistance to the tetracyclines is due to the ribosomal protection protein (Perez et al., 2007). The ribosomal protection protein is encoded by the tetracycline M gene and protects the ribosome from the action of tetracycline, minocycline and doxycline (Ribera et al., 2003).

Modification in the structure of the DNA gyrase decreases the affinity of the enzyme to quinolones (Seward & Towner, 1998); therefore *A. baumannii* becomes resistant to quinolones (Perez et al., 2007). Modifications of the lipopolysaccharides (LPS's) in A. *baumannii* cause the bacterium to become resistant to polymyxins (Perez et al., 2007).

Modifications to the LPS in *A. baumannii* include acylation, presence of antigens and acidification, which all interfere with the binding of the polymyxins to the cell membrane (Peterson et al., 1987).

9. Spread and control of *Acinetobacter baumannii*

Infection control is critical concerning *A. baumannii* given its ability to cause outbreaks (Boyce & Pittet, 2002; Pittet, 2004). Contact precautions, hand washing and alcohol hand decontamination are rarely applied however are universally encouraged and important (Boyce & Pittet, 2002; Pittet, 2004). However, the applications of meticulous environmental decontamination and aggressive chlorhexidine baths as temporary measures to control outbreaks are the favourable approach (Maragakis et al., 2004; Wilks et al., 2006). However these methods are expensive, labour-intensive and must be clinically proven through trials (Maragakis et al., 2004; Wilks et al., 2006). The key to infection control measures lies within preventing dissemination of MDR clones (Maragakis et al., 2004; Wilks et al., 2006). The use of molecular tools for investigation of outbreaks to establish clonality among isolates allows for a more effective implementation of infection control measures and aids in the identification of environmental sources (Maragakis et al., 2004; Wilks et al., 2006). Polymerase Chain Reaction followed by electronspray ionization mass spectrometry and base composition analysis are used to determine clonality (Ecker et al., 2006; Hujer et al., 2006). Restriction of the use of especially broad-spectrum activity antibiotics is necessary for infection control strategies (Chakravarti et al., 2000; Hughes, 2003). The refinement of genomic and proteomic techniques represents hope for the discovery of new antimicrobials active against MDR organisms and for the development of vaccines (Chakravarti et al., 2000; Hughes, 2003). The success of these and other approaches for the containment of MDR *A. baumannii* depends on the commitment of clinical practitioners, scientists, hospitals and public health administrators and on the support of the informed public (Chakravarti et al., 2000; Hughes, 2003).

10. Diagnosis and detection of *Acinetobacter baumannii*

Monitoring the geographical spread of virulent or epidemic pathogens is achieved through the identification and typing of bacteria (Grundmann et al., 1997). Traditional methods for the identification of *A. baumannii* are unsatisfactory (Gerner-Smidt et al., 1991), due to the difficulty in distinguishing *A. baumannii* from *A. calcoaceticus* phenotypically (Giamarellou et al., 2008). *Acinetobacter baumanni* is predominantly diagnosed from sputum, blood, central venous catheter tips, pleural fluid, wound pus, bronchial washing and urine (Hsueh et al., 2002).

10.1 Direct phenotypic detection of *Acinetobacter baumannii*

Phenotypic methods of detecting *A. baumannii* include growing the isolates on fluorescence-lactose-denitrification media (FLN) in order to determine the amount of acid produced by the metabolism of glucose (http://microbewiki.kenyon.edu/index.php/Acinetobacter baumannii). This method is used to differentiate the respective species within the *Acinetobacter* genus (http://microbewiki.kenyon.edu/index.php/Acinetobacter_baumannii). Crude enzyme extracts and β-lactamase activity assays are other phenotypic methods used to detect antibiotic resistant strains of *A. baumannii* (Takahashi et al., 2000). Biochemical tests used to differentiate *A. baumannii* from other species of the *Acinetobacter* genus include the following: haemolysis test (-), histamine assimilation test (-), glucose oxidation test, citrate assimilation test (+), gelatin liquefaction test (-) (Prashanth & Badrinath, 2000).

10.1.1 Automated detection of *Acinetobacter baumannii*

A Vitek GNI card (bio Mérieux, France) is used for the detection of carbapenemase activity in clinical isolates. The results of the Vitek test are confirmed using the API 20NE system (bio Mérieux, France) (Clinical and Laboratory Standards Institute, 2009).

10.1.2 Manual methods of detection of *Acinetobacter baumannii*

The E-test (AB Biodisk, Sweden) is used to identify metallo-β-lactamase production by determining the minimum inhibitory concentration (MIC), which allows for the detection of the production of VIM or IMP enzymes (Walsh, 2005). Susceptibility testing can be performed using broth microdilution according to Clinical and Laboratory Standards Institute standards (2009) and the Kirby-Bauer double disk synergy test (Peleg et al., 2005). The disk approximation test with 2-mercaptopropionic acid or EDTA is used to screen for metallo-β-lactamase producers (Arakawa, 2000; Yong et al., 2006). Ethylenediaminetetraacetic acid (EDTA) is a chelator of Zn^{2+} and other divalent cations and therefore inhibits the metallo-β-lactamases that have zinc ions in their active sites (Lim et al., 1988).

The imipenem (IMP)-EDTA double-disk synergy test (DDST) can distinguish metallo-β–lactamase producing from metallo-β–lactamase non-producing Gram-negative bacilli (Lee et al., 2001). However, occasional isolates show false negative results due to a deficiency of zinc within the isolate's active site (Yigit et al., 2001). The test can be improved by using an IMP disk to which 10 µl of 50 mM zinc sulfate (140 µg/disk) has been added, to compensate for the lack of zinc or by using Mueller-Hinton agar to which zinc sulfate has been added to a final concentration of 70 $\mu g.ml^{-1}$ (Yigit et al., 2001).

The Hodge test is a simple method for screening metallo-β-lactamase producing isolates of Gram-negative bacilli (Lee et al., 2001). The Hodge test/cloverleaf test is a microbiological assay of carbapenemase activity, where an extract of the whole cell or the suspected isolates are tested against imipenem on an agar plate (Hornstein et al., 1997). It is unnecessary to test an isolate for a carbapenemase using the modified Hodge test when all of the carbapenems that are reported by a laboratory test are either intermediate or resistant (Clinical and Laboratory Standards Institute, 2009). However, the modified Hodge test is used for infection control and epidemiological purposes (Clinical and Laboratory Standards Institute, 2009). The imipenem disk test is a poor screening method for carbapenemases (Clinical and Laboratory Standards Institute, 2009).

10.2 Molecular detection of *Acinetobacter baumannii*

Molecular methods based on PCR for the detection of carbapenemase producing genes are used due to the problems with the direct phenotypic detection methods e.g. difficulty in distinguishing between species of the *Acinetobacter* genus (Vaneechoutte, 1996). The molecular methods include a PCR with primers for detecting OXA-23, OXA-24, OXA-51,

OXA-58, IMP-1, IMP-2, IMP-4, VIM-1, VIM-2, SPM-1, GIM-1, and SIM-1 genes can be used to detect all families and subgroups of the presumed carbapenemases (Petropoulou et al., 2006). The genotypic tests used to determine the clonal relatedness of the isolates include, Random amplified polymorphism DNA (RAPD PCR)-fingerprinting with the primers M13, Enterobacterial Repetitive Intergenic Consensus (ERIC2) and Pulsed Field Gel Electrophoresis (PFGE) using the *ApaI* enzyme can be performed (Seifert et al., 2005). The main advantages of the molecular techniques in comparison with the traditional phenotypic methods are high reproducibility and applicability to a wide variety of bacteria and time saving (Grundmann et al., 1997).

10.3 Indirect diagnosis of *Acinetobacter baumannii*

Gram-negative bacteria contain lipopolysaccharides (LPS's) on their outer membranes, which consist of covalently linked lipid A (anchors the LPS into the outer membrane) and the core polysaccharide (O-polysaccharide or O-antigen), which is linked to the lipid A (Pantophlet et al., 1999). The type of LPS found within *A. baumannii* has the smooth or S-form phenotype and can be used in clinical microbiology laboratories for clinical research purposes (Pantophlet et al., 1999).

11. Materials and methods

Ninety-seven imipenem/meropenem resistant *A. baumannii* isolates were collected between March and April 2009 from a Tertiary Academic hospital. These isolates were all given a unique number. The *A. baumannii* isolates were analysed by the Diagnostic Division of the department of Medical Microbiology, National Health Laboratory service (NHLS) at the University of Pretoria. The isolates were identified as *A. baumannii* and underwent susceptibility testing. The Vitek 2 (bioMérieux, France) automated system was used to phenotypically test for the presence of carbapenemases within the *A. baumannii* isolates. Ninety-seven imipenem/meropenem resistant isolates were streaked out onto 5% sheep blood agar plates (Diagnostics Media Products, NHLS, South Africa). The plates were incubated (Horo incubator) overnight at 37°C. Gram-staining was performed for each isolate. (2002). Brain-Heart infusion broth (Biolab, Wadeville, South Africa) was prepared and aliquoted into Bijou culture bottles before sterilization. The broth bottles were inoculated from overnight plate cultures of *A. baumannii* grown on 5% sheep blood agar (Diagnostic Media Products, NHLS, South Africa) by adding 3 to 4 colonies of an isolate into the broth. The inoculated broths were incubated in a Labcon shake incubator at 37°C overnight. A volume of 900 µl of the inoculated turbid broth and 900 µl of sterile glycerol was added to a sterilized cryotube and were stored at -70°C. The CLSI (2009) guidelines for the performance of the modified Hodge test and for the double disk synergy test were followed for the detection of carbapenemase production.

A MagNA Pure Compact Nucleic Acid Isolation Kit 1 (Roche, Germany) was used to perform automated whole cell DNA extraction according to the manufacturer's guidelines. A volume of 400 µl of each of the *A. baumannii* broth culture samples was added to a Magna Pure sample tube for automated DNA extraction. Sealed cartridges with the necessary reagents were added to each lane. The purified nucleic acids (100 µl of pure *A. baumannii*

DNA) were eluted and stored at -20°C for further analysis. The Nanodrop Spectrophotometer ND-1000 instrument was used to measure the DNA concentration for each of the samples.

Two multiplex PCR assays: 1) Multiplex PCR I reaction of OXA-23, OXA-24, OXA-51 and OXA-58 genes (Woodford et al., 2006) and 2) Multiplex PCR II reaction of IMP, VIM, GIM-1, SPM-1 and SIM-1 genes (Ellington et al., 2007) were performed using the QIAGEN Multiplex PCR 1000 kit (Promega, Madison, USA), which was set up according to the manufacturer's guidelines. The QIAGEN Multiplex PCR 1000 kit contains Multiplex PCR Master mix, RNAse free water and Q solution. The thermocycling was performed using the Eppendorf, Mastercycler epgradient S (Hamburg, Germany). The DNA gel electrophoresis (Elite 300 power pack, Wealtec, South Africa) was performed on a 2% agarose gel (Whitehead Scientific, Brackenfell, Cape Town), which contained 0.5 $\mu g.ml^{-1}$ ethidium bromide (Promega, Madison, USA). The loading dye used was Fermentas 6X orange loading dye solution (Fermentas UAB, Lithuania). The ready to use 100 bp ladder (Promega, Madison, USA) was used as a molecular size marker. A 10% solution of TBE buffer 10X (Promega, Madison. USA) was used for the preparation and running of the gels.

12. Prevalence of antibiotic resistance genes in *Acinetobacter baumannii* isolates in a clinical setting in the Pretoria area, South Africa

The origins of the *Acinetobacter baumannii* isolates collected in this study were 58% (56/97) from sputum specimens, 7% (7/97) from urine specimens, 11% (11/97) from blood cultures and 24% (23/97) from diverse specimens. The *A. baumannii* isolates collected for this study were both imipenem and meropenem resistant with a minimum inhibitory concentration (MIC) of >=16. The 97 *A. baumannii* isolates were subjected to susceptibility testing using the Vitek 2 instrument. The panel consisted of 18 antibiotics to determine the overall pattern of resistance. The selection of *A. baumannii* isolates used in this study was based on the Vitek 2 instrument. Both imipenem and meropenem resistant *A. baumannii* isolates were included in this study. All of the *A. baumannii* isolates showed 100% resistance to the following antibiotics in the panel: ampicillin; amoxicillin/clavulanic acid; cefuroxime; cefuroxime axetil; cefepime; imipenem; meropenem; nitrofurantoin and trimethoprim/sulfamethoxazole. The *A. baumannii* clinical isolates were all susceptible (0% resistance) to colistin (Table 2).

The Hodge test showed that 74% (72/97) of the *A. baumannii* isolates were positive for carbapenemase production and 26% (25/97) of the *A. baumannii* isolates were negative for carbapenemase production (Figure 2). These results are similar to the findings of the study conducted in Korea by Lee et al. (2003), which reported a prevalence of 66% positive for carbapenemase production, 26% negative for carbapenemase production and 8% data unknown.

The Cloverleaf or Hodge test is cumbersome and imperfect. False positives occur due to AmpC and impermeability, not due to β-lactamase production. Weak false positives occur due to AmpC hyperproducers. AmpC hydrolysing β-lactams are produced by Gram-negative bacteria [Presentation by David Livermore on "Detecting carbapenemases" at the 49th Interscience conference on antimicrobial agents and chemotherapy (ICAAC)]. Some *A. baumannii* isolates are resistant to ertapenem, but are rarely resistant to any of the other

Antibiotic Tested	Percentage resistance
Ampicillin	100% (97/97)
Amoxicillin/Clavulanic acid	100% (97/97)
Piperacillin/Tazobactam	99% (96/97)
Cefuroxime	100% (97/97)
Cefuroxime Axetil	100% (97/97)
Cefotaxime	99% (96/97)
Ceftazidime	49% (48/97)
Cefepime	100% (97/97)
Imipenem	100% (97/97)
Meropenem	100% (97/97)
Amikacin	25% (24/97)
Gentamicin	89% (86/97)
Tobramycin	5% (5/97)
Nalidixic acid	95% (92/97)
Ciprofloxacin	91% (88/97)
Nitrofurantoin	100% (97/97)
Colistin	0% (0/97)
Trimethoprim/sulfamethoxazole	100% (97/97)

Table 2. Antibiotic resistance patterns in *Acinetobacter baumannii* isolates from a Tertiary Academic Hospital

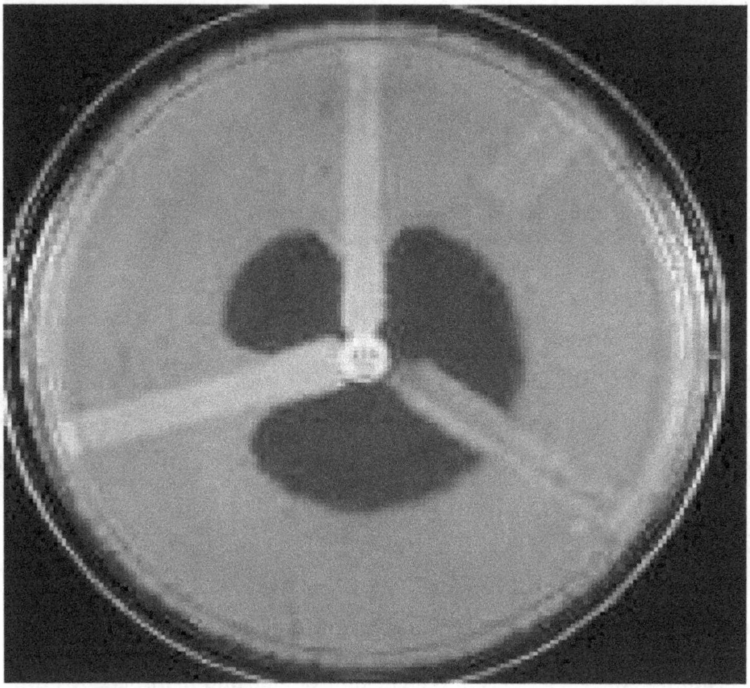

Fig. 2. Hodge or cloverleaf test of three *Acinetobacter baumannii* isolates

carbapenems. The Hodge test is very time consuming to set up and the reading of the results is subjective. Some strains produce bacteriocins, which kill the indicator organism [Presentation by David Livermore on "Detecting carbapenemases" at the 49th Interscience conference on antimicrobial agents and chemotherapy (ICAAC)]. Beta-lactamase production affects the porins of the outer membrane, thus making *A. baumannii* impermeable to antibiotics and therefore resistant to antibiotics e.g. carbapenems [Presentation by David Livermore on "Detecting carbapenemases" at the 49th Interscience conference on antimicrobial agents and chemotherapy (ICAAC)]. The class of carbapenemase cannot be determined by the results of the Modified Hodge test. Some isolates show a slight indentation, but do not produce carbapenemase (Standard operating procedure of the Department of Health and Human Services, Centres for Disease Control and Prevention: "Modified Hodge Test for Carbapenemase Detection in Enterobacteriaceae").

The double disk synergy test showed that 33% (32/97) of the *A. baumannii* isolates were susceptible to both ertapenem and EDTA and 19% (18/97) of the isolates did not grow (Figure 3). A prevalence of 45% (44/97) was recorded for *A. baumannii* isolates that were ertapenem resistant and EDTA susceptible and a prevalence of 3% (3/97) was recorded for both ertapenem and EDTA resistance. These findings are lower than the results of the study conducted in Korea by Lee et al. (2003), which reported a prevalence of 94% (75/80) of *A. baumannii* isolates susceptible for both imipenem and EDTA; all the isolates grew in that study; 5% (5/97) of the *A. baumannii* isolates were resistant to imipenem and susceptible to EDTA and 0% (0/97) isolates were resistant to both imipenem and EDTA.

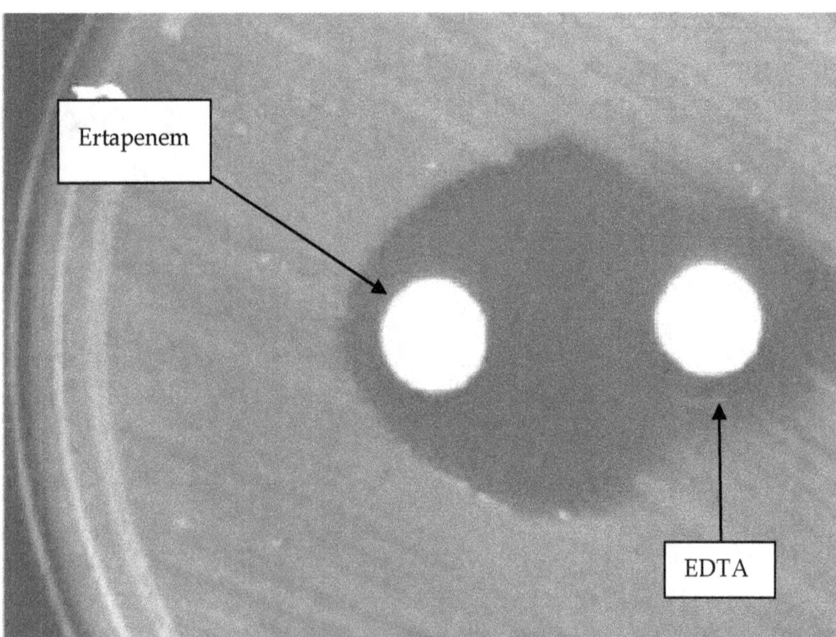

Fig. 3. Double disk synergy test of one *Acinetobacter baumannii* isolate

EDTA permeabilizes the bacterial cell, is a chelator of zinc and disrupts OXA dimers, which may be stabilized by zinc [Presentation by David Livermore on "Detecting carbapenemases" at the 49th Interscience conference on antimicrobial agents and chemotherapy (ICAAC)]. Therefore EDTA disrupts the function of the carbapenemase producing genes and hence the *A. baumannii* isolates are more susceptible to ertapenem in the presence of EDTA than without EDTA. The discrepancies in the results of this study compared to the results of the study conducted by Lee et al. (2003) were due to the use of different carbapenems. Ertapenem was used in this study, while Lee et al. used imipenem in their study conducted in 2003. Imipenem disks perform poorly as a screen for carbapenemases (Clinical and Laboratory Standards Institute, 2009) and thus ertapenem was used in this study.

The *A. baumannii* clinical specimens were cultured and two different multiplex PCR assays were performed on the extracted DNA sample of each isolate. The first multiplex PCR assay (Multiplex PCR I) was performed to screen for the presence of the OXA-group genes (OXA-23, OXA-24, OXA-51 and OXA-58). The second Multiplex PCR assay (Multiplex PCR II) screened for the presence of the Metallo-β-lactamase genes (IMP, VIM, SIM, SPM and GIM). Multiplex PCR I showed that 80% (78/97) of the *A. baumannii* isolates were positive for OXA-51, 52% (50/97) were positive for OXA-23, 1% (1/97) were positive for OXA-58 and 2% (2/97) were positive for OXA-24 (Figure 4). Figure 5 showed the gel electrophoresis pattern of the OXA-51, OXA-23, OXA-58 and OXA-24 genes.

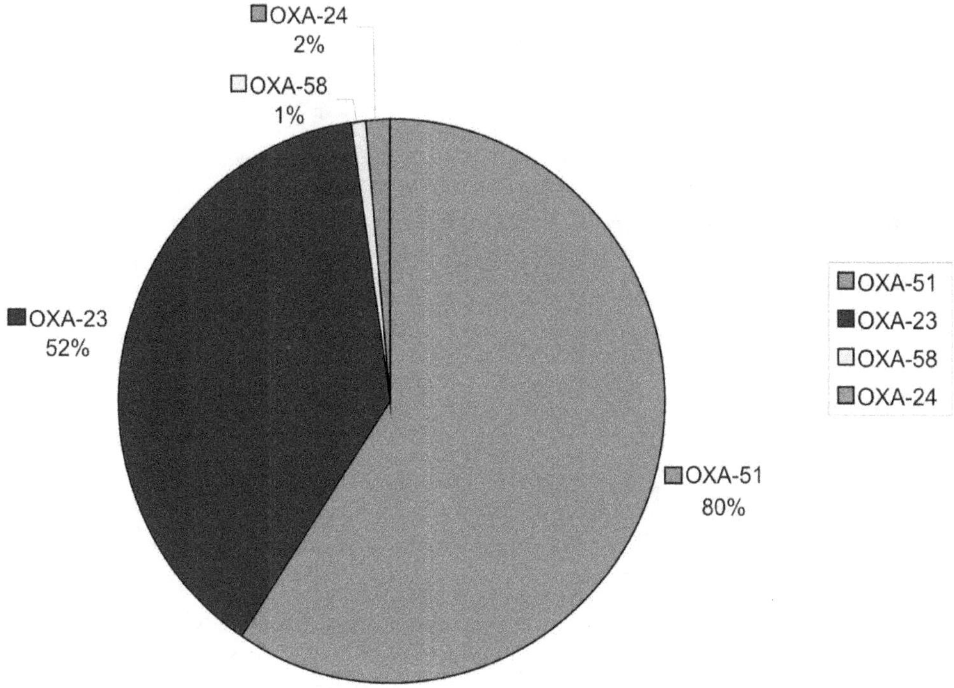

Fig. 4. Pie chart showing the results of the Multiplex PCR I for the prevalence of the OXA genes in the 97 *Acinetobacter baumannii* isolates obtained from a Tertiary Academic Hospital

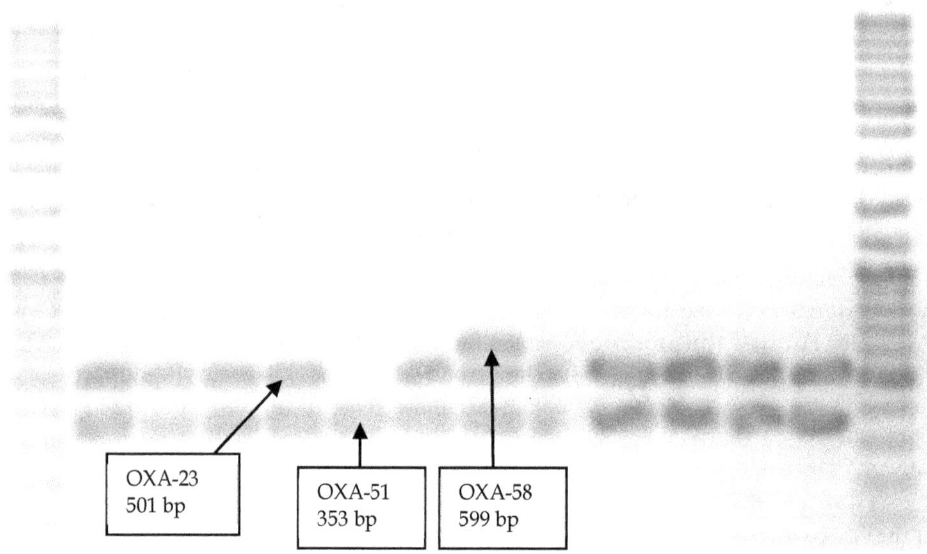

Fig. 5. Results obtained after Multiplex PCR I was performed, using a 2% agarose gel for the detection of OXA genes in the *Acinetobacter baumannii* isolates. Lanes 2, 3, 4, 5, 7, 9, 10, 11, 12 and 13 were positive for both OXA 51 and OXA-23. Lane 6 was positive only for OXA-51. Lane 8 was positive for OXA-23, OXA-51 and OXA-58. Lanes 1 and 14 contain the molecular weight markers (100 bp DNA ladder).

The multiplex PCR I results showed there were four distinctive strains of *A. baumannii* circulating in a Tertiary Academic hospital in Gauteng, South Africa. The first group of strains were positive for both OXA-51 and OXA-23 (52%). The second group of strains was positive for OXA-51 (26%) alone. The third group of strains were positive for both OXA-51 and OXA-24 (2%) and the fourth group of strains were positive for both OXA-51 and OXA-58 (1%) (Figure 6).

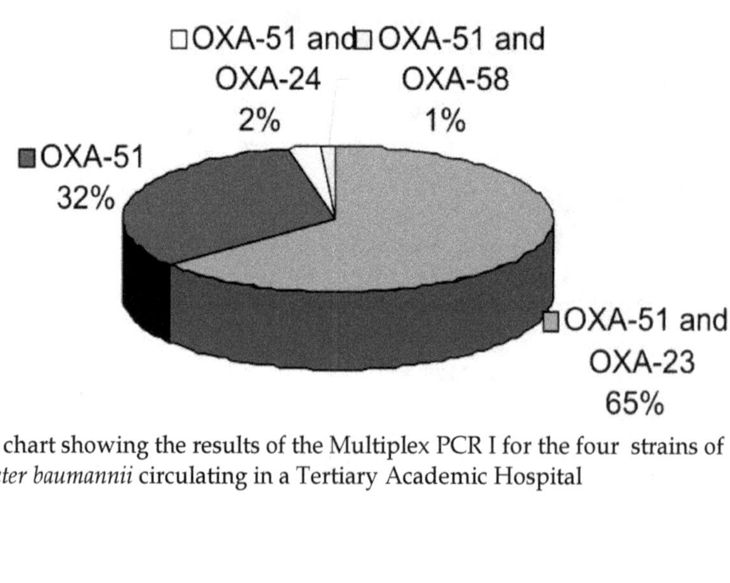

Fig. 6. Pie chart showing the results of the Multiplex PCR I for the four strains of *Acinetobacter baumannii* circulating in a Tertiary Academic Hospital

OXA-51 is an abiquitous or naturally occurring gene within *A. baumannii* (Merkier & Centron, 2006). OXA-51 is a chromosomally located gene, which needs to be regulated upstream by IS_{Aba1} to provide resistance [Presentation by David Livermore on "Detecting carbapenemases" at the 49th Interscience conference on antimicrobial agents and chemotherapy (ICAAC)]. The prevalence of OXA-51 in clinical isolates of *A. baumannii* in this study was 80% (78/97). This figure is lower than the findings of a study conducted in Iran by Feizabadi and colleagues (2008), which reported a 100% prevalence of the OXA-51 gene in clinical isolates of *A. baumannii.*

The prevalence of OXA-23 in clinical isolates of *A. baumannii* in this study was 52% (50/97). This finding was similar to the OXA-23 prevalence of 66.5% in the Asia Pacific nations (India, China, Thailand, Singapore, Hong kong and Korea) (Mendes et al., 2009). However, based on other studies conducted in Iran by Feizabadi and colleagues (2008) who reported a prevalence of 36.5% in clinical isolates of *A. baumannii* the prevalence of OXA-23 varies worldwide. OXA-23 forms part of the class D metallo-β-lactamases and is an acquired carbapenemase gene, thus a varied prevalence is observed as not all *A. baumannii* isolates will obtain the gene compared to OXA-51 which is a chromosomal carbapenemase gene occuring naturally in *A. baumannii* (Merkier & Centron, 2006). The carbapenemase gene occurs in widespread clones and contributes to the multidrug resistant nature of *A. baumannii* [Presentation by David Livermore on "Detecting carbapenemases" at the 49th Interscience conference on antimicrobial agents and chemotherapy (ICAAC)].

The OXA-24 genes also form part of the class D metallo-β-lactamases and are acquired carbapenemase genes, which occur within widespread clones [Presentation by David Livermore on "Detecting carbapenemases" at the 49th Interscience conference on antimicrobial agents and chemotherapy (ICAAC)]. The prevalence of OXA-24 in A. *baumannii* in this study was 2% (2/97). This finding was similar to the OXA-24 prevalence of 5.6% in *A. baumannii* clinical isolates from a study conducted in Thailand, Taiwan and Indonesia in 2008 (Mendes et al., 2008). However, a prevalence of 26% of OXA-24 was reported in the study conducted by Feizabadi and colleagues in Iran in 2008. The varied prevalence results are due to OXA-24 being an acquired gene within *A. baumannii* and thus not all isolates will contain the gene (Merkier & Centron, 2006).

The prevalence of OXA-58 in clinical isolates of *A. baumannii* in this study was 1% (1/97). This finding was lower than the OXA-58 prevalence of 15% in *A. baumannii* isolates in the study conducted by Feizabadi and colleagues in Iran in 2008. The differences in the results of this study and other studies are due to OXA-58 being an acquired carbapenemase gene and the presence of this gene within widespread clones Presentation by David Livermore on "Detecting carbapenemases" at the 49th Interscience conference on antimicrobial agents and chemotherapy (ICAAC)].

No metallo-β-lactamase genes were detected in any of the *A. baumannii* isolates. IMP, VIM, SIM, SPM and GIM genes belong to the class B metallo-β-lactamases and are acquired carbapenemase genes. IMP (primarily detected in South Korea) and VIM (previously detected in China) are the two metallo-β-lactamase genes, which are the most frequently detected genes in *A. baumannii* isolates (Coelho et al., 2006). The prevalence of the metallo-β-lactamase genes is generally low within *A. baumannii* isolates as illustrated in a study by Mendes and colleagues (2009) where the prevalence was 0.8% in Taiwan. VIM, SIM, SPM, IMP and GIM have not been detected in South Africa yet. Therefore the results of this study compared with the literature in that the selected *A. baumannii* isolates were negative for all metallo-β-lactamase genes.

13. Conclusions

Acinetobacter baumannii is an important opportunistic pathogen and causes a variety of nosocomial infections especially within the ICU of the Tertiary Academic Hospital in Gauteng, South Africa. The results of the phenotypic analysis in the form of the Hodge test and Double disk synergy test were similar to the results obtained from the study conducted by Lee et al. in Korea in 2003. The discrepancies with the results of the two studies can be largely due to the use of different carbapenem antibiotic disks. The Hodge test is imperfect as false positives occur due to AmpC production and impermeability of the bacterium to antibiotics due to β-lactamase ability to affect the porins of the outer membrane.

After completion of this study it is evident that the OXA group of genes (class D carbapenemases) are a problem in clinical isolates of *A. baumannii* from the Tertiary Academic Hospital. It was found that OXA-51 genes (80%) and OXA-23 genes (52%) were highly prevalent in this study and these prevalence rates were similar to the worldwide prevalence of OXA genes, which are widespread in *A. baumannii* throughout the world (Feizabadi et al., 2008). Metallo-β-lactamase (MBL) genes were not prevalent in the selected clinical isolates of *A. baumannii* due to the contained spread of the genes and thus no metallo-β-lactamase has been detected in South Africa thus far. According to Livermore molecular tests are definitive, but a few isolates with strong carbapenemase activity were negative in all molecular tests [Presentation by David Livermore on "Detecting carbapenemases" at the 49th Interscience conference on antimicrobial agents and chemotherapy (ICAAC)].

The multiplex PCR assays proved to be a rapid technique for antimicrobial susceptibility testing, however, there is much work to be done in order to investigate the possibilities of multiplex PCR assays as an alternative to current antimicrobial susceptibility testing. Continuous research and surveillance is necessary to monitor the prevalence of antibiotic resistance genes associated with *A. baumannii* in clinical settings. The ability of *A. baumannii* to grow in biofilms poses a threat concerning the possibilities of the spread of both the bacteria and the antibiotic resistance genes, which should be investigated in future research.

14. References

Allen KD & Green HT (1987) Hospital outbreak of multi-resistant *Acinetobacter anitratus*: an airborne mode of spread? *Journal of Hospital Infections* 9:110-119

Ambler R P, Coulson A F W, Frere J M, Ghuysen J M, Joris B, Forsman M, Levesque R C, Tiraby G & Waley S G (1991) A standard numbering scheme for the class A -β-lactamases. *Biochemistry Journal* 276:269–270

Appleman MD, Belzberg H, Citron DM, Heseltine PN, Yellin AE, Murray J & Berne TV (2000) In vitro activities of nontraditional antimicrobials against multiresistant *Acinetobacter baumannii* strains isolated in an intensive care unit outbreak. *Antimicrobial Agents and Chemotherapy* 44:1035–1040

Arakawa Y, Shibata N, Shibayama K, Kurokawa H, Yagi T, Fujiwara H & Goto M (2000) Convenient test for screening metallo-β-lactamase-producing gram-negative bacteria by using thiol compounds. *Journal of Clinical Microbiology* 38:40–43

Aubert D, Poirel L, Chevalier J, Leotard S, Pages JM & Nordmann P (2001) Oxacillinase-mediated resistance to cefepime and susceptibility to ceftazidime in *Pseudomonas aeruginosa. Antimicrobial Agents and Chemotherapy* 45:1615–1620

Aubron C, Poirel L, Ash RJ & Nordmann P (2005) Carbapenemase-producing *Enterobacteriaceae*, U.S rivers. *Emerging Infectious Diseases* 11:260–264

Beck-Sagué CM, Jarvis WR, Brook JH, Culver DH, Potts A, Gay E, Shotts BW, Hill B, Anderson RL & Weinstein MP (1990) Epidemic bacteremia due to *Acinetobacter baumannii* in five intensive care units. *American Journal of Epidemiology* 132: 723-733

Bergogne-Berezin E & KJ Towner (1996) *Acinetobacter* spp. as nosocomial pathogens: microbiological, clinical, and epidemiological features. *Clinical Microbiology Reviews* 9:148–165

Bernards AT, Beauford AJ, Dijkshoorn L and van Boven CPA (1997) Outbreak of septicemia in neonates caused by *Acinetobacter junii* investigated by amplified ribosomal DNA restriction analysis (ARDRA) and four typing methods. *Journal of Hospital Infections* 35: 129-140

Blot S, Vandewoude K & Colardyn F (2003) Nosocomial bacteremia involving *Acinetobacter baumannii* in critically ill patients: a matched cohort study. *Intensive Care Medicine* 29:471–475

Bou G, Cervero G, Dominguez MA, Quereda C & Martinez-Beltran J (2000) Characterization of a nosocomial outbreak caused by a multiresistant *Acinetobacter baumannii* strain with a carbapenem-hydrolyzing enzyme: high-level carbapenem resistance in *A. baumannii* is not due solely to the presence of beta-lactamases. *Journal of Clinical Microbiology* 38:3299–3305

Bouvet PJM & Grimont PAD (1986) Taxonomy of the genus *Acinetobacter* with the recognition of *Acinetobacter baumannii* sp. nov., *Acinetobacter haemolyticus* sp. nov., *Acinetobacter johnsonii* sp. nov,. *Acinetobacter junii* sp. nov. & emended description of *Acinetobacter calcoaceticus* and *Acinetobacter lwoffii*. *International Journal of Systematic Bacteriology* 36: 228-240

Boyce JM & Pittet D (2002) Guideline for hand hygiene in health-care settings: recommendations of the Healthcare Infection Control Practices Advisory Committee and the HICPAC/SHEA/APIC/IDSA Hand Hygiene Task Force. *Infection Control and Hospital Epidemiology* 23:S3–40

Bradley JS (1997) Meropenem: A new, extremely broad-spectrum beta-lactam antibiotic for serious infections in pediatrics. *The Pediatric Infectious Disease Journal* 16:263-268

Brown S, Bantar C, Young H & Amyes S (1996) An outbreak of imipenem resistance in *Acinetobacter* strains from Buenos Aires, Argentina, abstract C-122, p 56 In Abstracts of the 36th Interscience Conference on Antimicrobial Agents and Chemotherapy. American Society for Microbiology, Washington, DC

Brown S & Amyes SG (2005) The sequences of seven class D β-lactamases isolated from carbapenem-resistant *Acinetobacter baumannii* from four continents. *Clinical Microbiology and Infectious Diseases* 11:326-329

Brown S, Young HK & Amyes SG (2005) Characterisation of OXA-51, a novel class D carbapenemase found in genetically unrelated clinical strains of *Acinetobacter baumannii* from Argentina. *Clinical Microbiology and Infectious Diseases* 11: 15-23

Brown S & Amyes S (2006) OXA-β-lactamases in *Acinetobacter*: the story so far. *Journal of Antimicrobial Chemotherapy* 57:1-3

Bush K (1988) Recent developments in lactamase research and their implications for the future. *Reviews of Infectious Diseases* 10:681–690; 739–743

Bush K, Jacoby GA & Medeiros AA (1995) A functional classification scheme for beta-lactamases and its correlation with molecular structure. *Antimicrobial Agents and Chemotherapy*. 39:1211-1233

Cappelli G, Sereni L, Scialoja MG, Morselli M, Perrone S, Ciuffreda A, Bellesia M, Inguaggiato P, Albertazzi A & Tetta C (2003) Effects of biofilm formation on haemodialysis monitor disinfection. *Nephrology Dialysis Transplantation* 18:2105–2111.

Cefai C, Richards J, Gould FK & McPeake P (1990) An outbreak of *Acinetobacter* respiratory tract infection resulting from incomplete disinfection of ventilatory equipment. *Journal of Hospital Infections* 15: 177-182

Chakravarti DN, Fiske MJ, Fletcher LD, & Zagursky RJ (2000) Application of genomics and proteomics for identification of bacterial gene products as potential vaccine candidates. *Vaccine* 19:601–612

Cisneros JM, Reyes MJ & Pachón J (1996) Bacteremia due to *Acinetobacter baumannii*: Epidemiology, clinical and prognostic features. *Clinical Infectious Diseases* 22: 1026-1032

Cisneros JM & Rodriguez-Bano J (2002) Nosocomial bacteremia due to *Acinetobacter baumannii*: epidemiology, clinical features and treatment. *Clinical Microbiology and Infection* 8: 687-693

Clark RB (1996) Imipenem resistance among *Acinetobacter baumannii*: association with reduced expression of a 33-36-kDa outer membrane protein. *Journal of Antimicrobial Chemotherapy* 38: 245-51

Clinical and Laboratory Standards Institute (2009) Performance standards for antimicrobial susceptibility testing, Nineteenth informal supplement. CLSI document M100-S-19. Clinical and Laboratory Standards Institute, Wayne, Pennsylvania

Cloete TE (2003) Resistance mechanisms of bacteria to antimicrobial compounds. *International Biodeterioration and Biodegradation* 51: 277-282

Coelho J, Woodford N, Turton J & Livermore D M (2004) Multiresistant *Acinetobacter* in the UK: how big a threat? *Journal of Hospital Infections* 58:167–169

Coelho J, Woodford N, Afzal-Shah M & Livermore D (2006) Occurrence of OXA-58-like carbapenemases in *Acinetobacter* spp. collected over 10 years in three continents. *Antimicrobial Agents and Chemotherapy* 50:756–758

Collis CM, Kim JM, Stokes HW & Hall RM (2002) Integron-encoded Intl integrases preferentially recognize the adjacent cognate attl site in recombination with a 59-be site. *Molecular Microbiology* 46: 1415-1427

Corbella X, Pujol M & Ayats J (1996) Relevance of digestive tract colonization in the epidemiology of nosocomial infections due to multiresistant *Acinetobacter baumannii*. *Clinical Infectious Diseases* 23:329-334

Corbella X, Ariza J, Ardanuy C, Vuelta M, Yubau F, Sora M, Pujol M & Gudiol F (1998) Efficacy of sulbactam alone and in combination with ampicillin in nosocomial infections caused by multiresistant *Acinetobacter baumannii*. *Journal of Antimicrobial Chemotherapy* 42: 793-802

Cucarella C, Solano C, Valle J, Amorena B, Lasa I & Penades JR (2001) Bap, a *Staphylococcus aureus* surface protein involved in biofilm formation. *Journal of Bacteriology* 183:2888–2896

Cuhna BA. *Acinetobacter* (2007) http://www.emedicine.com/MED/topic3456.htm

Dalla-Costa LM, Coelho JM, Souza HAPHM, Castro MES, Stier CJN, Bragagnolo KL, Rea-Neto A, Penteado-Filho SR, Livermore DM & Woodford N (2003) Outbreak of carbapenem-resistant *Acinetobacter baumannii* producing the OXA-23 enzyme in Curitiba, Brazil. *Journal of Clinical Microbiology* 41:3403–3406

D'Agata EMC, Thayer V & Schaffner W (2000) An outbreak of *Acinetobacter baumannii*: the importance of cross-transmission. *Infection Control of Hospital Epidemiology* 21: 588-591

Devaud M, Kayser FH & Bachi B (1982) Transposon-mediated multiple antibiotic resistance in *Acinetobacter* strains. *Antimicrobial Agents and Chemotherapy* 22:323–329

Dijkshoorn L, Aucken HM, Gerner-Smidt P, Janssen P, Kaufmann ME, Garaizar J, Ursing J & Pitt TL (1996) Comparison of outbreak and non-outbreak *Acinetobacter baumannii* strains by genotypic and phenotypic methods. *Journal of Clinical Microbiology* 34: 1519-1525

Dima S, Kritsotakis EI, Roumbelaki M, Metalidis S, Karabinis A, Maguina N, Klouva F, Levidiotou S, Zakynthinos E, Kioumis J & Gika A (2007) Device-associated nosocomial infection rates in intensive care units in Greece. *Infection Control and Hospital Epidemiology* 28:602–605

Dupont M, Pages JM, Lafitte D, Siroy A & Bollet C (2005) Identification of an OprD homologue in *Acinetobacter baumannii*. *Journal of Proteome Research* 4:2386–2390

Ecker JA, Massire C, Hall TA, Ranken R, Pennella TT, Ivy CA, Blyn LB, Hofstadler SA, Endy TP, Scott PT, Lindler L, Hamilton T, Gaddy C, Snow K, Pe M, Fishbain J, Craft D, Deye G, Riddell S, Milstrey E, Petruccelli B, Brisse S, Harpin V, Schink A, Ecker DJ, Sampath R & Eshoo MW (2006) Identification of *Acinetobacter* species and genotyping of *Acinetobacter baumannii* by multilocus PCR and mass spectrometry. *Journal of Clinical Microbiology* 44:2921–2932

Ellington MJ, Kistler J, Livermore DM and Woodford N (2007) Multiplex PCR for rapid detection of genes encoding acquired metallo-β-lactamases. *Journal of Antimicrobial Chemotherapy* 59: 321-322

Euzéby JP (2008) List of prokaryotic names with standing in nomenclature http://www.bacterio.cict.fr/classificationac.html#*Acinetobacter*

Falagas ME, Bliziotis IA, & Siempos II (2006) Attributable mortality of *Acinetobacter baumannii* infections in critically ill patients: a systematic review of matched cohort and case-control studies. *Critical Care* 10:R48

Feizabadi MM, Fathollahazadeh B, Taherikalani M, Rasoolinejad M, Sadeghifard N, AligholiM, Soroush S & Mohammadi-Yegane S (2008) Antimicrobial susceptibility patterns and distribution of bla_{OXA} genes among *Acinetobacter* spp isolated from patients at Tehran hospitals. *Japanese Journal of Infectious Diseases* 61: 274-278

Fernandez-Cuenca F, Martinez-Martinez L, Conejo MC, Ayala JA, Perea EJ & Pascual A (2003) Relationship between beta-lactamase production, outer membrane protein and penicillin-binding protein profiles on the activity of carbapenems against clinical isolates of *Acinetobacter baumannii*. *Journal of Antimicrobial Chemotherapy* 51:565–574

Fournier PE, Vallenet D, Barbe V, Audic S, Ogata H, Poirel L, Richet H, Robert C, Mangenot S, Abergel C, Nordmann P, Weissenbach J, Raoult D & Claverie JM (2006) Comparative genomics of multidrug resistance in *Acinetobacter baumannii*. *PLoS Genetics*. 2:e7

Frere J M, Galleni M, Bush K & Dideberg O (2005) Is it necessary to change the classification of lactamases? *Journal of Antimicrobial Chemotherapy* 55:1051–1053

Fritsche TR, Stilwell MG, and Jones RN (2005) Antimicrobial activity of doripenem (S-4661): a global surveillance report (2003). *Clinical Microbiology and Infect*ions 11:974–984

Garcia-Garmendia JL, Ortiz-Leyba C, Garnacho-Montero J, Jimenez-Jimenez FJ, Perez-Paredes C, Barrero-Almodovar AE & Gili-Miner M (2001) Risk factors for *Acinetobacter baumannii* nosocomial bacteremia in critically ill patients: a cohort study. *Clinical Infectious Diseases*. 33:939–946

Garrity GM, Brenner DJ, Krieg RN & Staley JT (2005) Bergey's Manual of Systematic Bacteriology, Volume 2: The Proteobacteria, Part B: The Gammaproteobacteria, pg 415-435. Springer, New York, USA

Gerischer U (2008) *Acinetobacter* Molecular Biology 1st edition, Caister Academic Press ISBN 987-1-904455-20-2

Gerner-Smidt P (1987) Endemic occurrence of *Acinetobacter calcoaceticus* biovar anitratus in an intensive care unit. *Journal of Hospital Infections*. 10: 265-272

Gerner-Smidt P, Tjernberg I & Usring J (1991) Reliability of phenotypic tests for identification of *Acinetobacter species*. *Journal of Clinical Microbiology* 29: 277-282

Getchell-White SI; Donowitz LG & Groeschel DHM (1989) The inanimate environment of an intensive care unit as a potential source of nosocomial bacteria: evidence for long survival of *Acinetobacter calcoaceticus*. *Infection Control and Hospital Epidemiology* 10: 402-407

Giamarellou H, Antoniadou A & Kanellakopoulou (2008) Review: *Acinetobacter baumannii:* a universal threat to public health? *International Journal of Antimicrobial Agents* 32: 106-119

Go ES, Urban C, Burns J, Kreiswirth B, Eisner W & Mariano NF (1994) Clinical and molecular epidemiology of *Acinetobacter* infections sensitive only to polymyxin B and sulbactam. *Lancet* 12:1329-1332

Go J and Cuhna BA (1999) *Acinetobacter baumannii:* Infection control implications. *Infectious Disease Practices* 23: 65-68

Goldstein FW, Labigne-Roussel A, Gerbaud G, Carlier C, Collatz E & Courvalin P (1983) Transferable plasmid-mediated antibiotic resistance in *Acinetobacter. Plasmid* 10:138–147

Grundmann HJ, Towner KJ, Dijkshoorn L, Gerner-Smidt P, Maher M, Seifert H & Vaneechoutte M (1997) Multicenter study using standardized protocols and reagents for evaluation of reproducibility of PCR-based fingerprinting of *Acinetobacter* spp. *Journal of Clinical Microbiology* 35: 3071-3077

Guardabassi L, Dijkshoorn L, Collard JM, Olsen JE & Dalsgaard A (2000) Distribution and *in vitro* transfer of tetracycline resistance determinants in clinical and aquatic *Acinetobacter* strains. *Journal of Medical Microbiology* 49: 929-936

Heritier C, Dubouix A, Poirel L, Marty N & Nordmann P (2005a) A nosocomial outbreak of *Acinetobacter baumannii* isolates expressing the carbapenem-hydrolysing oxacillinase OXA-58. *Journal of Antimicrobial Chemotherapy* 55: 115-118

Heritier C, Poirel L, Fournier, Claverie J, Raoult D & Nordmann P (2005b) Characterization of the naturally occurring oxacillinase of *Acinetobacter baumannii. Antimicrobial Agents and Chemotherapy* 49: 4174-4179

Heritier C, Poirel L & Nordmann P (2006) Cephalosporinase overexpression resulting from insertion of IS*Aba1* in *Acinetobacter baumannii. Clinical Microbiology and Infection* 12:123–130

Hogg GM, Barr JG & Webb CH (1998) *In-vitro* activity of the combination of colistin and rifampicin against multidrug-reistant strains of *Acinetobacter baumannii. Journal of Antimicrobial Chemotherapy* 41: 494-495

Hornstein M, Sautjeau-Rostoker C, Peduzzi J, Vessieres A, Hong LT, Barthelemy M, Scavizzi M & Labia R (1997) Oxacillin-hydrolyzing lactamase involved in resistance to imipenem in *Acinetobacter baumannii. FEMS Microbiology Letters* 153:333–339

Hsueh P-R, Teng L-J, Chen C-Y, Chen W-H, Yu C-J, Ho S-W & Luh K-T (2002) Pandrug-Resistant *Acinetobacter baumannii* causing nosocomial infections in a University in Taiwan. *Emerging Infectious Diseases* 8: 827-832

Hughes D (2003) Exploiting genomics, genetics and chemistry to combat antibiotic resistance. *Nature Reviews Genetics* 4:432–441

Hujer KM, Hujer AM, Hulten EA, Bajaksouzian S, Adams JM, Donskey CJ, Ecker DJ, Massire C, Eshoo MW, Sampath R, Thomson JM, Rather PN, Craft DW, Fishbain JT, Ewell AJ, Jacobs MR, Paterson DL & Bonomo RA (2006) Analysis of antibiotic resistance genes in multidrug-resistant *Acinetobacter* sp. isolates from military and civilian patients treated at the Walter Reed Army Medical Center. *Antimicrobial Agents and Chemotherapy* 50:4114–4123

Huys G, Cnockaert M, Vaneechoutte M, Woodford N, Nemec A, Dijkshoorn L & Swings J (2005) Distribution of tetracycline resistance genes in genotypically related and unrelated multiresistant *Acinetobacter baumannii* strains from different European hospitals. *Research in Microbiology* 156: 348-355

Jacobs RF: Imipenem-cilastatin (1986) The first thienamycin antibiotic *The Pediatric Infectious Disease Journal* 5:444-448

Jawad A, Hawkey PM, Herritage J & Snelling AM (1994) Description of Leeds *Acinetobacter* Medium, a new selective and differential medium for isolation of clinically important *Acinetobacter* spp and comparison with Herellea agar and Holton's agar. *Journal of Clinical Microbiology*. 32: 2353-2358

Jawad A, Heritage J, Snelling AM, Gascoyne-Binzi DM & Hawkey PM (1996) Influence of relative humidity and suspending menstrual on survival of *Acinetobacter* spp on dry surfaces. *Journal of Clinical Microbiology* 34: 2881-2887

Jeon B, Jeong SH, Bae IK, Kwon SB, Lee K, Young D, Lee JH, Song JS & Lee SH (2005) Investigation of a nosocomial outbreak of imipenem- resistant *Acinetobacter baumannii* producing the OXA-23-lactamase in Korea. *Journal of Clinical Microbiology* 43:2241–2245

Joly-Guillou ML (2005) Clinical impact and pathogenicity of *Acinetobacter. Clinical Microbiology and Infection* 11:868–873

Jones RN, Huynh HK, Biedenbach DJ, Fritsche TR & Sader HS (2004) Doripenem (S-4661), a novel carbapenem: comparative activity against contemporary pathogens including bactericidal action and preliminary in vitro methods evaluations. *Journal of Antimicrobial Chemotherapy* 54:144- 154

Jones RN, Sader HS & Fritsche TR (2005) Comparative activity of doripenem and three other carbapenems tested against Gram-negative bacilli with various beta-lactamase resistance mechanisms. *Diagnostic Microbiology and Infectious Disease* 52:71–74

Kahlmeter G., Brown DF, Goldstein FW, MacGowan AP, Mouton JW, Odenholt I, Rodloff A, Soussy CJ, Steinbakk M, Soriano F & Stetsiouk O (2006) European Committee on Antimicrobial Susceptibility Testing (EUCAST) technical notes on antimicrobial susceptibility testing. *Clinical Microbiology and Infection* 12:501–503

Kramer A, Schwebke I & Kampf G (2006) How long do nosocomial pathogens persist on inanimate surfaces? A systematic review. *BMC Infectious Diseases* 6:130

Kuo L, Teng L, Yu C, Ho S and Hsueh P (2004) Dissemination of a clone of unusual phenotype of pandrug-resistant *Acinetobacter baumannii* at a University Hospital in Taiwan. *Journal of Clinical Microbiology* 42: 1759-1763

Landman D, Quale J M, Mayorga D, Adedeji A, Vangala K, Ravishankar J, Flores C & Brooks S (2002) Citywide clonal outbreak of multiresistant *Acinetobacter baumannii* and *Pseudomonas aeruginosa* in Brooklyn, NY: the preantibiotic era has returned. *Archives of Internal Medicine* 162:1515–1520

Laraki N, Franceschini N, Rossolini GM, Santucci P, Meunier C, de Pauw, Amicosante G, Frère JM & Galleni (1999) Biochemical characterization of the *Pseudomonas aeruginosa* 101/1477 metallo-β-lactamase IMP-1 produced by *Escherichia coli*. *Antimicrobial Agents and Chemotherapy* 43: 902-906

Lauretti L, Riccio ML, Mazzariol A, Cornaglia G, Amicosante G, Fontana R & Rossolini GM (1999) Cloning and characterization of bla_{VIM}, a new integron-borne metallo-lactamase gene from a *Pseudomonas aeruginosa* clinical isolate. *Antimicrobial Agents and Chemotherapy* 43:1584– 1590

Lee K, Chong Y, Shin HB, Kim YA, Yong D & Yum JH (2001) Modified Hodge test and EDTA-disk synergy tests to screen metallo-ß-lactamase-producing strains of *Pseudomonas* and *Acinetobacter* species. *Clinical Microbiology and Infection* 7:88-91

Lee K, Lee WG, Uh Y, Ha GY, Cho J, Chong Y & the Korean Nationwide Surveillance of Antimicrobial Resistance group (2003) VIM- and IMP-Type Metallo-β-lactamase-Producing *Pseudomonas* spp. and *Acinetobacter* spp. in Korean Hospitals. *Emerging Infectious Diseases* 9: 868–871

Lee K, Yum JH, Yong D, Lee HM, Kim HD, Docquier JD, Rossolini GM & ChongY (2005) Novel acquired metallo-beta-lactamase gene, bla_{SIM-1}, in a class 1 integron from *Acinetobacter baumannii* clinical isolates from Korea. *Antimicrobial Agents and Chemotherapy* 49:4485–4491

Lim HM, Pene JJ & Shaw RW (1988) Cloning, nucleotide sequence, and expression of the *Bacillus cereus* 5/B/6-lactamase II structural gene. *Journal of Bacteriology* 170:2873–2878

Limansky AS, Mussi MA & Viale AM (2002) Loss of a 29-kilodalton outer membrane protein in *Acinetobacter baumannii* is associated with imipenem resistance. *Journal of Clinical Microbiology* 40:4776–4778

Livermore DM & Woodford N (2006) The lactamase threat in *Enterobacteriaceae*, Pseudomonas and *Acinetobacter*. *Trends in Microbiology* 14:413–420

Lolans K, Rice TW, Munoz-Price LS & Quinn JP (2006) Multicity outbreak of carbapenem-resistant *Acinetobacter baumannii* isolates producing the carbapenemase OXA-40. *Antimicrobial Agents and Chemotherapy* 50:2941- 2945

Loukili NH, Granbastien B, Faure K, Guery B, and Beaucaire G (2006) Effect of different stabilized preparations of peracetic acid on biofilm. *Journal of Hospital Infections* 63:70–72

Lorenz MG & Wackernagel W (1994) Bacterial gene transfer by natural genetic transformation in the environment. *Microbiological Reviews* 58:563- 602

Ma JF, Hager PW, Howell ML, Phibbs PV & Hasset D (1998) Cloning and characterization of *Pseudomonas aeruginosa* zwf gene encoding glucose-6-phosphate dehydrogenase, an enzyme important in resistance to methyl viologen (paraquat). *Journal of Bacteriology* 180: 1741-1749

Majiduddin FK & Palzkill T (2003) Amino acid sequence requirements at residues 69 and 238 for the SME-1-lactamase to confer resistance to-lactam antibiotics. *Antimicrobial Agents and Chemotherapy* 47:1062–1067

Maragakis LL, Cosgrove SE, Song X, Kim D, Rosenbaum P, Ciesla N, Srinivasan A, Ross T, Carroll K & Perl TM (2004) An outbreak of multidrug-resistant *Acinetobacter baumannii* associated with pulsatile lavage wound treatment. *Journal of the American Medical Association* 292:3006–3011

Marchand I, Damier-Piolle L, Courvalin P & Lambert T (2004) Expression of the RND-type efflux pump AdeABC in *Acinetobacter baumannii* is regulated by the AdeRS two-component system. *Antimicrobial Agents and Chemotherapy* 48:3298–3304

Marque S, Poirel L, Heritier C, Brisse S, Blasco MD, Filip R, Coman G, Naas T & Nordmann P (2005) Regional occurrence of plasmid mediated carbapenem-hydrolyzing oxacillinase OXA-58 in *Acinetobacter* spp. in Europe. *Journal of Clinical Microbiology* 43:4885–4888

McDonald LC, Banerjee SN, Jarvis WR & the National Nosocomial Infections Surveillance System (1999) Seasonal variation of *Acinetobacter* infections: 1987-96. *Clinical Infectious Diseases* 29: 1133-1137

Mendes RE, Bell JM, Turnidge JD, Castanheira M & Jones RN (2009) Emergence and widespread dissemination of OXA-23, -24/40 and -58 carbapenemases among *Acinetobacter* spp in Asia-Pacific nations: report from the SENTRY Surveillance Program. *Journal of Antimicrobial Chemotherapy* 63: 55-59

Merkier AK & Centròn D (2006) *bla*$_{OXA-51}$-type β-lactamase genes are ubiquitous and vary within a strain in *Acinetobacter baumannii*. *International Journal of Antimicrobial Agents* 28: 110-113

Metzgar D, Bacher JM, Pezo V, Reader J, Doring V, Schimmel P, Marliere P & de Crecy-Lagard V (2004) *Acinetobacter* sp. ADP1: an ideal model organism for genetic analysis and genome engineering. *Nucleic Acids Research* 32:5780–5790

Mulin B, Talon D & Viel JF (1995) Risk factor for nosocomial colonization with multiresistant *Acinetobacter baumannii*. *European Journal of Clinical Microbiology and Infectious Diseases* 14: 569-576

Mushtaq S, Ge Y & Livermore DM (2004) Comparative activities of doripenem versus isolates, mutants, and transconjugants of *Enterobacteriaceae* and *Acinetobacter* spp. with characterized beta-lactamases. *Antimicrobial Agents and Chemotherapy* 48:1313–1319

Mussi MA, Limansky AS & Viale AM (2005) Acquisition of resistance to carbapenems in multidrug-resistant clinical strains of *Acinetobacter baumannii*: natural insertional inactivation of a gene encoding a member of a novel family of beta-barrel outer membrane proteins. *Antimicrobial Agents and Chemotherapy* 49:1432–1440

Naas T, Levy M, Hirschauer C, Marchandin H & Nordmann P (2005) Outbreak of carbapenem-resistant *Acinetobacter baumannii* producing the carbapenemase OXA-23 in a tertiary care hospital of Papeete, French Polynesia. *Journal of Clinical Microbiology* 43:4826-4829

Nikaido H (1996) Multidrug efflux pumps of Gram-negative bacteria. *Journal of Bacteriology* 178: 5853-5859

Nordmann P, Mariotte S, Naas T, Labia R & Nicolas M-H (1993) Biochemical properties of a carbapenem-hydrolyzing-lactamase for *Enterobacter cloacae* and cloning of the gene into *Escherichia coli*. *Antimicrobial Agents and Chemotherapy* 37:939–946

Nordmann, P & Poirel L (2002) Emerging carbapenemases in Gram negative aerobes. *Clinical Microbiology and Infection* 8:321–331

Nordmann, P (2004) *Acinetobacter baumannii,* the nosocomial pathogen par excellence. *Pathologie Biologie* 52:301–303

Pajkos A, Vickery K & Cossart Y (2004) Is biofilm accumulation on endoscope tubing a contributor to the failure of cleaning and decontamination? *Journal of Hospital Infections* 58:224–229

Palmen R & Hellingwerf KJ (1997) Uptake and processing of DNA by *Acinetobacter calcoaceticus*—a review. *Gene* 192:179–190

Pantophlet R, Brade L & Brade H (1999) Identification of *Acinetobacter baumannii* strains with monoclonal antibodies against the O antigens of their lipopolysaccharides. *Clinical and Diagnostic Laboratory Immunology* 6: 323-329

Paton R, Miles RS and Hood J (1993) ARI-1: β-lactamase mediated imipenem resistance in *Acinetobacter baumannii. International Journal of Antimicrobial Agents* 2: 81-88

Patterson JE, Vecchio J, Pantelick EL, Farrel P, Mazon D, Zervos MJ & Heirholzer WJ Jr (1991) Association of contaminated gloves with transmission of *Acinetobacter calcoaceticus* var *anitratus* in an intensive care unit. *American Journal of Medicine* 91: 479-483

Peleg AY, Franklin C, Bell J & Spelman DW (2005) Dissemination of the metallo-β-lactamase gene bla_{IMP-4} amongst Gram negative pathogens in a clinical setting in Australia. *Clinical Infectious Diseases* 41:1549-1556

Perez F, Hujer AM, Hujer KM, Decker BK, Rather PN & Bonomo RA (2007) Minireview: Global challenge of mulidrug-resistant *Acinetobacter baumannii. Antimicrobial Agents and Chemotherapy* 51: 3471-3484

Peterson AA, Fesik SW & McGroarty EJ (1987) Decreased binding of antibiotics to lipopolysaccharides from polymyxin-resistant strains of *Escherichia coli* and *Salmonella typhimurium. Antimicrobial Agents and Chemotherapy* 31: 230-237

Petropoulou D, Tzanetou K, Syriopoulou VP, Daikos GL, Ganteris G & Malamou-Lada E (2006) Evaluation of imipenem/imipenem EDTA disk method for detection of metallo-lactamase-producing *Klebsiella pneumoniae* isolated from blood cultures. *Microbial Drug Resistance* 12:39–43

Pittet D (2004) The Lowbury lecture: behaviour in infection control. *Journal of Hospital Infection* 58:1–13

Poirel L, Cabanne L, Vahaboglu H, & Nordmann P (2005) Genetic environment and expression of the extended-spectrum Beta-lactamase bla_{PER-1} gene in gram-negative bacteria. *Antimicrobial Agents and Chemotherapy* 49:1708–1713

Poirel L & Nordmann P (2006) Carbapenem resistance in *Acinetobacter baumannii*: mechanisms and epidemiology. *Clinical Microbiology and Infection* 12:826–836

Poole K (2005) Efflux-mediated antimicrobial resistance. *Journal of Antimicrobial Chemotherapy* 56:20–51

Pottumarthy S, Moland ES, Jeretschko S, Swanzy SR, Thomson KS and Fritsche TR (2003) NmcA carbapenem-hydrolyzing enzyme in *Enterobacter cloacae* in North America. *Emerging Infectious Diseases* 9:999–1002

Pournaras S, Markogiannakis A, Ikonomidis A, Kondyli L, Bethimouti K, Maniatis AN, Legakis NJ & Tsakris A (2006) Outbreak of multiple clones of imipenem-resistant *Acinetobacter baumannii* isolates expressing OXA-58 carbapenemase in an intensive care unit. *Journal of Antimicrobial Chemotherapy* 57:557–561

Prashanth K & Badrinath S (2000) Simplified phenotypic tests for identification of *Acinetobacter spp* and their antimicrobial susceptibility status. *Journal of Medical Microbiology* 49: 773-778

Projan SJ (2004) Small molecules for small minds? The case for biologic pharmaceuticals. *Expert Opinion on Biological Therapy* 4: 1345-1350

Radice M, Power P, Gutkind G, Fernandez K, Vay C, Famiglietti A, Ricover N & Ayala J (2004) First class A carbapenemase isolated from *Enterobacteriaceae* in Argentina. *Antimicrobial Agents and Chemotherapy* 48:1068– 1069

Rahal J (2006) Novel antibiotic combinations against infections with almost completely resistant *Pseudomonas aeruginosa* and *Acinetobacter* species. *Clinical Infectious Diseases* 43: 95-99

Rasmussen B A, Bush K, Keeney D, Yang Y, Hare R, O'Gara C & Medeiros A A (1996) Characterization of IMI-1 β-lactamase, a class A carbapenem-hydrolyzing enzyme from *Enterobacter cloacae*. *Antimicrobial Agents and Chemotherapy* 40:2080–2086

Ribera A, Ruiz J & Vila J (2003) Presence of the Tet M determinant in a clinical isolate of *Acinetobacter baumannii*. *Antimicrobial Agents and Chemotherapy* 47: 2310-2312

Robenshtok E, Paul M, Leibovici L, Fraser A, Pitlik S, Ostfeld I, Samra Z, Perez S, Lev B & Weinberger M (2006) The significance of *Acinetobacter baumannii* bacteraemia compared with *Klebsiella pneumoniae* bacteraemia: risk factors and outcomes. *Journal of Hospital Infection* 64: 282-287

Rodriguez-Hernańdez MJ, Pachoń J & Pichardo C (2000) Imipenem, doxycycline and amikacin in monotherapy and in combination in *Acinetobacter baumannii* experimental pneumonia. *Journal of Antimicrobial Chemotherapy* 45: 493-501

Santillana E, Beceiro A, Bou G & Romero A (2007) Crystal structure of the carbapenemase OXA-24 reveals insights into the mechanism of carbapenem hydrolysis. *Proceedings of the National Academy of Science USA* 104:5354–5359

Savov E, Chankova D, Vatcheva R & Dinev N (2002) In vitro investigation of the susceptibility of *Acinetobacter baumannii* strains isolated from clinical specimens to ampicillin/sulbactam alone and in combination with amikacin. *International Journal of Antimicrobial Agents* 20:390–392

Scaife W, Young HK, Paton RH & Amyes SG (1995) Transferable imipenem-resistance in *Acinetobacter* species from a clinical source. *Journal of Clinical Microbiology* 36: 585-586

Scerpella EG, Wanger AR, Armitige L, Anderlini P and Ericsson CD (1995) Nosocomial outbreak caused by a multiresistant clone of *Acinetobacter baumannii*: results of the case control and molecular epidemiologic investigations. *Infection Control and Hospital Epidemiology* 16: 92-97

Schreckenberger PC & Von Graevenitz A (2000) *Acinetobacter*, *Achromobacter*, *Acaligenes*, *Moraxella*, *Methylobacterium* and other non-fermentative Gram-negative rods, pg 539-560. In Murray PR, Baron EJ, Pfaller MA, Tenover FC and Yolken RH (ed), Manual of clinical Microbiology, 7th ed. ASM Press, Washington DC, USA

Seifert H, Strate A & Pulverer G (1995) Nosocomial bacteremia due to *Acinetobacter baumannii*, clinical features, epidemiology and predictors of mortality. *Medicine* 74: 340-349

Seifert H, Dijkshoorn L, Gerner-Smidt P, Pelzer N, Tjernberg I & Vaneechoutte A (1997) Distribution of *Acinetobacter* species on human skin: comparison of phenotypic and genotypic identification methods. *Journal of Clinical Microbiology* 35: 2819-2825

Seifert H, Dolzani L & Bressan R (2005) Standardization and interlaboratory reproducibility assessment of pulsed-field gel electrophoresis-generated fingerprints of *Acinetobacter baumannii*. *Journal of Clinical Microbiology* 43:4328–35

Segal H, Garny S & Elisha BG (2005) Is IS (ABA-1) customized for *Acinetobacter*. *FEMS Microbiology Letters* 243:425–429

Seward, R. J (1999) Detection of integrons in worldwide nosocomial isolates of *Acinetobacter* spp. *Clinical Microbiology and Infection* 5:308–318

Seward RJ & Towner KJ (1998) Molecular epidemiology of quinolone resistance in *Acinetobacter spp*. *Clinical Microbiology and Infection* 4: 248-254

Sheretz RJ & Sullivan ML (1985) An outbreak of infections with *Acinetobacter calcoaceticus* in burn patients: contamination of patients' mattresses. *Journal of Infectious Diseases* 151: 252-258

Siroy A, Molle V, Lemaitre-Guillier C, Vallenet D, Pestel-Caron M, Cozzone AJ, Jouenne T & De E (2005) Channel formation by CarO, the carbapenem resistance-associated outer membrane protein of *Acinetobacter baumannii*. *Antimicrobial Agents and Chemotherapy* 49:4876–4883

Smith MG, Des Etages SG & Snyder M (2004) Microbial synergy via an ethanol-triggered pathway. *Molecular and Cellular Biology* 24:3874–3884

Smith MG, Gianoulis TA, Pukatzki S, Mekalanos JJ, Ornston LN, Gerstein M & Snyder M (2007) New insights into *Acinetobacter baumannii* pathogenesis revealed by high-density pyrosequencing and transposon mutagenesis. *Genes and Development* 21:601–614

Sougakoff W, L'Hermite G, Pernot L, Naas T, Guillet V, Nordmann P, Jarlier V & Delettre J (2002) Structure of the imipenem-hydrolyzing class A-lactamase SME-1 from *Serratia marcescens*. *Acta Crystallographica Section D Biological Crystallography Journal* 58:267–274

Swenson JM, Killgore GE & Tenover FC (2004) Antimicrobial susceptibility testing of *Acinetobacter* spp. by NCCLS broth microdilution and disk diffusion methods. *Journal of Clinical Microbiology* 42:5102–5108

Takahashi A, Yomoda S, Kobayashi I, Okubo T, Tsunoda M & Iyobe S (2000) Detection of carbapenemase-producing *Acinetobacter baumannii* in a hospital. *Journal of Clinical Microbiology* 38: 526-529

Talbot GH, Bradley J, Edwards JE Jr, Gilbert D, Scheld M, & Bartlett JG (2006) Bad bugs need drugs: an update on the development pipeline from the Antimicrobial Availability Task Force of the Infectious Diseases Society of America. *Clinical Infectious Disease* 42:657–668

Thongpiyapoom S, Narong MN, Suwalak N, Jamulitrat S, Intaraksa P, Boonrat J, Kasatpibal N & Unahalekhaka A (2004) Device-associated infections and patterns of antimicrobial resistance in a medical-surgical intensive care unit in a university hospital in Thailand. *Journal of the Medical Association of Thailand* 87:819–824

Turton JF, Kaufmann ME, Glover J, Coelho JM, Warner M, Pike R & Pitt TL (2005) Detection and typing of integrons in epidemic strains of *Acinetobacter baumannii* found in the United Kingdom. *Journal of Clinical Microbiology* 43:3074–3082

Turton JF, Woodford N, Glover J, Yarde S, Kaufmann ME & Pitt TL (2006) Identification of *Acinetobacter baumannii* by detection of the $bla_{\text{OXA-51-like}}$ carbapenemase gene intrinsic to this species. *Journal of Clinical Microbiology* 44: 2974-2976

Ullah JH, Walsh TR, Taylor IA, Emery DC, Verma CS & Gamblin SJ (1998) The crystal structure of the L1 metallo-β-lactamase from *Stenotrophomonas maltophilia* at 1.7 resolution. *Journal of Molecular Biology* 284: 125-136

Vahaboglu H, Budak F, Kasap M, Gacar G, Torol S, Karadenizli A, Kolayli F & Eroglu C (2006) High prevalence of OXA-51-type class D Beta-lactamases among ceftazidime-resistant clinical isolates of *Acinetobacter* spp.: co-existence with OXA-58 in multiple centers. *Journal of Antimicrobial Chemotherapy* 58:537–542

Van Dessel H, Dijkshoorn L, Van der Reijden T, Bakker N, Paauw A & Van de Broek E (2004) Identification of a new geographically widespread multiresistant *Acinetobacter baumannii* clone from European hospitals. *Research in Microbiology* 155: 105-112

Vaneechoutte M (1996) DNA fingerprinting techniques for microorganisms. A proposal for classification and nomenclature. *Molecular Biotechnology* 6: 115-142

Villegas MV & Hartstein AI (2003) *Acinetobacter* outbreaks, 1977–2000. *Infection Control and Hospital Epidemiology* 24:284–295

Villers D, Espaze E, Coste-burel M, Giauffret F, Ninin E, Nicolas F & Richet H (1998) Nosocomial *Acinetobacter baumannii* infections: Microbiological and clinical epidemiology. *Annals of Internal Medicine* 129: 182-189

Walsh T, Toleman M, Poirel L & Nordmann P (2005) Metallo-β-lactamases: the quiet before the storm? *Clinical Microbiological Reviews* 18:306-325

Walsh TR (2005) The emergence and implications of metallo-beta-lactamases in Gram-negative bacteria. *Clinical Microbiology and Infection* 11(Suppl. 6):2–9.

Walther-Rasmussen J & Hoiby N (2006) OXA-type carbapenemases. *Journal of Antimicrobial Chemotherapy* 57:373–383

Wang JT, McDonald LC, Chang SC & Ho M (2002) Community-Acquired *Acinetobacter baumannii* bacteremia in adult patients in Taiwan. *Journal of Clinical Microbiology* 40: 1526-1529

Watanabe M, Iyobe S, Inoue M & Mitsuhashi S (1991) Transferable imipenem resistance in *Pseudomonas aeruginosa*. *Antimicrobial Agents and Chemotherapy* 35:147–151

Weernink A, Severin WPJ, Tjernberg I & Dijkshoorn L (1995) Pillows an unexpected source of *Acinetobacter*. *Journal of Hospital Infections*. 29: 189-199

Wilks M, Wilson A, Warwick S, Price E, Kennedy D, Ely A & Millar MR (2006) Control of an outbreak of multidrug-resistant *Acinetobacter baumannii-calcoaceticus* colonization and infection in an intensive care unit (ICU) without closing the ICU or placing patients in isolation. *Infection Control and Hospital Epidemiology* 27:654–658

Wilson SJ, Knipe CJ, Zieger MJ, Gabehart KM, Goodman JE, Volk HM & Sood R (2004) Direct costs of multidrug-resistant *Acinetobacter baumannii* in the burn unit of a public teaching hospital. *American Journal of Infection Control* 32:342–344

Wise R (1986) In vitro and Pharmacokinetic properties of the carbapenems. *Antimicrobial Agents and Chemotherapy* 30:343-349

Wisplinghoff H, Bischoff T, Tallent SM, Seifert H, Wenzel RP & Edmond MB (2004) Nosocomial bloodstream infections in US hospitals: analysis of 24 179 cases from a prospective nationwide surveillance study. *Clinical Infectious Diseases* 39: 309-317

Wood CA & Reboli AC (1993) Infections caused by carbapenem-resistant *Acinetobacter calcoaceticus* biotype anatraus. *Journal of Infectious Diseases* 167: 448-451

Woodford N, Ellington MJ, Coehlo JM, Turton JF, Ward ME, Brown S, Amyes SGB & Livermore DM (2006) Multiplex PCR for genes encoding prevalent OXA carbapenemases in *Acinetobacter spp. International Journal of Antimicrobial Agents* 27: 351-353

Yang Y, Wu P & Livermore D M (1990) Biochemical characterization of a lactamase that hydrolyzes penems and carbapenems from two *Serratia marcescens* isolates. *Antimicrobial Agents and Chemotherapy* 34:755–758

Yigit H, Queenan AM, Anderson GJ, Domenech-Sanchez A, Biddle JW, Steward CD, Alberti S, Bush K & Tenover F C (2001) Novel carbapenem-hydrolyzing-lactamase, KPC-1, from a carbapenem-resistant strain of *Klebsiella pneumoniae. Antimicrobial Agents and Chemotherapy* 45:1151- 1161

Yong D, Choi YS, Roh KH, Kim CK, Park YH, Yum JH, Lee K and Chong Y (2006) Increasing prevalence and diversity of metallo-β-lactamases in *Pseudomonas* spp., *Acinetobacter* spp., and *Enterobacteriaceae* from Korea. *Antimicrobial Agents and Chemotherapy* 50:1884–1886

Young DM. & Ornston LN (2001) Functions of the mismatch repair gene *mut*S from *Acinetobacter* sp. strain ADP1. *Journal of Bacteriology* 183: 6822–6831

Yu Y-S, Du X-X, Zhou Z-H, Chen Y-G & Li L-J (2006) First isolation of *bla*IMI-2 in an *Enterobacter cloacae* clinical isolate from China. *Antimicrobial Agents and Chemotherapy* 50:1610–1611

Yum JH, Yi K, Lee H, Yong D, Lee K, Kim JM, Rossolini GM & Chong Y (2002) Molecular characterization of metallo-beta-lactamase-producing *Acinetobacter baumannii* and *Acinetobacter* genomospecies 3 from Korea: identification of two new integrons carrying the bla_{VIM-2} gene cassettes. *Journal of Antimicrobial Chemotherapy* 49:837–840.

Zarrilli R, Crispino M, Bagattini M, Barretta E, Popolo A. D, Triassi M & Villari P (2004) Molecular epidemiology of sequential outbreaks of *Acinetobacter baumannii* in an intensive care unit shows the emergence of carbapenem resistance. *Journal of Clinical Microbiology* 42:946–953

10

Staphylococcal Infection, Antibiotic Resistance and Therapeutics

Ranginee Choudhury[1], Sasmita Panda[1], Savitri Sharma[2,*] and Durg V. Singh[1,*]
[1]*Infectious Disease Biology, Institute of Life Sciences, Bhubaneswar*
[2]*Ocular Microbiology Service, LV Prasad Eye Institute, Bhubaneswar*
India

1. Introduction

Staphylococcus spp. are a challenge for the modern day medicine due to the complexity of disease process and presence and expression patterns of their respective virulence factors. The members of this genus possess many known toxins, multiple immunoavoidance mechanisms and adherence factors, most of which demonstrate transient, timed, and disease-specific expression. They cause different types of infections in a host that are either planktonic, biofilm mediated or both. Sepsis and pneumonia are mainly caused by planktonic forms whereas, a whole range of diseases, namely, endophthalmitis, osteomyelitis, endocarditis, chronic skin infections, indwelling medical device infections, chronic rhino-sinusitis, and dental implantits are caused by the biofilmic form of the bacteria. Abscess can be caused by both of the forms (Harro et al., 2010). Staphylococci are human pathogen, known for their ability to become resistant to antibiotics. They have been associated, besides causing ophthalmic infections, with skin infections and sepsis. Methicillin resistant *S. aureus* (MRSA), in addition to resistance to other drugs, have emerged as a widespread cause of community infection as well. In this chapter, we describe the epidemiology and antibiotic resistance among *S. aureus* and other species with special reference to ophthalmic infections and focus on newer approaches for treatment of staphylococcus infection like phage therapy and vaccines.

2. Staphylococcus in wound and eye infections

Staphylococcus aureus, a gram-positive bacterium, discovered in 1880's has been shown to be a potential pathogen causing infections such as minor skin infections and post-operative wound infection. Since the introduction of penicillin for the treatment, the mortality rate of individuals caused by *S. aureus* infection was about 80%. After emergence of penicillin resistance and introduction of methicillin in 1961, *S. aureus* developed resistance to methicillin due to acquisition of the *mecA* gene. During last 47 years, various hospital-associated methicillin-resistant *S. aureus* (HA-MRSA) and later virulent community-associated MRSA (CA-MRSA) clones characterised by the presence of toxin Panton-Valentine-leukocidin (PVL), were reported (Deurenberg and Stobberingh, 2008).

Staphylococci have a special relationship with the eye. On one hand, almost all species of staphylococci may be present in the lid margins or conjunctiva as normal commensals without causing disease and on the other hand, they may cause severe eye infections which may result in irreversible blindness. Colonization by resident bacteria on the ocular surface can provide a defense by inhibiting the growth of virulent bacterial strains (Iskeleli et al., 2005). However, in cases of trauma, or alteration of ocular tissue, indigenous flora may cause significant external and internal ocular infection (Speaker et al., 1991). In previous studies, native ocular flora has been shown to be predominantly *Staphylococcus* species (Iskeleli et al., 2005). While normal ocular flora has been well established in the developed world, there have been very few publications from rest of the world. In a study of the normal conjunctiva from Rajasthan, India, 86% of eyes were culture positive for bacteria and 12% positive for fungi. The most common bacterial isolates were *S. albus* (32%) followed by *S. aureus* (28%) (Tomar et al., 1971). In another study from Masungbo, Sierra Leone where analysis of conjunctival swabs obtained from healthy eyes of 276 residents showed presence of coagulase-negative staphylococci (28.6%), fungus (26.0%) and *S. aureus* (19.9%) (Capriotti et al., 2009). Many studies have not speciated the staphylococci from normal lids and conjunctiva, however, *S. epidermidis* is reported to be the most common species (McCulley et al., 1982).

Both coagulase negative and positive staphylococci are responsible for a variety of anterior and posterior segment of eye infections such as blepharitis, canaliculitis, dacryocystitis, conjunctivitis, keratitis, scleritis, endophthalmitis, preseptal and orbital cellulitis etc. Important attributes of organisms causing ocular infections include virulence, invasiveness, numbers of organism entering the host tissues and the site of entry. Coagulase, lipase and esterase are important bacterial enzymes produced by staphylococci associated with blepharitis. Several characteristics of the host also determine the effect of bacterial virulence and development of disease. Age, use of drugs and contact lens use, trauma, surgery etc. may also influence the effect of virulence factors besides presence of risk factors e.g., dry eye states, chronic nasolacrimal duct obstruction, previous ocular disease etc. Tissue injury can result from direct action of bacteria and their toxins, as well as from bacteria induced inflammation. Immunopathologic activities include recruitment of polymorphonuclear cells, macrophages and lymphocytes. Mediators of inflammation such as histamine, tumour necrosis factor, cytokines, leukotrienes, prostaglandins etc. play important role in interaction with the bacteria and their removal or proliferation.

Type of endophthalmitis	Geographic area	Duration of study	No. of patients	No, of isolates	% of CoNS	References
Posttraumatic	India	7 years	182	139	17.3	(Kunimoto et al., 1999b)
Postoperative	India	7 years	206	176	46.0	(Kunimoto et al., 1999a)
Postoperative	Singapore	5 years	34	21	57.0	(Wong and Chee, 2004)
Postoperative	India	--	80	37	62.6	(Srinivasan et al., 2002)
Postoperative	USA	5 years	278	313	49.9	(Benz et al., 2004)

Table 1. Prevalence of *Staphylococcus* species in endophthalmitis in various studies

Inflammation of the lid margin or blepharitis may be anterior or posterior, the former involving the lash line and the latter meibomian glands. Both the conditions may be associated with skin diseases such as dermatitis (seborrhoeic or atopic) and rosacea. The anterior blepharitis with lash collarettes, crusting, lid ulceration and folliculitis is usually associated with *S. aureus.* The most common form of bacterial conjunctivitis is the acute mucopurulent form of *S. aureus.* This may be associated with obstruction of the Naso-lacrimal duct. *S. aureus* conjunctivitis can become chronic due to its affinity for the eyelid margin and the resultant blepharitis. Coagulase negative staphylococci (CoNS), characteristically the endogenous flora of the ocular surface, are most of the common cause of postoperative endophthalmitis world over (Callegan et al., 2002; Kunimoto et al., 1999a, Benz et al., 2004, Wong and Chee, 2004). CoNS also rank first among bacteria causing posttraumatic endophthalmitis of which 45.3% isolates belong to gram positive cocci and 17.3% of these were belong to gram positive bacilli (Kunimoto et al., 1999b). Whereas CoNS do not commonly cause endogenous endophthalmitis, *S. aureus* have been reported from such infection (Callegan et al., 2002). **Table 1.** shows the prevalence of *Staphylococcus* species in patients with endophthalmitis.

Microbial keratitis is a serious infection of the cornea that may be caused by a variety of organisms including staphylococci. Most of the studies from developed countries such as the USA (Liesegang and Forster, 1980, Ormerod et al., 1987, Asbell and Stenson, 1982) (except southern USA) and Australia (McClellan et al., 1989) have listed *S. epidermidis* or coagulase negative staphylococci as the leading cause of bacterial keratitis. In India, the leading cause of bacterial keratitis varies; however, some investigators have listed staphylococci as the commonest bacteria (Gopinathan et al., 2009). It is possible that some investigators may have considered *S. epidermidis* or coagulase negative staphylococci as a normal commensal of the conjunctiva and underreported the isolation of these organisms from corneal samples. Few studies have recommended application of certain criteria to determine significance of a positive culture from corneal scrapings (Gopinathan et al., 2009). Since *S. epidermidis* form the commonest commensal of the extraocular surfaces, it is highly probable that these organisms invade corneal tissues compromised by antimicrobial and / or corticosteroid therapy or trauma.

For treatment of eye infections, antibiotics are usually administered topically as eye drops or intraocular injections, depending on the clinical condition. Other routes of administration such as subconjunctival injection are rarely used. Topically administered drugs have major advantage of localized drug effects, avoidance of hepatic first pass metabolism, and convenience. The disadvantage is low bioavailability to intraocular tissues, estimated to be only 1-10% (Davies, 2000). A large number of eye drops for topical therapy are available for extraocular eye infections, that include fluoroquinolones, macrolides, aminoglycosides, glycopeptides, tetracyclines, chloramphenicol, Neosporin (bacitracin, neomycin, polymyxin).

A broad range of three generations of fluoroquinolones are available such as ciprofloxacin (0.3%), ofloxacin (0.3%), levofloxacin (0.5% and 1.5%) , gatifloxacin (0.3%) and moxifloxacin (0.5%, preservative free) as eye drops also. Gatifloxacin and moxifloxacin, the newer fourth generation fluoroquinolones that target both DNA gyrase and topoisomerase IV are highly effective against gram positive bacteria including staphylococci in human and animal corneal ulcer model (Romanowski et al., 2005, Aliprandis et al., 2005). However, gatifloxacin was shown to be more effective than moxifloxacin against staphylococci (Reddy et al., 2010).

Fluoroquinolone eye drops are widely used for prophylaxis before eye surgery to prevent postoperative infection, most commonly caused by CoNS. Recently, intracameral injection of moxifloxacin has been found to be safe and effective in reducing the rate of postoperative endophthalmitis following cataract surgery (Lane et al., 2008).

Historically, the aminoglycosides have been the mainstay in the treatment of ocular infections. However, increasing resistance has limited their use in recent years in the treatment of staphylococcal infections. Glycopeptides such as vancomycin and teicoplanin the bactericidal antibiotics which inhibit peptidoglycan synthesis in the bacterial cell wall by complexing with cell wall precursors are highly effective against staphylococci including methicillin resistant staphylococci. However, eye drops are not yet available. Injectable vancomycin is routinely used for intravitreal injection (1mg/0.1ml) for the treatment of bacterial endophthalmitis. Emergence of vancomycin resistance has been reported in CoNS (Schwalbe et al., 1987). Topical ocular formulations of erythromycin are effective for conjunctivitis and blepharitis, however clarithromycin and azithromycin are derivatives that offer significant advantage over erythromycin owing to their expanded spectra (Barry et al., 1988).

Systemic infection with methicillin resistant *S. aureus* (MRSA) is known to cause morbidity and mortality. The prevalence of MRSA in ocular infections varies in different studies. While it is reported to be as low as 3% in England (Shanmuganathan et al., 2005), it is high (25-64%) in Japan (Fukuda et al., 2002). However, Indian workers have also reported increasing prevalence of MRSA over the years (Bagga et al., 2010). These authors showed decreased susceptibility to fluoroquinolones among MRSA from ocular infections. Shanmuganathan et al. (2005) found the MRSA susceptible to chloramphenicol and gentamicin and resistant to third generation fluoroquinolones (ciprofloxacin and ofloxacin) and cefazolin. Topical administration of fortified cefazolin (5%) was recommended for the treatment of staphylococcal keratitis based on in vitro susceptibility of *S. aureus* and CoNS (Sharma et al., 1999, Sharma et al., 2004). In an ongoing study, 4 of the 45 isolates (8.9%) of *S. aureus* from eye infections were MRSA (Kar et al., 2010). Using microbroth dilution and E test, a high level of resistance to fluoroquinolones but susceptibility to cefazolin, vancomycin and chloramphenicol was found among both MRSA and MSSA strains (Kar et al., 2010).

3. Antibiotic resistance

Antibiotics that are used against *Staphylococcus* spp. basically target cell wall synthesis, protein synthesis, nucleic acid synthesis and other metabolic pathways. The selection pressure applied by the antibiotics that are used in clinical and agricultural settings has promoted the evolution and spread of genes that confer resistance (Allen et al., 2010). Resistance to various antibiotics can be either internal or acquired by horizontal gene transfer via various mobile genetic elements like plasmids, transposons, integrons, etc. Internal mechanisms include mutational modification of gene targets, over expression of various efflux pumps; whereas acquired resistance involves enzymatic inactivation of the drug and bypassing of the target.

Exposure to antibiotics may lead to the formation of persister cells, small colony variants (SCVs), biofilms and over-expression of efflux pumps (Lewis, 2008, Singh et al., 2009, Proctor et al., 1998, Kwon et al., 2008, Martinez et al., 2009b) (Fig. 1). Persisters are dormant, multidrug tolerant variants of regular cells that are formed through a combination of stochastic and deterministic events in microbial populations (Lewis, 2010). Persisters over express genes such as chromosomal toxin-antitoxin modules that shut down their cellular functions, therefore, antibiotictarget inducing dormant cell to become tolerant to the lethal action of antibiotics (Keren et al., 2004, Singh et al., 2009). Another major problem posed by persister cells is they hide at various niches evading the host immune system, such as central nervous system (*Treponema pallidum*), macrophages or granulomas (*Mycobacterium tuberculosis*), stomach (*Helicobacter pylori*), gallbladder (*Salmonella typhi*) etc. (Jayaraman, 2008).

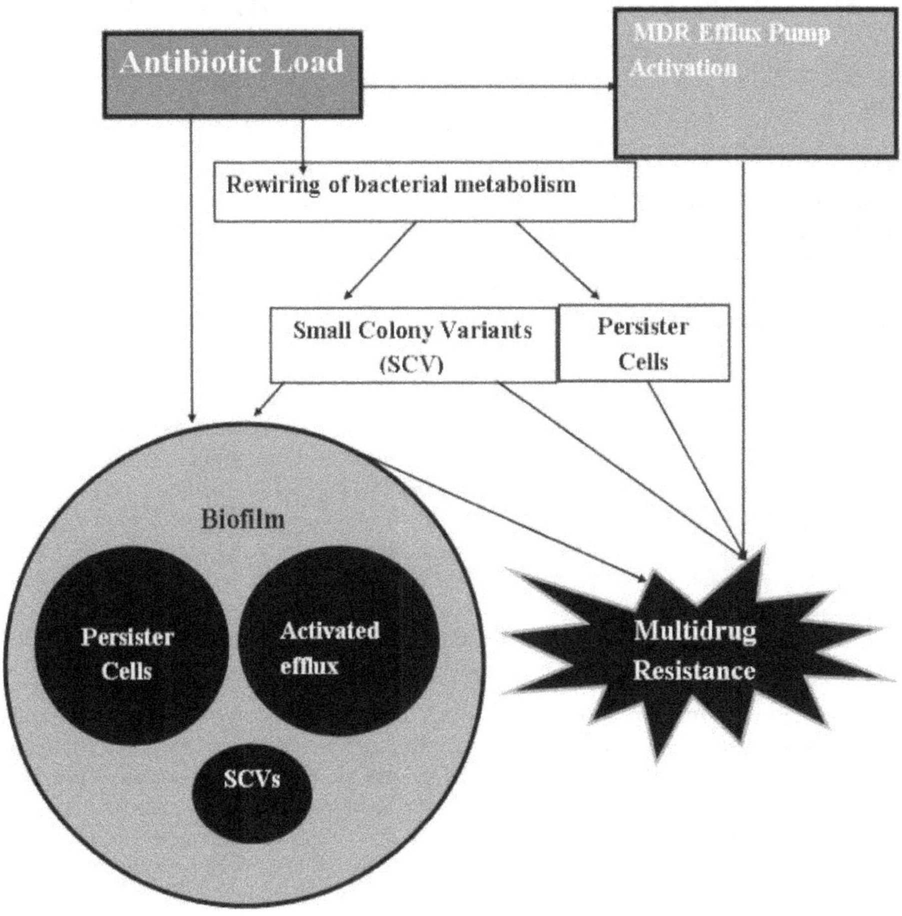

Fig. 1. Sub-inhibitory concentrations of antibiotics lead to formation of persister cells (Lewis, 2010), small colony variants (Proctor et al., 1998), biofilms (Kwon et al., 2008) and over-expression of efflux pumps (Martinez et al., 2009b). Biofilms are known to harbor cells with these kinds of modifications (Singh et al., 2010, Allegrucci and Sauer, 2007, Kvist et al., 2008). SCVs have enhanced biofilm forming capability (Singh et al., 2010). Each of these mechanisms may lead to multidrug resistance or it may be the combinatorial effect of all the above-mentioned processes.

SCVs constitute a slow-growing subpopulation of bacteria with distinctive phenotype and pathogenic traits (Proctor, 2006). They differ from the normal phenotype in their colony size, growth rate, pigmentation, haemolysis, expression of virulence factors, haemin and menadione auxotrophy, aminoglycosides and cell wall inhibitors action (Singh et al., 2009). Defective respiratory activity serves as the biochemical basis for the development of SCVs (Proctor et al., 1998). SCV of *S. epidermidis* may play a role in the pathogenesis of prosthetic valve endocarditis (Baddour and Christensen, 1987), and catheter-induced endocarditis (Baddour et al., 1988). Several findings mandate the investigation of small colony variants for persistent infections (Proctor et al., 1994, Proctor et al., 1998, Spearman et al., 1996, Kahl et al., 1998, Abele-Horn et al., 2000).

Bacteria in biofilms can tolerate ten to thousand fold higher levels of antibiotics than the genetically equivalent planktonic bacteria (Resch et al., 2005). Staphylococcal biofilms cause biomaterial-associated infections which do not respond to antimicrobial treatment often requiring removal of the same leading to substantial morbidity and mortality (Gotz and Peters, 2000). It has also been observed that biofilms harbour persister cells and small colony variants (Singh et al., 2010, Allegrucci and Sauer, 2007) (Fig. 1). Whereas planktonic persisters are eliminated by the immune system *in vivo*, persisters in biofilms serve as a shield evading the immune response (Lewis, 2010). According to Levin and Rozen (Levin and Rozen, 2006), a reservoir of such shielded persisters is a potential source for the emergence of heritable antibiotic resistance.

Kvist et al., (2008) reported the enhanced activity of efflux pumps in the bacteria residing in the biofilms (Fig. 1). The authors argued that the cramped environment in the biofilm demands better waste management leading to escalation of efflux pumps thereby increasing the antibiotic resistance of the biofilm cells. Reduction in biofilm formation was observed with the addition of efflux pump inhibitors (Kvist et al., 2008). Under physiological conditions, efflux pumps are involved in housekeeping activities like detoxification of intracellular metabolites, cell homeostasis, intracellular signal trafficking and bacterial virulence in animal and plant hosts. However, in the presence of high concentration of antibiotics and other environmental factors, they can shift their functional roles (Martinez et al., 2009a).

Antibiotics and their resistance genes were evolved in non-clinical environments in the pre-antibiotic usage era. Some antibiotics which may serve signalling purposes at the low concentration are probably found in natural ecosystems. Resistance determinants to these antibiotics were originally selected in their hosts for metabolic purposes or signal trafficking. Other antibiotic-resistance genes have been obtained by virulent bacteria through horizontal gene transfer (Martinez et al., 2009a). For example, *S. aureus mecA* gene is located on a mobile genetic element, the staphylococcal cassette chromosome *mec* (SCCmec) (Tsubakshita et al., 2010), horizontally acquired from other staphylococcal species *S. sciuri* (Couto et al., 1996) and *S. fleurettii* (Katayama et al., 2000). Also high level of vancomycin resistance is associated with carriage of *vanA* cluster encoded by Tn1546 transposon, first reported in *Enterococcus* species (Uttley et al., 1988). VRSA isolates from Michigan and Pennsylvania were found to harbor plasmids of 57.9Kb and 120Kb respectively carrying the transposon (Weigel et al., 2003, Tenover et al., 2004).

Resistance to fluoroquinolones offer a classic example of point mutations (e.g., *gyrA&B*, *grlA&B*) and efflux mediated resistance (Morar and Wright, 2010). Point mutations in particular regions of each enzyme subunit, known as Quinolone-Resistance-Determining-Region (QRDR) makes the enzyme less susceptible to inhibition by fluoroquinolones. The level of resistance increases in a stepwise manner each time with an additional mutation in target enzyme (Hooper, 2001). Selection pressure exerted by enhanced use of quinolones have led to the emergence of resistant strains carrying mutations within the endogenous transport system that improve affinity of the efflux system for quinolones (Ohshita et al., 1990, Chopra, 1992). The quinolone resistance in *S. aureus* also involves enhanced efflux by the Nor family of multidrug efflux pumps (McCallum et al., 2010). Several reports have linked increased expression of NorA to reduced susceptibility to chloramphenicol, beta-lactams, tetracycline, puromycin and some dyes, such as ethidium bromide (McCallum et al., 2010, Hooper, 2001, Ruiz, 2003). Point mutations in *norA* gene have been associated with reduced uptake of norfloxacin by the cell (Ohshita et al., 1990). NorB and NorC are the other members of Nor family encoding fluroquinolone resistance (Truong-Bolduc et al., 2006).

Although fluoroquinolones are considered first-line treatment of ocular infections, 85% of MRSA are resistant to ophthalmic fluoroquinolones (McDonald and Blondeau, 2010). This rise in resistance mandates the need for new agents. Basifloxacin, a novel fluoroquinolone was approved as a topical agent for treatment of bacterial conjunctivitis in May 2009 demonstrated rapid bactericidal activity against isolates that showed in vitro resistance to other fluoroquinolones, beta-lactams, macrolides and aminoglycosides (Haas et al., 2010). Moreover, basifloxacin lack systemic counterpart, thereby eliminating the contribution of systemic use of this drug to the emergence of resistance, although cross resistance from other systemic fluoroquinolones is possible (McDonald and Blondeau, 2010).

The direct relationship between the development of Linezolid (the last-line agent) resistance and prolonged exposure of the drug among cystic fibrosis patients was reported by Endimiani et al., (2011). Linezolid resistance in *S. aureus* is uncommon though there are reports of mutations in 23S rRNA and ribosomal protein L3 and L4 encoded by *rplD* gene and *rplC* genes (Locke et al., 2009). However, the most worrisome mechanism involving acquisition of the methytransferase *cfr* that methylates the 23S rRNA associated with mobile genetic elements had first been identified in 16.5 kb multi-drug resistance plasmid in *Staphylococcus sciuri* (Kehrenberg et al., 2005).

4. Therapeutics & therapy

With the ample evidence of strong association between antibiotic resistance and antibiotic consumption the scientific community should also come up with alternative means of antibacterial therapies, besides legitimately using available antibiotics, which can be used either alone or in conjunction with the antibiotics. Here we discuss some of the alternative strategies including vaccine development, phage therapy, use of lytic enzymes and plant-derived antibacterials. There are some reports on the use of nanoparticles as an efficient means of delivering antibacterials.

4.1 Staphylococcal vaccines

S. aureus has devised various mechanisms to evade the immune system. (i) two immunoglobulin binding proteins (protein A and Sbi), (ii) immune cell lysing toxins (Hlg, PVL), (iii) proteins interfering with complement activation (SCIN- staphylococcal complement inhibitor) and (iv) chemotaxis of neutrophils inhibiting peptides. Production of superantigens by *S. aureus* leads to allergy and immunosuppression. *S. epidermidis* relies primarily on cell-surface polymers and the ability to form a biofilm to survive in the host (Foster, 2005). However, protective role of antistaphylococcal antibodies from staphylococcal infection has been well documented in literature (Dryla et al., 2005). Holtfreter and Broker (2005) reported that carriers have high titers of neutralizing antibodies specific for those superantigens that are expressed by their colonizing strain. This carriage status confers strain specific humoral immunity, which may contribute to protection during *S. aureus* septicemia. Substantial controversy exists as to whether staphylococcal infections may be prevented by vaccination and, if so, which antigens should be selected and patients targeted for vaccination. In a comprehensive review on immune-therapeutics for staphylococcal infections by Ohlsen and Lorenz (2010) described the necessity for the development of both passive and active immunotherapies against *Staphylococcus*. The underlying criteria for the selection of targets e.g. gene products or toxins, should be conservability and expression in most of the clinical isolates.

4.1.1 MSCRAMM (Microbial Surface Component Recognizing Adhesive Matrix Molecules)

Some of the surface proteins of *S. aureus* have been exploited for immunotherapy. MSCRAMM protein family represents prototype of targets because of their exposed location and virulence involvement (Ohlsen and Lorenz, 2010, Flock, 1999). The best characterized MSCRAMM proteins include (i) clumping factor B (clfB), (ii) collagen-binding protein (Cna), and (ii) fibronectin-binding protein (FnBPA) (Ohlsen and Lorenz, 2010, Garcia-Lara et al., 2005). Veronate (Inhibitex) was developed by including anti-clfA and SdrG (*S. epidermidis* protein) from selected human donors (Patti, 2005), but failed to reach its target endpoints for the protection because of low birth weight babies at clinical trial III (Ohlsen and Lorenz, 2010).

Aurexis® is a humanized monoclonal antibody that recognizes clumping factor A (ClfA), a cell surface protein expressed by virtually all strains of *S. aureus*. Aurexis® binds with high affinity and specificity and interferes with *S. aureus* ability to colonize and spread to fibrinogen containing substrates such as wound sites, biomaterial coated implants, and damaged endovascular tissues. Inhibitex is actively seeking a corporate partner(s) for the continued clinical development of Aurexis® (http://www.inhibitex.com/Pipeline/Partnerships.html). Antibodies against clumping factor B (clfB) (Schaffer et al., 2006), Cna (Mamo et al., 2000), FnBPA (Zhou et al., 2006) have shown promising results. However, antibodies against against these targets have not yet been included in clinical trials (Ohlsen and Lorenz, 2010). Stranger-Jones et al., (2006) reported that the combination of four surface proteins IsdA, IsdB, SdrB, and SdrE afforded high level of protection against invasive disease or lethal challenge with human clinical *S. aureus* isolates.

4.1.2 Capsule

Capsular polysaccharides (CPs) represent the best established targets for vaccine-induced immunity to bacterial cells. About 70%-80% of *S. aureus* strains produce one of two CP antigens e.g. CP5 or CP8 (Skurnik et al., 2010). Nabi pharmaceuticals developed a vaccine StaphVax™ conjugating CP5 and CP8 to detoxified *Pseudomonas aeruginosa* exoprotein A, that failed to protect haemodialysis patients against *S. aureus* infections (Ohlsen and Lorenz, 2010,

Shinefield et al., 2002). To enhance the efficacy of StaphVax™, Pentastaph™ -pentavalent *S. aureus* vaccine was developed that included surface polysaccharide component 336, PVL and alpha-toxin to eliminate *S. aureus* by phagocytosis and neutralizing bacterial toxins. This vaccine has been evaluated in Phase II for safety and immunogenicity (Ohlsen and Lorenz, 2010).

4.1.3 Biofilm as the vaccine target

Although the significance of biofilm in infections has been recognized, there has not been much effort to develop vaccine targeting biofilms. The possible target sites for vaccine development may be the bacterial cells within the biofilm and/or biofilm matrix (Harro et al., 2010). Cerca et al., (2007) reported that an antibody developed against *Staphylococcus* Poly-N-acetyl glucosamine (PNAG) was found effective against different strains of *E. coli*. In another report, effectiveness of PNAG as vaccine candidate in *S. aureus* mediated skin abcesses and lethal *E. coli* peritonitis was demonstrated (Gening et al., 2010). However, PNAG may not be an ideal vaccine candidate against those strains possessing *icaADBC* locus because it is not produced in all biofilm-producing staphylococcal strains (Harro et al., 2010, Rohde et al., 2001). Therefore, it was suggested that vaccine studies should be focussed on the cell embedded in the matrix rather than the matrix. A proteomic approach of looking into the comparative proteomes of the planktonic and biofilm cells may be an interesting area to start with (Harro et al., 2010).

4.1.4 Whole cell vaccine

Vaccine Research International (http://www.vri.org.uk/) is developing a vaccine (SA75) using chloroform killed whole cells of *S. aureus*. Phase I clinical trials have been successfully completed. The whole cell preparation could provide a broad spectrum of *S. aureus* antigens in a single vaccine some of which had immune-stimulatory affect and act as an adjuvant generating higher antibody response against protective antigens. However, the mechanism of action is unknown and down-regulation of immune pathways by components of the vaccine cannot be ruled out (Ohlsen and Lorenz, 2010).

4.1.5 Staphylococcal enterotoxin as a vaccine candidate

Virulence factor-specific antibodies derived from vaccination or employed as therapeutics represent a potential defense against bacterial diseases (Larkin et al., 2010). Staphylococcal enterotoxins are considered potential biowarfare agents that can be spread through ingestion or inhalation (Drozdowski et al., 2010). Staphylococcal enterotoxins (SEs) and related toxic shock syndrome toxin-1 (TSST-1) act as superantigens. These protein toxins can cause acute gastroenteritis and toxic shock syndrome. There are more than twenty different SEs described to date with varying amino acid sequences, common conformations, and similar biological effects. Picomolar concentrations of these superantigenic toxins activate specific T-cell subsets after binding to major histocompatibility complex class II. Activated T-cells vigorously proliferate and release proinflammatory cytokines plus chemokines that can elicit fever, hypotension, and other ailments which include a potentially lethal shock (Larkin et al., 2009, Varshney et al., 2010).

Studies on the protective effect of non-toxic mutant GST–mTSST-1 fusion protein against staphylococcal infection, was purified and tested. Mice were immunized with the GST–mTSST-1 plus alum adjuvant and challenged with viable *S. aureus*. The results indicate the efficacy of this protein in the elimination of bacterial load from the organs as well as in the inhibition of production of pro-inflammatory cytokines due to TSST-1 in the splenic cells. Furthermore immunization with GST–mTSST-1 strongly induced the production of TSST-1 specific antibodies, especially immunoglobulin G1 and immunoglobulin G2b (Cui et al., 2005).

Varshney et al., 2010 showed that four murine monoclonal antibodies bind to conformational epitopes that are destroyed by deletion of the distal C-terminal 11 Amino acids (Varshney et al., 2010). This study, for the first time, showed that MRSA derived SEB (staphylococcal enterotoxin B) contains a deletion in the C-terminal, which affects binding of certain protective Abs. This study also demonstrated enhanced protection against SEBILS (SEB induced Lethal Shock) when two non-protective mAbs were combinedly administered *in vivo*.

Drozdowski et al., (2010) generated high-affinity SEB-specific antibodies capable of neutralizing SEB *in* vitro as well as *in vivo* in a mouse model. They described for the first time recombinantly-derived human monoclonal antibodies against SEB that possess high affinity, target specificity, and therapeutic potential for superantigen-induced toxic shock. These antibodies prevent intoxication by interfering with toxin binding to MHC II and/or TCR. In addition to potential applications for treating toxic shock syndrome, human monoclonal antibodies recognizing SEB or other bacterial superantigens may be useful if employed as an adjunct therapy with antibiotics in treating *S. aureus* infections.

STEBvax is a new vaccine developed against toxic shock syndrome. It is currently under clinical trial phase I. The vaccine is being tested for prophylactic and therapeutic use (http://clinicaltrials.gov/ct2/show/NCT00974935).

Larkin et al., (2010) selected human monoclonal antibodies from a phage display library, using a recombinant SEB vaccine (STEBVax) incorporating site-specific mutations that prevent MHC II interactions. This group discovered that some antibody clones cross-react with SEC1, SEC2, and streptococcal pyrogenic exotoxin C (SpeC), while others were highly specific for SEB. Many of the antibodies effectively inhibited T-cell activation by SEB in vitro, bound to toxin with nanomolar affinity, and prevented SEB-induced toxic shock in vivo. This recombinantly-derived, human monoclonal antibodies against SEB had high affinity, target specificity, and therapeutic potential for superantigen-induced toxic shock. These antibodies prevented intoxication by interfering with toxin binding to MHC II and/or T-cell antigen receptors. The author suggested the potential applications for treating toxic shock syndrome, human monoclonal antibodies recognizing SEB or other bacterial superantigens may be useful if employed as an adjunct therapy along with antibiotics in treating difficult *S. aureus* infections (Larkin et al., 2010).

4.1.6 Future perspectives in vaccine development

As discussed earlier, comparative proteomic analysis of planktonic and biofilm cells is an interesting area to look for vaccines against biofilm. Another important strategy is to look for immunodominant antigens. This strategy has led to the identification of a wide range of surface and extracellular target antigens such as IsdB, GrfA, IsaA, IsaB, Atl, IsdA, IsdH,

FmtB, SspA, SspB and Lip (Lorenz et al., 2000, Etz et al., 2002, Clarke and Foster, 2006). The rationale behind such a strategy is that the patients may develop antibodies against specific staphylococcal antigens during infection that may be critical for combating the infections (Ohlsen and Lorenz, 2010).

Another promising strategy is the reduction of nasal colonization by *S. aureus* as several studies have shown that nasal carriers have increased risk of developing infections by endogenous strains (von Eiff et al., 2001, Wertheim et al., 2004). Vaccination with clumping factor B, iron-responsive surface determinants (Isd) A and H, teichoic acid and capsular polysaccharides have been reported to reduce the nasal colonization with *S. aureus* (Dryla et al., 2005, Clarke and Foster, 2006).

4.2 Phage therapy

The rise of multidrug resistant bacteria has enforced the resurgence of phage therapy in the West, though this mode of therapy is being practiced for several years in Eastern Europe. Some of the success stories on phage therapy are described here. The Eliava Institute in Tbilisi, Republic of Georgia, has developed a highly virulent, monoclonal staphylococcal bacteriophage active against 80-95% of *S. aureus* strains including MRSA. This product was used for local and generalized infections, including neonatal sepsis, osteomyelitis, wound infections, pneumonia etc. (Hanlon, 2007). There are some polyvalent obligate lytic *S. aureus* phages e.g. phage phi812, phageK and phage44AHJD which have been successfully tested for their efficacy in killing *S. aureus* including MRSA strains (Mann, 2008). Evaluation of phageK showed marked reduction of pathogenic and antibiotic resistant coagulase positive and negative staphylococci associated with bovine and human infections that included *S. aureus, S. epidermidis, S. saprophyticus, S. chromogenes, S. capitis, S. hominis, S. haemolyticus, S. caprae,* and *S. hyicus*. The modified phage generated by passing through less susceptible target strain can be used in combination with phageK to increase the host range. This study had also shown the potential of delivering the phage in the form of handwash or antistaphylococcal cream (O'Flaherty et al., 2005b). Merabishvili and colleagues (2009), demonstrated laboratory-based production and quality control of a cocktail, currently under evaluation, consisting of exclusively lytic bacteriophages for the treatment of *Pseudomonas aeruginosa* and *S. aureus* infections of burn wound.

Curtin and Donlan (2006), reported use of phage *e.g.* phage456, in reducing the biofilm formation and adherence of *S. epidermidis* biofilms on both hydrogel-coated and serum/hydrogel coated silicone catheters. The presence of divalent cations in the growth medium (Mg^{++}, Ca^{++}) further increased the efficacy of phage456 in reducing biofilm formation. Polyvalent *Staphylococcus* phage combined with highly efficient *Pseudomonas* T7-like phage (phage phiIBB-PF7A) effectively showed reduction in dual species biofilms, killing and finally removal of bacteria from the host substratum (Sillankorva et al., 2010).

There were efforts to engineer bacteriophage by over-expressing proteins to target gene networks, particularly non-essential genes, to enhance bacterial killing by antibiotics. Using this approach, Lu and Collins (2007), engineered a T7 phage which significantly reduced *Escherichia coli* biofilm. They claim that this combinatorial approach may reduce the incidence of antibiotic resistance and enhance bacterial killing.

There are many advantages of using phage in therapeutics. (i) Dysbiosis can be avoided due to their specificity, (ii) Multiple administrations are not required because phage replicates at the site of infection, (iii) Phage could select resistant mutants of the selected bacteria, and (iv) Selection of new phages is rapid compared to the development of new antibiotic which may take several years. However, the disadvantage is that the causal organism needs to be identified before administering the phage (Sulakvelidze et al., 2001). Moreover, prior to the extensive therapeutic use of phages it is prudent to ensure the safety of therapeutic phages. The phages should not carry out generalized transduction and possess gene sequences having significant homology with known antibiotic resistances, phage-encoded toxins and other bacterial virulence factors (Sulakvelidze et al., 2001).

4.3 Antistaphylococcal lytic enzymes

Antistaphylococcal lytic enzymes can be broadly divided into two groups: (i) Staphylococcal phage lysins (endolysins) and (ii) Bacteriocins (e.g. Lysostaphin) (Borysowski and Gorski, 2009a).

4.3.1 Lysins

Lysins are enzymes, consist of N-terminal catalytic domain and C-terminal bacterial cell-wall binding domain, and are produced by bacteriophage that digests the bacterial cell wall (Fischetti, 2010, Borysowski and Gorski, 2009a). LysK, highly specific for the genus *Staphylococcus*, was obtained from phageK, has been effectively used in the treatment of staphylococcal infections (O'Flaherty et al., 2005a). Interestingly MV-L derived from bacteriophage phiMRII was found specific to *S. aureus* and *S. simulans* infection (Rashel et al., 2007). This phage also acted synergistically with glycopeptide antibiotics against VISA and MRSA. Moreover, MV-L induced antibodies could not abolish the bacteriolytic activity. Endolysin from another phi11 showed elimination of *S. aureus* NCTC8325 biofilm but not of *S. epidermidis* O-47 biofilm (Sass and Bierbaum, 2007). Purified endolysin (MW 53.3kDa) from virulent *S. aureus* bacteriophage Twort, *plyTW*, demonstrated cleavage of staphylococcal peptidoglycan. Upstream of *plyTW* there is Twort holin gene, *holTW*, which produces unspecific holes in the bacterial cytoplasmic membrane, degrade staphylococcal peptidoglycan through hydrolysis of alanine amino bonds (Loessner et al., 1998). CHAP (cysteine-histidine dependent amidohydrolase/ peptidase) exhibits lytic activity against staphylococcal isolates including MRSA, was identified by deletion analysis of LysK domain. CHAP can be used as single domain for therapeutic purposes over the whole enzyme as this may lower the risk of immunogenic response (Horgan et al., 2009).

4.3.2 Synergistic effect of lysins

Manoharadas et al., (2009) constructed a chimeric endolysin (P16-17) consisting of N-terminal D-alanyl-glycyl endopeptidase domain and C-terminal P16 endolysin domain and P17 minor coat protein, targeting cell wall of *S. aureus* phage. This domain swapping approach and subsequent purification resulted in finding soluble P16-17 protein, which exhibited antimicrobial activity against *S. aureus*. This protein further augmented the antimicrobial efficacy of gentamicin suggesting synergistic effect in reducing effective dose of aminoglycosides. Synergistic effect of nisin and LysH5, the endolysin encoded by phi-SauS-IPLA88 was demonstrated (Garcia et al., 2010). It was suggested that better lytic enzymes can be constructed by using methods like protein engineering, domain swapping and gene shuffling. Owing to the non-existence of bacterial resistance to lysins someday phage lytic enzymes could be an essential strategy to combat pathogenic bacteria (Fischetti et al., 2010).

4.3.3 Lysostaphin as a therapeutic agent

Lysostaphin, a 25kDa protein possessing two functional domains: N-terminal catalytic domain and C-terminal cell wall binding domain B, is a plasmid-encoded extracellular enzyme produced by *S. simulans* biovar *staphylolyticus* (Borysowski and Gorski, 2009b). It is a Zn-containing endopeptidase that specifically cleaves the bonds between the glycine residues in the interpeptide cross-bridges of the staphylococcal peptidoglycan resulting in the hypotonic lysis of the bacterial cell (Kumar, 2008). There are several reports of lysostaphin mediated lysis of clinically relevant antibiotic resistant staphylococcal strains. Lysostaphin which is readily absorbed onto catheter surfaces without losing lytic property shows promise in the prevention of catheter-related bloodstream infections caused by CoNS and *S. aureus* (Shah et al., 2004, Borysowski and Gorski, 2009a). Lysostaphin has successfully eradicated nasal colonization of MSSA, MRSA and mupirocin-resistant *S. aureus* in experimental cotton rats (Kokai-Kun et al., 2003). In combination with lysostaphin, oxacillin or vancomycin, showed increased efficacy against MRSA (Kokai-Kun et al., 2007, Patron et al., 1999). Several workers demonstrated the effectiveness of lysostaphin in the treatment of biofilms formed by *S. aureus* and *S. epidermidis* and disruption of biofilms on glass and plastic surfaces (King et al., 1980, Walencka et al., 2005, Wu et al., 2003). Evaluation of PEGylation potential in improving lysostaphin pharmacokinetics showed substantial increase in serum drug half-life and reduced binding to anti-lysostaphin antibodies while maintaining the enzyme's lytic activity (Walsh et al., 2003).

4.3.4 Lysostaphin therapy in ocular infections

Lysostaphin was also tested as a potential means of treating some ocular infections, especially endophthalmitis and keratitis. Dajcs et al., (2001) demonstrated the effect of lysostaphin on MRSA endophthalmitis in the rabbit model. Lysostaphin when administered twice after 8h and 24h post-infection showed 88% and 50% sterilization compared to 0% sterilization in untreated controls. However, the severity of ocular inflammation could be controlled only on 8h post-infection treatment models. Lysostaphin as a probable immunizing agent was also investigated. In this study, rabbits were immunized with lysostaphin by subcutaneous, intranasal or intraocular route that showed successful retention of bactericidal activity in vivo, in spite of the high titre of anti-lysostaphin antibodies (Dajcs et al., 2002, Balzli et al., 2010).

4.3.5 Synergistic effects

Synergistic inhibition by ranalexin (a cationic peptide) in combination with lysostaphin resulted in an enhanced bactericidal effect. This finding, therefore, suggested that dressings could be impregnated with ranalexin and lysostaphin to treat wound infections caused by MRSA (Graham and Coote, 2007, Desbois et al., 2010). Furthermore lysozyme has been reported enhancing lysostaphin activity (Cisani et al., 1982). Combinatorial action of various beta-lactam antibiotics or mupirocin or gentamicin enhancing lysostaphin activity was reported by various groups (Polak et al., 1993, Climo et al., 2001, Kiri et al., 2002, LaPlante, 2007). Thus, it is concluded that lysostaphin is an effective agent as pre- and post-treatment option for staphylococcal infections though CoNS showed generally weaker effect than *S. aureus* (Borysowski and Gorski, 2009a). This was because of presence of higher amount of serine than glycine in peptidoglycan of coagulase-negative staphylococci (Kumar, 2008).

4.4 Plant-derived antibacterials

Plant-derived antibacterials are of three types: (i) traditional antibiotics, (ii) antibacterials that target bacterial virulence, and (iii) inhibitors of MDR pump. The first two categories have not been explored in detail (Lewis and Ausubel, 2006). The details of third category of compounds obtained from plant sources, their properties as MDR/ EPI inhibitors and its use as antibacterial against staphylococcal infection are summarized in Table 2.

Identification of EPIs from natural sources is still in infancy. However, the chemical diversity of plants and microorganisms and their requirement for nutrients to synthesize such compounds should make the search for EPIs from such sources an attractive option (Stavri et al., 2007).

4.5 Nature's backyard

Resistance of microbial pathogens to antibiotics is a serious threat to the well-being of mankind. Recently, two small molecules, platensimycin, identified from strain of *Streptomyces platensis* isolated from soil sample in South Africa, by using antisense differential sensitivity whole-cell screening program, targeting the fatty acid biosynthesis pathway of gram-positive bacteria. The platensimycin ($C_{24}H_{27}NO_7$, MW 441.47) comprises of two distinct structural element connected by an amide bond, is active against MRSA, VISA, Vancomycin-resistant enterococci and linezolid and macrolide resistant pathogens (Wang et al., 2006) (Fig. 2A).

Continued screening led to the discovery of platencin ($C_{24}H_{27}NO_6$, MW 425.2), a novel product that is chemically and biologically related to platensimycin which exhibits broad-spectrum antibacterial activity against gram positive bacteria which inhibit fatty acid biosynthesis (Fig. 2B). These molecule targets two essential proteins, beta-ketoacyl synthase II (FabF) and III (FabH) (Wang et al., 2007). These studies reflect upon the fact that nature holds the treasure trove of antibiotics which are yet to be explored.

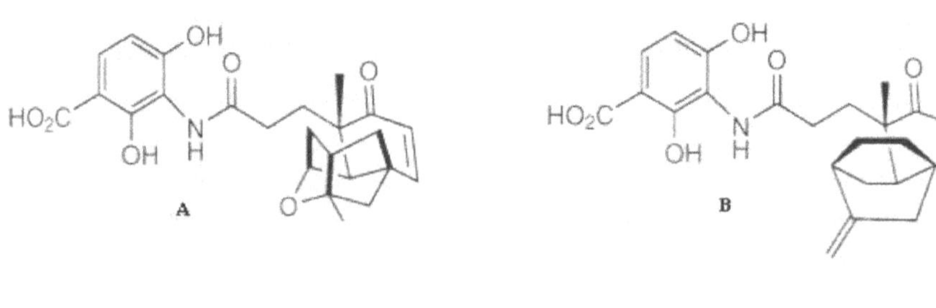

Fig. 2. Chemical structure of Platensimycin (A) and Platencin (B).

	Common name & plant species name	Compound	Properties	Total effect	Synergistic effect	References
1	Barberry & *Berberis* species	Berberine & 5′-methoxyhydnocarpin	Hydrophobic cation increases membrane permeability and intercalate DNA	Inhibit MDR	Antibacterial	(Stermitz et al., 2000)
2	Golden seal & *Hydrastis canadensis*	Berberine & 5′-methoxyhydnocarpin	5′-methoxyhydnocarpin-linking of berberine to INF_{55}	Inhibit MDR	Antibacterial	(Ball et al., 2006)
3	Silvery lupine & *Lupinus argenteus*	Isoflavones	Enhances activity of berberine and norfloxacin	Inhibit MDR	Antibacterial	(Morel et al., 2003)
4	Fabaceae & *Dalea versicolor*	Phenolic metabolites	Enhances activity of berberine, erythromycin and tetracycline	Inhibit MDR	Antibacterial	(Belofsky et al., 2004)]
5	Smoke tree & *Dalea spinosa*	2-arylbenzofuran aldehyde & Phenolic compounds; SpinosanA, Pterocarpan & Isoflavone	Enhances activity of berberine	Inhibit MDR	Antibacterial	(Belofsky et al., 2006)
6	Tea	Epicatechin gallate & Epigallocatechin gallate	Enhances activity of norfloxacin and tetracycline	Inhibit MDR	Antibacterial	(Gibbons et al., 2004, Sudano Roccaro et al., 2004)
7	Rosemery & *Rosmarinus officinalis*	Diterpines, Carnosic acid & Carnesol	Potentiate activity of tetracycline and erythromycin	Inhibit MDR	Antibacterial	(Oluwatuyi et al., 2004)
8	Gipsywort & *Lycopus europaeus*	Lipophilic extract	Potentiate activity of tetracycline and erythromycin	Inhibit MDR	Antibacterial	(Gibbons et al., 2003)
9	Grapefruit oil & *Citrus paradisi*	Coumarin derivative: Bergamottin epoxide & Coumarin epoxide	Enhances activity of ethidium bromide and norfloxacin	Inhibit MDR	Antibacterial	(Abulrob et al., 2004)
10	Piperine & *Piper nigrum* & *Piper longum*	Piperine	Potentiating action of piperine in combination with ciprofloxacin	Inhibit MDR	Antibacterial	(Khan et al., 2006)

Table 2. Properties of MDR/ EPI inhibitors isolated from medicinal plants and its use as antibacterial agent against Staphylococcal infection.

5. Conclusions

Extensive applied and basic research is needed to come up with strategies combating the major challenges of staphylococcal infections. Recently, folic acid tagged chitosan nanoparticles were effectively used to deliver vancomycin. It proved to be an efficient method to increase the bioavailability of the same (Chakraborty et al., 2010). Researchers have developed Nitric oxide releasing nanoparticles as treatment for skin and soft tissue infections successfully tested in murine models (Han et al., 2009, Englander and Friedman, 2010).

Use of vaccines and phages for the treatment and control staphylococcal infections might be a sustainable alternative to antibiotics. The advent of high throughput sequencing has led to the analysis of phage genomes and better understanding of phage evolution, phage-host interaction, bacterial pathogenicity, phage ecology and origin of phages (O'Flaherty et al., 2009). With the background knowledge of phage genomics, it will be possible to approach phage therapeutics cautiously and effectively. Future research should focus on multidisciplinary approach on the development of alternative/conjunctive strategies for treatment and prevention of staphylococcal infections.

6. Acknowledgement

This study, in part, was supported by Department of Science and Technology, New Delhi, grant no: SR/SO/HS-117/2007 to SS and DVS, DST-WOS-A grant no: SR/WOS-A/208/2009 to RC, and fund contributed by Department of Biotechnology, New Delhi to Institute of Life Sciences, Bhubaneswar. Junior Research Fellowship awarded by Department of Science and Technology, New Delhi to SP is gratefully acknowledged.

7. References

Abele-horn, M.; Schupfner, B.; Emmerling, P.; Waldner, H. & Goring, H. (2000). Persistent wound infection after herniotomy associated with small-colony variants of *Staphylococcus aureus*. *Infection*, Vol.28, pp. 53-54, ISSN: 0300-8126

Abulrob, AN.; Suller, MT.; Gumbleton, M.; Simons, C. & Russell, AD. (2004). Identification and biological evaluation of grapefruit oil components as potential novel efflux pump modulators in methicillin-resistant *Staphylococcus aureus* bacterial strains. *Phytochemistry*, Vol.65, pp. 3021-3027, ISSN: 0031-9422

Aliprandis, E.; Ciralsky, J.; Lai, H.; Herling, I. & Katz, HR. (2005). Comparative efficacy of topical moxifloxacin versus ciprofloxacin and vancomycin in the treatment of *P. aeruginosa* and ciprofloxacin-resistant MRSA keratitis in rabbits. *Cornea*, Vol.24, pp. 201-205, ISSN: 0277-3740

Allegrucci, M. & Sauer, K. (2007). Characterization of colony morphology variants isolated from *Streptococcus pneumoniae* biofilms. *J Bacteriol*, Vol.189, pp. 2030-2038, ISSN: 0021-9193

Allen, HK.; Donato, J.; Wang, HH.; Cloud-hansen, KA.; Davies, J. & Handelsman, J. (2010). Call of the wild: antibiotic resistance genes in natural environments. *Nat Rev Microbiol*, Vol.8, pp. 251-259, ISSN: 1740-1526

Asbell, P. & Stenson, S. (1982). Ulcerative keratitis. Survey of 30 years' laboratory experience. *Arch Ophthalmol*, Vol.100, pp. 77-80, ISSN: 0003-9950

Baddour, LM. & Christensen, GD. (1987). Prosthetic valve endocarditis due to small-colony staphylococcal variants. *Rev Infect Dis*, Vol.9, pp. 1168-74, ISSN: 0162-0886

Baddour, LM.; Simpson, WA.; Weems, JJ Jr.; Hill, MM. & Christensen, GD. (1988). Phenotypic selection of small-colony variant forms of *Staphylococcus epidermidis* in the rat model of endocarditis. *J Infect Dis*, Vol.157, pp. 757-763, ISSN: 0022-1899

Bagga, B.; Reddy, AK. & Garg, P. (2010). Decreased susceptibility to quinolones in methicillin-resistant *Staphylococcus aureus* isolated from ocular infections at a tertiary eye care centre. *Br J Ophthalmol*, Vol.94, pp. 1407-1408, ISSN: 0007-1161

Ball, AR.; Casadei, G.; Samosorn, S.; Bremner, JB.; Ausubel, FM.; Moy, TI. & Lewis, K. (2006). Conjugating berberine to a multidrug efflux pump inhibitor creates an effective antimicrobial. *ACS Chem Biol*, Vol.1, pp. 594-600, ISSN: 1554-8929

Balzli, CL.; McCormick, CC.; Caballero, AR. & O' Callaghan, RJ. (2010). Sustained anti-staphylococcal effect of lysostaphin in the rabbit aqueous humor. *Curr Eye Res*, Vol.35, pp. 480-486, ISSN: 0271-3683

Barry, AL.; Jones, RN. & Thornsberry, C. (1988). In vitro activities of azithromycin (CP 62.;993).; clarithromycin; erythromycin.; roxithromycin.; and clindamycin. *Antimicrob Agents Chemother*, Vol.32, pp. 752-754, ISSN: 1502-2307

Belofsky, G.; Carreno, R.; Lewis, K.; Ball, A.; Casadei, G. & Tegos, GP. (2006). Metabolites of the "smoke tree".; *Dalea spinosa*.; potentiate antibiotic activity against multidrug-resistant *Staphylococcus aureus*. *J Nat Prod*, Vol.69, pp. 261-264, ISSN: 0163-3864

Belofsky, G.; Percivill, D.; Lewis, K.; Tegos, GP. & Ekart, J. (2004). Phenolic metabolites of *Dalea versicolor* that enhance antibiotic activity against model pathogenic bacteria. *J Nat Prod*, Vol.67, pp. 481-484, ISSN: 0163-3864

Benz, MS.; Scott, IU.; Flynn, HW Jr.; Unonius, N. & Miller D. (2004). Endophthalmitis isolates and antibiotic sensitivities: a 6-year review of culture-proven cases. *Am J Ophthalmol*, Vol.137, pp. 38-42, ISSN: 0002-9394

Borysowski, A. & Gorski, A. (2009a). Enzybiotics and their potential applications in medicine, In: *Enzybiotics: Antibiotic Enzymes as Drugs and Therapeutics*, Villa, TG. & Patricia Veiga Crespo, PV. (Ed.)., pp. 1-26 ISBN: 978-0-470-37655-3, John Wiley and Sons, Inc., Hoboken, NJ, USA

Borysowski, A. & Gorski, A. (2009b). Anti-staphylococcal lytic enzymes, In: *Enzybiotics: Antibiotic Enzymes as Drugs and Therapeutics*, Villa, TG. & Crespo, PV. (Ed.)., pp. 149-172 ISBN: 978-0-470-37655-3, John Wiley and Sons, Inc., Hoboken, NJ, USA

Callegan, MC.; Engelbert, M.; Parke, DW 2nd.; Jett, BD. & Gilmore, MS. (2002). Bacterial endophthalmitis: epidemiology.; therapeutics.; and bacterium-host interactions. *Clin Microbiol Rev*, Vol.15, pp. 111-124, ISSN: 0893-8512

Capriotti, JA.; Pelletier, JS.; Shah, M.; Caivano, DM. & Ritterband, DC. (2009). Normal ocular flora in healthy eyes from a rural population in Sierra Leone. *Int Ophthalmol*, Vol.29, pp. 81-84, ISSN: 0165-5701

Cerca, N.; Maira-litran, T.; Jefferson, KK.; Grout, M.; Goldmann, DA. & Pier GB. (2007). Protection against *Escherichia coli* infection by antibody to the *Staphylococcus aureus* poly-N-acetylglucosamine surface polysaccharide. *Proc Natl Acad Sci U S A*, Vol.104, pp. 7528-7533, ISSN: 1091-6490

Chakraborty, SP.; Sahu, SK.; Mahapatra, SK.; Santra, S.; Bal, M.; Roy, S. & Pramanik P. (2010). Nanoconjugated vancomycin: new opportunities for the development of anti-VRSA agents. *Nanotechnology*, Vol.21, pp. 1-9, ISSN: 0957-4484

Chopra, I. (1992). Efflux-based antibiotic resistance mechanisms: the evidence for increasing prevalence. *J Chemother*, Vol.30, pp. 737-739, ISSN: 1502-2307

Cisani, G.; Varaldo, PE.; Grazi, G. & Soro, O. (1982). High-level potentiation of lysostaphin anti-staphylococcal activity by lysozyme. *Antimicrob Agents Chemother*, Vol.21, pp. 531-535, ISSN: 1502-2307

Clarke, SR. & Foster, SJ. (2006). Surface adhesins of *Staphylococcus aureus*. *Adv Microb Physiol*, Vol.51, pp. 187-224, ISSN: 0065-2911

Climo, MW.; Ehlert, K. & Archer GL. (2001). Mechanism and suppression of lysostaphin resistance in oxacillin-resistant *Staphylococcus aureus*. *Antimicrob Agents Chemother*, Vol.45, pp. 1431-1437, ISSN: 1502-2307

Couto, I.; de Lencastre, H.; Severina, E.; Kloos, W.; Webster, JA.; Hubner, RJ.; Sanches, IS. & Tomasz, A. (1996). Ubiquitous presence of a *mecA* homologue in natural isolates of *Staphylococcus sciuri*. *Microb Drug Resist*, Vol.2, pp. 377-391, ISSN: 1076-6294

Cui , JC.; Hu, DL.; Lin, YC.; Qian, AD. & Nakane, A. (2005). Immunization with glutathione S-transferase and mutant toxic shock syndrome toxin 1 fusion protein protects against *Staphylococcus aureus* infection. *FEMS Immunol Med Microbiol*, Vol.45, pp. 45-51, ISSN: 0928-8244

Curtin, JJ. & Donlan, RM. (2006). Using bacteriophages to reduce formation of catheter-associated biofilms by *Staphylococcus epidermidis*. *Antimicrob Agents Chemother*, Vol.50, pp. 1268-1275, ISSN: 1502-2307

Dajcs, JJ.; Thibodeaux, BA.; Girgis, DO.; Shaffer, MD.; Delvisco, SM. & O'Callaghan, RJ. (2002). Immunity to lysostaphin and its therapeutic value for ocular MRSA infections in the rabbit. *Invest Ophthalmol Vis Sci*, Vol.43, pp. 3712-3716, ISSN: 0146-0404

Dajcs, JJ.; Thibodeaux, BA.; Hume, EB.; Zheng , X.; Sloop, GD. & O'Callaghan RJ. (2001). Lysostaphin is effective in treating methicillin-resistant *Staphylococcus aureus* endophthalmitis in the rabbit. *Curr Eye Res*, Vol.22, pp. 451-457, ISSN: 0271-3683

Davies, NM. (2000). Biopharmaceutical considerations in topical ocular drug delivery. *Clin Exp Pharmacol Physiol*, Vol.27, pp. 558-562, ISSN: 0305-1870

Desbois , AP.; Gemmell, CG. & Coote, PJ. (2010). In vivo efficacy of the antimicrobial peptide ranalexin in combination with the endopeptidase lysostaphin against wound and systemic meticillin-resistant *Staphylococcus aureus* (MRSA) infections. *Int J Antimicrob Agents*, Vol.35, pp. 559-565, ISSN: 0924-8579

Deurenberg, RH. & Stobberingh, EE. (2008). The evolution of *Staphylococcus aureus*. *Infect Genet Evol*, Vol.8, pp. 747-763, ISSN: 1567-1348

Drozdowski, B.; Zhou, Y.; Kline, B.; Spidel, J.; Chan, YY.; Albone, E.; Turchin, H.; Chao, Q.; Henry, M.; Balogach, J.; Routhier, E.; Bavari, S.; Nicolaides, NC.; Sass, PM. & Grasso, L. (2010). Generation and characterization of high affinity human monoclonal antibodies that neutralize staphylococcal enterotoxin B. *J Immune Based Ther Vaccines*, Vol.8, pp. 1-9, ISSN: 1476-8518

Dryla, A.; Prustomersky, S.; Gelbmann, D.; Hanner, M.; Bettinger, E.; Kocsis, B.; Kustos, T.; Henics, T.; Meinke, A. & Nagy, E. (2005). Comparison of antibody repertoires against *Staphylococcus aureus* in healthy individuals and in acutely infected patients. *Clin Diagn Lab Immunol*, Vol.12, pp. 387-398, ISSN: 1071-412X

Endimiani, A.; Blackford, M.; Dasenbrook, EC.; Reed, MD.; Bajaksouszian, S.; Hujer, AM.; Rudin, SD.; Hujer, KM.; Perreten, V.; Rice, LB.; Jacobs, MR.; Konstan, MW. & Bonomo, RA. (2011). Emergence of linezolid-resistant *Staphylococcus aureus* after prolonged treatment of cystic fibrosis patients in Cleveland. *Antimicrob Agents Chemother*, epub. 24 January 2011, ISSN: 1502-2307

Englander, L. & Friedman, A. (2010). Nitric oxide nanoparticle technology: a novel antimicrobial agent in the context of current treatment of skin and soft tissue infection. *J Clin Aesthet Dermatol*, Vol.3, pp. 45-50, ISSN: 1941-2789

Etz, H.; Minh, DB.; Henics, T.; Dryla, A.; Winkler, B.; Triska, C.; Boyd, AP.; Sollner, J.; Schmidt, W.; Von Ahsen, U.; Buschle, M.; Gill, SR.; Kolonay, J.; Khalak, H.; Fraser, CM.; von Gabain, A.; Nagy, E. & Meinke, A. (2002). Identification of in vivo expressed vaccine candidate antigens from *Staphylococcus aureus*. *Proc Natl Acad Sci U S A*, Vol.99, pp. 6573-6578, ISSN: 1091-6490

Fischetti, VA. (2010). Bacteriophage endolysins: a novel anti-infective to control Gram-positive pathogens. *Int J Med Microbiol*, Vol.300, pp. 357-362, ISSN: 0022-2615

Flock, JI. (1999). Extracellular-matrix-binding proteins as targets for the prevention of *Staphylococcus aureus* infections. *Mol Med Today*,Vol.5 pp. 532-537, ISSN: 1357-4310

Foster, TJ. (2005). Immune evasion by staphylococci. *Nat Rev Microbiol*, Vol.3, pp. 948-958, ISSN: 1740-1526

Fukuda, M.; Ohashi, H.; Matsumoto, C.; Mishima, S. & Shimomura, Y. (2002). Methicillin-resistant *Staphylococcus aureus* and methicillin-resistant coagulase-negative *Staphylococcus* ocular surface infection efficacy of chloramphenicol eye drops. *Cornea*, Vol.21, pp. S86-89, ISSN: 0277-3740

Garcia-Lara, J.; Masalha, M. & Foster, SJ. (2005). *Staphylococcus aureus*: the search for novel targets. *Drug Discov Today*, Vol.10, pp. 643-651, ISSN: 1359-6446

Garcia, P.; Martinez, B.; Rodriguez, L. & Rodriguez, A. (2010). Synergy between the phage endolysin LysH5 and nisin to kill *Staphylococcus aureus* in pasteurized milk. *Int J Food Microbiol*, Vol.141, pp. 151-155, ISSN: 0168-1605

Gening, ML.; Maira-Litran, T.; Kropec, A.; Skurnik, D.; Grout, M.; Tsvetkov, YE.; Nifantiev, NE. & Pier, GB. (2010). Synthetic {beta}-(1->6).-linked N-acetylated and nonacetylated oligoglucosamines used to produce conjugate vaccines for bacterial pathogens. *Infect Immun*, Vol.78, pp. 764-772, ISSN: 0019-9567

Gibbons, S.; Moser, E. & Kaatz, GW. (2004). Catechin gallates inhibit multidrug resistance (MDR). in *Staphylococcus aureus*. *Planta Med*, Vol.70, pp. 1240-1242, ISSN: 0032-0943

Gibbons, S.; Oluwatuyi, M. & Kaatz, GW. (2003). A novel inhibitor of multidrug efflux pumps in *Staphylococcus aureus*. *J Antimicrob Chemother*, Vol.51, pp. 13-17, ISSN: 0305-7453

Gopinathan, U.; Sharma, S.; Garg, P. & Rao, GN. (2009). Review of epidemiological features.; microbiological diagnosis and treatment outcome of microbial keratitis: experience of over a decade. *Indian J Ophthalmol*, Vol.57, pp. 273-279, ISSN: 0301-4738

Götz, F., and Peters, G. (2000). Colonization of medical devices by coagulase-negative staphylococci, In: *Infections Associated with Indwelling Medical Devices,* Waldvogel, FA. & Bisno, AL. (Ed.)., pp. 55 - 88, ASM Press, ISBN: 978-1555811778, Washington DC, USA

Graham, S. & Coote, PJ. (2007). Potent.; synergistic inhibition of *Staphylococcus aureus* upon exposure to a combination of the endopeptidase lysostaphin and the cationic peptide ranalexin. *J Antimicrob Chemother*, Vol.59, pp. 759-762, ISSN: 0305-7453

Haas, W.; Pillar, CM.; Hesje, CK.; Sanfilippo, CM. & Morris, TW. (2010). Bactericidal activity of besifloxacin against staphylococci.; *Streptococcus pneumoniae* and *Haemophilus influenzae*. *J Antimicrob Chemother*, Vol.65, pp. 1441-1447, ISSN: 0305-7453.

Han, G.; Martinez, LR.; Mihu, MR.; Friedman, AJ.; Friedman, JM. & Nosanchuk, JD. (2009). Nitric oxide releasing nanoparticles are therapeutic for *Staphylococcus aureus* abscesses in a murine model of infection. *PLoS One*, Vol.4, e7804, ISSN: 1932-6203

Hanlon, GW. (2007). Bacteriophages: an appraisal of their role in the treatment of bacterial infections. *Int J Antimicrob Agents*, Vol.30, pp. 118-128, ISSN: 0924-8579

Harro, JM.; Peters, BM.; O'May, GA.; Archer, N.; Kerns, P.; Prabhakara, R. & Shirtliff, ME. (2010). Vaccine development in *Staphylococcus aureus*: taking the biofilm phenotype into consideration. *FEMS Immunol Med Microbiol*, Vol.59, pp. 306-323, ISSN: 0928-8244

Holtfreter, S. & Broker, BM. (2005). Staphylococcal superantigens: do they play a role in sepsis? *Arch Immunol Ther Exp (Warsz)*, Vol.53, pp. 13-27, ISSN: 0004-069X

Hooper, DC. (2001). Emerging mechanisms of fluoroquinolone resistance. *Emerg Infect Dis*, Vol.7, pp. 337-341, ISSN: 1080-6059

Horgan, M.; O'Flynn, G.; Garry, J.; Cooney, J.; Coffey, A.; Fitzgerald, GF.; Ross, RP. & Mcauliffe, O. (2009). Phage lysin LysK can be truncated to its CHAP domain and retain lytic activity against live antibiotic-resistant staphylococci. *Appl Environ Microbiol*, Vol .5, pp. 872-874, ISSN: 0099-2240

Iskeleli, G.; Bahar, H.; Eroglu, E.; Torun, MM. & Ozkan, S. (2005). Microbial changes in conjunctival flora with 30-day continuous-wear silicone hydrogel contact lenses. *Eye Contact Lens*, Vol.31, pp. 124-126, ISSN: 1542-2321

Jayaraman, R. (2008). Bacterial persistence: some new insights into an old phenomenon. *J Biosci*, Vol.33, pp. 795-805, ISSN 0250-5991

Kahl, B.; Herrmann, M.; Everding, AS.; Koch, HG.; Becker, K.; Harms, E.; Proctor RA. & Peters, G. (1998). Persistent infection with small colony variant strains of *Staphylococcus aureus* in patients with cystic fibrosis. *J Infect Dis*, Vol.177, pp. 1023-1029, ISSN: 0022-1899

Kar, S.; Panda, S.; Sharma, S.; Singh, DV.; Das, S. & Sahu, SK. (2010). Antibiogram of methicillin resistant and sensitive *Staphylococcus aureus* isolates from ocular infections. *Proceedings of MICROCON 2010 34th Annual conference of Indian Association of Medical Microbiologists*, Kolkata, India, November 26-28, 2010

Katayama, Y.; Ito, T. & Hiramatsu, K. (2000). A new class of genetic element.; staphylococcus cassette chromosome mec.; encodes methicillin resistance in *Staphylococcus aureus*. *Antimicrob Agents Chemother*, Vol.44, pp. 1549-1555, ISSN: 1502-2307

Kehrenberg, C.; Schwarz, S.; Jacobsen, L.; Hansen, LH. & Vester, B. (2005). A new mechanism for chloramphenicol, florfenicol and clindamycin resistance: methylation of 23S ribosomal RNA at A2503. *Mol Microbiol*, Vol.57, pp. 1064-1073, ISSN: 0950-382X

Keren, I.; Kaldalu, N.; Spoering, A.; Wang, Y. & Lewis, K. (2004). Persister cells and tolerance to antimicrobials. *FEMS Microbiol Lett*, Vol.230, pp. 13-18, ISSN: 0378-1097

Khan, IA.; Mirza, ZM.; Kumar, A.; Verma, V. & Qazi, GN. (2006). Piperine.; a phytochemical potentiator of ciprofloxacin against *Staphylococcus aureus*. *Antimicrob Agents Chemother*, Vol.50, pp. 810-812, ISSN: 1502-2307

King, BF.; Biel, ML. & Wilkinson, BJ. (1980). Facile penetration of the *Staphylococcus aureus* capsule by lysostaphin. *Infect Immun*, Vol.29, pp. 892-896, ISSN: 0019-9567

Kiri, N.; Archer, G. & Climo, MW. (2002). Combinations of lysostaphin with beta-lactams are synergistic against oxacillin-resistant *Staphylococcus epidermidis*. *Antimicrob Agents Chemother*, Vol.46, pp. 2017-2020, ISSN: 1502-2307

Kokai-Kun, JF.; Chanturiya, T. & Mond, JJ. (2007). Lysostaphin as a treatment for systemic *Staphylococcus aureus* infection in a mouse model. *J Antimicrob Chemother*, Vol.60, pp. 1051-1059, ISSN: 0305-7453

Kokai-Kun, JF.; Walsh, SM.; Chanturiya, T. & Mond, JJ. (2003). Lysostaphin cream eradicates *Staphylococcus aureus* nasal colonization in a cotton rat model. *Antimicrob Agents Chemother*, Vol.47, pp. 1589-1597, ISSN: 1502-2307

Kumar, JK. (2008). Lysostaphin: an antistaphylococcal agent. *Appl Microbiol Biotechnol*, Vol.80, pp. 555-561, ISSN: 0175-7598

Kunimoto, DY.; Das, T.; Sharma, S.; Jalali, S.; Majji, AB.; Gopinathan, U.; Athmanathan, S.; Rao, TN. (1999a). Microbiologic spectrum and susceptibility of isolates: part I. Postoperative endophthalmitis. Endophthalmitis Research Group. *Am J Ophthalmol*, Vol.128, pp. 240-242, ISSN: 0002-9394

Kunimoto, DY.; Das, T.; Sharma, S.; Jalali, S.; Majji, AB.; Gopinathan, U.; Athmanathan, S.; Rao, TN. (1999b). Microbiologic spectrum and susceptibility of isolates: part II. Posttraumatic endophthalmitis. Endophthalmitis Research Group. *Am J Ophthalmol*, Vol.128, pp. 242-244, ISSN: 0002-9394

Kvist, M.; Hancock, V. & Klemm, P. (2008). Inactivation of efflux pumps abolishes bacterial biofilm formation. *Appl Environ Microbiol*, Vol.74, pp. 7376-7382, ISSN: 0099-2240

Kwon, AS.; Park, GC.; Ryu, SY.; Lim, DH.; Lim, DY.; Choi, CH.; Park, Y. & Lim, Y. (2008). Higher biofilm formation in multidrug-resistant clinical isolates of *Staphylococcus aureus*. *Int J Antimicrob Agents*, Vol.32, pp. 68-72, ISSN: 0924-8579

Lane, SS.; Osher, RH.; Masket, S. & Belani, S. (2008). Evaluation of the safety of prophylactic intracameral moxifloxacin in cataract surgery. *J Cataract Refract Surg*, Vol.34, pp. 1451-1459, ISSN: 0886-3350

Laplante, KL. (2007). In vitro activity of lysostaphin.; mupirocin.; and tea tree oil against clinical methicillin-resistant *Staphylococcus aureus*. *Diagn Microbiol Infect Dis*, Vol.57, pp. 413-418, ISSN: 0732-8893

Larkin, EA.; Carman, RJ.; Krakauer, T. & Stiles, BG. (2009). *Staphylococcus aureus*: the toxic presence of a pathogen extraordinaire. *Curr Med Chem*, Vol.16, pp. 4003-4019, ISSN: 0929-8673

Larkin, EA.; Stiles, BG. & Ulrich, RG. (2010). Inhibition of toxic shock by human monoclonal antibodies against staphylococcal enterotoxin B. *PLoS One*, Vol.5, e13253, ISSN: 1932-6203

Levin, BR. & Rozen, DE. (2006). Non-inherited antibiotic resistance. *Nat Rev Microbiol*, Vol.4, pp. 556-562, ISSN: 1740-1526

Lewis, K. (2010). Persister cells. *Annu Rev Microbiol*, Vol.64, pp. 357-372, ISSN: 0066-4227

Lewis, K. (2008). Multidrug tolerance of biofilms and persister cells. *Curr Top Microbiol Immunol*, Vol.322, pp. 107-131, ISSN: 0070-217X

Lewis, K. & Ausubel, FM. (2006). Prospects for plant-derived antibacterials. *Nat Biotechnol*, Vol.24, pp. 1504-1507, ISSN: 1087-0156

Liesegang, TJ. & Forster, RK. (1980). Spectrum of microbial keratitis in South Florida. *Am J Ophthalmol*, Vol.90, pp. 38-47, ISSN: 0002-9394

Locke, JB.; Hilgers, M. & Shaw, KJ. (2009). Novel ribosomal mutations in *Staphylococcus aureus* strains identified through selection with the oxazolidinones linezolid and torezolid (TR-700). *Antimicrob Agents Chemother*, Vol.53, pp. 5265-5274, ISSN: 1502-2307

Loessner, MJ.; Gaeng, S.; Wendlinger, G.; Maier, SK. & Scherer, S. (1998). The two-component lysis system of *Staphylococcus aureus* bacteriophage Twort: a large TTG-start holin and an associated amidase endolysin. *FEMS Microbiol Lett*, Vol.162, pp. 265-274, ISSN: 0378-1097

Lorenz, U.; Ohlsen, K.; Karch, H.; Hecker, M.; Thiede, A. & Hacker, J. (2000). Human antibody response during sepsis against targets expressed by methicillin resistant *Staphylococcus aureus*. *FEMS Immunol Med Microbiol*, Vol.29, pp. 145-153, ISSN: 0928-8244

Lu, TK. & Collins, JJ. (2007). Dispersing biofilms with engineered enzymatic bacteriophage. *Proc Natl Acad Sci U S A*, Vol.104, pp. 11197-11202, ISSN: 1091-6490

Mamo, W.; Froman, G. & Muller, HP. (2000). Protection induced in mice vaccinated with recombinant collagen-binding protein (CnBP) and alpha-toxoid against intramammary infection with *Staphylococcus aureus*. *Microbiol Immunol*, Vol.44, pp. 381-384, ISSN: 0385-5600

Mann, NH. (2008). The potential of phages to prevent MRSA infections. *Res Microbiol*, Vol.159, pp. 400-405, ISSN: 0923-2508

Manoharadas, S.; Witte, A. & Blasi, U. (2009). Antimicrobial activity of a chimeric enzybiotic towards *Staphylococcus aureus*. *J Biotechnol*, Vol.139, pp. 118-123, ISSN: 0168-1656

Martinez, JL.; Fajardo, A.; Garmendia, L.; Hernandez, A.; Linares, JF.; Martinez-Solano, L. & Sanchez, MB. (2009a). A global view of antibiotic resistance. *FEMS Microbiol Rev*, Vol.33, pp. 44-65, ISSN: 0168-6445

Martinez, JL.; Sanchez, MB.; Martinez-Solano, L.; Hernandez, A.; Garmendia, L.; Fajardo, A. & Alvarez-Ortega, C. (2009b). Functional role of bacterial multidrug efflux pumps in microbial natural ecosystems. *FEMS Microbiol Rev*, Vol.33, pp. 430-449, ISSN: 0168-6445

McCallum, N.; Berger-Bachi, B. & Senn, MM. (2010). Regulation of antibiotic resistance in *Staphylococcus aureus*. *Int J Med Microbiol*, Vol.300, pp. 118-129, ISSN: 0022-2615

McClellan, KA.; Bernard, PJ. & Billson, FA. (1989). Microbial investigations in keratitis at the Sydney Eye Hospital. *Aust N Z J Ophthalmol*, Vol.17, pp. 413-416, ISSN: 0814-9763

McCulley, JP.; Dougherty, JM. & Deneau, DG. (1982). Classification of chronic blepharitis. *Ophthalmology*, Vol.89, pp. 1173-1180, ISSN: 0161-6420

McDonald, M. & Blondeau, JM. (2010). Emerging antibiotic resistance in ocular infections and the role of fluoroquinolones. *J Cataract Refract Surg*, Vol.36, pp. 1588-1598, ISSN: 0886-3350

Merabishvili, M.; Pirnay, JP.; Verbeken, G.; Chanishvili, N.; Tediashvili, M.; Lashkhi, N.; Glonti, T.; Krylov, V.; Mast, J.; Van Parys, L.; Lavigne, R.; Volckaert, G.; Mattheus, W.; Verween, G.; De Corte, P.; Rose, T.; Jennes, S.; Zizi, M.; De Vos, D. & Vaneechoutte, M. (2009). Quality-controlled small-scale production of a well-defined bacteriophage cocktail for use in human clinical trials. *PLoS One*, Vol.4, e4944, ISSN: 1932-6203

Morar, M. & Wright, GD. (2010). The genomic enzymology of antibiotic resistance. *Annu Rev Genet*, Vol.44, pp. 25-51, ISSN: 0066-4197

Morel, C.; Stermitz, FR.; Tegos, G. & Lewis, K. (2003). Isoflavones as potentiators of antibacterial activity. *J Agric Food Chem*, Vol.51, pp. 5677-5679, ISSN: 0021-8561

O'Flaherty, S.; Coffey, A.; Meaney, W.; Fitzgerald, GF. & Ross, RP. (2005a). The recombinant phage lysin LysK has a broad spectrum of lytic activity against clinically relevant staphylococci.; including methicillin-resistant *Staphylococcus aureus*. *J Bacteriol*, Vol.187, pp. 7161-7164, ISSN: 0021-9193

O'Flaherty, S.; Ross, RP. & Coffey, A. (2009). Bacteriophage and their lysins for elimination of infectious bacteria. *FEMS Microbiol Rev*, Vol.33, pp. 801-819, ISSN: 0168-6445

O'Flaherty, S.; Ross, RP.; Meaney, W.; Fitzgerald, GF.; Elbreki, MF. & Coffey, A. (2005b). Potential of the polyvalent anti-Staphylococcus bacteriophage K for control of antibiotic-resistant staphylococci from hospitals. *Appl Environ Microbiol*, Vol.71, pp. 1836-1842, ISSN: 0099-2240

Ohlsen, K. & Lorenz, U. (2010). Immunotherapeutic strategies to combat staphylococcal infections. *Int J Med Microbiol*, Vol.300, pp. 402-410, ISSN: 0022-2615

Ohshita, Y.; Hiramatsu, K. & Yokota, T. (1990). A point mutation in *norA* gene is responsible for quinolone resistance in *Staphylococcus aureus*. *Biochem Biophys Res Commun*, Vol.172, pp. 1028-1034, ISSN: 0006-291X

Oluwatuyi, M.; Kaatz, GW. & Gibbons, S. (2004). Antibacterial and resistance modifying activity of *Rosmarinus officinalis*. *Phytochemistry*, Vol.65, pp. 3249-3254, ISSN: 0031-9422

Ormerod, LD.; Hertzmark, E.; Gomez, DS.; Stabiner, RG.; Schanzlin, DJ. & Smith, RE. (1987). Epidemiology of microbial keratitis in southern California. A multivariate analysis. *Ophthalmology*, Vol.94, pp. 1322-1333, ISSN: 0161-6420

Patron, RL.; Climo, MW.; Goldstein, BP. & Archer, GL. (1999). Lysostaphin treatment of experimental aortic valve endocarditis caused by a *Staphylococcus aureus* isolate with reduced susceptibility to vancomycin. *Antimicrob Agents Chemother*, Vol.43, pp. 1754-1755, ISSN: 1502-2307

Patti, JM. (2005). Vaccines and immunotherapy for staphylococcal infections. *Int J Artif Organs*, Vol.28, pp. 1157-1162, ISSN: 0391-3988

Polak, J.; Della Latta, P. & Blackburn, P. (1993). In vitro activity of recombinant lysostaphin-antibiotic combinations toward methicillin-resistant *Staphylococcus aureus*. *Diagn Microbiol Infect Dis*, Vol.17, pp. 265-270, ISSN: 0732-8893

Proctor, RA.; Balwit, JM. & Vesga, O. (1994). Variant subpopulations of *Staphylococcus aureus* as cause of persistent and recurrent infections. *Infect Agents Dis*, Vol.3, pp.302-312, ISSN: 1056-2044

Proctor, RA.; Kahl, B.; von Eiff, C.; Vaudaux, PE.; Lew, DP. & Peters, G. (1998). Staphylococcal small colony variants have novel mechanisms for antibiotic resistance. *Clin Infect Dis*, Vol.27 Suppl 1, pp. S68-74, ISSN: 1058-4838

Proctor, RA. (2006). Respiration and small-colony variants of *Staphylococcus aureus*, In: *Gram Positive Pathogens*, V.A. Fischetti, VA., Novick, RP., Ferretti, DA., Portnoy, DA. & Rood, JI. (Ed.)., pp. 434-442, ASM Press, ISSN: 978-1-55581-343-7, Washington, DC, USA

Rashel, M.; Uchiyama, J.; Ujihara, T.; Uehara, Y.; Kuramoto, S.; Sugihara, S.; Yagyu, K.; Muraoka, A.; Sugai, M.; Hiramatsu, K.; Honke, K. & Matsuzaki, S. (2007). Efficient elimination of multidrug-resistant *Staphylococcus aureus* by cloned lysin derived from bacteriophage phi MR11. *J Infect Dis*, Vol.196, pp. 1237-1247, ISSN: 0022-1899

Reddy, AK.; Garg, P.; Alam, MR.; Gopinathan, U.; Sharma, S. & Krishnaiah, S. (2010). Comparison of in vitro susceptibilities of Gram-positive cocci isolated from ocular infections against the second and fourth generation quinolones at a tertiary eye care centre in South India. *Eye (Lond)*, Vol.24, pp. 170-174, ISSN: 0950-222X

Resch, A.; Fehrenbacher, B.; Eisele, K.; Schaller, M. & Gotz, F. (2005). Phage release from biofilm and planktonic *Staphylococcus aureus* cells. *FEMS Microbiol Lett*, Vol. 252, pp. 89-96, ISSN: 0378-1097

Rohde, H.; Knobloch, JK.; Horstkotte, MA. & Mack, D. (2001). Correlation of biofilm expression types of *Staphylococcus epidermidis* with polysaccharide intercellular adhesin synthesis: evidence for involvement of *icaADBC* genotype-independent factors. *Med Microbiol Immunol*, Vol.190, pp. 105-112, ISSN: 0300-8584

Romanowski, EG.; Mah, FS.; Yates, KA.; Kowalski, RP. & Gordon, YJ. (2005). The successful treatment of gatifloxacin-resistant *Staphylococcus aureus* keratitis with Zymar (gatifloxacin 0.3%). in a NZW rabbit model. *Am J Ophthalmol*, Vol.139, pp. 867-877, ISSN: 0002-9394

Ruiz, J. (2003). Mechanisms of resistance to quinolones: target alterations.; decreased accumulation and DNA gyrase protection. *J Antimicrob Chemother*, Vol.51, pp. 1109-1117, ISSN: 0305-7453

Sass, P. & Bierbaum, G. (2007). Lytic activity of recombinant bacteriophage phi11 and phi12 endolysins on whole cells and biofilms of *Staphylococcus aureus*. *Appl Environ Microbiol*, Vol.73, pp. 347-352, ISSN: 0099-2240

Schaffer, AC.; Solinga, RM.; Cocchiaro, J.; Portoles, M.; Kiser, KB.; Risley, A.; Randall, SM.; Valtulina, V.; Speziale, P.; Walsh, E.; Foster, T. & Lee, JC. (2006). Immunization with *Staphylococcus aureus* clumping factor B.; a major determinant in nasal carriage.; reduces nasal colonization in a murine model. *Infect Immun*, Vol.74, pp. 2145-2153. ISSN: 0019-9567

Schwalbe, RS.; Stapleton, JT. & Gilligan, PH. (1987). Emergence of vancomycin resistance in coagulase-negative staphylococci. *N Engl J Med*, Vol.316, pp. 927-931, ISSN: 0028-4793

Shah, A.; Mond, J.& Walsh, S. (2004). Lysostaphin-coated catheters eradicate *Staphylococcus aureus* challenge and block surface colonization. *Antimicrob Agents Chemother*, Vol.48, pp.2704-277, ISSN: 1502-2307

Shanmuganathan, VA.; Armstrong, M.; Buller, A. & Tullo, AB. (2005). External ocular infections due to methicillin-resistant *Staphylococcus aureus* (MRSA). *Eye (Lond)*, Vol.19, pp. 284-291, ISSN: 0950-222X

Sharma, S.; Kunimoto, DY.; Rao, NT.; Garg, P. & Rao, GN. (1999). Trends in antibiotic resistance of corneal pathogens: Part II. An analysis of leading bacterial keratitis isolates. *Indian J Ophthalmol*, Vol. 47, pp. 101-109, ISSN: 0301-4738

Sharma, V.; Sharma, S.; Garg, P. & Rao, GN. (2004). Clinical resistance of *Staphylococcus keratitis* to ciprofloxacin monotherapy. *Indian J Ophthalmol*, Vol.52, pp. 287-292, ISSN: 0301-4738

Shinefield, H.; Black, S.; Fattom, A.; Horwith, G.; Rasgon, S.; Ordonez, J.; Yeoh, H.; Law, D.; Robbins, JB.; Schneerson, R.; Muenz, L.; Fuller, S.; Johnson, J.; Fireman, B.; Alcorn, H. & Naso, R. (2002). Use of a *Staphylococcus aureus* conjugate vaccine in patients receiving hemodialysis. *N Engl J Med*, Vol.346, pp. 491-496, ISSN: 0028-4793

Sillankorva, S.; Neubauer, P. & Azeredo, J. (2010). Phage control of dual species biofilms of *Pseudomonas fluorescens* and *Staphylococcus lentus*. *Biofouling*, Vol.26, pp. 567-575, ISSN: 0892-7014

Singh, R.; Ray, P.; Das, A. & Sharma, M. (2010). Enhanced production of exopolysaccharide matrix and biofilm by a menadione-auxotrophic *Staphylococcus aureus* small-colony variant. *J Med Microbiol*, Vol.59, pp. 521-527, ISSN: 0022-2615

Singh, R.; Ray, P.; Das, A. & Sharma, M. (2009). Role of persisters and small-colony variants in antibiotic resistance of planktonic and biofilm-associated *Staphylococcus aureus*: an in vitro study. *J Med Microbiol*, Vol.58, pp. 1067-1073, ISSN: 0022-2615

Skurnik, D.; Merighi, M.; Grout, M.; Gadjeva, M.; Maira-Litran, T.; Ericsson, M.; Goldmann, DA.; Huang, SS.; Datta, R.; Lee, JC. & Pier, GB. (2010). Animal and human antibodies to distinct *Staphylococcus aureus* antigens mutually neutralize opsonic killing and protection in mice. *J Clin Invest*, Vol.120, pp. 3220-33, ISSN: 0021-9738

Speaker, MG.; Milch, FA.; Shah, MK.; Eisner, W. & Kreiswirth, BN. (1991). Role of external bacterial flora in the pathogenesis of acute postoperative endophthalmitis. *Ophthalmology*, Vol.98, pp. 639-649, discussion 650, ISSN: 0161-6420

Spearman, P.; Lakey, D.; Jotte, S.; Chernowitz, A.; Claycomb, S. & Stratton, C. (1996). Sternoclavicular joint septic arthritis with small-colony variant *Staphylococcus aureus*. *Diagn Microbiol Infect Dis*, Vol.26, pp. 13-15, ISSN: 0732-8893

Srinivasan, R.; Tiroumal, S.; Kanungo, R. & Natarajan, MK. (2002). Microbial contamination of the anterior chamber during phacoemulsification. *J Cataract Refract Surg*, Vol.28, pp. 2173-2176, ISSN: 0886-3350

Stavri, M.; Piddock, LJ. & Gibbons, S. (2007). Bacterial efflux pump inhibitors from natural sources. *J Antimicrob Chemother*, Vol.59, pp. 1247-1260, ISSN: 0305-7453

Stermitz, FR.; Lorenz, P.; Tawara, JN.; Zenewicz, LA. & Lewis, K. (2000). Synergy in a medicinal plant: antimicrobial action of berberine potentiated by 5'-methoxyhydnocarpin.; a multidrug pump inhibitor. *Proc Natl Acad Sci U S A*, Vol.97, pp. 1433-1437, ISSN: 1091-6490

Stranger-Jones, YK.; Bae, T. & Schneewind, O. (2006). Vaccine assembly from surface proteins of *Staphylococcus aureus*. *Proc Natl Acad Sci U S A*, Vol.103, pp. 16942-16947, ISSN: 1091-6490

Sudano Roccaro, A.; Blanco, AR.; Giuliano, F.; Rusciano, D. & Enea, V. (2004). Epigallocatechin-gallate enhances the activity of tetracycline in staphylococci by inhibiting its efflux from bacterial cells. *Antimicrob Agents Chemother*, Vol.48, pp. 1968-1973, ISSN: 1502-2307

Sulakvelidze, A.; Alavidze, Z. & Morris, JG Jr. (2001). Bacteriophage therapy. *Antimicrob Agents Chemother*, Vol.45, pp. 649-659, ISSN: 1502-2307

Tenover, FC.; Weigel , LM.; Appelbaum, PC.; McDougal, LK.; Chaitram, J.; McAllister, S.; Clark, N.; Killgore, G.; O'hara, CM.; Jevitt, L.; Patel, JB. & Bozdogan, B. (2004). Vancomycin-resistant *Staphylococcus aureus* isolate from a patient in Pennsylvania. *Antimicrob Agents Chemother*, Vol.48, pp. 275-280, ISSN: 1502-2307

Tomar, VP.; Sharma, OP. & Joshi, K. (1971). Bacterial and fungal flora of normal conjunctiva. *Ann Ophthalmol*, Vol.3, pp. 669-671, ISSN: 0042-465x

Truong-Bolduc, QC.; Strahilevit, J. & Hooper, DC. (2006). NorC, a new efflux pump regulated by MgrA of *Staphylococcus aureus*. *Antimicrob Agents Chemother*, Vol.50, pp. 1104-1107, ISSN: 1502-2307

Tsubakishita, S.; Kuwahara-Arai, K.; Sasaki, T. & Hiramatsu, K. (2010). Origin and molecular evolution of the determinant of methicillin resistance in staphylococci. *Antimicrob Agents Chemother*, Vol.54, pp. 4352-4359, ISSN: 1502-2307

Uttley, AH.; Collins, CH.; Naidoo, J. & George, RC. (1988). Vancomycin-resistant enterococci. *Lancet*, Vol.1, pp. 57-58, ISSN: 0140-6736

Varshney, AK.; Wang, X.; Cook, E.; Dutta, K.; Scharff, MD.; Goger, MJ. & Fries, BC. (2010). Generation.; characterization and epitope mapping of neutralizing and protective monoclonal antibodies against staphylococcal enterotoxin B induced lethal shock. *J Biol Chem*, Vol.286, pp. 9737-9747, ISSN: 0021-9258

von Eiff, C.; Becker, K.; Machka, K.; Stammer, H. & Peters, G. (2001). Nasal carriage as a source of *Staphylococcus aureus* Bacteremia Study Group. *N Engl J Med*, Vol.344, pp. 11-16, ISSN: 0028-4793

Walencka, E.; Sadowska, B.; Rozalska, S.; Hryniewicz, W. & Rozalska, B. (2005). Lysostaphin as a potential therapeutic agent for staphylococcal biofilm eradication. *Pol J Microbiol*, Vol. 54, pp. 191-200, ISSN: 1733-1331

Walsh, S.; Shah, A. & Mond, J. (2003). Improved pharmacokinetics and reduced antibody reactivity of lysostaphin conjugated to polyethylene glycol. *Antimicrob Agents Chemother*, Vol.47, pp. 554-558, ISSN: 1502-2307

Wang, J.; Kodali, S.; Lee, SH.; Galgoci, A.; Painter, R.; Dorso, K.; Racine, F.; Motyl, M.; Hernandez, L.; Tinney, E.; Colletti, SL.; Herath, K.; Cummings, R.; Salazar, O.; Gonzalez, I.; Basilio, A.; Vicente, F.; Genilloud, O.; Pelaez, F.; Jayasuriya, H.; Young, K.; Cully, DF. & Singh, SB. (2007). Discovery of platencin.; a dual FabF and FabH inhibitor with in vivo antibiotic properties. *Proc Natl Acad Sci U S A*, Vol.104, pp. 7612-7616, ISSN: 1091-6490

Wang, J.; Soisson, SM.; Young, K.; Shoop, W.; Kodali, S.; Galgoci, A.; Painter, R.; Parthasarathy, G.; Tang, YS.; Cummings, R.; Ha, S.; Dorso, K.; Motyl, M.; Jayasuriya, H.; Ondeyka, J.; Herath, K.; Zhang, C.; Hernandez, L.; Allocco, J.; Basilio, A.; Tormo, JR.; Genilloud, O.; Vicente, F.; Pelaez, F.; Colwell, L.; Lee, SH.; Michael, B.; Felcetto, T.; Gill, C.; Silver, LL.; Hermes, JD.; Bartizal, K.; Barrett, J.; Schmatz, D.; Becker, JW.; Cully, D. & Singh, SB. (2006). Platensimycin is a selective FabF inhibitor with potent antibiotic properties. *Nature*, Vol.441, pp. 358-361, ISSN: 0028-0836

Weigel, LM.; Clewell, DB.; Gill, SR.; Clark, NC.; McDougal, LK.; Flannagan, SE.; Kolonay, JF.; Shetty, J.; Killgore, GE. & Tenover, FC. (2003). Genetic analysis of a high-level vancomycin-resistant isolate of *Staphylococcus aureus*. *Science*, Vol.302, pp. 1569-1571, ISSN: 1095-9203

Wertheim, HF.; Vos, MC.; Ott, A.; van Belkum, A.; Voss, A.; Kluytmans, JA.; van Keulen, PH.; Vandenbroucke-Grauls, CM.; Meester, MH. & Verbrugh, HA. (2004). Risk and outcome of nosocomial *Staphylococcus aureus* bacteraemia in nasal carriers versus non-carriers. *Lancet*, Vol.364, pp. 703-705, ISSN: 0140-6736

Wong, TY. & Chee, SP. (2004). The epidemiology of acute endophthalmitis after cataract surgery in an Asian population. *Ophthalmology*, Vol.111, pp. 699-705, ISSN: 0161-6420

Wu, JA.; Kusuma, C.; Mond, JJ. & Kokai-Kun, JF. (2003). Lysostaphin disrupts *Staphylococcus aureus* and *Staphylococcus epidermidis* biofilms on artificial surfaces. *Antimicrob Agents Chemother*, Vol.47, pp. 3407-3414, ISSN: 1502-2307

Zhou, H.; Xiong, ZY.; Li, HP.; Zheng, YL. & Jiang, YQ. (2006). An immunogenicity study of a newly fusion protein Cna-FnBP vaccinated against *Staphylococcus aureus* infections in a mice model. *Vaccine*, Vol.24, pp. 4830-4837, ISSN: 0264-410X

11

Antibiotic Resistance in *Staphylococcus* Species of Animal Origin

Miliane Moreira Soares de Souza[1], Shana de Mattos de Oliveira Coelho[1], Ingrid Annes Pereira[2], Lidiane de Castro Soares[3], Bruno Rocha Pribul[1] and Irene da Silva Coelho[1]

[1]*Institute of Veterinary, Microbiology and Immunology Department, Federal Rural University of Rio de Janeiro,*
[2]*Institute Osvaldo Cruz Foundation, Rio de Janeiro,*
[3]*University Severino Sombra, Rio de Janeiro,*
Brazil

1. Introduction

Staphylococcus is a genus of worldwide distributed bacteria correlated to several infectious of different sites in human and animals. Its importance is not only because of its distribution and pathogenicity but especially due to its ability to overcome antimicrobial effects. The goal of this chapter is to report data obtained from a decade of research in animal science field concerning to staphylococci antimicrobial resistance.

2. Characteristics and distribution of Staphylococci species in animals: An overview

The genus *Staphylococcus* is in the bacterial family Staphylococcaceae (Ludwig, 2009). Staphylococci are Gram-positive spherical bacteria that occur in clusters resembling grapes due to its perpendicular division planes where cells remains attached to one another following each successive division.

The genotypic standards for assigning an organism to the genus *Staphylococcus* include determination of guanine plus cytosine (G+C) content of 30-39mol% and phylogenetic trees constructed by comparison of 16S rRNA or 23R rRNA sequences (Takahashi et al., 1999). The phenotypic criteria is based on the ultrastructure and chemical composition of the cell wall, typical form Gram positive bacteria and catalase reaction positive for all species, except for *S. aureus* subsp *anaerobius* and *S. saccharolyticus*, which are strictly anaerobic. This genus comprises more than 50 species separated into two distinct groups based on their ability to produce coagulase. This topic approaches *Staphylococcus* spp distribution considering that different animal species have specific staphylococcal microbiota. Otherwise some clonal strains can colonize different animal species as is the case of methicillin-resistant *Staphylococcus aureus* (MRSA). Molecular techniques have been used to relate clonal groups of MRSA isolated from different animal species in order to understand its model of dissemination.

2.1 Coagulase-positive Staphylococci

This group includes the major pathogenic *Staphylococcus* species. *Staphylococcus aureus* is considered the most pathogenic one, especially due to its ability to produce a large range of virulence factors that enables it to colonize different tissues of a large range of animal species. The coagulase protein has the ability to turn fibrinogen into fibrin threads by a mechanism different from natural clotting (Palma et al., 1999). This protein is codified by the gene *coa* which possess a conserved and a repeated polymorphic region that can be used to measure relatedness among *Staphylococcus* coagulase positive isolates (Reinoso et al., 2006). The variable region of *coa* is comprised of 81-bp tandem short sequence repeats (SSRs) that are variable in both number and sequence, as determined by restriction fragment length polymorphism analysis of PCR products (Goh et al., 1992).

Staphylococcal protein A is a membrane-bound exoprotein characterized and well known for its ability to bind to the Fc region of immunoglobulins of most mammalian species. This protein is encoded by the *spaA* gene with a polymorphic (X) and a conserved region. The polymorphic X region consists of a variable number of repeated 24 pairs of bases located in the coding region for the cellular wall C-terminal extremity (Koreen et al., 2004). The diversity of the *spaA* short sequence repeat region seems to arise from deletion and duplication of the repetitive units and also by point mutation and this variation can be used in epidemiological studies. Frenay et al. (1994) reported epidemic MRSA strains with more than seven repeats and Montesinos et al. (2002) described isolates with 11 repeats as the most common type involved in an epidemic human outbreak caused by MRSA. The *coa* typing can be used to enhance the value of *spa* typing by providing more supported inferences on strain lineage and clonality among isolates with similar or identical *spa* repeat organization (Tenover et al., 1994). The use of more than one genetic marker for relating strains is desirable and likely to become increasingly important because recombination will eventually diversify resistant staphylococcal species to the extent that clonal types within a given region can no longer be distinguished by a single locus.

Staphylococcus aureus also produces others exoproteins that contribute to its ability to colonize host tissues such as slime and hemolysins. The adherence and fixation of *S. aureus* on biological surfaces represent the fundamental step in the development of infections. The production of slime mediates adhesion to implanted surfaces acting as a cementing matrix making bacteria less accessible to the host's defense system (Coelho et al, 2009). Slime production is controlled by the *ica* operon (*icaADBC*) and the co-expression of the *icaA* and *icaD* genes leads to a significant increase in such production (Arciola et al., 2001).

The alpha and beta hemolysins are important factors in the pathogenesis of Staphylococcal infections. The beta-toxin is an Mg^{2+}-dependent sphingomyelinase C which degrades sphingomyelin in the outer phospholipid layer of the membrane (Linehan et al., 2003).

The *agr* (*accessory gene regulator*) operon (*agrA, agrB, agrC agrD* and *hld)* is recognized as a quorum-sensing gene cluster that up-regulates production of secreted virulence factors such as alpha and beta-hemolysins, proteases, DNAses and sphingomyelinase. This same cluster also down-regulates the production of cell-associated virulence factors in a cell density-dependent manner in *S. aureus* (Lyon et al., 2000). The *agr* locus comprises two divergent transcriptional units under the control of the promoters P2 (RNA II) and P3 (RNA III). The

P3 transcript, an RNA III molecule, mediates the up-regulation of secreted virulence factors as well as the down-regulation of surface proteins (Novick, 2000).

Coelho et al. (2011) evaluated the presence of some *Staphylococcus aureus* virulence genes, including *coa, spaA, hla* e *hlb* in order to understand the distribution of *S. aureus* strains in dairy farms at Rio de Janeiro, Brazil, and contribute to the establishment of preventive strategies to reduce the spread of infection.

In veterinary medicine, others coagulase-positive staphylococci are reported as important pathogens, such as *Staphylococcus intermedius,* whose reclassification was proposed by Devriese et al. (2005), creating the *S. intermedius* group (SIG) including *S. intermedius,* a new specie *S. pseudintermedius* and *S. delphini.* Like *S. aureus,* the *S. intermedius* strains isolated from animals have been reported to produce an array of virulence factors, including leukotoxin, enterotoxin, and hemolysins, together with elements essential for biofilm formation (Futagawa-Saito et al., 2006). Besides SIG, others significative coagulase-positive in animals are *S. schleiferi* subsp. *coagulans, S. aureus* subsp. *anaerobius.*

2.2 Coagulase-negative Staphylococci

This group comprises the majority of *Staphylococcus* species. Coagulase-negative staphylococci (CNS), which were traditionally considered to be minor infectious pathogens, have become more common (Huxley et al., 2002). Several CNSs have been isolated from animal clinical specimens such as *Staphylococcus epidermidis, Staphylococcus simulans, Staphylococcus xylosus, Staphylococcus chromogenes, Staphylococcus warneri, Staphylococcus haemolyticus, Staphylococcus sciuri, Staphylococcus saprophyticus, Staphylococcus hominis, Staphylococcus caprae, Staphylococcus cohnii* subsp. *cohnii, Staphylococcus cohnii* subsp. *urealyticus, Staphylococcus capitis* subsp. *capitis* and *Staphylococcus capitis* subsp. *urealyticus* (Lilenbaum et al., 2000; Pereira et al., 2009; Pyöräla et al., 2009; Soares et al., 2008).

The conventional methods for CNS identification were primarily developed for human strains and their poor performance for identifying strains of animal origin seems to be related to a limited number of veterinary strains in databases (Bes et al., 2000). Additionally, the reference method developed by Bannerman (2003) is costly and too time consuming to be used in a clinical laboratory. Several molecular targets have been exploited for the molecular identification of *Staphylococcus* species, including the *groEL* gene (Goh et al., 1996). This gene, which encodes a 60-kDa polypeptide (known as GroEL, 60-kDa chaperonin, or HSP60 for heat shock protein 60) has the potential to serve as a general phylogenic marker because of its ubiquity and conservation in nature (Segal & Ron, 1996). Also it was proven to be an ideal universal DNA target for identification to the species level because it has well-conserved DNA sequences within a given species, but with sufficient sequence variations to allow for species-specific identification (Goh et al., 1996). Santos et al., (2008) had successfully used the *groEL* gene as a tool for the identification of the main *Staphylococcus* coagulase-negative species by PCR restriction fragment length polymorphism (RFLP). This group investigated 54 cows from 23 dairy herds located in the Brazilian States of Minas Gerais, Rio de Janeiro and São Paulo, between 1995 and 2003 and concluded that this gene constitutes a reliable and reproducible molecular method for identification of CNS species responsible for bovine mastitis.

2.3 Staphylococcal infections in animals

Reports of the importance of *Staphylococcus* species as pathogens in animal infections have been described and appear to be increasing. Among coagulase-positive species, *Staphylococcus aureus* is a cause of mastitis, dermatitis and suppurative conditions in several animal species. *S. aureus* causing mastitis is widely distributed in cattle, goats and sheep. The infection is often subclinical in cattle, leading to reduced milk production and milk quality, but acute catarrhal or even gangrenous inflammation may also occur.

For a long time, *S. intermedius* had been majorly considered a primary cause of pyoderma in dogs. It has also been reported to be involved in other diseases, such as pyometra, otitis externa and purulent infections of the joints, eyelids and conjunctiva (Werckenthin et al., 2001). Nowadays, a new classification was proposed by Devriese et al. (2005), creating the *S. intermedius* group (SIG) including *S. intermedius,* a new specie *S. pseudintermedius* and *S. delphini*. According to Sasaki et al. (2007), *S. pseudintermedius* is actually the major specie involved in this pathology. Futhermore, according to these authors, *S. intermedius* is restricted to feral pigeons and *S. delphini* which was usually described as the cause of suppurative skin lesions in dolphins is now considered to be involved in a larger spectrum of infectious animal diseases. *S. aureus* subsp. *anaerobius* has been implicated in lymphadenitis in sheep and *S. schleiferi* subsp. *coagulans* in external otitis in dogs.

Coagulase Negative Staphylococci (CNSs) have also been studied considering its potential pathogenicity for human and animals. Nowadays these bacteria are of great interest in veterinary medicine because they are currently considered emerging pathogens of bovine mastitis. Although CNS are not as pathogenic as the other principal mastitis pathogens and infection mostly remains subclinical, they can cause persistent infections, which result in increased milk somatic cell count (SCC) and decreased milk quality (Pyorala & Taponen, 2009). The prevalence of CNS mastitis is higher in primiparous cows than in older cows. Also this agent is implicated in the etiology of infectious diseases in household pets (Pereira et al., 2009). The most frequently isolated CNS species vary according to the geographical region under scrutiny and sample origin. In Brazil, Soares et al. (2008) detected prevalence of *S.xylosus* in mastitic milk samples, despite *S. chromogenes*, *S. simulans* and *S. epidermidis*, in general, appear to be the most frequently isolated CNS from mammary secretion samples worldwide (De Vliegher et al., 2003; Taponen et al., 2006).

Besides, *S. hyicus*, a variable coagulase producer, but mainly coagulase-negative, causes exudative epidermitis ("greasy pig disease") and an often acute generalized skin infection in piglets. Systemic forms of the disease which result in the death of the animals are also seen. Poor hygienic conditions as well as ec

toparasitic infestations favour the onset of the *S. hyicus* infection. Surviving piglets show retarded growth rates. In adult pigs, subacute skin infections, mastitis or metritis, but also septic arthritis may be caused by *S. hyicus* (Brückler et al., 1994). In goats and sheep however, enzootic acute gangrenous mastitis is commonly seen.

3. Antimicrobial resistance in Staphylococci of animal origin

Antibiotic resistance is the most puzzling question of public healthy in the earlier decade of this 21st century. Among bacteria this question seems to be more alarming due to its short generation time and efficient gene recombination mechanisms. *Staphylococcus aureus* is the most representative example of how antibiotic resistance is a serious threatening worldwide. Nevertheless, all others coagulase-positive staphylococci are also able to develop resistance mechanisms to a large range of antimicrobials. Furthermore, the strains of several CNS species were also found to have high levels of resistance to various antibiotics.

This topic will discuss features of the resistance of staphylococci to antimicrobials, specially methicillin (oxacillin) and vancomicin, its mechanisms and epidemiology. Crucial questions about the use or abolishment of antibiotics used as "growth promoters" to food animal production will also be discussed.

3.1 Methicillin resistance

ß-lactamic antibiotics are the most frequently used in anti-staphylococcal infection therapy. Bacterial resistance mechanisms to this class of antibiotics include production of ß-lactamases and low-affinity penicillin-binding protein 2a (PBP2a) determined by the presence of the chromosomal genes *bla* and *mecA*, respectively. The latter, designated for methicillin resistance, precludes therapy with any of the currently available ß-lactam antibiotics, and may predict resistance to several classes of antibiotics (Moon et al., 2007). The isolation of *Staphylococcus aureus* methicillin- resistant (MRSA) from animals was first reported in 1972 following its detection in milk from mastitic cows (Devriese et al., 1972). Recent works reports a low incidence of MRSA mastitis and low prevalence of methicillin resistance among bovine *S. aureus* isolates (Juhász-Kaszanyitzky et al., 2007; Lee, 2003; Moon et al., 2007) so clinically it can be concluded that MRSA does not appear to be an important bovine mastitis pathogen. Nevertheless, the importance of epidemiological data concerns about MRSA in animals is reasonable and requires careful study in order to understand its emergence and dissemination. The long-term low prevalence of MRSA mastitis is quite surprising given the number of years since the first identification of MRSA in cattle and the close contact of humans with the udders of dairy cattle. Otherwise, several reports have been published showing MRSA infection in domestic animals, including dogs, cats, cattle, sheep, chickens, rabbits, and horses as an increasing trend (Goni et al., 2004; Hartmann et al., 1997; Lee, 2003; O'Mahony et al. 2005; Rich & Roberts 2004; Weese, 2005; Weese et al., 2006).

It is certain that animals are a source of human MRSA infection in some circumstances, but humans may also serve as sources of infection in animals. Exposure of household pets to MRSA was probably inevitable due to its increasingly prevalence in humans. Changes in the epidemiology of MRSA in unique specie may be reflected in changes in other species. The true scope of MRSA in animals and its impact on human health are still only superficially understood, but it is clear that MRSA is a potentially important veterinary and public health concern that requires a great deal more study to enhance understanding and effective response (Weese & Van Duijkeren, 2010). While most animals with MRSA are merely colonized, a wide range of clinical infections can occur. As would be expected with staphylococci, most MRSA infections in pets affect the skin and soft tissue. Wound infections, surgical site infections, pyoderma, otitis, and urinary tract infections are most common, but various other opportunistic infections have been reported (Baptiste et al., 2005; Griffeth & Morris, 2008). In a research developed by our team, 8% of MRSA was detected in a hundred of clinical specimens from different sites of household pets evaluated (Pereira et al., 2009).

Recently, a new MRSA was identified using high throughput DNA microarray screening. Complete genome sequencing revealed that this strain is distinctly different to previously described MRSA. It carries a new type of SCC*mec* encoding highly divergent genes that are very different to any described previously in MRSA or in any other organism. It was found to belong to the genetic lineage clonal complex 130 (CC130), which has previously only been associated with MSSA from cows and other animals, but not humans, strongly suggesting that the new MRSA originated in animals. (Gárcia-Alvarez et al., 2011)

Staphylococcal cassette chromosome *mec* (SCC*mec*) is a mobile genetic element composed by *mec* and *ccr* genes complex, which encodes methicillin resistance and the recombinases responsible for its mobility, respectively (Katayama et al., 2000). The expression of PBP-2a is controlled by regulator elements encoded by *mecR1* and *mecI* which are located adjacent to *mecA* on the chromosome. Deletion or mutation which occurred in *mec* regulator gene is considered to be associated with constitutive production of PBP-2a. Hence *Staphylococcus* spp possessing intact *mecRI* and *mecI* as well as *mecA* are phenotypically methicillin susceptible because of the repression of PBP-2a production by *mec* regulator elements. Such genomic changes in *mec* regulator genes are considered to alter or remove their repressor function on *mecA* gene transcription, which may lead to constitutive production of PBP-2a. The *mec* gene complex has been classified into four classes, and the *ccr* gene complex has been classified into three allotypes. Different combinations of *mec* and *ccr* gene complex types have so far defined six types of SCC*mec* elements (type I, II, III, IV, V) (Ito et al., 2004). It is important to analyze the genomic diversity found in *mec* regulator genes of staphylococci in order to understand the molecular basis for methicillin resistance.

The detection of methicillin resistance in routine clinical laboratories has been problematic ever since the emergence of MRSA during the 1960s and the difficulties are associated mainly with heterogeneous expression of resistance in most staphylococal strains currently prevalent (Witte et al., 2007). Misidentification of methicillin resistance can have serious adverse clinical consequences. False-susceptibility may result in treatment failure and in the spread of resistant *Staphylococcus* spp making it difficult to apply control measures and leading to the increasing of healthcare costs and may lead to overuse of glycopeptides (Velasco et al., 2005).

3.2 Vancomicin resistance

The glycopeptide vancomycin was first released in 1958. Vancomycin is an inhibitor of cell wall synthesis in *S. aureus* and other gram-positive organisms. While beta-lactam antibiotics inhibit cell wall synthesis by binding to the transpeptidase active site of penicillin binding proteins, vancomycin acts by a completely different mechanism so it has been the treatment of choice for serious infections caused by MRSA (Howden et al., 2010), but increase in vancomycin use has led to the emergence of two types of glycopeptide-resistant *S. aureus*. The first one, designated vancomycin intermediate resistant *S. aureus* (VISA) and the vancomycin-resistant S. aureus (VRSA).

The first report of clinical *S.aureus* isolate with reduced vancomycin susceptibility (VISA) was made by Hiramatsu et al. (1997) and generated great concern in the medical community. From there on, reports of strains of *S. aureus* (predominately MRSA) demonstrating the heterogeneous VISA (hVISA) or VISA phenotype have now been reported for many countries including the United States, Japan, Australia, France, Scotland, Brazil, South Korea, Hong Kong, South Africa, Thailand, Israel, and others (Bierbaum et al. 1999; Chang et al., 2003; Denis et al. 2002; Ferraz et al., 2000 Gemmell, 2004; Howden et al., 2010; Kim et al., 2000; Perichon & Courvalin, 2006; Sng et al.,2005; Song et al., 2004; Tenover et al., 2004; Weigel et al., 2007)

Nowadays it is conceivable that VISA phenotype is related to the bacterial cell wall thickening, a passive resistance mechanism that reduces vancomycin access to its active site, which is localized in the cytoplasmic membrane in the division septum (Howden et al., 2010). It results in accumulation of acyl-D-alanyl-D-alanine (X-DAla-D-Ala) targets in the periphery that sequester glycopeptides (Cui et al., 2003).

Since 2002, nine methicillin-resistant *Staphylococcus aureus* (MRSA) strains that are also resistant to vancomycin (VRSA) have been reported in the United States. The fully vancomicin-resistant *Staphylococcus aureus* phenotype (VRSA) is due to acquisition from *Enterococcus* spp. of the *vanA* operon, carried by transposon Tn1546, resulting in high-level resistance (Arthur et al., 1993, Patel et al., 1997).

The emergence of enterococci vancomicin-resistant strains has been related to the use of avoparcin as growth promoter in swine culture (Aarestrup et al., 1996). Studies report the transfer of glycopeptide- and macrolide-resistance genes by transconjugation among enterococci and from *Enterococcus faecalis* to *S. aureus* (Młynarczyk et al., 2002). The vancomycin-resistance gene acquisition by *S. aureus* from *E. faecium* in the clinical environment has also been reported by Weigel et al. (2007). Recently, Tiwari & Sen (2006) have reported a VRSA which is *van* gene-negative.

In veterinary medicine, vancomycin-resistant enterococci were isolated from the feces of poultry and pig herds. It has significant impact in public healthy cause dissemination via contaminated animal food products possible (Aarestrup, 1995). These vancomycin-resistant *E. faecium* isolates from animals had decreased susceptibilities to avoparcin, a glycopeptide antibiotic widely used as a growth promoter in Western Europe and Australasia. Avoparcin is a fermentation product from a strain of *Streptomyces candidus* and is closely related to vancomycin (Aarestrup et al., 1996). Aarestrup et al (1996) showed that *E. faecium* isolates coresistant to vancomycin and avoparcin are commonly found in the feces of pigs and poultry in Denmark.

3.3 Others antimicrobials resistance

In Veterinary Medicine, clindamycin has been chosen as an antimicrobial alternative for the treatment of infections in dogs and cats caused by methicillin-resistant *Staphylococcus aureus* (MRSA) (Walther et al., 2008; Weese et al., 2006) and methicillin-resistant *Staphylococcus pseudintermedius* (MRSP) (Schwarz et al., 2008; Wettstein et al., 2008). However, an inducible form of clindamycin-resistance may be present in some staphylococci. These staphylococcal strains appear susceptible on routine antimicrobial susceptibility testing, but resistance can be induced during treatment, possibly resulting in treatment failure (Swenson et al., 2007; Yilmaz et al., 2007).

Azithromycin have a remarkable application due to its superior pharmacokinetics properties and broad spectrum activity, including Gram-positive and negative bacteria species, intracellular pathogens and protozoan parasites. The principal characteristic that supported its prescription and clinical significance is that it can be administrated by oral and parental routes, only by a single daily dose in short period of treatment facilitating veterinary therapy. Nevertheless, most of the knowledge that supports its use in veterinary therapy was based on studies that proved its therapeutic efficacy in human infections. Empirical antimicrobial chemotherapy without previous accomplishment of bacterial identification and antimicrobial susceptibility assays contributes to increase of antimicrobial resistance prevalence in pet animal reservoirs (Guardabassi et al., 2004; Morgan et al.; 2008).

Pereira et al. (2009) evaluated azithromycin resistance among 100 staphylococci isolates from pet animals infections. It was detected a percentual of resistant isolates of 54% to *Staphylococcus intermedius*, 67% of *S. aureus*, 38% of *S. hyicus*, 67% of coagulase-negative *Staphylococcus* spp through disc diffusion test. The variability of azithromycin susceptibility pattern is different to what is observed in humans infections whereas *Staphylococcus aureus* is the classical isolated pathogen. Broth dilution test detected azithromycin $MIC_{50}/_{90}$ values of 16µg/mL, 64µg/mL in staphylococci isolates, respectivally, and 256µg/mL in Gram-negative rods (GNR). Agar dilution azithromycin $MIC_{50}/_{90}$ values corresponded to 32µg/mL and 256µg/mL in staphylococci and >512µg/mL in GNR. Crescent azithromycin resistance rate has been previously reported. A study from 90's decade, detected azithromycin $MIC_{50/90}$ >128 µg/mL of MRSA isolated from human clinical samples (Neu, 1991). When comparing human MIC values reported in literature to data obtained from pet animal samples in the present study, azithromycin activity pattern may vary from different bacteria species and hosts, leading to therapeutic failures when classical human pathogens are adopted as reference to calculate dose and drug concentration. This justify microbiologic and pharmacokinetic assays to determine the specific azithromycin susceptibility breakpoints and therapeutic drug concentration to different bacteria species detected from animal disease.

It is important to point that MIC_{50} values varied among different staphylococci species, such as, *Staphylococcus intermedius* (32µg/mL), *S. hyicus* (32µg/mL), CNS (32µg/mL), from that value detected in *S. aureus* (16µg/mL) isolated from pet animal specimens.

Pereira et al. (2009) also evaluated the genetic markers of *Staphylococcus* spp azithromycin resistance by PCR technique and detected a 39% prevalence of *erm* genes, being *ermC* gene the most detected, showing a prevalence of 24% among all *Staphylococcus* isolates, followed by 12% *ermA* and 3% of *ermB*. No isolates were positive to *mefA* gene, what may support the theory about methylase ribossomal modification as the principal resistance mechanism associated to macrolide resistance among staphylococci. The expression of *erm* genes can be inducible or constitutive. When expression is constitutive, the staphylococci are resistant to all macrolide, lincosamide and streptogramin B (MLS_B) antimicrobials (Schmitz et al., 2000). In this study, it was detected MLS_B resistance in 14% constitutive azithromycin-resistant *Staphylococcus* spp. Inducible resistance phenotype, expressed by a "D zone" next to clindamycin disc was available in 5% (5/100) of *Staphylococcus* spp.

Most of the knowledge applied to define microbiologic use and dose of azithromycin was based on *Staphylococcus aureus* assays, because this specie acts as classical pathogen of human infections, but the frame of etiology and antimicrobial susceptibility pattern change when animal pathogens are considered.

Gentamicin is one of the most used antibiotics in dairy farm cattle. It is especially used as a prophylactic measure of mastitis control through intramammary injection. Its principal resistance mechanism is mediated by the production of enzymes which transform aminoglycosides into inactive derivatives, such as acetyltranspherases, adenylyltranspherases and phosphotransferases. Modified aminoglycosides lose the ability to bind ribosomes and inhibit bacterial protein synthesis (Watanabe et al., 2009). Specific staphylococcal resistance to gentamicinis mediated by a bifuntional enzyme that acts as both acetyltranspherase and adenylyltranspherase. This enzyme is codified by the genes *aac* (*6'*)-*Ie* + *aph* (2") which are transported in transposon Tn4001 located in plasmids of pSK1 family, conjugative plasmids pSK23 and in the chromosome (Udo & Dashti, 2000). Genetic elements Tn4001 are disseminated in *S. aureus* and CNSs. There is little information about its occurrence in staphylococci of animal origin (Lange et al., 2003).

3.4 Growth promoters

Antibiotic use in sub therapeutic levels as growth promoters is still common in Brazilian animal production. Defenders of this model believe that antimicrobial abolishment will result in higher morbidity, with a consequent raise of antimicrobial therapeutic use and consequently higher mortality. Also they think that it will directly implicate the efficiency of productivity as animals without growth promoters have a higher food consumer to achieve the same weight gain.

On the other hand, the European Economic Community established severe restrictions for products presenting antimicrobial residues defending the idea that this sub therapeutic use contributes to a positive selective pressure and to the spread of antimicrobial resistance genes between different pathogens. European Market defends that efficient animal handling is sufficient to control the infectious diseases and that avoid the probability of antimicrobial therapeutic failure. It is a highly controversial subject of extreme importance in a world concerned to the need of the improvement of food production. The experience of avoparcin use as growth promoter in some European countries and the consequent dissemination of a crossed-resistance to vancomicin in *Enterococcus faecium* and *E. faecalis* seems to be related to the adoption of these restrictive measures (Aarestrup et al., 1996)

Since 2003, Brazil instituted a work group in order to analyze and evaluate the use of substances such as carbadox, olaquindox, bacitracin zinc, spiramycin, virginiamycin and tylosin phosphate as animal feed additives products. In 2005, it also included the evaluation of avilamycin, flavomycin, enramycin, monensin and maduramycin.

The most efficient alternative to the antimicrobial indiscriminate use are probiotics. Probiotic acts in a significantly different mechanism from antimicrobials. They are thought to improve intestinal microbial balance through favoring the elimination of pathogenic bacteria and the proliferation of non pathogenic organisms. As a consequence it contributes to growth promotion without enhance antimicrobial resistance.

4. Advances in the field of nucleic acid-based techniques for the identification/typing and detection of antibiotic resistant *Staphylococcus* species

The importance of being able to identify staphylococci species routinely in clinical laboratories is increasing. However, the exact identification of CNS is not easy, because the biochemical traits of the species are very similar and many clinical isolates show intermediate traits. Additionally, the use of commercial identification kits to identify staphylococci does not include all *Staphylococcus* species, and their reliability for certain species is not sufficient. Molecular methods of identification seem to be the key to fulfill these spaces, as gene specific markers are being recognized. In the same way, molecular techniques have been developed in order to improve the detection of antibiotic resistant bacterial strains. So, nucleic acid-based detection systems offer rapid and sensitive methods to detect the presence of resistance genes and play a critical role in the elucidation of resistance mechanisms. This topic will discuss the variety of nucleic-based techniques used for diagnostic applications and demonstrate that no universal technique exists which is optimal for detection of specific genes. The choice of a particular technique is also dependent on the information required or the targets under consideration, but some techniques are more favored than others.

The advantages of genotypic detection of antibiotic resistance and bacterial characterization include: (i) The search for a defined resistance determinant; (ii) Independence upon phenotypic categories such as susceptibility, intermediate susceptibility and resistance for which breakpoints may vary between countries; (iii) Detection of low-level resistance which is difficult to detect using phenotypic methods; (iv) Reduction of the detection time through its performance directly with clinical specimens. This is particularly important for difficult-to-culture organisms; (v) Reduction in detection time of slow growth of the organism; (vi) More precise and fast therapeutic predictions; (vii) Minor biohazard risk once it is not necessary to propagate by culture of a microorganism (Sundsfjord et al., 2004).

On the other hand, the genotypic approach contains certain limitations and pitfalls: (i) It is based on screening for resistance determinants whereas antimicrobial therapy is preferably based on the detection of susceptibility; (ii) You can only screen for what you already know so it does not take into account new resistance mechanisms; (iii) There are silent genes and pseudogenes that may cause false-positive results. (iv) It may detect not clinically relevant resistance genotypes; (v) Mutations in primer binding sites can generate false-negative results; (vi) It presents low clinical sensitivity when performed directly on mixed microbial samples due to inhibition of nucleic acid amplification or a limited number of targets; (vii) Regulatory mutations that affect gene expression are not detected unless a quantitative measurement of the specific mRNA is targeted; (viii) Unlike for conventional culture-based susceptibility test methods, no standards exist for performing genetic testing methods (Sundsfjord et al., 2004).

Nucleic acid-based technology can be divided into hybridization systems and amplification systems, although most amplification technologies are also partly based on hybridization technology.

In hybridization, the DNA in a sample is rendered single stranded and allowed to combine with a single-stranded probe. Early hybridizations were performed with target DNA immobilized on a nitrocellulose membrane, but nowadays a variety of different solid supports are used. After binding of the target, the probe can hybridize. Probes can be labeled with a variety of reporters, including radioactive isotopes, antigenic substrates, enzymes or chemiluminescent compounds. Current modalities of hybridization DNA or RNA that have been used to detection of antimicrobial resistance in *Staphylococcus* spp. are Southern and Northern Blotting, FISH (Fluorescence *In Situ* Hybridization), microarray and Branched DNA (bDNA).

In Southern blotting, DNA becomes immobilized on a membrane and can be used as a substrate for hybridization analysis with labelled DNA or RNA probes that specifically target individual restriction fragments in the blotted DNA (Southern, 1975). The major difference between Southern and Northern blotting is that in the latter, RNA, rather than DNA, is immobilized in the membrane. The Southern blotting techniques was utilized to detect *mec*A gene in *Staphylococcus aureus* and to evaluate the efficiency of the techniques as PCR (Bignardi et al., 1996; Lan Mo & Qi-nan Wang, 1997).

Fluorescence *In Situ* Hybridization (FISH) is a technique originally developed for clinical diagnosis (Levsky & Singer, 2003). This approach applies the principle of hybridization involving the penetration of a fluorescent labeled sequence-specific nucleic acid probe into fixed cells, followed by specific binding to the complementary sequences of the target nucleic acid. It allows rapid simultaneous detection of structurally intact target genes while they are with the associated organism or particle (Bottari et al., 2006). It involves direct detection of the DNA without amplification of the target sequence and can be especially useful to detect specific bacterial community and antibiotic resistance gene (Rahube & Yost, 2010). A peptide nucleic acid fluorescence in situ hybridization (PNA FISH) (AdvanDx, Woburn, MA, USA) assay was development to rapidly detect *Staphylococcus aureus* (Forrest et al., 2006; Lawson et al., 2011). Peptide nucleic acid (PNA) molecules are pseudopeptides that obey Watson-Crick base-pairing rules for hybridization to complementary nucleic acid targets (RNA and DNA) (Nielsen et al., 1994). Due to their uncharged, neutral backbones, PNA probes exhibit favorable hybridization characteristics such as high specificities, strong affinities, and rapid kinetics, resulting in improved hybridization to highly structured targets such as rRNA. In addition, the relatively hydrophobic character of PNA compared to that of DNA oligonucleotides enables PNA probes to penetrate the hydrophobic cell wall of bacteria following mild fixation conditions that do not lead to disruption of cell morphology (Stefano & Hyldig-Nielsen, 1997).

DNA microarrays are based on the principle of hybridization which allow the mass screening of sequences. The method is based upon gene-specific probes (oligonucleotides or PCR amplicons) deposited on a solid surface like glass or a silicon chip. The test DNA is extracted, labelled and hybridized to the array. Target-probe duplexes are detected with a reporter system. Probe-target hybridization is usually detected and quantified by detection of fluorophore-, silver-, or chemiluminescence-labeled targets to determine relative abundance of nucleic acid sequences in the target (Schena et al., 1995). Microarray technology enables detection of a large number of resistance genes in a single experiment and has the potential for significant automation in a microchip format. However, a cost-effective and user-friendly format for application in antimicrobial susceptibility testing remains to be developed (Sundsfjord et al., 2004). There are many examples of the use of DNA microarray for detection of antibiotic resistance genes in staphylococcal (Cui et al., 2005; Frye et al., 2006; Garneau et al., 2010; Monecke et al., 2007; Zhu et al., 2007a). Recently, a team of scientists at the University of Dublin, the Irish National MRSA Reference Laboratory and the University of Dresden and Alere Technologies in Germany identified a new MRSA strain using high throughput DNA microarray screening. The new strain is not detected as MRSA by routine conventional and real time DNA-based polymerase chain reaction (PCR) assays commonly used to screen patients for MRSA (Shore et al., 2011).

Branched DNA (bDNA) was developed by Chiron Corp. and uses multiple hybridization sites for enzyme-coupled probes (Nolte, 1998). Target-specific probes bound to a solid surface are allowed to capture target ssDNA. A second probe is allowed to hybridize with the target. This probe has a 5′ extension that does not hybridize with the target. This extension can hybridize with a bDNA probe. This probe has a bristle-like structure. At least 15 bristles are attached to each probe, and as many as three alkaline phosphatase reporter molecules can bind to each bristle. A signal is generated by the addition of a chemiluminescent substrate. Branched DNA was used to detect *mecA* gene in *Staphylococcus* spp. culture and from blood (Kolbert et al., 1998; Zheng et al., 1999).

The amplification systems include, but are not limited to, simple and multiplex PCR, PCR-RFLP, PCR-single-strand conformation polymorphism (PCR-SSCP), DNA sequencing and real-time PCR. Amplification methods are more easily adapted in the laboratory compared to DNA probe assays and are the preferred methods for genetic detection of resistance determinants. An internal amplification control for both sample preparation and amplification is recommended to exclude false-negative results using consensus 16S rDNA primers or a more genus-or species-specific target; e.g. the *nuc* gene for *Staphylococcus aureus* (Brakstad et al., 1992; Hoorfar et al., 2004; Vannuffel et al., 1995). It is also critical that negative controls without template DNA and positive controls with defined targets be included to check for false-positive and false-negative results, respectively.

The Polymerase Chain Reaction (PCR) was first described by Mullis et al. (1987), and its first diagnostic application was published by Saiki et al. (1988). The technique became broadly used after the introduction of a thermostable DNA polymerase from *Thermus aquaticus* (Taq DNA polymerase) (Saiki et al., 1988) and the development of automated oligonucleotide synthesis and thermocyclers. PCR involves cycles of heating the sample for denaturing, annealing of the primers, and elongation of the primers. It has been the most commonly used nucleic acid amplification technique in the detection of antimicrobial genes, including *Staphylococcus aureus* (Simeoni et al., 2008).

Multiplex Polymerase Chain Reaction (Multiplex PCR) is a modification of PCR that have also been used to detection of antimicrobial genes in *Staphylococcus aureus* (Amghalia, et al., 2009; Braoios et al., 2009; Zhang et al., 2005) which consists of multiple primer sets within a single PCR mixture to produce amplicons of varying sizes that are specific to different DNA sequences. By targeting multiple genes at once, additional information may be gained from a single test run that otherwise would require several times the reagents and more time to perform.

The specificity of the amplicon can be confirmed by various methods such as restriction fragment length polymorphism (RFLP) analysis, single-strand conformational polymorphism (SSCP) analysis or DNA sequencing.

Restriction Fragment Length Polymorphism, or RFLP is a technique that exploits variations in homologous DNA sequences. It refers to a difference between samples of homologous DNA molecules that come from different locations of restriction enzyme sites. In PCR-RFLP analysis, the PCR product is digested by restriction enzymes and the resulting *restriction* fragments are separated according to their lengths by gel electrophoresis. It has been used to detect *groEL* gene in order to differentiate CNS species (Santos et al., 2007).

In PCR-single-strand conformation polymorphism (PCR-SSCP), the PCR amplication product is denatured into two single-stranded molecules and subjected to nondenaturing polyacrylamide gel electrophoresis. Under nondenaturing conditions, the single-stranded DNA (ssDNA) molecule has a secondary structure that is determined by the nucleotide sequence, buffer conditions, and temperature. PCR-SSCP is capable of detecting more than 90% of all single-nucleotide changes in a 200-nucleotide fragment (Hayashi, 1992).

DNA sequencing is almost universally performed by dideoxysequencing (Sanger et al., 1977) and is a well-known technique. Technological developments brought DNA sequencing within the capabilities of at least some diagnostic laboratories. The latest developments in nucleic acid sequence techniques, the pyrosequencing, have made the detection of mutational resistance easier by rapid DNA sequence analysis (Ronaghi et al., 1998). This technique has been used in the detection of linezolid resistance in enterococci, and to identify point mutations in 23S rRNA genes of linezolid-resistance *Staphylococcus aureus* and *Staphylococcus epidermis* (Sinclair et al., 2003; Zhu et al., 2007b) as well as rapid bacterial identification (Ronaghi et al., 2002).

The laborious post-PCR work and problems with carry-over contamination have been largely removed by the advent of real-time PCR, a powerful improvement on the basic PCR technique (Higuchi et al., 1993). The combination of fluorescent detection strategies with appropriate instrumentation enables a more accurate quantification of nucleic acids. This quantification is achieved by the measure ofthe increase in fluorescence during the exponential phase of PCR. The use of fluorescent agents and probes that only generate a fluorescence signal on binding to their target enables real-time amplification assays to be carried out in sealed tubes, eliminating the risk of carryover contamination. Different techniques are available to monitor real-time amplification. The amplification process can be monitored using nonspecific double-stranded deoxyribonucleic acid (DNA) binding dyes or specific fluorescent hybridization probes.

Four different chemistries, SYBR® Green (Molecular Probes), TaqMan® (Applied Biosystems, Foster City, CA, USA), Molecular Beacons and Scorpions® are available for real-time PCR.

Real-time PCR techniques have permitted the development of routine diagnostic applications for the microbiology laboratory (Espy et al., 2006; Mackay, 2004). Several reports have described the use of these techniques for detection of resistance determinants and surveillance of antimicrobial-resistant *Staphylococcus* spp. (Fang & Hedin, 2003; Huletsky et al., 2004; Palladino et al., 2003; Paule et al., 2005; Thomas et al., 2007; Volkmann et al., 2004). The ability to monitor the accumulating amplicon in real time is based on labelled primers, oligonucleotide probes and/or fluorescing amplicons producing a detectable quantitative signal related to the amount and specificity of the amplicon. Several improvements have been introduced. Reduced amplicon size, shorter cycling times and removal of separate post-PCR detection systems have allowed automation, reduced the detection time, and minimized the risk for carry-over contamination. Other significant technical developments include multiplex PCR assays using more than one primer set for simultaneous detection of several antimicrobial resistance genes (Depardieu et al., 2004; Martineau et al., 2000a; Sabet et al., 2006; Šeputienė et al., 2010; Suhaili et al., 2009).

4.1 Molecular Identification/Typing of *Staphylococcus* species

Earlier studies on the taxonomy of *Staphylococcus* species based on DNA-DNA reassociation indicated that in the genus there were nine distinct species groups, represented by *S. epidermidis*, *S. saprophyticus*, *S. simulans*, *S. intermedius*, *S. hyicus*, *S. sciuri*, *S. auricularis*, S. *aureus*, and *Staphylococcus caseolyticus* (Kloos & George, 1991). Several molecular targets have been exploited for the molecular identification of *Staphylococcus* species, including the 16S rRNA gene (De Buyser et al., 1992), the tRNA gene intergenic spacer (Maes et al., 1997), the heat shock protein 60 (HSP60) gene (Kwok et al., 1999), and the *femA* gene (Vannuffel et al., 1999). These targets, however, have been exploited through the technology of molecular probe hybridization, and therefore, they are useful only in laboratories that have the complete panel of probes and then only for identifying recognized *Staphylococcus* species. Further molecular targets that have been identified include the *nuc* gene, which occurs only in *S. aureus* (Brasktad et al., 1992), and a chromosomal DNA fragment specific for *Staphylococcus epidermidis* (Martineau et al., 1996).

The *rpoB*, gene encoding the highly conserved β subunit of the bacterial RNA polymerase, has previously been demonstrated to be a suitable target on which to base the identification of enteric bacteria (Mollet et al.,1997), spirochetes (Renesto et al.,2000), bartonellas (Renesto et al.,2001), and rickettsias (Drancourt & Raoult, 1999). The gene has been shown to be more discriminative than the 16S ribosomal DNA (rDNA) gene, which has also been used for identifying staphylococal bacteria (Mollet et al., 1997). In contrast to the probe hybridization technique and the RFLP approach, sequencing enables any isolate to be characterized, including new species by their phylogenetic relationships.

Other suitable targets for the molecular identification of *Staphylococcus* species that have been proposed include the *femA* gene, which was used in a multiplex PCR-reverse hybridization approach to identify 55 clinical isolates (Vannuffel et al.,1999). These, however, included only five *Staphylococcus* species, namely *S. aureus*, *S. epidermidis*, *S. hominis*, *S. saprophyticus*, and *S. simulans*. Finally, molecular identification methods for the identification of one or only a few *Staphylococcus* species have been reported for *S. saprophyticus* (Martineau et al., 2000b), *S. aureus* (Benito et al., 2000), and *S. epidermidis* (Wieser & Busse, 2000). Whole-genome DNA-DNA hybridization analysis (Svec et al., 2004) allows species identification, but the method is not suitable for routine use.

Accurate and rapid typing of *Staphylococcus aureus* is crucial to the control of infectious organisms (Naffa et al., 2005), and many different pheno- and genotyping methods have been used to distinguish their strains. Typing methods should have high and relevant discriminatory power and typeability, good reproducibility, applicability to all organisms of interest, ease of use, portability and low cost (Struelens et al., 1996). The common phenotyping techniques used for discriminating between bacteria from a single species are serotype, biotype, bacteriophage typing, or antibiogram. Techniques DNA-based such as pulsed field gel electrophoresis (PFGE), amplified fragment length polymorphism (AFLP), and multilocus sequence typing (MLST) have been many used (Melles et al., 2004; Murchan et al., 2003; Tenover et al., 1994). Other common techniques use the Polymerase Chain Reaction (PCR) targeted to specific sequences, for example ERIC-PCR; the resulting reactions yield fragments of different sizes, which can be used to discriminate between bacterial types. Sequencing an entire bacterial genome, and, using micro-array technologies, comparing strains to a reference strain (comparative genomic hybridization) is now technically feasible; however, the cost and time required limits the applicability for most epidemiologic studies (Foxman et al., 2005).

PFGE is the most commonly used method when studying local or short-term *S. aureus* epidemiology (Chung et al., 2000). PFGE involves embedding organisms in agarose, lysing the organisms in situ, and digesting the chromosomal DNA with restriction endonucleases that cleave infrequently (Finey, 1993; Goering & Winters, 1992). Slices of agarose containing the chromosomal DNA fragments are inserted into the wells of an agarose gel, and the restriction fragments are resolved into a pattern of discrete bands in the gel by an apparatus that switches the direction of current according to a predetermined pattern. The DNA restriction patterns of the isolates are then compared with one another to determine their relatedness. Multicentre studies using PFGE are now possible due to recent advances in the standardization of electrophoresis conditions (Chung et al., 2000; Oliveira et al., 2001) and the development of normalization and analysis software (Duck et al., 2003). Interpretative criteria for use in comparing complex PFGE patterns in outbreaks have been applied to non-outbreak situations to track the national and international dissemination of *S. aureus* clones (Tenover et al., 1995). The use of PFGE typing with adjusted interpretation criteria for grouping patterns with < 7 bands difference has been shown to correspond to clonal assignments made by other methods (Denis et al., 2004). The main criticisms of this technique for *S. aureus* are that PFGE may, on occasion, be too discriminatory for other than local or short-term epidemiological analyses, the arbitrary nature of the interpretive criteria used and the requirement for occasional subjective analysis of complex band patterns (Murchan et al., 2004).

Amplified fragment length polymorphism (AFLP) (Vos et al., 1995), a typing method, also documents the contribution of "accessory genetic elements" next to genome-core polymorphisms. AFLP scans for polymorphism in actual restriction sites and the nucleotides bordering these sites. As such it documents nucleotide sequence variation, insertions and deletions across entire genomes (Vos et al., 1995).

Multilocus sequence typing (MLST) (Maiden et al., 1998) has had a large impact on the field of bacterial typing and it has been used as an investigatory tool in many studies of *S. aureus* evolution and epidemiology (Aires de Sousa et al., 2003, Coombs et al., 2004, Enright et al., 2002; Mato et al., 2004). MLST characterizes bacterial isolates on the basis of sequence polymorphism within internal fragments of seven housekeeping genes, representing the stable "core" of the staphylococcal genome. Each gene fragment is translated into a distinct allele, and each isolate is classified as a sequence type (ST) by the combination of alleles of the seven housekeeping loci (Enright et al., 2002). MLST has a major advantage over PFGE as a reference method due to the unambiguous nature of DNA sequences which can be stored easily along with corresponding clinical information on each isolate in internet-linked databases. The *S. aureus* MLST website (www.mlst.net) currently contains information on > 1500 isolates from humans and animals from 40 different countries and represents a useful global resource for the study of the epidemiology of this species and the surveillance of hyper-virulent and / or antibiotic resistant clones.

The variety of molecular techniques used for diagnostic applications demonstrate that no universal technique exists which is optimal for detection of nucleic acids. The choice of a particular technique is also dependent on the information required or the targets under consideration, but some techniques are more favored than others. Hence, the genetic approach based on today's test principles cannot substitute for phenotypic methods in routine antimicrobial susceptibility testing. Novel resistance mechanisms will arise continuously or unknown pre-existing resistance genes will be mobilized from environmental reservoirs and spread under antimicrobial selection (Barlow et al., 2004). Thus, the role of traditional susceptibility testing will continue to be important. Rather the rationale for genetic assays is to complement conventional phenotypic analyses (Sundsfjord et al., 2004). Challenges that remain include the variety of point mutations or genes leading to resistance and the labor-intensive nature of current amplification methods. DNA chip technology combined with automated amplification techniques has the potential to meet these challenges. However, the development of DNA chips containing a broad range of resistance markers that are usable for many different species remains a formidable challenge and requires a broader knowledge of resistance markers than is currently available (Sundsfjord et al., 2004).

5. The relevance of surveillance for the prediction of antibiotic resistance

This topic discusses the relevance and limitations of surveillance initiatives in veterinary practice. Antibiotic resistance surveillance is based on the identification of new challenges, detection of new resistance mechanisms, monitoring the impact of new empiric antibiotic prescribing, identification of outbreaks of resistant organisms, detection of bacterial misidentification and promotion of the establishment of standards and **guidelines** for **education** and training for veterinaries, animal keepers, animal owners and the general public.

Cats and dogs represent potential sources of spread of antimicrobial resistance due to the extensive use of antimicrobial agents in these animals and their close contact with humans. Modern society has contributed to radical changes in the relationship between companion animals and humans through the years, with a significant raise in cats and dogs population and to a closer contact with humans (Guardabassi et al., 2004).

The introduction of a new drug, especially an antibiotic, has to be monitored in order to achieve its real benefit to the target audience. Recently, azithromycin was introduced to Brazilian pet market claiming to be an advantageous antimicrobial alternative to dogs and cats infections such as pyodermitis, external otitis, respiratory and urinary tract disturbs. Azithromycin have a remarkable application due to its superior pharmacokinetics properties and broad spectrum activity, including Gram-positive and negative bacteria species, intracellular pathogens and protozoan parasites· Pereira et al. (2009) evaluated the resistance to azithromycin of 225 clinical samples from different infectious sites of pet animals in order to establish the benefits of introducing this drug in veterinary therapy in Brazil since it has already been used for human therapy. Azithromycin resistance can be caused by several mechanisms, such as target modification mediated by a 23S rRNA methylase, presence of efflux pumps and drug inactivation (Lim et al., 2002). These resistance mechanisms were identified in a wide range of Gram-positive and negative bacteria, such as, *Staphylococcus* spp, *Streptococcus* spp, *Enterococcus faecium, Corynebacterium* spp, *Pseudomonas aeruginosa, Escherichia coli* and *Bacteroides* spp, all of them implicated in the etiology of household pets infections. Among them, *Staphylococcus* spp, a resident member of the normal cutaneous and mucosal microbiota of humans and animals, stands out as an important pathogen involved in several animals infectious diseases due to its wide range of virulence factors and ability to overcome antimicrobial effects (Garber, 2001). Predominant staphylococci azithromycin resistance mechanisms are that mediated to *erm*(A) and *erm*(C) determinants of 23S rRNA methylase and *mef* genes that encode efflux pumps. The *erm*(A) genes are mostly spread in methicillin-resistant strains and are borne by transposons related to Tn*554*, whereas *erm*(C) genes are mostly responsible for macrolide resistance in methicillin-susceptible strains and are borne by plasmids (Lim et al., 2002). Most of the knowledge applied to define microbiologic use and dose of azithromycin was based on *Staphylococcus aureus* assays, because this specie acts as a classical pathogen of human infections, but the frame of etiology and antimicrobial susceptibility pattern change when animal pathogens are considered.

Otherwise, gentamicin, even being the most utilized antimicrobial in bases for intramammary use, keeps its effectiveness against staphylococci isolated from mastitic milk. Those data support the idea of the importance of monitoring the impact of new/old empiric antibiotic prescribing

6. Concluding remarks

- *Staphylococcus* species distribution considers that different animal species have a different staphylococcal microbiota divided into coagulase-positive and coagulase-negative groups. In veterinary medicine, besides *S. aureus*, others coagulase-positive species are reported as important pathogens, such as *Staphylococcus intermedius*, the new specie *S. pseudintermedius*, *S. delphini*, *S. schleiferi* subsp. *coagulans* and *S. aureus* subsp. *anaerobius*. Several Coagulase-negative Staphylococci have been isolated from animal clinical specimens such as *Staphylococcus epidermidis*, *Staphylococcus simulans*, *Staphylococcus xylosus*, *Staphylococcus chromogenes*, *Staphylococcus warneri*, *Staphylococcus haemolyticus*, *Staphylococcus sciuri*, *Staphylococcus saprophyticus*, *Staphylococcus hominis*, *Staphylococcus caprae*, *Staphylococcus cohnii* subsp. *cohnii*, *Staphylococcus cohnii* subsp. *urealyticus*, *Staphylococcus capitis* subsp. *capitis* and *Staphylococcus capitis* subsp. *urealyticus*.
- *Staphylococcus aureus* is considered the most pathogenic specie, especially due to its ability to produce a large range of virulence factors that enables it to colonize different tissues of a large range of animal species, such as coagulase, slime, protein A, hemolysins. Otherwise, like *S. aureus*, the *S. intermedius* strains isolated from animals have been reported to produce an array of virulence factors, including leukotoxin, enterotoxin, and hemolysins, together with elements essential for biofilm formation.
- The epidemiological and clinical importance of Staphylococcal species is not only because of its distribution and pathogenicity but especially due to its ability to overcome antimicrobial effects. So there is a need for continued vigilance and systematic study to enlarge the understanding of its dynamic. Considering the spread of MRSA strains it is necessary to determine risk factors for animal infections, especially for household pets that live in strict contact to men, the relationship between animal and human carriage, and the genetic relationship of animal and human strains.
- hVISA or VISA phenotype, mostly MRSA, have now been reported for many countries and it is considered to be related to the bacterial cell wall thickening, a passive resistance mechanism that reduces vancomycin access to its active site. Also MRSA strains that are also VRSA have been reported in the United States. VRSA phenotype is

due to acquisition from *Enterococcus* spp. of the *vanA* operon, carried by transposon Tn1546, resulting in high-level resistance. The emergence of enterococci vancomicin-resistant strains has been related to the use of avoparcin as growth promoter in swine culture and it seemed to arise in staphylococci due to the transfer of glycopeptide- and macrolide-resistance genes by transconjugation among enterococci and from *Enterococcus faecalis* to *S. aureus.*

- The large range of molecular techniques available for use demonstrates that no universal technique exists which is optimal for detection of nucleic acids. The choice of a particular technique is also dependent on the information required or the targets under consideration. Hence, the genetic approach based on today's test principles cannot substitute for phenotypic methods in routine identification and antimicrobial susceptibility testing.
- Antibiotic resistance surveillance is based on the identification of new challenges, detection of new resistance mechanisms, monitoring the impact of new empiric antibiotic prescribing, identification of outbreaks of resistant organisms, detection of bacterial misidentification and promotion of the establishment of standards and **guidelines** for **education** and training for veterinaries, animal keepers, animal owners and the general public.

7. Future challenges

Tenover (2008) in his article "Vancomicin-resistant *Staphylococcus aureus*: a Perfect but Geographically Limited Storm?" gives us a clue that antibitioc resistance issue is not so simple answer. Science is a creative activity that request exploration and gambling. We have to be open-minded to understand that some evolutionary steps are more successful than others and the pathways to resistance are not so predictable. As Tenover (2008) said: "Predicting which resistant strains will ultimately survive and disseminate is virtually impossible; predicting that at least some strains will disseminate broadly is a certainty." The biggest challenge is keep researching in order to enhance our knowledge of the mechanisms beyond resistance, the evolutionary pathways of resistance among microorganisms, and selective pressure factors that contribute to the expression of underlying genes.

8. Acknowledgments

We are grateful to FAPERJ for Grants No. E-26/103.076/2008 and E-26/111.147/20108 and CNPq for Grant No 473140/2008-0. We express our sincere thanks to Professor Cristina Bogni and Professor Mirta Demo, Department of Microbiology, University of Rio Cuarto, Cordoba, Argentina, for providing us with technical conditions for the development of part of this work. We have no words to express our deep gratitude to Professor Elina Reinoso, Department of Microbiology, University of Rio Cuarto, Cordoba, Argentina, and Dr. José Ivo Baldani, EMBRAPA - Agrobiologia, Brazil, for helping us performing the initial PCR experiments for Shana Coelho tesis.

9. References

Aarestrup, F. M. (1995). Occurrence of glycopeptide resistance among *Enterococcus faecium* isolates from conventional and ecological poultry farms. *Microbiological Drug Resistance*. Vol.1, pp. 255–257.

Aarestrup, F.M.; Ahrens, P.; Madsen,M.; Pallesen,L.V.; Poulsen, R.L. & Westh, H. (1996). Glycopeptide susceptibility among Danish *Enterococcus faecium* and Enterococcus faecalis isolates of animal and human origin and PCR identification of genes within the *VanA* cluster. *Antimicrobial Agents and Chemotherapy*. Vol. 40, No. 8, pp. 1938-1940.

Aires de Sousa, M.; Bartzavali, C.; Spiliopoulou, I.; Sanches, I.S.; Crisostomo, M.I. & H. de Lencastre. (2003). Two international methicillin-resistant *Staphylococcus aureus* clones endemic in a university hospital in Patras, Greece. *Journal of Clinical Microbiology*. Vol. 41, pp. 2027-2032.

Amghalia, E.; Nagi, A.A.; Shamsudin, M.N.; Radu, S.; Rosli, R.; Neela, V. & Rahim, R.A. (2009). Multiplex PCR Assays for the Detection of Clinically Relevant Antibiotic Resistance Genes in *Staphylococccus aureus* Isolated from Malaysian Hospitals. *Research Journal of Biological Sciences*. Vol. 4, No. 4, pp. 444-448.

Arciola, C.R.; Baldassarri, L. & Montanaro, L. (2001). Presence of *icaA* and *icaD* genes and slime production in a collection of staphylococcal strains from catheter-associated infections. *Journal of Clinical Microbiology*. Vol.39, No.6, pp. 2151–2156.

Arthur, M.; Molinas, C.; Depardieu, F. & Courvalin, P. (1993). Characterization of Tn1546, a Tn3-related transposon conferring glycopeptide resistance by synthesis of depsipeptide peptidoglycan precursors in *Enterococcus faecium* BM4147. Journal of Bacteriology. Vol. 175, pp. 117-127.

Bannerman, T.M. *Staphylococcus*, *Micrococcus* and other catalase-positive cocci that grow aerobically. (2003). In: P. R. Murray (Ed.). *Manual of Clinical Microbiology*, Eighth Edition. Washington, DC: ASM Press, Vol. 1, pp. 384-404.

Baptiste, K.E.; Williams, K.; Willams, N.J.; Wattret, A.; Clegg, P.D.; Dawson, S.; Corkill, J.E. & O'Neill, T. (2005) Methicillin-resistant staphylococci in companion animals. *Emerging Infectious Disease Journal*. Vol. 11, pp. 1942-1944.

Barlow, R.S.; Pemberton, J.M.; Desmarchelier, P.M. & Gobius, K.S. (2004). Isolation and characterization of integron-containing bacteria without antibiotic selection. *Antimicrobial Agents and Chemotherapy*.Vol. 48, pp.838–842.

Benito, M.J.; Rodriguez, M.M.; Cordoba, M.G.; Aranda, E. & Cordoba, J.J. (2000). Rapid differentiation of *Staphylococcus aureus* from *Staphylococcus* spp. by arbitrarily primed-polymerase chain reaction. *Letters of Applied Microbiology*. Vol. 31, pp. 368-373.

Bes, V.; Guérin-Faublée, H.; Meugnier, J.; Etienne & Freney, J. (2000). Improvement of the identification of staphylococci isolated from bovine mammary infections using molecular methods, *Veterinary Microbiology*. Vol.71, pp. 287–294.

Bierbaum, G., Fuchs, K.; Lenz, W.; Szekat, C. & Sahl, H. G. (1999). Presence of *Staphylococcus aureus* with reduced susceptibility to vancomycin in Germany. *European Journal of Clinical Microbiology and Infectious Diseases*. Vol. 18, pp. 691–696.

Bignardi, G.E.; Woodford, N.; Chapman, A.; Johnson A.P. & Speller, D.C.E. (1996). Detection of the *mecA* gene and phenotypic detection of resistance *in Staphylococcus aureus* isolates with borderline or low-level methicillin Resistance. *Journal of Antimicrobial Chemotherapy*. Vol. 37, pp. 53-63.

Bottari, B.; Ercolini, D.; Gatti, M. & Neviani, E. (2006). Application of FISH technology for microbiological analysis: current state and prospects. *Applied Microbiology and Biotechnology*.Vol 73, pp. 485-494

Brakstad, O.G.; Aasbakk, K. & Maeland, J.A. (1992). Detection of *Staphylococcus aureus* by polymerase chain reaction amplification of the *nuc* gene. *Journal of Clinical Microbiology*. Vol. 30, pp. 1654-1660.

Braoios, A.; Fluminhan, J.A. & Pizzolitto, A.C. (2009) Multiplex PCR use for *Staphylococcus aureus* identification and oxacillin and mupirocin resistance evaluation. *Revista de Ciências Farmacêuticas Básica Aplicada*. Vol 30, No.3, pp. 303-307.

Brückler, J.; Schwarz, S. & Untermann, F. (1994) Staphylokokken-Infektionen und Enterotoxine Band II/I. *Handbuch der bakteriellen Infektionen bei Tieren, 2. Auflage*, Gustav Fischer Verlag Jena, Stuttgart.

CDC (1997). Reduced susceptibility of *Staphylococcus aureus* to vancomycin - Japan, 1996.*MMWR Morb Mortal Wkly Rep*. Vol. 46, pp. 624–626.

CDC (2004). Brief report: vancomycin-resistant *Staphylococcus aureus* - New York. *MMWR Morb Mortal Wkly Rep*. Vol. 53, pp. 322–323.

Chang, S.; Sievert, D.M.; Hageman, J.C.; Boulton, M.L.; Tenover, F.C.; Downes, F.P.; Shah, S.; Rudrik, J.T.; Pupp, G.R.; Brown, W.J.; Cardo, D. & Fridkin, S.K. (2003). Infection with vancomycin-resistant *Staphylococcus aureus* containing the *vanA* resistance gene. *The New England Journal of Medicine*. Vol. 348, pp. 1342-1347.

Chung, M., Lencastre, H.; Matthews, P.; Tomasz,A.; Adamsson,I.; Sousa, M.A.; Camou, T.; Cocuzza, C.; Corso,A.; Couto,I.; Dominguez, A.; Gniadkowski, M.; Goering,R.; Gomes,A.; Kikuchi, K.; Marchese,A.; Mato,R.; Melter,O.; Oliveira,D.; Palacio,R.; Sa-Leao, R.; Sanches, I.S.; Song, J.H.; Tassios, P.T. & Villari, P. (2000). Molecular typing of methicillin-resistant *Staphylococcus aureus* by pulsed-field gel electrophoresis: comparison of results obtained in a multilaboratory effort using identical protocols and MRSA strains. *Microbial Drug Resistance*. Vol. 6, pp.189-198.

Coelho, S.M.O.; Reinoso, E.; Pereira, I.A.; Soares, L.C.; Demo, M.; Bogni, C. & Souza, M.M.S. (2009). Virulence factors and antimicrobial resistance of *Staphylococcus aureus* isolated from bovine mastitis in Rio de Janeiro. *Pesquisa Veterinária Brasileira*. Vol. 29, No.5, pp. 369-374.

Coelho, S.M.O; Pereira, I.A.; Soares, L.C.; Pribul B.R. & Souza, M.M.S. (2011). Profile of virulence factors of *Staphylococcus aureus* isolated from subclinical bovine mastitis in the state of Rio de Janeiro, Brazil. *Journal of Dairy Science*. Vol. 94, No. 7, pp. 3305-3310.

Coombs, G. W.; Nimmo, G.R.; Bell, J.M.; Huygens, F.; O'Brien, G.; Malkowski, F. M. J.; Pearson, J. C. ; Stephens, A.J. & Giffard, P.M. (2004) Genetic diversity among community methicillin-resistant *Staphylococcus aureus* strains causing outpatient infections in Australia. *Journal of Clinical Microbiology*. Vol. 42, pp. 4735–4743.

Cui, L., Ma, X.; Sato, K.; Okuma, K.; Tenover, F.C.; Mamizuka, E.M.; Gemmell, C.G.; Kim, M.N.; Ploy, M. C.; El-Solh, N.; Ferraz, V. & Hiramatsu, K. (2003). Cell wall thickening is a common feature of vancomycin resistance in *Staphylococcus aureus*. *Journal of Clinical Microbiology*. Vol.41, pp. 5-14.

Cui, L.; Lian, J-Q.; Neoh, H.; Reyes, E. & Hiramatsu, K. (2005). DNA Microarray-Based Identification of Genes Associated with Glycopeptide Resistance in *Staphylococcus aureus*. Antimicrobial Agents and Chemotherapy. Vol. 49, No.8, pp. 3404–3413.

De Buyser, M. L.; Morvan, A.; Aubert, S.; Dilasser, F. & El Solh, N. (1992). Evaluation of ribosomal RNA gene probe for the identification of species and sub-species within the genus *Staphylococcus*. *Journal of Genetic Microbiology*. Vol. 138, pp. 889-899.

De Vliegher, S.; Laevens, H.; Devriese, L.A.; Opsomer, G.; Leroy, J.L.; Barkema, H.W. & De Kruif,A. (2003). Prepartum teat apex colonization with *Staphylococcus chromogenes* in dairy heifers is associated with low somatic cell count in early lactation. *Veterinary Microbiology*. Vol. 92, pp. 245–252.

Denis, O.; Nonhoff, C.; Byl, B.; Knoop, C.; Bobin-Dubreux, S. & Struelens, M. J. (2002). Emergence of vancomycin-intermediate *Staphylococcus aureus* in a Belgian hospital: microbiological and clinical features. *Journal of Antimicrobial Chemotherapy*. Vol.50, pp. 383–391.

Denis, O., Deplano, A.; Nonhoff, N.; De Ryck, R.; de Mendonca, R.; Rottiers, S.; Vanhoof, R. & Struelens, M.J. (2004). National surveillance of methicillin-resistant Staphylococcus aureus in Belgian hospitals indicates rapid diversification of epidemic clones. *Antimicrobial Agents of Chemotherapy*.Vol. 48, pp. 3625-3629.

Depardieu, F.; Perichon, B. & Courvalin, P. (2004). Detection of the *van* alphabet of enterococci and staphylococci at the species level by multiplex PCR. *Journal of Clinical Microbiology*. Vol. 42, pp. 5857–5860.

Devriese, L.A.; Vandamme, L.R. & Fameree, L. (1972). Methicillin-resistant *Staphylococcus aureus* strains isolated from bovine mastitis cases. *Zentralblatt fur Veterinarmedizin*. Vol.19, pp. 598-605.

Devriese, L.A.; Vancanneyt, M. & Baele, M. (2005). *Staphylococcus intermedius* sp. nov., a coagulase positive species from animals. *International Journal of Systematic and Evironmental Microbiology*, Vol. 55, pp. 1569-1573.

Drancourt, M. & Raoult, D. (1999). Characterization of mutations in the *rpoB* gene in naturally rifampin-resistant *Rickettsia* species. *Antimicrobial Agents of Chemotherapy*. Vol. 43, pp. 2400-2403.

Duck, W.M.; Steward, C.D.; Banerjee, S.N.; McGowan Jr., J.E. & Tenover, F. C. (2003). Optimization of computer software settings improves accuracy of pulsed-field gel electrophoresis macrorestriction fragment pattern analysis. *Journal of Clinical Microbiology*. Vol. 41, pp. 3035-3042.

Enright, M.C.; Robinson, D.A.; Randle, G.; Feil, E.; Grundmann, J.H. & Spratt B. G. (2002). The evolutionary history of methicillin-resistant *Staphylococcus aureus* (MRSA). *Proceedings of the National Academy of Sciences USA*. Vol. 99, pp. 7687–7692.

Espy, M.J.; Uhl, J. R.; Sloan, L. M.; Buckwalter, S.P.; Jones, M.F.; Vetter, E.A.; Yao, J.D.C.; Wengenack, N.L.; Rosenblatt, J.E.; Cockerill III, F.R. & Smith, T.F. (2006). Real-Time PCR in Clinical Microbiology: Applications for Routine Laboratory Testing. *Clinical Microbiology Reviews*. pp. 165–256.

Fang, H. & Hedin, G. (2003). Rapid screening and identification of methicillin-resistant *Staphylococcus aureus* from clinical samples by selective-broth and Real-Time PCR Assay. *Journal of Clinical Microbiology*. Vol.41, pp.2894–2899.

Ferraz, V.; Duse, A. G.; Kassel, M.; Black, A. D.; Ito, T. & Hiramatsu, K. (2000). Vancomycin-resistant *Staphylococcus aureus* occurs in South Africa. *South African Medical Journal*. Vol.90, pp.1113.

Forrest, G.N.; Mehta, S.; Weekes, E.; Lincalis, D.P.; Johnson, J.K. & Venezia, R.A. (2006). Impact of rapid in situ hybridization testing on coagulase-negative staphylococci positive blood cultures. *Journal of Antimicrobial Chemotherapy*. Vol. 58, pp.154–158.

Foxman, B.; Zhang, L.; Koopman.; James, S.K.; Manning, S.D. & Marrs, C.F. (2005). Choosing an appropriate bacterial typing technique for epidemiologic studies. *Epidemiologic Perspectives & Innovations*. Vol. 2, pp.10.

Frenay, H.M.E.; Theelen, J.P.G.; Schouls, L.M.; Vandenbroucke-Grauls, C.M.J.; Verhoef, J.; Van-Leeuwen, W.J. & Mooi, F.R. (1994). Discrimination of epidemic and nonepidemic methicillin-resistant *Staphylococcus aureus*, strains on the basis of protein A gene polymorphism. *Journal of Clinical Microbiology*. Vol.32, pp.846-847.

Frye, J.G.; Jesse, T.; Long, F.; Rondeau, G.; Porwollik, S.; McClelland, M.; Jackson, C.R.; Englen, M. & Fedorka-Cray, P.J. (2006). DNA microarray detection of antimicrobial resistance genes in diverse bacteria. *International Journal of Antimicrobial Agents*. Vol. 27, pp. 138–151.

Futagawa-Saito, K.; Ba-Thein, W.; Sakurai, N. &. Fukuyasu, T. (2006). Prevalence of virulence factors in *Staphylococcus intermedius* isolates from dogs and pigeons. *BMC Veterinary Research*. Vol. 2, p. 4.

Garber, R. (2001). In: Inteligência Competitiva de Mercado. Ed. Madras editora, pp. 248-249, São Paulo

García-Alvarez, L.; Holden, M.; Lindsay, H.; Webb, C.R.; Brown, D.F.J.; Curran, M.D.; Walpole, E.; Brooks, K.; Pickard, D.; Teale, M.; Parkhill, J.; Bentley, S.D.; Edwards, G.; Girvan, E.K.; Kearns, A.M.; Pichon, B.; Hill, R.L.R.; Larsen, A.R.; Skov, R.; Peacock S.J.; Maskell, D. & Holmes, M.A. (2011). Meticillin-resistant *Staphylococcus aureus* with a novel *mecA* homologue in human and bovine populations in the UK and Denmark: a descriptive study. *The Lancet Infectious Diseases*. Vol. 11, pp. 70126-70128.

Garneau, P.; Labrecque, O.; Maynard, C.; Messier, S.; Masson, L. & Harel, J. (2010). Use of a Bacterial Antimicrobial Resistance Gene Microarray for the Identification of Resistant *Staphylococcus aureus*. *Zoonoses and Public Health*. Vol. 57, pp. 94-99.

Gemmell, C. G. (2004). Glycopeptide resistance in *Staphylococcus aureus*: is it a real threat? Journal of Infectious Chemotherapy. Vol.10, pp. 69–75.

Goh, S.H.; Byrne, S.K.; Zhang, J.L. & Chow, A.W. (1992). Molecular typing of *Staphylococcus aureus* on the basis of coagulase gene polymorphisms. *Journal of Clinical Microbiology*. Vol. 30, pp. 1642-1645.

Goh, S.H.; Potter, S.; Wood, J.O.; Hemmingsen, S.M.; R Eynolds R.P. & Chow, A.W. (1996). HSP60 gene Sequences as Universal Targets for Microbial Species Identification: Studies with Coagulase-Negative Staphylococci. *Journal of Clinical Microbiology*. Vol. 34, No. 4, pp. 818-823.

Goni, P.; Vergara, Y.; Ruiz, J.; Albizu, I.; Vila,J. & Gomez-Lus, R. (2004). Antibiotic resistance and epidemiological typing of *Staphylococcus aureus* strains from ovine and rabbit mastitis. *International Journal of Antimicrobial Agents*. Vol. 23, pp. 268–272.

Griffeth, C. & Morris, D.O. (2008). Screening for skin carriage of methicillin-resistant coagulase-positive staphylococci and *Staphylococcus schleiferi* in dogs with healthy and inflamed skin. *Veterinary Dermatology*. Vol.19, pp. 142–149.

Guardabassi, L.; Loeber, M.E. & Jacobson, A. (2004) Transmission of multiple antimicrobial-resistant *Staphylococcus intermedius* between dogs affected by deep pyoderma and their owners. *Veterinary Microbiology*. Vol.98, pp. 23-27.

Hartmann, F.A.; Trostle, S.S. & Klohnen, A.A.O. (1997). Isolation of methicillin-resistant *Staphylococcus aureus* from a postoperative wound infection in a horse. *Journal of the American Veterinary Medical Association*. Vol. 211, No.5, pp. 590-592.

Hayashi, K. (1992). PCR-SSCP: a method for detection of mutations. *Genetic Analysis Techniques and Applications*. Vol. 9, pp. 73–79.

Higuchi, R.; Fockler, C.; Dollinger, G. & Watson, R. (1993). Kinetic PCR analysis: real-time monitoring of DNA amplification reactions. *Biotechnology*. Vol.11, pp.1026–1030.

Hiramatsu, K.; Aritaka, N.; Hanaki, H.; Kawasaki, S.; Hosoda, Y.; Kobayashi, I. (1997). Dissemination in Japanese hospitals of strains of *S.aureus* heterogeneously resistant to vancomycin. *The Lancet*. Vol. 350, pp. 1670-1673.

Hoorfar, J.; Malorny, B.; Abdulmawjood, A.; Cook, N.; Wagner, M. & Fach, P. (2004). Practical considerations in design of internal amplification controls for diagnostic PCR assays. *Journal of Clinical Microbiology*. Vol.42, pp.1863–1868.

Howden,B. P; Davies, J. K.; Johnson, P. D. R.; Stinear, T. P. & Lindsay Grayson, M. (2010). Reduced Vancomycin Susceptibility in *Staphylococcus aureus*, Including Vancomycin-Intermediate and Heterogeneous Vancomycin-Intermediate Strains: Resistance Mechanisms, Laboratory Detection, and Clinical Implications. *Clinical Microbiology Reviews*. Vol. 23, pp. 99–139

Huletsky, A.; Giroux, R.; Rossbach, V.; Gagnon, M.; Vaillancourt, M.; Bernier, M.; Gagnon, F.; Truchon, K.; Bastien, M.; Picard, F.J.; Van Belkum, A.; Ouellette, M.; Roy, P.H. & Bergeron, M.G.(2004). New Real-Time PCR assay for rapid detection of methicillin-resistant *Staphylococcus aureus* directly from specimens containing a mixture of staphylococci. *Journal of Clinical Microbiology*. Vol. 42, pp.1875–84.

Huxley, J.N.; Greent, M.J.; Green, L.E. & Bradley, A.J. (2002). Evaluation of the efficacy of an internal teat sealer during the dry period. *Journal of Dairy Science*. Vol. 85, pp. 551–561.

Ito, T.; Ma, X.X.; Takeuchi, F.; Okuma, K.; Yuzawa, H.; Hiramatsu, K. (2004). Novel type V staphylococcal cassette chromosome *mec* driven by a novel cassette chromosome recombinase, *ccrC*. *Antimicrobial Agents of Chemotherapy*. Vol. 48, pp.2637-2651.

Juhász-Kaszanyitzky, E.; Janosi, S.; Somogyi, P.; Dan, A.; Van Der, L.; Bloois, G.; Van Duijkeren, E. & Wagenaar, J.A. (2007). MRSA Transmission between Cows and Humans. *Emmerging Infection Disease*. Vol.13, pp. 630–632.

Katayama, Y.; Ito, T.; Hiramatsu, K. (2000). A new class of genetic element, staphylococcus cassette chromosome *mec*, encodes methicillin resistance in *Staphylococcus aureus*. *Antimicrobial Agents of Chemotherapy*. Vol. 44, No.6, pp. 1549-55.

Kim M.N.; Pai C.H. & Woo JH (2000). Vancomycin intermediate *Staphylococcus aureus* in Korea. *Journal of Clinical Microbiology*. Vol.38, pp. 3879-3881.

Kloos, W.E. & George, C.G. (1991). Identification of *Staphylococcus* species and subspecies with the Microscan Pos ID and rapid Pos ID panel systems. *Jounal of Clinical Microbiology*. Vol. 29, pp. 738-744.

Kolbert, C.P.; Arruda, J.; Varga-Delmore, P.; Zheng, X.; Lewis, M.; Kolberg, J. & Persing, D.H. (1998) Branched-DNA assay for detection of the *mecA* gene in oxacillin-resistant and oxacillin-sensitive staphylococci. *Journal of Clinical Microbiology*. Vol.36, pp.2640–2644.

Koreen L.; Ramaswamy, S.V.; Graviss, E.A.; Naidich, S.; Musser, J.M. & Kreiswirth, B.N. (2004). *Spa* typing method for discriminating among *Staphylococcus aureus* isolates: implications for use of a single marker to detect genetic micro- and macrovariation. *Journal of Clinical Microbiology*. Vol. 42, pp.792-799.

Kwok, A.Y., Su, S.C. ; Reynolds, R .P. ; Bay, S.J.; Av-Gay, Y. ; Dovichi, N. J. & Chow, A.W. (1999). Species identification and phylogenetic relationships based on partial HSP60 gene sequences within the genus *Staphylococcus*. *International. Journal of Systematic Bacteriology*. Vol. 49, pp. 1181-1192.

Lan Mo, M.D. & Qi-nan Wang, M.D. (1997). Rapid Detection of Methicillin-Resistant Staphylococci Using Polymerase Chain Reaction. *International Journal of Infectious Disease*. Vol. 2, pp.15-20.

Lange, C. C.; Werckenthin, C. & Schwarz, F. (2003). Molecular analysis of the plasmid-borne *aacA/aphD* resistance gene region of coagulase-negative staphylococci from chickens. *Journal of Antimicrobial Chemotherapy* . Vol. 51, pp.1397–1401.

Lawson, T.; Connally, R.E.; Iredell, Jonathan, R. Vemulpad, S. & Piper, J.A. (2011). Detection of *Staphylococcus aureus* With a Fluorescence In Situ Hybridization That Does Not Require Lysostaphin. *Journal of Clinical Laboratory Analysis.* Vol. 25, pp. 142–147.

Lee, J. H. (2003). Methicillin (oxacillin)-resistant *Staphylococcus aureus* strains isolated from major food animals and their potential transmission to humans. *Applied Environmental Microbiology.* Vol. 69, pp. 6489–6494.

Levsky, J.M. & Singer, R.H. (2003). Fluorescence in situ hybridization: past, present and future. *Journal of Cell Science.* Vol.116, pp. 2833-2838.

Lilenbaum, W.; Veras, M.; Blum, E. & Souza, G.N. (2000) Antimicrobial susceptibility of staphylococci isolated from otitis externa in dogs. *Letters of Applied Microbiology.* Vol 31, pp. 42-45.

Lim, J.A.; Kwon, A.R.; Kim, S.K.; Chomg, Y.; Lee, K. & Choi, E.C. (2002). Prevalence of resitance to macrolide, lincosamide and streptrogramine antibiotics in Gram-positive cocci isolated in Koream hospital. *Journal of Antimicrobial Chemotheraty.* Vol.49, pp. 489-495.

Linehan, D.; Etienne, J. & Sheehan D. (2003). Relationship between haemolytic and sphingomyelinase activities in a partially purified β-like toxin from *Staphylococcus schleiferi. FEMS Immunology and Medical Microbiology* . Vol. 36, No.1, pp. 95-102.

Ludwig, W.; Schleifer, K-H. & Whitman, W. B. 2009. Revised Road Map to the Phylum *Firmicutes. http://www.bergeys.org/outlines/Bergeys_Vol_3_Outline.pdf, pp. 1-32*

Lyon, G. J.; Mayville, P.; Muir, T.W.R. & Novick, P. (2000). Rational design of a global inhibitor of virulence response in *Staphylococcus aureus*, based in part on localization of the site of inhibition to the receptor-histidine kinase, *AgrC. The Proceedings of the National Academy of Sciences of the United States of America.*Vol. 97, pp. 13330-13335.

Mackay, I.M. (2004). Real-time PCR in the microbiology laboratory. *Clinical Microbiology and Infection.* Vol.10, pp.190–212.

Maes, N.; De Gheldre, Y.; DeRyck, R.; Vaneechoutte, M.; Meugnier, H.; Etienne, J. & Struelens, M. J. (1997). Rapid and accurate identification of *Staphylococcus* species by tRNA intergenic spacer length polymorphism analysis. *Jounal of Clinical Microbiology.* Vol 35, pp. 2477-2481.

Maiden, M.C.; Bygraves, J.A.; Feil, E.; Morelli, G.; Russell, J.E.; Urwin, R.; Zhang, Q.; Zhou, J.; Zurth, K.; Caugant, D.A; Feavers, I.M.; Achtman, M. & Spratt, B.G. (1998). Multilocus sequence typing: a portable approach to the identification of clones within populations of pathogenic microorganisms. *Proceedings of the National Academy of Sciences* USA. Vol. 95, pp. 3140–3145.

Martineau, F.; Picard, F.J. & Lansac, N. (2000). Correlation between resistance genotype determined by multiplex PCR assays and the antibiotic susceptibility patterns of *Staphylococcus aureus* and *Staphylococcus epidermidis. Antimicrobial Agents of Chemotherapy.* Vol. 44, pp.231–238.

Martineau, F.; Picard, F. J.; Menard, C.; Roy, P. H.; Ouellette, M. & Bergeron, M. G. (2000). Development of a rapid PCR assay specific for *Staphylococcus saprophyticus* and application to direct detection from urine samples. *Journal of Clinical Microbiology.* Vol. 38, pp. 3280-3284.

Martineau, F.; Picard, F.J.; Roy, P. H.; Ouellette, M. & Bergeron, M.G. (1996). Species-specific and ubiquitous DNA-based assays for rapid identification of *Staphylococcus epidermidis. Journal of Clinical Microbiology.* Vol. 34, pp. 2888-2893.

Mato, R.; Campanile, F.; Stefani, S.; Crisostomo, M.I.; Santagati, M.; Sanches, S.I. & Lencastre, H. (2004). Clonal types and multidrug resistance patterns of methicillin-resistant *Staphylococcus aureus* (MRSA) recovered in Italy during the 1990s. *Microbial Drug Resistance*. Vol. 10, pp. 106-113.

Melles, D.C.; Gorkink, R.F.; Boelens, H.A.; Snijders, S.V.; Peeters, J.K.; Moorhouse, M.J.; Van Der Spek, P.J.; Van Leeuwen, W.B.; Simons, G.; Verbrugh, H.A. & Van Belkum, A. (2004). Natural population dynamics and expansion of pathogenic clones of *Staphylococcus aureus*. *The Journal of Clinical Investigation*. Vol. 114, pp. 1732-1740.

Młynarczyk, A.; Młynarczyk, G. & Łuczak, M. (2002). Conjugative transfer of glycopeptide and macrolide resistant genes among enterococci and from *Enterococcus faecalis* to *Staphylococcus aureus*. *Med Dosw Mikrobiol*. Vol. 54, pp. 21-28.

Mollet, C.; Drancourt, M. & Raoult, D. (1997). *rpoB* gene sequence analysis as a novel basis for bacterial identification. *Molecular Microbiology*. Vol. 26, pp. 1005-1011.

Monecke, S.; Kuhnert, P.; Hotzel, H.; Slickers, P. & Ehricht, R. (2007). Microarray based study on virulence-associated genes and resistance determinants of *Staphylococcus aureus* isolates from cattle. *Veterinary Microbiology*. Vol.125, pp. 128-140.

Montesinos I.; Salido, E.; Delgado, T.; Cuervo, M. & Sierra, A. (2002). Epidemiological genotyping of methicillin resistant *Staphylococcus aureus* by pulsed field gel electrophoresis at a university hospital and comparison with antibiotyping and protein A and coagulase gene polymorphisms. *Journal of Clinical Microbiology*. Vol. 40, pp. 2119-2125.

Moon, J.S.; Lee, A.R.; Kang, H.M.; Lee, E.S.; Kim, M.N.; Paik, Y.H.; Park, Y.H.; Joo, Y.S. & Koo, H.C. (2007). Phenotypic and genetic antibiogram of methicillin-resistant staphylococci isolated from bovine mastitis in Korea. *Journal of Dairy Science*. Vol. 90, pp. 1176-1185.

Morgan, M. (2008). Methicillin-resistant *Staphylococcus aureus* and animals: zoonotic or humanosis. *Journal of Antimicrobial Chemotherapy* 62, 1181-1187.

Mullis, K.B. & Faloona, F. A. (1987). Specific synthesis of DNA *in vitro* via a polymerase-catalyzed chain reaction. *Methods in Enzymology*. Vol.155, pp. 335-350.

Murchan, S.; Kaufmann, M.E.; Deplano, A.; De Ryck, R.; Struelens, M.; Zinn, C.E.; Fussing, V.; Salmenlinna, S.; Vuopio-Varkila, J.; El Solh N.; Cuny, C.; Witte, W.; Tassios, P.T.; Legakis N.; Van Leeuwen, W.; Van Belkum, A.; Vindel A.; Laconcha, I.; Garaizar, J.; Haeggman, S.; Olsson-Liljequist, B.; Ransjo, U.; Coombes G. & Cookson, B. (2003). Harmonization of pulsed-field gel electrophoresis protocols for epidemiological typing of strains of methicillin-resistant *Staphylococcus aureus*: a single approach developed by consensus in 10 European laboratories and its application for tracing the spread of related strains. *Journal of Clinical Microbiology*. Vol 41, pp. 1574-1585.

Murchan, S.; Aucken, H.M.; O'Neill, G.L.; Ganner, M. & Cookson, B.D. (2004). Emergence, spread, and characterization of phage variants of epidemic methicillin-resistant *Staphylococcus aureus* 16 in England and Wales. *Journal of Clinical Microbiology. Vol.* 42, pp. 5154-5160.

Naffa, R.G.; Bdour, S.M.; Migdadi, & Shehabi, A.A. (2006). Enterotoxicity and genetic variation among clinical *Staphylococcus aureus* isolates in Jordan. *Journal of Medical Microbiology*. Vol. 55, No. 2, pp.183-187.

Neu, H.C. (1991). Clinical Microbiology of Azithromycin. *The American Journal of Medicine*. 91(3A), 3A-12S.

Nielsen, P. E.; Egholm, M. & Buchard, O. (1994). Peptide nucleic acids (PNA). A DNA mimic with a peptide backbone. *Bioconjugate Chemestry*. Vol. 5, pp. 3–7.

Nolte, F. S. (1998). Branched DNA signal amplification for direct quantitation of nucleic acid sequences in clinical specimens. *Advances in Clinical Chemistry*. Vol. 33, pp. 201–235.

Novick, R.P. (2000). Pathogenicity factors and their regulation. In Gram-Positive Pathogens. Fischetti, V.A., Novick, R.P.; Ferreti, J.J.; Portnoy, D.A. & Rood, J.I. (eds). *Washington, DC: American Society for Microbiology Press*. pp. 392–407.

O'Mahony, R.; Abbott, Y.; Leonard, F.C.; Markey, B.K.; Quinn, P.J.; Pollock, P.J.; Fanning, S. & Rossney, A.S. (2005) Methicillin-resistant *Staphylococcus aureus* (MRSA) isolated from animals and veterinary personnel in Ireland. *Veterinary Microbiology*. Vol. 109, pp. 285-296.

Oliveira, D.C.; Tomasz, A. & Lencastre, H. (2001). The evolution of pandemic clones of methicillin-resistant *Staphylococcus aureus*: identification of two ancestral genetic backgrounds and the associated *mec* elements. Microbial Drug Resistance. Vol. 7, pp.349-361.

Palladino, S.; Kay, I.D.; Flexman, J.P.; Boehm, I.; Costa, A.M.G; Lambert, E.J. & Christiansen, K.J. (2003). Rapid detection of *vanA* and *vanB* genes directly from clinical specimens and enrichment broths by Real-Time multiplex PCR assay. *Journal of Clinical Microbiology*. Vol. 41, pp. 2383–2386.

Palma M,; Haggar A. & Flock J. (1999). Adherence of *Staphylococcus aureus* is enhanced by an endogenous secreted protein with broad binding activity. *Journal of Bacteriology*. Vol.181, pp. 2840–2845.

Patel, R.; Uhl, J.R.; Kohner, P.; Hopkins, M.K. & Cockerill, F.R. (1997). Multiplex PCR detection of *vanA, vanB, vanC-1*, and *vanC2/3* genes in enterococci. *Journal of Clinical Microbiology*. Vol. 35, pp. 703–707.

Paule, S.M.; Pasquariello, A.C.; Thomson, R.B.; Kaul, K.L. & Peterson, L.R. (2005). Real-Time PCR Can Rapidly Detect Methicillin-Susceptible and Methicillin-Resistant *Staphylococcus aureus* Directly From Positive Blood Culture Bottles. *American Journal of Clinical of Pathology*. Vol. 124, pp. 404-407.

Pereira, I.A.; Soares, L.C.; Coelho, S.M.O.; Pribul, B.R. & Souza, M.M.S. (2009). Suscetibilidade à azitromicina de isolados bacterianos de processos infecciosos em cães e gatos. *Pesquisa Veterinária Brasileira*. Vol. 29, No. 2, pp.153-159.

Perichon, B. & Courvalin, P. (2006). Synergism between beta-lactams and glycopeptides against vanA-type methicillin-resistant *Staphylococcus aureus* and heterologous expression of the *vanA* operon. *Antimicrobial Agents of Chemotherapy*. Vol.50, pp. 3622–3630.

Pyorala,S. & Taponen, S. (2009). Coagulase-negative staphylococci: Emerging mastitis pathogens. *Veterinary Microbiology*, Vol. 134, pp. 3-8.

Rahube, T.O. & Yost, C.K. (2010). Antibiotic resistance plasmids in wastewater treatment plants and their possible dissemination into the environment. *African Journal of Biotechnology*. Vol. 9, No.54, pp 9183-9190.

Reinoso, E.B.; El-Sayed, A.; Lämmler, C.; Bogni, C. & Zschöck M. (2006). Genotyping of *Staphylococcus* aureus isolated from humans, bovine subclinical mastitis and food samples in Argentina. *Microbiological Research*. Vol. 163, pp. 314-22.

Renesto, P.; Lorvellec-Guillon, K.; Drancourt, M. & Raoult, D. (2000). *rpoB* gene analysis as a novel strategy for identification of spirochetes from the genera *Borrelia, Treponema*, and *Leptospira*. *Journal of Clinical Microbiology*. Vol. 38, pp. 2200-2203

Renesto, P.; Gouvernet, J.; Drancourt, M.; Roux, V. & Raoult, D. (2001). Use of *rpoB* gene analysis for detection and identification of *Bartonella* species. *Journal of Clinical Microbiology*. Vol. 39, pp. 430-437.

Rich, M. & Roberts, L. (2004). Methicillin-resistant *Staphylococcus aureus* isolates from companion animals. *Veterinary Research*. Vol.154, pp.310.

Ronaghi, M.; Uhlen, M. & Nyren, P. (1998). A sequencing method based on real-time pyrophosphate. *Science*, Vol. 281, pp. 363–365.

Ronaghi, M. & Elahi, E. (2002). Pyrosequencing for microbial typing. *Journal of Chromatography*. Vol. 782, pp. 67–72.

Sabet, N.S.; Subramaniam, G.; Navaratnam, P. & Sekaran, S.D. (2006). Simultaneous species identification and detection of methicillin resistance in staphylococci using triplex real-time PCR assay. *Diagnostic Microbiology and Infectious Disease*. Vol.56, pp. 13–18.

Saiki, R.K.; Gelfand, D.H.; Stoffel, S.; Scharf, S.J.; Higuchi,R.; Horn, G.T.; Mullis, K.B. & Ehrlich, H.A. (1988). Primer-directed enzymatic amplification with a thermostable DNA polymerase. *Science* Vol. 239, pp. 487–491.

Sanger, F.; Nicklen, S. & Coulson, A.R. (1977). DNA sequencing with chain-terminating inhibitors. *Proceedings of the National Academy of Sciences*. Vol. 74, pp. 5463–5467.

Santos, O.C.S.; Barros,E.M.; Bastos, M.C.F.; Santos,K.R.N.; Giambiagi-Demarval, M. (2008). Identification of coagulase-negative staphylococci from bovine mastitis using RFLP-PCR of the *groEL* gene. *Veterinary Microbiology*. Vol.130, N°1-2, pp. 134-140.

Sasaki, S.; Kikuchi,K.; Tanaka,Y.; Takahashi, N.; Kamata, S. & Hiramatsu, K. (2007). Methicillin-resistant Staphylococcus *pseudintermedius* in a veterinary teaching hospital. *Journal of Clinical Microbiology*. Vol.45, pp. 1118–1125.

Schena, M.; Shalon, D.; Davis, R.W. & Brown, P.O. (1995). Quantitative monitoring of gene expression patterns with a complementary DNA microarray. *Science*. Vol. 270, pp. 467–470.

Schmitz, F.J.; Sadurski, R.; Kray, A.; Boos, M.; Geisel, R.; Köhrer, K.; Verhoef, J.; Fluit, A.C. (2000). Prevalence of macrolide-resistance genes in *Staphylococcus aureus* and *Enterococcus faecium* isolates from 24 european University hospitals. *Journal of Antimicrobial Chemotherapy*. Vol. 45, pp. 891-894.

Schwarz, S.; Kadlec, K. & Strommenger, B. (2008). Methicillin-resistant *Staphylococcus aureus* and *Staphylococcus pseudintermedius* detected in the BfT-GermVet monitoring programme 2004–2006 in Germany. *Journal of Antimicrobial Chemotherapy*. Vol. 61, pp. 282–285.

Segal & Ron, E.Z. (1996). Regulation and organization of the *groE* and *dnaK* operons in eubacteria, *FEMS. Microbiology Letters*. Vol.138, pp. 1–10.

Šeputienė, V.; Vilkoicaitė, A.; Armalytė, J.; Pavilonis, A. & Sužiedėlienė, E. (2010). Detection of Methicillin-Resistant *Staphylococcus aureus* using Double Duplex Real-Time PCR and Dye Syto 9. *Folia Microbiologica*. Vol. 55 , No.5, pp. 502–507.

Shore,A.C.; Deasy, E.C.; Slickers, P.; Brennan,G.; O'Connell, B.; Monecke,S.; Ehricht,R. & Coleman, D.C. (2011). Detection of Staphylococcal Cassette Chromosome *mec* Type XI Carrying Highly Divergent *mecA*, *mecI*, *mecR1*, *blaZ*, and *ccr* Genes in Human Clinical Isolates of Clonal Complex 130 Methicillin-Resistant *Staphylococcus aureus*. *Antimicrobial Agents and Chemotherapy*. Vol. 55, No. 8, pp. 3765-3773.

Simeoni, D.; Rizzottia, L.; Cocconcelli, P.; Gazzola, S.; Dellaglio, F. & Torriani, S. (2008). Antibiotic resistance genes and identification of staphylococci collected from the production chain of swine meat commodities. *Food Microbiology*. Vol. 25, pp. 196–201.

Sinclair, A.; Arnold, C. & Woodford, N. (2003). Rapid detection and estimation by pyrosequencing of 23S rRNA genes with a single nucleotide polymorphism conferring linezolid resisistance in enterococci. *Antimicrobial Agents of Chemotherapy*. Vol. 47, pp. 3620–3622.

Sng, L. H.; Koh, T. H.; Wang, G. C.; Hsu, L. Y.; Kapi, M. & Hiramatsu, K. (2005). Heterogeneous vancomycin-resistant *Staphylococcus aureus* (hetero-VISA) in Singapore. *International Jounal of Antimicrobial Agents*. Vol. 25, pp. 177–179.

Soares, L. C.; Pereira, I. A.; Coelho, S.M.O.; Cunha, C.M.M.; Oliveira, D.F.B.; Miranda, A.F. & Souza, M.M.S. (2008). Caracterização fenotípica da resistência a antimicrobianos e detecção do gene *mecA* em *Staphylococcus* spp. coagulase-negativos isolados de amostras animais e humanas. *Ciência Rural*. Vol. 38, No. 5, pp. 1346-1350.

Song, J. H., Hiramatsu, K.; Suh, J. Y.; Ko, K. S. ; Ito, T.; Kapi, M.; Kiem, S.; Kim, Y. S.; Oh, W. S.; Peck, K. R. & Lee, N. Y. (2004). Emergence in Asian countries of *Staphylococcus aureus* with reduced susceptibility to vancomycin. *Antimicrobial Agents Chemotherapy*. Vol. 48, pp. 4926–4928.

Southern, E.M. (1975) Detection of specific sequences among DNA fragments separated by gel electrophoresis. *Journal of Molecular Biology*. Vol. 98, pp. 503–517.

Stefano, K. & J. J. Hyldig-Nielsen. (1997). Diagnostic applications of PNA oligomers. *In* S. A. Minden & L. M. Savage (ed.), Diagnostic gene detection & quantification technologies. IBC Library Series, Southborough, Mass.

Struelens, M. J. (1996). Consensus guidelines for appropriate use and evaluation of microbial epidemiologic typing systems. *Clinical Microbiology Infectious*. Vol.2, pp.2-11.

Suhaili, Z.; Johari, S.A.; Mohtar, M.; Abdullah, A.R.T.; Ahmad, A. & Ali, A.M. (2009). Detection of Malaysian methicillin-resistant *Staphylococcus aureus* (MRSA) clinical isolates using simplex and duplex real-time PCR. *World Journal of Microbiology & Biotechnology*. Vol. 25, pp. 253–258.

Sundsfjord, A.; Simonsen, G.S.; Haldorsen, B.C.; Haaheim, H.; Hjelmevoll, S.O.; Littauer, P. & Dahl, K.H. (2004) Genetic methods for detection of antimicrobial resistance. *Acta Pathologica, Microbiologica. et Immunologica Scandinavica*. Vol. 112, No. 11-12, pp. 815-837.

Svec, P.; Vancanneyt,M.; Sedlacek, I.; Engelbeen, K.; Stetina, V.; Swings, J. & Petras, P. (2004). Reclassification of *Staphylococcus pulvereri* Zakrzewska-Czerwinska et al. 1995 as a later synonym of *Staphylococcus vitulinus* Webster et al. 1994. *Internartional Journal of Systematic and Evolutionary Microbiology*. Vol.54, pp. 2213-2215.

Swenson, J.M.; Lonsway, D.; McAllister, S.; Thompson, A.; Jevitt, L. & Patel, J.B. (2007). Detection of *mec*A-mediated resistance using cefoxitin disk diffusion (DD) in a collection of *Staphylococcus aureus* expressing *borderline* oxacillin MICs. *Diagnostic Microbiology and Infectious Disease*. Vol. 58, pp. 33-39.

Takahashi, T.; Satoh, I. & Kikuchi, N. (1999). Phylogenetic relationships of 38 taxa of the genus *Staphylococcus* based on 16S rRNA gene sequence analysis. *International Journal of Systematic Bacteriology* Vol. 49, pp. 725–728.

Taponen, S.; Simojoki, H.; Haveri, M.; Larsen, H.D. & Pyorala, S. (2006). Clinical characteristics and persistence of bovine mastitis caused by different species of coagulase-negative staphylococci identified with API or AFLP. *Veterinary Microbiology*. Vol. 115, pp. 199-207.

Tenover, F.C.; Arbeit, R.; Archer G.; Biddle, J.; Byrne, S.; Goering, R.; Hancock, G.; Hebert, G.A.; Hill, B. & Hollis, R. (1994). Comparison of traditional and molecular methods of typing isolates of *Staphylococcus aureus*. *Journal of Clinical Microbiology*. Vol. 32, pp. 407–415.

Tenover, F.C.; Arbeit, R.D.; Goering, R.V.; Mickelsen, P.A.; Murray, B.E.; Persing, D.H. & Swaminathan, B. (1995). Interpreting chromosomal DNA restriction patterns produced by pulsed-field gel electrophoresis: criteria for bacterial strain typing. *Journal of Clinical Microbiology*. Vol. 33, pp. 2233-2239.

Tenover, F.C.; Weigel, L.M.; Appelbaum, P.C.; McDougal, L.K.; Chaitram, J.; McAllister, S.; Clark, N. Killgore, G.; O'Hara, C.M.; Jevitt,L.; Patel, J.B. & Bozdogan, B. (2004). Vancomycin-resistant *Staphylococcus aureus* isolate from a patient in Pennsylvania. *Antimicrobial Agents and Chemotherapy*. Vol. 48, pp. 275-280.

Tenover, F. C. (2008). Vancomycin-resistant *Staphylococcus aureus*: a perfect but geographically limited storm? *Clinical Infection Disease*; Vol. 46, pp. 675–677.

Thomas, L.C.; Gidding, H.F.; Ginn, A.N.; Olma, T. & Iredell, J. (2007). Development of a real-time *Staphylococcus aureus* and MRSA (SAM-) PCR for routine blood culture. *Journal of Microbiological Methods*. Vol.68, pp. 296–302.

Tiwari, H.K. & Sen, M.R. (2006). *Emergence of vancomycin resistant Staphylococcus aureus (VRSA) from a tertiary care hospital from northern part of India. Infection Disease*, Vol.6, pp. 156.

Udo, E.E., & Dashti, A.A. (2000). Detection of genes encoding aminoglycoside-modifying enzymes in staphylococci by polymerase chain reaction and dot blot hybridization. *International Journal of Antimicrobial Agents*. Vol. 13, pp. 273-279.

Vannuffel, P., Heusterspreute, M.; Bouyer, M.; Vandercam, B.; Philippe, M. & Gala, J.L. (1999). Molecular characterization of *femA* from *Staphylococcus hominis* and *Staphylococcus saprophyticus*, and *femA*-based discrimination of staphylococcal species. *Research Microbiology*. Vol. 150, pp. 129-141.

Vannuffel, P.; Gigi, J.; Ezzedine, H.; Vandercam, B.; Delmee, M. & Wauters, G.; Gala, J.L. (1995). Specific detection of methicillin-resistant *Staphylococcus* species by multiplex PCR. *Journal of Clinical Microbiology*. Vol. 33, pp.2864–2867.

Velasco, D.; Tomas, M.M.; Cartelle, M.; Beceiro, A.; Perez, A.; Molina, F.; Moure, R.; Villanueva, R. & Bou, G. (2005). Evaluation of different methods for detecting methicillin (oxacillin) resistance in *Staphylococcus aureus*. *J. Antimicrobial Chemotherapy*. Vol.55, No.3, pp. 379-382.

Volkmann, H.; Schwartz, T.; Bischoff, P.; Kirchen, S. & Obst, U. (2004). Detection of clinically relevant antibiotic-resistance genes in municipal wastewater using real-time PCR (TaqMan). *Journal of Microbiological Methods*. Vol.56, pp.277– 286.

Vos, P.R.; Hogers, M.; Bleeker, M.; Van De Lee Reijans, T.; Hornes, M.; Fritjers, A.; Pot, J.; Peleman, J.; Kuiper, M.; Zabeau, M. (1995). AFLP: A new concept for DNA fingerprinting. *Nucleic Acids Research*. Vol. 23, pp. 4407-4414.

Walther, B.; Wieler, L.; Friedrich, A.; Hanssen, A.; Kohn, B.; Brunnberg, L. & Lübke-Becker, A. (2008). Methicillin-resistant *Staphylococcus aureus* (MRSA) isolated from small and exotic animals at a university hospital during routine microbiological examinations. *Veterinary Microbiology*. Vol. 127, pp. 171–178.

Watanabe, S.; Kobayashi, N.; Quiñones, D.; Nagashima, S.; Uehara, N. & Watanabe, N. (2009). Genetic diversity of enterococci harboring the high-level gentamicin resistance gene *aac*(6')-Ie-*aph*(2'')-Ia or *aph*(2'')-Ie in a Japanese hospital. *Microbial Drug Resistance*. Vol.15, pp.185-94.

Weese, J.S. (2005) Methicillin-resistant *Staphylococcus aureus*: An emerging pathogen in small animals. *Journal of the American Animal Hospital Association*. Vol.41, pp. 150-157.

Weese J.; Caldwell, F.; Willey, B.; Kreiswirth, B.; McGeer, A.; Rousseau J. & Low, D. (2006). An outbreak of methicillin-resistant *Staphylococcus aureus* skin infections resulting from horse to human transmission in a veterinary hospital. *Veterinary Microbiology*. Vol. 114, pp. 160–164.

Weese, J.S. & Van, Duijkeren, E. (2010). Methicillin-resistant *Staphylococcus aureus* and *Staphylococcus pseudintermedius* in veterinary medicine. *Veterinary Microbiology*. Vol. 140, pp. 418-29.

Weigel, L.M.; Donlam, R.M.; Shin, D.H.; Jensen,B.; Clark, N.C.; McDougal, L.K.; Zhu, W.; Musser, K.A.; Thompson, J.; Kohlerschmidt, D.; Dumas, N.; Limberger, R.J. & Patel, J.B. (2007). High-level vancomycin resistant *Staphylococcus aureus* isolates associated with a polymicrobial biofilm. *Antimicrobial Agents of Chemotherapy*.Vol. 51, pp. 231–238

Werckenthin, C.; Cardoso, M.; Martel, J.L. & Schwarz, S. (2001). Antimicrobial resistance in staphylococci from animals with particular reference to bovine *Staphylococcus aureus*, porcine *Staphylococcus hyicus*, and canine *Staphylococcus intermedius*. *Veterinary Research*. Vol. 32, pp. 341–362.

Wettstein, K.; Descloux, S.; Rossano, A. & Perreten, V. (2008). Emergence of methicillin-resistant *Staphylococcus pseudintermedius* in Switzerland: three cases of urinary tract infection in cats. *Schweiz Arch Tierheilk*. Vo.150, pp. 339–343.

Wieser, M. & Busse, H.J. (2000). Rapid identification of *Staphylococcus epidermidis*. *International Journal of Systematic and Evolutionary Microbiology*. Vol. 50, pp. 1087-1093.

Witte, W.; Pasemann, B.; Cuny, C. (2007). Detection of low-level oxacillin resistance in *mec*A-positive *Staphylococcus aureus*. *Clinical Microbiological and Infection. Vol.* 13, No. 4, pp. 408-412.

Yilmaz, G.; Aydin, K.; Iskender, S.; Caylan, R. & Koksal, I. (2007). Detection and prevalence of inducible clindamycin resistance in staphylococci. *Journal of Medical Microbiology*. Vol. 56, pp. 342–345.

Zhang, K.; McClure, J.; Elsayed, S.; Louie, T. & Conly, J.M. (2005). Novel Multiplex PCR Assay for Characterization and Concomitant Subtyping of Staphylococcal Cassette Chromosome mec Types I to V in Methicillin-Resistant *Staphylococcus aureus*. *Journal of Clinical Microbiology*. pp. 5026–5033.

Zheng, X.; Kolbert, C.P.; Varga-Delmore, P.; Arruda, J.; Lewis, M.; Kolberg, J.; Cockerill, F.R. & Persing, D. H. (1999). Direct *mecA* Detection from Blood Culture Bottles by Branched-DNA Signal Amplification. *Journal of Clinical Microbiology*. Vol.37, pp. 4192-4193.

Zhu, L.X.; Zhang, Z.-W.; Wang, C.; Yang, H.-W.; Jiang, D.; Zhang, Q.; Mitchelson, K. & Cheng, J. (2007). Use of a DNA microarray for simultaneous detection of antibiotic resistance genes among staphylococcal clinical isolates. *Journal of Clinical Microbiology*. Vol.45, pp. 3514-3521.

Zhu, W.; Tenover, F.C.; Limor, J.; Lonsway, D.; Prince, D.; Dunne, W.M. Jr & Patel, J.B. (2007). Use of pyrosequencing to identify point mutations in domain V of 23S rRNA genes of linezolid-resistant *Staphylococcus aureus* and *Staphylococcus epidermidis*. *European Journal of Clinical Microbiology Infection Disease*. Vol. 26, No.3, pp.161-165.

Current Trends of Emergence and Spread of Vancomycin-Resistant Enterococci

Guido Werner
Robert Koch-Institute, Wernigerode Branch, Germany

1. Introduction

Enterococci are intestinal colonizers in many mammals including man, birds, reptiles and even invertebrates and are also found in diverse environments such as sewage, soil and water. They have been used for decades for food fermentation and preservation due to their metabolic properties and their capability to produce bacteriocins active against food contaminants like *Listeria*. Within the last two decades enterocococci became prominent as important hospital-acquired pathogens. Isolates of *Enterococcus faecalis* and *E. faecium* are the third- to fourth-most prevalent nosocomial pathogen worldwide. Among ICU-acquired bloodstream infections enterococci ranked second most prevalent according to data from an European project on Healthcare-Associated Infections.[1] Infections with enterococci hit the very young, the elderly and immuno-compromised patients and are thus mostly restricted to specific hospital wards like haemato-oncological, paediatric, and intensive care units. The growing number of patients at risk of acquiring an enterococcal infection is linked to an aging population, especially in industrialised countries, and an increasing application of invasive medical treatment options.

Non-susceptibility to glycopeptide antibiotics like vancomycin and teicoplanin is the key resistance characteristic in enterococci. Acquired resistance to vancomycin is mediated by various mechanisms (types VanA/B/D/E/G/L; Table 1); the *vanA* and *vanB* resistance genotypes are by far the most prevalent. The reservoir for *vanA*- and *vanB*-type resistance in humans is in *E. faecium* (Christiansen et al., 2004; Willems and van Schaik W. 2009; Johnson et al., 2010; Willems et al., 2011). Consequently, increasing rates of VRE in several European countries are due to an increasing prevalence of vancomycin-resistant *E. faecium* (VREfm). Ampicillin- and/or vancomycin-resistant *E. faecalis* (VREfs) are still rare. Defined clonal groups of *E. faecium* show an enhanced capacity to disseminate in the nosocomial setting and are thus called epidemic or hospital-acquired (Top et al., 2008a; Willems and van Schaik W. 2009; EARSS 2009; Willems et al., 2011). These strains can be assigned to distinct clonal groups or complexes based on various molecular typing schemes and subsequent phylogenetic analyses (Willems and van Schaik W. 2009; Willems et al., 2011). Hospital-acquired *E. faecium* are mostly ampicillin-resistant, partly high-level ciprofloxacin-resistant

[1] http://www.ecdc.europa.eu/en/publications/Publications/1011_SUR_Annual_Epidemiological_Report_on_Communicable_Diseases_in_Europe.pdf

and possess additional genomic content (accessory genome), which includes putative virulence traits such as a gene for an enterococcal surface protein, *esp*, genes encoding different cell wall-anchored surface proteins, a putative hyaluronidase gene, hyl_{Efm} and a gene encoding a collagen-binding protein, *acm* (Willems et al., 2001; Leavis et al., 2007; Hendrickx et al., 2007; Hendrickx et al., 2008; Heikens et al., 2008; Sillanpaa et al., 2008; Nallapareddy et al., 2008; Hendrickx et al., 2009; van Schaik et al., 2010; Laverde Gomez et al., 2010; van Schaik and Willems 2010).

2. Natural antibiotic resistances in *E. faecium* and *E. faecalis*

Besides their huge arsenal of insusceptibilities to physicochemical and environmental stresses (Murray 1990; Facklam et al., 2002) *E. faecalis* and *E. faecium* possess a broad spectrum of natural antibiotic resistances (Klare et al., 2003; Arias and Murray 2008).

All enterococci are naturally (intrinsically) resistant to the following agents: semisynthetic penicillins (e.g., oxacillin), cephalosporins of all classes, monobactams and polymyxins. Aminoglycosides show insusceptibility at a low level, most probably due to a reduced uptake. At least, isolates of *E. faecalis* and *E. faecium* show clindamycin insusceptibility; in *E. faecalis* this is known to be associated with the expression of an ABC porter designated Lsa (Singh et al., 2002; Singh and Murray 2005). Presence of Lsa also mediates resistance to streptogramin A which in the consequence also leads to resistance to the streptogramin A/B combination (quinupristin/dalfopristin). Insusceptibility to fluoroquinolones, for instance to ciprofloxacin, is most probably associated with expression of chromosomal *qnr* homologues (functionally proven only for *E. faecalis,* (Arsene and Leclercq 2007; Rodriguez-Martinez et al., 2008). Isolates of *E. faecalis* are also resistant to mupirocin, a property that can be used to differentiate them from other enterococcal species. Although not reaching the level of what is defined as resistance, penicillins are generally less active against enterococci than against streptococci and in addition, *E. faecium* is less susceptible than *E. faecalis* (Murray 1990).

3. Acquired antibiotic resistances in *E. faecium* and *E. faecalis*

The already tremendous spectrum of intrinsic insusceptibilities of *E. faecalis* and *E. faecium* is accompanied by the potential to acquire resistance to all antimicrobial drugs available (Tenover and McDonald 2005; Rice 2006). Therapeutically important are resistance properties against penicllin/ampicillin, gentamicin/streptomycin and glycopeptides (vancomycin/teicoplan) as well as resistances against antibiotics of last resort quinupristin/dalfopristin [*E. faecium*], linezolid and tigecycline (maybe also daptomycin).

3.1 Penicillin resistance

Penicillin resistance in *E. faecalis* is rare and if occurring linked to certain clonal lineages expressing beta-lactamases similar or identical to the *S. aureus* penicillinase (Nallapareddy et al., 2005; Ruiz-Garbajosa et al., 2006; McBride et al., 2007). Penicillin resistance in *E. faecium* is mediated via point mutations in the housekeeping *pbp5* gene leading to reduced penicillin binding to the expressed protein (Jureen et al., 2004; Rice et al., 2004; Rice et al., 2009). Mutated *pbp5'* was also found as an integral part of conjugative transposons, like Tn*5382,* thus encoding transferable ampicillin and VanB-type vancomycin resistance (Carias et al.,

1998; Valdezate et al., 2009). Results of a recent study suggested additional factors independent from pbp5′ contributing to acquired ampicillin resistance in hospital strains of *E. faecium* (Galloway-Pena et al., 2011).

3.2 Aminoglycoside resistance

Only the two aminoglycosides gentamicin and streptomycin exemplify a synergistic effect when given in combination with a cell-wall active agent like a penicillin or a glycopeptide (Murray 1990). Certain aminoglycoside-modifying enzymes mediate acquired high-level gentamicin and streptomycin resistance in *E. faecalis* and *E. faecium*. The *aac6′-aph2″* (*aac(6′)-Ie-aph(2″)-Ia*) gene encodes a bifunctional enzyme encoding high-level resistance to all aminoglycosides except streptomycin (Horodniceanu et al., 1979). It is the most prevalent form of acquired gentamicin resistance in both species and associated with homologues of transposon Tn*4001*/Tn*5281* flanked by two copies of IS*256* and most probably originating from staphylococci (Casetta et al., 1998; Hallgren et al., 2003; Saeedi et al., 2004). Gentamicin resistance may also be encoded by other determinants such as *aac(6′)-Ii*, *aph(2″)-Ie*, and *ant(6)-Ia* (Jackson et al., 2004; Jackson et al., 2005; Zarrilli et al., 2005; Mahbub et al., 2005). High-level streptomycin resistance is encoded by the *aadE* gene which is an integral part of a multi-resistance gene cluster *aadE-sat4-aphA* encoding streptomycin-streptothricin-kanamycin resistance. The *sat4* gene encoding streptothricin (nourseothricin) resistance has first been described in *Campylobacter coli* (Jacob et al., 1994; Bischoff and Jacob 1996). In staphylococci the *aadE-sat4-aphA* gene cluster is flanked by two copies of IS*1182* constituting transposon Tn*5405* (Derbise et al., 1996; Derbise et al., 1997). The *aadE-sat4-aphA* gene cluster is widespread among many Gram-positive genera and it remains to be speculative where this gene clusters originates from and subsequently spread to other bacteria. Strikingly, in *S. aureus* the *sat4* gene possesses a point mutation within the coding region leading to a pre-mature STOPP codon; whereas it is complete and functional in *C. coli* and enterococci encoding detectable streptothricin (nourseothricin) insusceptibility (Schwarz et al., 2001; Werner et al., 2001a; Teuber et al., 2003; Werner et al., 2003a).

3.3 Fluoroquinolone resistance

The targets of fluoroquinolones are topoisomerases II and IV, and mutational changes among genes encoding mainly subunits A and to a lesser extent also subunits B are associated with increased MICs to ciprofloxacin and other fluoroquinolones (Hooper 2002; Jacoby 2005). Topoisomerase II (DNA gyrase) appears to be the primary target in Gram-negative bacteria and topoisomerase IV is the primary target in Gram-positive bacteria. Corresponding in vitro selection models were also described for enterococci; however, results are somehow conflicting regarding the primary target in *Enterococcus* spp. and the necessity of specific mutations in one or both A subunit genes to confer what is specified as high-level ciprofloxacin resistance (Onodera et al., 2002; Oyamada et al., 2006a; Oyamada et al., 2006b). Molecular studies with high-level ciprofloxacin-resistant clinical isolates revealed mutations in both A subunits associated with different levels of ciprofloxacin resistance, whereas mutations in *gyrB* and *parE* alleles were only infrequently found (Woodford et al., 2003; Leavis et al., 2006; Valdezate et al., 2009; Werner et al., 2010a).

3.4 Resistance to macrolides, lincosamides and streptogramin B (MLS_B)

Resistance to MLS_B antibiotics is encoded by the widespread *erm*(B) gene and only occasionally via *erm*(A) or *erm*(C)(Roberts et al., 1999). Erm ("erythromycin resistance methylases") confer resistance by modifying nucleotide A2058 of the bacterial 23S rRNA (methylation) leading to resistance to MLS_B antibiotics. The resistance phenotype is partly overlapping with the spectrum of natural resistances in *Enterococcus* (lincosamides); however, *erm* genes are widespread among other Gram-positive bacteria such as streptococci, staphylococci, lactococci and lactobacilli where the corresponding resistance phenotype has been studied in detail (Shaw and Clewell 1985; Novick and Murphy 1985). Naturally, the expression of *erm* genes is induced with low levels of 14-membered macrolides (i.e. erythromycin) and results in cross-resistance to all 14-, 15- and 16-membered macrolides, lincosamides and streptogramin B antibiotics. Induction results from translational relief of attenuation (Horinouchi and Weisblum 1980). Constitutive expression of *erm*(A) and *erm*(C) in staphylococci results from deletions, duplications, and point mutations in the region of the leader peptide, and is selected for by the use of non-inducing antibiotics (Werckenthin et al., 1999; Werckenthin and Schwarz 2000; Schmitz et al., 2001). In enterococci *erm*(B) is constitutively expressed (Werner et al., 2000; Werner et al., 2002; Martel et al., 2003); however, corresponding modifications in the leader peptide could not be linked unambiguously to cause the corresponding phenotype in wildtype isolates (Rosato et al., 1999; Werner et al., 2002). Recent in vitro studies have linked point mutations rather than deletions and duplications to a corresponding *erm*(B) constitutive phenotype in enterococci (Min et al., 2008). The *erm*(B) determinant is widespread among enterococci, especially *E. faecium* and *E. faecalis* and is part of many multi-resistance plasmids and often linked to Tn*1546*-like *vanA* elements (Aarestrup et al., 2000a; Borgen et al., 2002; Werner et al., 2003a; Werner et al., 2003b; Manson et al., 2003b; Werner et al., 2006; Laverde Gomez et al., 2010). Another mechanism mediating macrolide (and streptogramin B) resistance is conferred by the *msrA-C* genes (Reynolds et al., 2003; Kerr et al., 2005) whereas *msrC* is discussed as a species-specific property in *E. faecium* (Singh et al., 2001; Werner et al., 2001b) shown to encode erythromycin and clarithromycin resistance when expressed in *S. aureus* (Reynolds and Cove 2005). Staphylococcal efflux pumps of the Vgb-type encoding for streptogramin type B resistance remain extremely rare among *E. faecium* (Werner et al., 2002).

3.5 Streptogramin A resistance

Two types of acetyltransferases VatD and VatE mediate resistance to streptogramin A in enterococci, mainly *E. faecium* (Werner et al., 2002). *E. faecalis* is naturally resistant to streptogramin A and thus the synergism of the A and B streptogramin combination is abolished (Werner et al., 2002; Singh et al., 2002). However, a few studies described also *vat* genes to be prevalent among related lactic acid bacteria (Gfeller et al., 2003) and *E. faecalis* isolates (Simjee et al., 2002; Jones and Deshpande 2004). Their relevance for increasing the level of streptogramin resistance in *E. faecalis* is unclear; nevertheless, resistance determinants could further spread to *E. faecium* and other enterococcal species thus rendering their level of streptogramin susceptibility. Staphylococcal efflux pumps of the Vga-type encoding for streptogramin type A resistance remain unknown to *E. faecium* (Werner et al., 2002); except for a single Korean *E. faecium* isolate described recently harbouring streptogramin A resistance genes *vgaD* and *vatG* on a plasmid fragment encoding for a new efflux pump type and a new streptogramin acetyltransferase, respectively (Jung et al., 2010).

3.6 Tetracycline resistance

Resistance to tetracyclines is mediated via different acquired *tet* genes encoding proteins mediating (a) ribosomal protection [*tet*(O)/(M)(S)] or efflux [tet(K)/(L)] [(Roberts 2005). Most wide-spread among enterococci and best studied are elements containing *tet*(M). The *tet*(M) gene mostly resides on conjugative transposons of the Tn*916*/Tn*1545*- or Tn*5397*-types that possess a very wide host range and can exist in several functional copies thus supporting flexibility and recombinational events within a given bacterial genome (Thal et al., 1997; Roberts et al., 2001; Agerso et al., 2006; Rice et al., 2007; Boguslawska et al., 2009; de Vries et al., 2009; Rice et al., 2010; Roberts and Mullany 2011).

3.7 Linezolid resistance

Linezolid is a synthetic oxazolidinone antibiotic of last resort active against multi- and vancomycin-resistant enterococci. It inhibits first steps of ribosome formation [108]. Although being fully synthetic, resistance is selected under therapy and is in relation to the duration of treatment (Prystowsky et al., 2001; Pai et al., 2002; Ruggero et al., 2003; Seedat et al., 2006). However, a few reports documented resistance detection independent from linezolid treatment (Rahim et al., 2003; Bonora et al., 2006). Resistance results from point mutations in 23S rRNA, preferably at position 2576 (G > T)(Sinclair et al., 2003; Werner et al., 2004; Qi et al., 2006; Werner et al., 2007a) and the level of resistance is dependent on the number of mutated alleles per genome (Marshall et al., 2002; Lobritz et al., 2003; Bourgeois-Nicolaos et al., 2007; Boumghar-Bourtchai et al., 2009). Once established, resistance levels quickly arise due to recombinational exchange of mutated 23S rDNA alleles under selective pressure (Willems et al., 2003; Boumghar-Bourtchai et al., 2009). In *Staphylococcus*, a Cfr methylase is able to modify 23S rRNA at position A2503 leading to cross-resistance to a number of antibiotics including oxazolidinones (Toh et al., 2007); however, the corresponding *cfr* gene has not been described in enterococci so far.

3.8 Tigecycline resistance

Tigecycline is a member of a new tetracycline antibiotic class containing a 9-tert-butylglycylamido group named glycylcyclines and acts similar to tetracyclines by inhibiting protein biosynthesis. Tigecycline is active against many Gram-negative and Gram-positive bacteria including isolates of Enterococcus. International surveillance studies revealed in general potent in vitro activity; non-susceptible isolates are very rare. A single resistance mechanism linked to an overexpression of an oxygen- and flavin-dependent monooxygenase, TetX, originating from anaerobic bacteria of the genus Bacteroides was described (Moore et al., 2005). A single tigecycline-non-susceptible *E. faecalis* isolate was reported recently and investigated in greater details; however, the underlying resistance mechanism could not been determined (Werner et al., 2008b).

3.9 Daptomycin resistance

Daptomycin is a cyclic lipopeptide antibiotic disrupting cell membrane composition, function and permeability (Straus and Hancock 2006a; Straus and Hancock 2006b). Daptomycin is active against many Gram-positive bacteria. Its in vivo activity against enterococci is still debatable (Canton et al., 2010). Daptomycin resistance developed under therapy in bacteria other than enterococci and was multifactorial and is still not understood completely (Fischer et al., 2011).

3.10 Vancomycin resistance

Glycopeptide antibiotics consist of a peptide ring to which several sugars are covalently linked. They are produced by actinomycetes and have a quite complex structure. This voluminous structure prevents penetration through the outer membrane of Gram-negative bacteria limiting their therapeutic use only to treat infections with Gram-positive bacteria. Two naturally produced antibiotics have been introduced into antimicrobial treatment, vancomycin and teicoplanin; the latter only outside North-America. Three semisynthetic progenitors designated as lipoglycopeptides or glycolipopeptides (dalbavancin, telavancin, oritavancin) are promising new candidate drugs partially active against multi-resistant and also vancomycin-(intermediate)resistant bacteria (Zhanel et al., 2010a). The primary target of glycopeptides is the C-terminal D-Alanyl-D-Alanine ending of the peptide side chain of the enterococcal peptidoglycan cell wall precursor. Due to steric hindrance the cell wall synthesis enzymes like transglycosylases, transpeptidases and D,D-carboxypeptidases cannot access their target and cell wall synthesis stops. Vancomycin and related glycopeptides act as dimers (Batchelor et al., 2010).

Enterococci were the first pathogens that showed acquired vancomycin resistance and corresponding strains have been isolated from clinical samples from patients in Europe and the USA in the late 1980s (Leclercq et al., 1988; Leclercq et al., 1989; Sahm et al., 1989). The corresponding resistance phenotypes which included inducible resistance to all known glycopeptides or vancomycin only were designated VanA and VanB, respectively. In fact, the structure, localization and functional interplay of the resistance determinants arranged in specific transposable elements in enterococci has been studied with some of the first identified VRE: *E. faecium* BM4147 (*vanA* genotype) from France (Leclercq et al., 1988) and *E. faecalis* V583 (*vanB* genotype) from the USA (Sahm et al., 1989). The latter became prominent as the first *Enterococcus* isolate that has been completely sequenced (Paulsen et al., 2003). To date eight types of acquired vancomycin resistance in enterocooci are known having a related mechanism of resistance and a similar resistance gene cluster composition but show major differences in prevalence (**Table 1** and **Figure 1;** see recent reviews for details: (Courvalin 2005; Courvalin 2006; Werner et al., 2008a; Werner et al., 2008c). Worldwide by far the most prevalent type is *vanA* followed by *vanB*. The *vanA* gene is an integrated part of Tn*1546* or derivatives of this transposon which are usually located on transferable plasmids (Werner et al., 2008a; Werner 2011). *vanB* could be subdivided into three different allele types (*vanB1-3*) with *vanB-2* the most prevalent type worldwide. The *vanB* alleles are part of Tn*1547* or the conjugative transposon Tn*1549/5382* which are mainly chromosomally located and less frequently, on plasmids (Werner et al., 2006; Zheng et al., 2009; Hegstad et al., 2010; Bjorkeng et al., 2011). The main clinical relevant reservoir of *vanA* and *vanB* elements is in *E. faecium*, at least in Europe, Northern and Latin America and Southeast Asia, although they have also been observed occasionally in other enterococcal species (see **Table 1** and below)(Zirakzadeh and Patel 2005; Werner et al., 2008a; Werner 2011).

4. The *van* alphabet in *Enterococcus* spp.

Non-susceptibility to glycopeptide antibiotics like vancomycin and teicoplanin is the key resistance characteristic in enterococci. Acquired resistance to vancomycin is mediated by

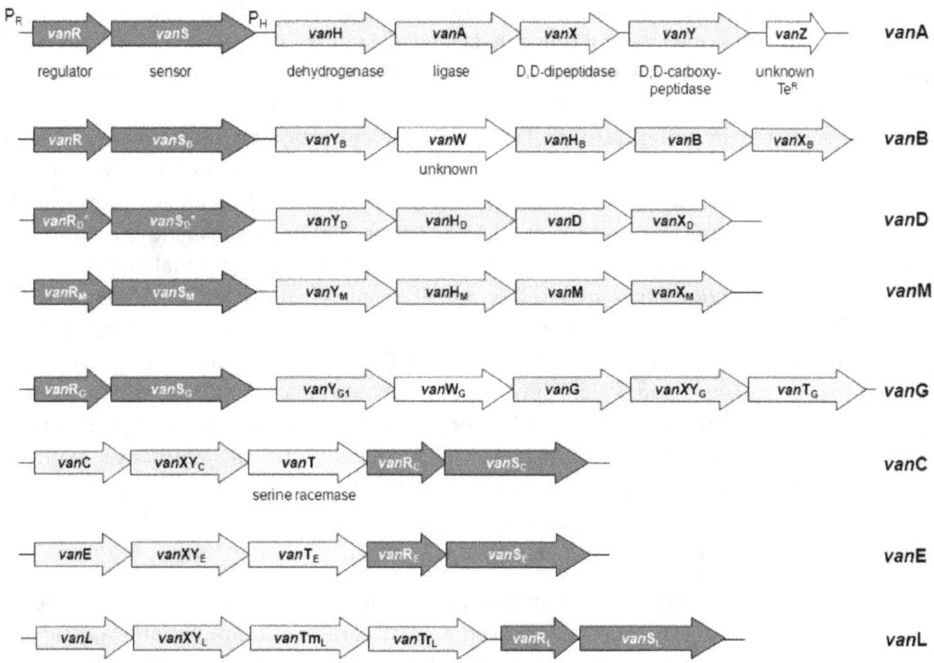

The image of the *vanC* cluster from naturally vancomycin-resistant *E. gallinarum* and *E. casseliflavus* were introduced for reasons of comparability. Arrows indicate genes and arrowheads show the direction of transcription. Colour codes represent functional groups: red, two-component regulatory system; yellow, core genes essential for resistance expression; grey, serine racemase; white, additional or unknown function. Arrow lengths are according to the size of the genes but are not drawn to scale. * denotes point mutations leading to constitutive expression of the VanD-type resistance. For further details see main text or references given there. P_R and P_H are promoters preceding *vanR* and *vanH*, respectively. Te^R, gene associated with decreased teicoplanin susceptibility. For references see legend of Table 1.

Fig. 1. **Structure and composition of the vancomycin resistance clusters *vanA-M*** (see also Table 1). Types *vanA, vanB, vanD* and *vanM* encode D-Ala-D-Lac mediated resistance; types *vanC, vanE, vanL* and *vanG* (also *vanN*, not shown) encode D-Ala-D-Ser mediated resistance (see text and Table for details)

various mechanisms (types VanA/B/D/E/G/L/M/N; **Table 1**); the *vanA* and *vanB* resistance genotypes are by far the most prevalent worldwide. Isolates of *E. gallinarum* and *E. casseliflavus* (= E. *flavescens*) are naturally (intermediate-)resistant to vancomycin at low levels (MIC = 8 mg/L) by a so-called VanC-1/-2 type.

4.1 The VanA resistance type

The original *vanA* gene cluster contains nine genes which are arranged in a transposon structure (Arthur et al., 1993)(Fig. 1). It is flanked by two incomplete inverted repeats and possesses two coding sequences located at the left end (ORFs 1 and 2 not shown in Fig. 1). Their putative proteins show similarity with resolvases and transposases of various transposons or plasmids. The entire element is 10,981 bp and designated Tn*1546,* belonging to transposons of the Tn*3*-family.

Expression of VanA type vancomycin resistance in enterococci is inducible via a complex mechanism. The consequences of a prevented cell wall synthesis are sensed by an as yet still unknown mechanism via a membrane-associated, Tn*1546*-encoded protein VanS possessing a histidine kinase in its cytoplasmatic C-terminus. The histidine kinase function of the VanS protein is activated by autophosphorylation and the corresponding phosphate moiety is transferred to a cytoplasmic response regulator called VanR also encoded on Tn*1546*. Phosphorylated VanR functions as a transcriptional activator binding at two promoters P_R and P_H in the *vanA* resistance gene cluster (Arthur et al., 1997). This leads to the expression of two transcripts of genes that are arranged in an operon structure and that are transcribed unidirectional: the *vanRS* genes themselves and the gene cluster *vanHAXYZ* (**Fig. 1**). The proteins VanH, VanA and VanX possess essential functions for the expression of glycopeptide resistance whereas VanY encodes a D,D-carboxypeptidase contributing to elevated resistance levels and a VanZ protein of unknown function but contributing by an unknown mechanism to low-level teicoplanin resistance (**Fig. 2**)(Arthur and Quintiliani, Jr. 2001). VanA type vancomycin resistance is mediated via an alternative pathway synthesizing cell wall precursors ending in D-Alanyl-D-Lactat (D-Ala-D-Lac) showing reduced glycopeptide binding and down-shifting of the regular cell wall synthesis by house-keeping enzymes (**Fig. 1**)(Arthur and Quintiliani, Jr. 2001).

Studies about characterizing the structure of *vanA* gene clusters in enterococci of different ecological and geographical sources displayed a great variety of point mutations, deletions (in/of non-essential genes), and insertions of additional DNA (mainly IS elements) leading to modified and fragmented Tn*1546* structures. This can be demonstrated in a phylogenetic tree of relatedness exemplifying elements typically identified in US hospital VRE, poultry VRE, pig/human commensal VRE, etc. (Willems et al., 1999; Werner et al., 2006). Typing of *vanA* gene clusters allows elucidating ways of spread of vancomycin resistance either via clonal spread of VRE or via horizontal gene transfer between different enterococci (Park et al., 2007; Sletvold et al., 2010).

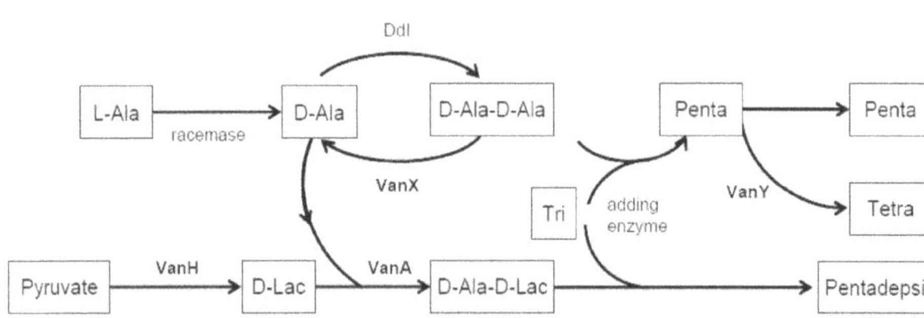

Ddl, D-Ala:D-Ala ligase; adding enzyme is a synthetase; Penta, L-Ala-γ-D-Glu-L-Lys-D-Ala-D-Ala; Pentadepsi, L-Ala-γ-D-Glu-L-Lys-D-Ala-D-Lac; Tetra, L-Ala-γ-D-Glu-L-Lys-D-Ala; Tri, L-Ala-γ-D-Glu-L-Lys. Penta, Tetra, Tri, Pentadepsi represent amino acid side chains linked to the enterococcal peptidoglycan disaccharide precursor N-acetyl-glucosamin-N-acetyl-muramic acid. Resistance enzymes encoded by the *vanA* cluster are shown in bold. [Figure adapted from (Courvalin 2006)].

Fig. 2. **VanA-type glycopeptide resistance.** Synthesis of an alternative, vancomycin-resistant pentadepsipeptide peptidoglycan precursor in VanA-type resistant strains.

4.2 The VanB resistance type

The typical VanB phenotype is characterized by inducible moderate vancomycin resistance levels (MICs of 8 - 64 mg/L) and teicoplanin susceptibility. *vanB* isolates with high-level vancomycin resistance have also been identified. Differences in the *vanB* gene were found and three different *vanB* ligase alleles were assigned which can be used for subtyping [*vanB*-1/-2/-3; (Dahl et al., 2003; Werner et al., 2006)]. However, the different *vanB* genotypes did not correlate with the level of vancomycin resistance. Despite being slightly different in nucleotide composition, the *vanB* cluster types 1 to 3 all resemble the core structure of the *vanA* gene cluster (**Fig. 1**). Genes of related composition and function are arranged in a similar manner, an equivalent to *vanZ* is lacking and an additional gene *vanW* of unknown function was found. Genes encoding the two-component regulatory system *vanR$_B$S$_B$* are only distantly related to their Tn*1546* counterparts and regulation of gene expression is different, because only vancomycin, but not teicoplanin, is an inducer of the *vanB* cluster. The entire transposon backbone of *vanB* clusters is different to *vanA*; distinct *vanB* cluster types are either flanked by certain IS elements or an integral part of larger mobile and/or conjugative elements that may be composed of several individual elements [Tn*1547*, Tn*1549*, Tn*5382*-like, Tn*vamp*; (Carias et al., 1998; Dahl and Sundsfjord 2003; Werner et al., 2006; Launay et al., 2006; Valdezate et al., 2009; Lopez et al., 2009)]. The conjugative *vanB* transposon Tn*1549* or its backbone is widely prevalent among *vanB* type enterococci and related Gram-positive bacteria such as *Clostridium* spp. (see chapter 5;(Launay et al., 2006; Tsvetkova et al., 2010)). Conjugative transposons have been known for a long time in *Enterococcus* and *Bacteroides* and were lately also identified in Gram-negatives. They have an important function for a wide distribution of (resistance) genes across species and genus barriers and for genomic rearrangements in bacteria in general (Rice et al., 2005; Roberts and Mullany 2009; Rice et al., 2010; Roberts and Mullany 2011).

Whereas teicoplanin does not induce VanB type resistance, constitutively resistant mutants quickly arose in vivo during therapy or in vitro after teicoplanin challenge (Baptista et al., 1999; Kawalec et al., 2001a; Kawalec et al., 2001b; San Millan et al., 2009b). Accordingly, teicoplanin treatment is not recommended for eradicating VanB VRE infections despite a correspondingly suggestive diagnostic result (teicoplanin susceptibility).

Expression via the VanB type two-component regulatory system VanR$_B$S$_B$ is differently regulated in various Gram-positive hosts. Naturally occurring VanB type *Streptococcus bovis/gallolyticus* isolates retained the VanB phenotype inducible by vancomycin only (Poyart et al., 1997; Mevius et al., 1998). Genetic constructs of *vanB* cluster elements in a *Bacillus subtilis* background did not show an inducible phenotype since VanS$_B$ was active also without vancomycin addition (San Millan et al., 2009a). In addition, it was shown that the phosphorylated regulator VanR$_B$-P was capable of binding to a number of promoter regions and thus controlling expression of genes commonly regulated by response regulators.

4.3 The VanC resistance type

The two motile species *E. gallinarum* and *E. casseliflavus* possess an intrinsic resistance to vancomycin at a low level designated VanC-1 and VanC-2, respectively. The corresponding *vanC*-type ligase gene possessed minor sequence diversity resulting in the two described subtypes *vanC*-1 and *vanC*-2 (Courvalin 2005; Courvalin 2006). The formerly third species *E.*

flavescens described as possessing a supposed *vanC*-3 gene was merged recently with the species *E. casseliflavus* (Naser et al., 2006b) thus leading to two subtypes of *E. casseliflavus* with slightly different *vanC-2/-3* subtype variants. Recently, another subtype *vanC-4* was described in another *E. casseliflavus* isolate with 93-95% nucleotide identity with *vanC-2/-3* (Naser et al., 2006a).

Resistance phenotype	VanA	VanB[2]	VanD[2]	VanE	VanG[2]	VanL	VanM	VanN[4]
MIC vancomycin in µg/ml	16 - 1000	4 - 32 (-1000)	16 - 512	8 - 32	16	8	>256	16
MIC teicoplanin in µg/ml	(4-) 16 - 512	0,5 - 1	0,5 - 64	0,5	0,5	S	0.75 / 96[3]	S
expression	inducible	inducible	constitutive	inducible	inducible	inducible	inducible	?
ligase	D-Ala-D-Lac	D-Ala-D-Lac	D-Ala-D-Lac	D-Ala-D-Ser	D-Ala-D-Ser	D-Ala-D-Ser	D-Ala-D-Lac	D-Ala-D-Ser
localization	plasmid/ chrom.	chrom./ plasmid	chrom.	chrom.	chrom.	chrom.?	plasmid	?
transferable by conjugation	+/-	+/-	-	-	+	-	+	?
Distribution among enterococcal species	*E. faecium* *E. faecalis* *E. durans* *E. hirae* *E. gallinarum*[1] *E. casseliflavus*[1] *E. raffinosus* *E. avium* *E. mundtii*	*E. faecium* *E. faecalis* *E. durans* *E. gallinarum*[1]	*E. faecium* *E. faecalis* *E. raffinosus* *E. gallinarum*[1]	*E. faecalis*	*E. faecalis*	*E. faecalis*	*E. faecium*	*E. faecium*

S, susceptible (no MIC given); [1] Acquisition of *vanA, vanB* or *vanD* genes in addition to vanC1/C2 genes - rare event; [2] subtypes exist (*vanB*1-3, *vanD*1-5, *vanG*1-2); [3] several strains exist with different teicoplanin MICs; [4] data from a presentation given by R. Leclercq, ESCMID conference on Enterococci, Barcelona/ES, 18.-20.11.2009.

Table 1. **Types of acquired vancomycin resistance in enterococci**

Nucleotide identity varied also along the other elements of the *vanC*-4 cluster with genes $vanXY_C$, $vanT_C$, $vanR_C$, and *vanSc* showing 88-93 % identity with corresponding genes of the *vanC-2/-3* cluster (see below and **Fig. 1**). VanC type resistance is mediated via a modified D-Ala-D-Ser moiety similar to VanE/G/L/N types reaching also a similar low level of resistance only (Arias et al., 2000). All these resistance types require activity of a serine racemase converting L-Ser into D-Ser, the first one of these enzymes/genes was described in *E. gallinarum* (Arias et al., 1999). The *vanC*-1 gene cluster of *E. gallinarum* contains a ligase gene *vanC*-1, a combined D-Ala-D-Ala dipeptidase/carboxypeptidase $vanXY_C$ gene, a *vanT* racemase gene and two genes encoding a sensor kinase/response regular two-component regulatory system $vanR_C$ and $vanS_C$ (Reynolds et al., 1999; Reynolds and Courvalin 2005). The *vanC*-2 cluster in *E. casseliflavus* showed a composition similar to the *vanC*-1 cluster in *E. gallinarum* (Dutta and Reynolds 2002). Due to the different VanC resistance mechanism a *vanH* equivalent is functionally not required and missing. Initially it was thought that VanC type resistance was always constitutively expressed as a species-specific property. However,

E. casseliflavus expressed an inducible resistance phenotype which was detected several hours after induction in vitro (Dutta and Reynolds 2002). *E. gallinarum* isolates expressing an inducible and constitutive phenotypes were identified; mutational changes in the amino acid sequences of the corresponding sensor histidine kinases $VanS_C$ in constitutive and inducible strains were demonstrated (Panesso et al., 2005). Acquisition of mobile *vanA, vanB* and *vanD* gene clusters additional to the natural *vanC*-1/-2 cluster in *E. gallinarum/casseliflavus* may lead to high-level vancomycin resistance in these strains; however, their prevalence remains low (Foglia et al., 2003; Mammina et al., 2005; Haenni et al., 2009; Neves et al., 2009).

4.4 The VanD resistance type

The basic organization of the *vanD* operons, which are located exclusively on the chromosome, is similar to that of the *vanA* and *vanB* clusters (Casadewall and Courvalin 1999; Boyd et al., 2000; Depardieu et al., 2003b; Depardieu et al., 2004; Boyd et al., 2004). Genes equivalent to *vanZ* or *vanW* are absent. The *vanD* resistance clusters appear as a remarkable example of how by certain mutational events regulatory networks adjust and finetune gene expression: VanD-type strains have negligible $VanX_D$ activity, an enzyme that normally shuts down synthesis of vancomycin-susceptible, housekeeping call wall precursors. This otherwise physiological drawback is compensated by an inactivated D-Ala-D-Ala ligase (deletions, point mutations, insertion) host enzyme, preventing synthesis of vancomycin-susceptible precursors ending in D-Ala-D-Ala. However, *vanD* expression and corresponding essential cell wall precursor synthesis would still request induction by glycopeptides (vancomycin dependence). Consequently all investigated VanD type *E. faecalis, E. faecium* and *E. avium* strains show a constitutive resistance phenotype resulting from different mutations in the $VanS_D$ sensor or $VanR_D$ regulator. Another unusual feature of VanD-type strains is their only slightly diminished susceptibility to teicoplanin (**Tab. 1**) which cannot be explained on the basis of already known DNA sequence diversities. Due to different strategies in establishing those complex and highly regulated networks independently and via different routes five different *vanD* cluster types had arranged and were characterized so far (Boyd et al., 2000; Depardieu et al., 2004). Up to now, VanD-type resistance still is a rare *van* resistance type among enterococci but has been described in a VanC type *E. gallinarum* N04-0414, too (Boyd et al., 2006b). In this strain the vancomycin resistance phenotype is constitutive but typical VanD strain features are lacking (mutations in $vanS_D$ linked to constitutive expression; shut-down of housekeeping D-Ala-D-Ala ligase activity, etc.). A *vanD* cluster was also described in *E. raffinosus* (Tanimoto et al., 2006). It showed almost identity to the *vanD4* gene cluster of *E. faecium* 10/96A and expressed all features of typical VanD type resistance such as an inducible resistance phenotype based on $VanS_D$ mutations.

Different VanD-type enterococci present a number of different combinations of mutations (mainly in $VanS_D$) suggesting an independent development and convergent evolution (Depardieu et al., 2009). These various modifications also led to a wide range of resistance phenotypes with low to high-level vancomycin resistant strains (16-512 mg/L) and susceptibility (0,5 mg/L) and low to high-level resistance to teicoplanin ($\leq$ 64 mg/L)(**Tab. 1**). Remarkably, VanD strain *E. faecium* BM4656 had a wildtype Ddl enzyme being the only VanD strain with a functional D-Ala-D-Ala ligase. In this strain, also enzymes $VanX_D$ and $VanY_D$ were active being essentiell for shutting down synthesis of glycopeptide-susceptible cell wall precursors in a background of an active host Ddl enzyme for mediating vancomycin resistance (**Fig. 3**) (Depardieu et al., 2009).

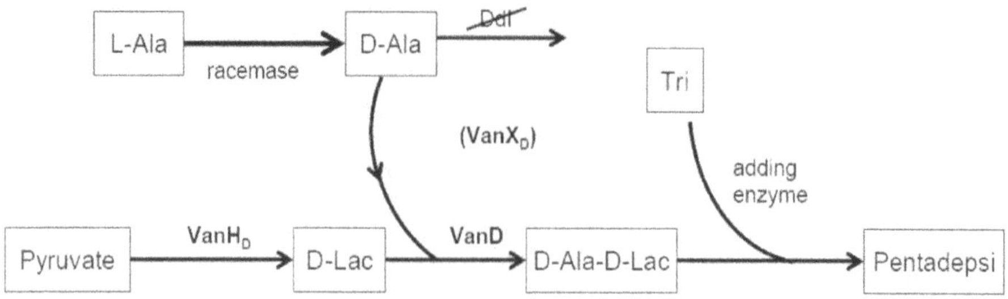

Ddl, D-alanine:D-alanine ligase; adding enzyme is a synthetase; Pentadepsi, L-Ala-γ-D-Glu-L-Lys-D-Ala-D-Lac; Tri, L-Ala-γ-D-Glu-L-Lys. Tri and Pentadepsi represent amino acid side chains linked to the enterococcal peptidoglycan disaccharide precursor N-acetyl-glucosamin-N-acetyl-muramic acid. Resistance enzymes encoded by the *vanD* cluster are shown in bold. [Figure adapted from (Courvalin 2006)].

Fig. 3. **VanD-type glycopeptide resistance.** Synthesis of peptidoglycan precursors in a VanD-type resistant strain. Dependence on the presence of vancomycin in a background of reduced VanX$_D$ activity (VanX$_D$) and a non-functional Ddl is compensated by mutations in VanR$_D$ or VanS$_D$ leading to a constitutive resistance phenotype (not demonstrated in details; see also main text and **Fig. 2**).

4.5 The VanE resistance type

Isolates representing a VanE resistance type were described in a few *E. faecalis* strains from Northern America and Australia (Fines et al., 1999; Abadia Patino et al., 2002; Boyd et al., 2002; Abadia Patino et al., 2004). The *vanE* resistance cluster resembles structures of the *vanC1* cluster naturally occurring in *E. gallinarum* (**Fig. 2**) and shows also highest similarities with the corresponding proteins. Therefore resistance is mediated by producing D-Ala-D-Ser-terminated cell wall precursors (**Tab. 1**). Due to that and as compared to the VanC resistance type, VanE type vancomycin resistance requires a VanT racemase converting L-Ser into D-Ser (Fines et al., 1999; Abadia Patino et al., 2002). VanE strains remain teicoplanin-susceptible and show moderate to low levels of inducible vancomycin resistance. Despite this phenotype, sequence determination suggested a putative non-functional VanS$_E$ protein indicating cross-talk between the VanR$_E$ response regulator and other functional membrane-located kinase activators. All five consecutive genes of the *vanE* gene cluster were cotranscribed from a single promoter (Abadia Patino et al., 2004). Downstream the *vanE* cluster in a single Canadian VanE-type *E. faecalis* an integrase gene is found, which may have been involved in the acquisition of this operon; however, when tested in vitro the *vanE* cluster was in all attempts not transferable (Boyd et al., 2002). Initially a *van* gene cluster designated *vanE* has been described in *Paenibacillus popilliae* showing 74-79 % protein sequence identity with the corresponding essential proteins VanH/A/X in *vanA* clusters (Patel et al., 2000; Patel 2000; Guardabassi et al., 2005; Guardabassi and Agerso 2006). This has later been renamed into *vanF* (see chapter 5).

4.6 The VanG resistance type

E. faecalis possessing a *vanG* cluster were low-level vancomycin-resistant and teicoplanin-susceptible (McKessar et al., 2000; Depardieu et al., 2003a; Boyd et al., 2006a). Resistance is mediated via inducible synthesis of D-Ala-D-Ser-terminated cell wall precursors. Only few isolates have been described and *vanG* gene clusters identified allow differentiation into two subtypes. The chromosomal *vanG* cluster consists of seven genes which according to its order and gene composition appear to be reassembled from different *van* operons (**Fig. 1**). In contrast to all the other *van* operons, the *vanG* cluster encodes three putative gene products with regulatory functions. Besides the common *van*R_G and *van*S_G determinants a *van*U_G gene encoding an additional putative transcriptional activator was identified (Depardieu et al., 2003a; Boyd et al., 2006a). The *vanY* gene is present but a frame-shift mutation resulting in premature termination of the encoded protein accounted for the lack of disaccharide-tetrapeptide prescursors in the cytoplasm (Depardieu et al., 2003a). VanG-type resistance was successfully transferred in vitro and acquisition of the *vanG* cluster was associated with a transfer of a 240 kb chromosomal fragment flanked by imperfect inverted repeats (Depardieu et al., 2003a). Crystallisation and X-ray analysis of the VanG D-Ala-D-Ser ligase in complex with ADP was described recently (Weber et al., 2009).

4.7 The VanL resistance type

A single *E. faecalis* isolate from Canada (N06-0364) expressed low level vancomycin resistance by a new mechanism called VanL (Boyd et al., 2008). The corresponding VanL gene mediates D-Ala-D-Ser ligation. The *vanL* gene cluster was similar in organization to the *vanC* operon, but the VanT serine racemase was encoded by two separate genes, *vanTm*$_L$ (membrane binding) and *vanTr*$_L$ (racemase) resembling the two functional domains of the otherwise combined *vanT* type racemase (**Fig. 1**)(Boyd et al., 2008). The putative VanL ligase exhibited 51 and 49% sequence identity to the VanE and VanC ligases, respectively. All attempts to transfer the *vanL* gene cluster in vitro failed. The *E. faecalis* isolate N06-0364 did not demonstrate plasmids assuming that the *vanL* gene cluster was chromosomally encoded.

4.8 The VanM resistance type

The *vanM* genotype was described in seven Chinese VRE isolates originating from a single hospital and revealing three different MLST (ST18, ST78, ST341) and five PFGE types/subtypes (Xu et al., 2010). A single VanM VRE was investigated in greater details. The translated sequence of VanM, the corresponding ligase, showed highest similarity to the VanA, the corresponding VanM gene product mediates ligation of the D-Ala-D-Lac peptide. The *vanM* gene cluster showed a gene arrangement similar to *vanB* and *vanD* with the D,D-carboxypeptidase gene *vanY*$_M$ preceding the ligase gene (**Fig. 1**). VanM type resistance was transferable by conjugation in vitro and plasmid-located. VanM phenotype showed in vitro resistance against vancomycin and tecioplanin in six of seven isolates investigated (the single ST341 isolate was susceptible to teicoplanin).

4.9 The vancomycin dependence phenotype

Soon after the first appearance of *vanA*- and *vanB*-type VRE, strains with unusual resistance phenotypes were notified including constitutively resistant strains and even vancomycin-dependent isolates of the species *E. faecalis, E. faecium* and *E. avium* (Woodford et al., 1994; Rosato et al., 1995; Sifaoui and Gutmann 1997). Features of in vitro selected strains were similar to variants identified from clinical cases mostly associated with long term vancomycin treatment. In vancomycin-dependent VRE the housekeeping D-Ala-D-Ala ligase (*ddl* gene) is not functional due to modifications in the coding sequence (point mutations, deletions, insertions). Consequently depletion of D-Ala-D-Ala dipeptides leads to an impaired cell wall synthesis. The effect could be complemented by providing the missing D-Ala-D-Ala dipeptide (Sng et al., 1998a) or similar di- or depsipeptides. Vancomycin is capable of inducing the VanA or VanB type resistance and thus providing D-Ala-D-Lac as the necessary substrate for a revived cell wall synthesis. These strains remain dependent on the inducing effect of vancomycin for an ongoing cell wall synthesis. Dependence on vancomycin could be circumvented by subsequent mutations targeting the two-component regulatory system of VanR and/or VanS. Mutations in the histidine kinase or the regulator may bypass the inducing property of the antimicrobial compound in leading to a constitutive resistance phenotype not requiring vancomycin anymore. This switch from inducible to constitutive vancomycin resistance phenotype may also appear independently from a previous vancomycin dependence phenotype (Sng et al., 1998b; Baptista et al., 1999). As described recently in a VanB type VRE, a mutation in the transcription terminator of the regulatory genes resulting in transcriptional readthrough of the resistance genes from the P_{RB} promoter in the absence of vancomycin may also circumvent vancomycin dependence and lead to a constitutive phenotype (San Millan et al., 2009b). Expression of vancomycin resistance comes along with a fitness burden under non-selective conditions (in the absence of glycopeptides). Accordingly VRE with a constitutive phenotype are less competitive under non-selective conditions (Foucault et al., 2010).

5. The *van* alphabet in non-enterococcal strains

5.1 The *van* alphabet in intestinal and environmental bacteria and glycopeptide producers

Prevalence studies revealed occurrence of different *van* genes like *vanB*, *vanD* and *vanG* in non-enterococcal, human intestinal colonizers of *Clostridium* spp., *Ruminococcus* spp. and others (Patel 2000; Stinear et al., 2001; Domingo et al., 2005; Ballard et al., 2005b; Domingo et al., 2007). One of these isolates was investigated further and a new, naturally vancomycin-resistant species, *Ruminococcus gauvreauii*, was identified possessing a *vanD* gene cluster (Domingo et al., 2008). In strains of *Clostridium symbiosum* an entire *vanB2* type Tn*1549* cluster was identified which was transferable in vitro and in vivo in the digestive tract of mice highlighting the important role that commensal, intestinal, non-enterococcal hosts may play for acquiring, preserving and distributing (vancomycin) resistance genes to nosocomial pathogens (Launay et al., 2006). The corresponding conjugative transposon Tn*1549* encodes all necessary functions for a successful transfer of the element across species and genus barriers also demonstrating its potential to transfer *vanB* type vancomycin resistance from *Enterococcus* to other important nosocomial pathogens like *Staphylococcus* spp, *C. difficile* and others (Tsvetkova et al., 2010). A large number of the *C. difficile* genome of the multi-drug resistant, clinical strain 630 consisted of mobile, genetic elements (11%) including a *tet*(M)-encoding self-conjugative transposon Tn*5397* (Sebaihia et al., 2006). Conjugative transposons like Tn*5397*/Tn*916* (and also Tn*1549*) are easily exchanged between members of different bacterial species and genera and are identified in a wide range of different, Gram-positive bacterial species capable of self-transfer and mobilisation of other, genetic elements (Roberts et al., 2001; Jasni et al., 2010; Roberts and Mullany 2011). *C. difficile* 630 also contained an element with similarity to a *vanG* type cluster; however, neither this cluster was complete nor was the strain vancomycin-resistant (Sebaihia et al., 2006). *Clostridium innocuum* is naturally intermediate-resistant to vancomycin (MIC = 8 mg/L). The mechanism of resistance was investigated in strain NCIB 10674 and found to be related due to the activity of two chromosomally encoded Ddl ligases and a racemase allowing the synthesis of a peptidoglycan precursor terminating in D-Ser similar to VanC/E/G/L type vancomycin resistance (David et al., 2004).

Certain vancomycin-resistant strains of fecal streptococci belonging to the *Streptococcus bovis* group (e.g., *S. gallolyticus, S. lutetiensis*) were found to contain *vanA* and *vanB* genes (Poyart et al., 1997; Mevius et al., 1998); however, these strains were not investigated in greater molecular details. Results of another study revealed that the entire *vanB2* type Tn*5397* conjugative transposon from a *S. lutetiensis* donor was capable to transfer into *E. faecium* and *E. faecalis* recipients in a *recA*-independent manner (Dahl and Sundsfjord 2003).

Strains of *Paenibacillus popilliae* and *Rhodococcus* spp. contain *vanA/B*-like resistance gene clusters originally called *vanE* in *P. popilliae* and later on designated *vanF* (Patel et al., 2000; Guardabassi et al., 2004; Guardabassi et al., 2005; Guardabassi and Agerso 2006). *P. popilliae* ATCC 14706 is high-level vancomycin-resistant and contained a gene cluster with $vanY_F$ and $vanZ_F$ preceding the *vanHFX* co-transcribed gene cluster. Two genes encoding a two-component regulatory system of the VanRS type were identified ca. 3kb upstream $vanY_F$ associated with an inducible VanF phenotype (Fraimow et al., 2005).

A number of *Lactobacillus, Pediococcus, Leuconostoc* and *Lactococcus* species are naturally resistant to vancomycin. This is an intrinsic property of certain species and, as known so far, mainly linked to a modified cell wall synthesis mediated via alternative precursors, functionally similar but not linked to an acquisition of any *van* gene cluster (Goffin et al., 2005). For instance , in *Leuconostoc mesenteroides* a Ddl enzyme with a residual D-Ala-D-Lac activity was identified allowing the production of vancomycin-resistant cell wall precursors (Kuzin et al., 2000). In *Lactobacillus plantarum* vancomycin resistance is also mediated via a species-specific Ddl ligase capable of synthesising D-Ala-D-Lac depsipeptides and, in addition, an intrinsic VanX-like D-Ala-D-Ala dipeptidase destroying vancomycin-susceptible cell wall precursors (Deghorain et al., 2007).

Certain soil bacteria produce glycopeptide antibiotics including vancomycin (*Amycolatopsis orientalis*) and teicoplanin (*Actinoplanes teichomyceticus*) as secondary metabolites. They prevent themselves from sensitivity against their own products by intrinsic resistance mechanisms similar but not identical to acquired resistance types in *Enterococcus* spp. (Marshall et al., 1997; Marshall et al., 1998; Patel 2000). It was speculated that enterococcal resistance genes originated from corresponding glycopeptide producers (Marshall et al., 1998; Patel 2000); however, comparably weak amino acid and nucleotide similarities among key genes and proteins involved in the resistance mechanism and the comparably high % GC of the VanRS regulatory system in the glycopeptide producers *Streptomyces toyocaensis* and *A. orientalis* suggested that a possible exchange between glycopeptide producers and nosocomial pathogens having acquired resistance properties did not happen recently (Courvalin 2005).

The anaerobic, Gram-positive, dehalogenating bacterium *Desulfitobacterium hafniense* Y51 was vancomycin-resistant by an inducible resistance phenotype (Patel et al., 2000). The strain contained a resistance Ddl enzyme with a preferred D-Ala-D-Lac ligase activity and a vancomycin resistance gene cluster showing a slightly different gene arrangement as compared with *vanA/B* clusters. The essential *vanH* homologue was missing in this cluster element; however, genome analysis of *D. hafniense* Y51 revealed at least four D-isomer-specific 2-hydroxyacid dehydrogenase genes capable in situ to perform the relevant vanH-type reaction. Nevertheless, the physiological role, the overall prevalence of this gene cluster and the phylogenetic relation to acquired resistance gene clusters in *Enterococcus* spp. remain unclear so far (Patel 2000).

It is known that intestinal colonisation could precede subsequent infections with VRE (Donskey 2004). Screening patients at risk for a colonisation with VRE is an important indicator in preventing and controlling VRE infections and outbreaks (Zirakzadeh and Patel 2006). Molecular assays provide certain advantages over microbiological tests in terms of time, sensitivity and accuracy. Prevalence of *van* genes, especially *vanB* in intestinal, non-enterococcal species impairs performance of rapid, molecular screening assays targeting the corresponding resistance genes only (Stamper et al., 2007; Mak et al., 2009; Usacheva et al., 2010). Results of a number of studies performed with various commercially available diagnostic assays in Northern America, Australia, Asia and different countries in Europe also revealed that *vanB* is generally prevalent among human intestinal colonizers and that this is not a specific property of human intestinal colonisers in certain parts of the world (Ballard et al., 2005a; Stamper et al., 2007; Mak et al., 2009; Usacheva et al., 2010; Lee et al., 2010; Marner et al., 2011; Werner et al., 2011c).

5.2 The *vanA* gene cluster in *Staphylococcus aureus*

Vancomycin is the antibiotic of choice for treating MRSA infected patients. Insusceptibility to vancomycin associated with treatment failure is insofar a matter of serious concern. Various microbiological changes could lead to reduced susceptibility against vancomycin including increased cell wall thickness, activated cell wall synthesis and reduced autolysis. The former changes are based on a modified host gene expression of determinants involved in cell wall synthesis leading to a so-called "trapping effect" where more unlinked cell wall precursors are present being able to bind (more) vancomycin ("to trap" the drug)(Cui et al., 2005; Werner et al., 2008c; Nannini et al., 2010). The Vancomycin intermediate-resistant phenotype (VISA) could be expressed homogeneously or only in a subset of investigated strains (1 of 10^5 cells = heterogeneous VISA - hVISA), the latter requires a sophisticated diagnostics via a population-based-analysis profiling (PAP)(Howden et al., 2010). VISA or hVISA phenotypes are not associated with (*van*) gene acquisition.

Early in vitro studies demonstrated the capability of a transfer of the enterococcal VanA type resistance into *S. aureus*/MRSA rendering descendents as vancomycin- and oxacillin-resistant (Noble et al., 1992). The first clinical *van*A-mediated high-level vancomycin-resistant MRSA (VRSA) was isolated from a dialysis patient in Michigan, USA (Weigel et al., 2003; Chang et al., 2003). Since then, less than a dozen additional cases have been described, nine in the United States (Michigan [n= 7], New York and Pennsylvania) and each one in India and in Iran (the latter two were not confirmed elsewhere) (Sievert et al., 2008; Finks et al., 2009; Nannini et al., 2010).

The US VRSA isolates showed high-level vancomycin resistance of >32 mg/L. All US patients affected by VRSA infections had a history of several underlying conditions and accordingly, all of them were treated extensively with antibiotics including vancomycin and most of them were co-colonized with VRE, respectively. The US VRSA isolates exhibited the *Sma*I macrorestriction patterns USA100, SCC*mec*II and USA800, SCC*mec*IV and all isolates could be assigned to sequence type 5 by multilocus sequence typing (MLST). Typing of corresponding strains, their resistance plasmids and corresponding Tn*1546*-like *vanA* clusters revealed that the isolates were unique and had evolved separately (see next paragraph).

From the first case patient a MRSA strain, a *vanA*-type *E. faecalis* and a *vanA*-type MRSA were isolated which allowed constructing a scenario where the MRSA received the *vanA* type resistance from the resistant co-colonising *E. faecalis*. This has been confirmed by molecular analysis of the corresponding *vanA*-type plasmids from related VRSA and MRSA isolates (Weigel et al., 2003; Clark et al., 2005; Zhu et al., 2008). The VRSA isolate contained a 58 kb conjugative plasmid pLW1043, the MRSA a ca. 47 kb pAM829 plasmid and the VRE two plasmids of 45 and 95 kb. Restriction digestion revealed similar patterns for the pLW1043 and pAM829 plasmids but not for the *E. faecalis* plasmids (Weigel et al., 2003). pLW1043 was fully sequenced and revealed a Tn*1546*-like *vanA* cluster integrated between the *blaZ* (beta-lactamase) and the *aacA-aphD* (gentamicin resistance) regions. It showed a mosaic-like structure, but the backbone was similar to staphylococcal type pSK41 plasmids and different from typical enterococcal plasmids suggesting acquisition of the *vanA* cluster by a resident staphylococcal-type plasmid (Kwong et al., 2008; Weaver et al., 2009). Interestingly, majority of other VRSA and co-colonising VRE isolates contained inc18-type *vanA* plasmids investigated in a follow up study (Zhu et al., 2008). The inc18-type plasmids represent broad-host range plasmids widely prevalent among Gram-positive bacteria of different enterococcal, staphylococcal and streptococcal species (Weaver et al., 2009). Plasmids from three VRSA cases were sequenced [plasmids pWZ7140 (47,277 bp), pWZ909 (42,602 bp), and pWZ1668 (48,365 bp)]. They were almost identical among each other and to a corresponding *vanA* plasmid from co-colonising *E. faecalis* strains revealing a possible direct transfer from an *E. faecalis* donor into MRSA (Zhu et al., 2008). Molecular studies with isogenic MRSA and VRSA isolates revealed that acquired VanA-type resistance was highly costly to the host, when induced (Foucault et al., 2009). In the absence of induction, the determined biological cost was minimal suggesting a serious potential for the dissemination of VRSA clinical isolates.

An comparison of US VRSA isolates (Michigan VRSA, Pennsylvania VRSA) to the *vanA*-type *E. faecalis* from the index patient, the possible donor of the resistance gene cluster for the Michigan VRSA, revealed interesting details on the resistance gene regulation and expression in different hosts (Perichon and Courvalin 2004). The Michigan VRSA was highly resistant to both glycopeptides, whereas the Pennsylvania VRSA displayed low-level resistance to vancomycin and reduced susceptibility to teicoplanin. Resistance genes were expressed at similarly high levels in the two VRSA and the *vanA*-type *E. faecalis*; however, resistance expression was notably delayed in the Pennsylvania strain. Resistance was lost at non-selective condition from the Pennsylvania VRSA. In contrast, it was stable in the Michigan VRSA and the VRE (Perichon and Courvalin 2004). Two Michigan VRSA isolates, designated VRSA-7 and VRSA-9 showed a vancomycin dependence phenotype. Molecular studies revealed a similar mechanism as known from enterococci with the corresponding resistance phenotype. VRSA-7 and VRSA-9 contained different mutations in the housekeeping D-Ala-D-Ala ligase leading to a decreased activity and dependence on the *vanA*-type D-Ala-D-Lac ligase for an ongoing cell wall synthesis (Moubareck et al., 2009; Meziane-Cherif et al., 2010). Strikingly, peptidoglycan precursors ending in D-Ala-D-Lac are not processed by PBP2a, the oxacillin-resistant penicillin binding protein encoded by *mecA* and consequently the VRSA-7 and VRSA-9 were fully susceptible to oxacillin, despite the production of a wild-type PBP2a (Moubareck et al., 2009). This also means that the combination of a beta-lactam and a glycopeptide antibiotic shows a synergistic effect for VRSA in general (Perichon and Courvalin 2006). Comparison of the two vancomycin-dependent VRSA isolates (VRSA-7/-9) indicated that the levels of vancomycin dependence and susceptibility to β-lactams correlate with the degree of D-Ala-D-Ala ligase impairment (Meziane-Cherif et al., 2010).

6. Prevalence of VRE among the hospital setting

Modern molecular typing techniques (AFLP, MLVA, MLST)[2] allow differentiating between commensal and hospital-associated/outbreak *E. faecium* isolates including vancomycin-resistant and vancomycin-susceptible variants (Willems and Bonten 2007; Willems and van Schaik W. 2009). Genomic diversity is higher in commensal *E. faecium* isolates (animal/human) as compared to hospital strains types that especially show a predominance of a number of specific MLST or MLVA types (Werner et al., 2007b; Werner et al., 2011a). Results of a comparative genome-based study revealed a distinct composition of the accessory genome in hospital-associated *E. faecium* strains (Leavis et al., 2007). Results have been confirmed by recent comparative analyses of completely sequenced *E. faecium* genomes (van Schaik et al., 2010; Palmer et al., 2010). The current model predicts that spread of ampicillin-resistant, hospital-associated *E. faecium* strains is a pre-requisite for successful establishment of VRE and further dissemination of vancomycin resistance among the hospital *E. faecium* population in general (Willems and Bonten 2007; Galloway-Pena et al., 2009; Willems and van Schaik W. 2009). To a larger or lesser extent, non-microbiological factors such as antibiotic consumption (particular classes and in general); "colonisation pressure", "understaffing", compliance with hand hygiene and other infection control measures also affect the role and number of enterococcal infections (Bonten et al., 1998; Cetinkaya et al., 2000; Murray 2000; Bonten et al., 2001; Panesso et al., 2010). Therefore, it might not come as a big surprise that despite having similar starting points and preconditions different countries experienced diverse trends in VRE prevalence. Already during the early and mid-1990s, epidemic clonal types of *E. faecium* were prevalent in hospitals in many countries, and this coincided in some European countries with a high prevalence of vancomycin resistance among *E. faecium* from animals and healthy volunteers linked to a widespread use of avoparcin as a growth promoter in commercial animal husbandry (Murray 1990; Murray 2000; Bonten et al., 2001; Panesso et al., 2010). However, VRE rates in clinical isolates increased in many countries and peaked only almost ten years later when glycopeptide resistance had already declined in the non-hospital reservoir. Retrospective epidemiological analyses in hospitals experiencing larger VRE outbreaks revealed that changes in specific procedures such as antibiotic policy, staffing, infection prevention and control regimes were, in some instances, significantly associated with increasing VRE rates, whereas in other settings this could not be shown. Increased VRE

---

[2] AFLP, Amplified-fragment length polymorphism; MLVA, Multiple Locus Variable number of tandem repeat Analysis; MLST, Multi-Locus Sequence Typing

prevalence is partly associated with spread of single, distinct epidemic clones or types (Klare et al., 2005; Top et al., 2007; Bonora et al., 2007; Werner et al., 2007c; Valdezate et al., 2009; Zhu et al., 2010; Johnson et al., 2010; Hsieh et al., 2010). In contrast, VRE outbreaks in single centres tend to be polyclonal suggesting a diverse population of hospital-acquired *E. faecium* strains and a highly mobile resistance determinant capable of spreading widely among suitable recipient strains (Yoo et al., 2006; Deplano et al., 2007; Kawalec et al., 2007; Borgmann et al., 2007; Werner et al., 2007c; Hsieh et al., 2009). Many facets of VRE and vancomycin resistance epidemiology are currently not fully understood and the question why vancomycin resistance is still mainly limited to *E. faecium* remains mainly unanswered (Garcia-Migura et al., 2007; Garcia-Migura et al., 2008; Werner et al., 2010b).

The main prevalent genotypes of acquired vancomycin resistance in enterococci worldwide are *vanA* and to a lesser extent *vanB*. The reservoir for *vanA/B* gene clusters is mainly in *E. faecium*; *vanA/B*-type resistant *E. faecalis* remain rare all over the world. Countries experiencing problems with increasing or significant higher rates of VRE always report about vancomycin-resistant *E. faecium*. Infections with members of other enterococcal species remain rare although also outbreaks with *vanA/B*-type resistant *E. faecalis, E. raffinosus or VanC-type E. gallinarum* were reported (Foglia et al., 2003; Kawalec et al., 2007; Neves et al., 2009; Shirano et al., 2010). In conclusion, the problem of VRE is mainly an issue of *vanA*-type vancomycin-resistant *E. faecium* (see the following).

6.1 Europe

Several national and European surveillance systems collect data on vancomycin resistance in enterococci. In some countries mandatory VRE surveillance is already established, in others coverage for the general population or selected settings is rather limited and the available data do not allow reliable statistical analyses and in some countries data are completely lacking. The most successful European antibiotic resistance surveillance scheme is the European Antimicrobial Resistance Surveillance System/network (EARSS/EARS-Net),[3] which was established in 1998 and is now funded by the European Centre for Disease Prevention and Control ECDC. EARS-Net collects data on antibiotic resistances in indicator bacteria exclusively from invasive (bloodstream) infections currently covering *Streptococcus pneumoniae, S. aureus, Escherichia coli, E. faecalis/E. faecium, Klebsiella pneumoniae* and *Pseudomonas aeruginosa*. In 2008 over 900 microbiological laboratories serving more than 1,500 hospitals from 33 countries provided susceptibility data from more than 700,000 invasive isolates. Inter-country comparison of collected data in the given setting reveals some drawbacks and limitations (not discussed here, see EARS reports and website). Accordingly, simple comparisons of surveillance data over time and between countries or even within single countries should be done carefully (see also chapter 4 in the EARS Annual Report 2008)(EARSS 2009). VRE surveillance within Europe has recently been reviewed and the reader is referred to this paper for any further details (Werner et al., 2008a). In the following only a short summary and, in addition, some new aspects to these previous reports are given.

[3] http://ecdc.europa.eu/en/activities/surveillance/EARS-Net/about_EARS-Net/Pages/about_network.aspx

VRE surveillance in the Nordic European countries, Norway, Denmark, Sweden, Finland and Iceland, is based on national public health programmes for containment of antimicrobial resistance, participation in EARS and in some countries case notification from laboratories and clinicians. The Nordic countries have traditionally had a low prevalence of antimicrobial resistance, and this is also true for VRE. Within the last years a recognisable reservoir of vancomycin resistance among animal enterococci was demonstrated despite the ban of using any antimicrobial growth promoter, especially avoparcin (Sorum et al., 2006; Nilsson et al., 2009a; Nilsson et al., 2009b). It is still unclear if and to what extent this reservoir influences the situation in the clinical setting. In Sweden, the situation has been stable with 18–53 cases of VRE infections and colonisations being reported annually between 2000 and 2007. However, the situation has changed rapidly with the predominant spread of a *vanB E. faecium* clone with 634 among 760 VRE cases described within a 20 months' period from 2007-2009 (Soderblom et al., 2010). General prevalence of VRE in a Swedish hospital during a post-outbreak situation was still low (Fang et al., 2010).

There is no single comprehensive surveillance scheme for monitoring VRE infections in the United Kingdom (UK). However, bacteraemia caused by VRE is monitored by four complementary surveillance programmes, with varying degrees of coverage and participation (Werner et al., 2008a). Numbers of VRE cases from invasive infections and general prevalence of vancomycin resistance in enterococci from the clinical setting is comparably high in relation to other European countries. Given the tremendous activities and partial success in reducing the MRSA burden in UK hospitals one might expect that these measures also lead to a reduction of VRE bacteraemia cases. Rates of vancomycin resistance among invasive *E. faecium* isolates varied between 33% (2005), 18% (2006), 21% (2007), 28% (2008), 13% (2009) (data from EARS-Net). The Department of Health mandatory glycopeptide-resistant enterococcal bacteraemia reporting scheme collects the total number of VRE bacteraemias in England each year. A supposed reduction in bacteraemia cases in both surveillance schemes conflicts with a possible reporting bias of participating hospitals and laboratories and it has to be shown that the supposed trends will be stable for the coming years[4]. The British Society for Antimicrobial Chemotherapy (BSAC) Bacteraemia Surveillance Programme reports data until 2008; however, a specific trend cannot be specified for "*E. faecium*" and "vancomycin resistance"[5].

Certain European countries (Netherlands, Denmark, Spain) showed a wide prevalence of hospital-associated clonal types of *E. faecium* but vancomycin resistance rates are still low (Oteo et al., 2007; Lester et al., 2008; Top et al., 2008b; Valdezate et al., 2009; Lester et al., 2009). In other countries rates of VRE remain at a comparably high rate such as Ireland and Portugal[5] (Novais et al., 2008; Morris-Downes et al., 2010). Decreasing rates were considered significant in countries like Italy, France, Israel and Greece; however, it has to be documented if these trends are indeed lasting and not biased by other, so far unknown factors (see EARS-Net data).

---

[4] http://www.hpa.org.uk/web/HPAwebFile/HPAweb_C/GGTSPU-vaccine-see.rki.de-11200-6823805-DAT/1278944284940

[5] http://www.bsacsurv.org/mrsweb/bacteraemia?organism=E.%20faecium&antimicrobial=van&year=All&country=All&summary=Enzyme%20Production&formname=bsac_bacteraemia&submit=Search%20%28%20this%20tab%20%29

Molecular typing of clinical enterococci sent to the German Focal Laboratory for Enterococcus revealed a significant increase in the number of *vanB*-type *E. faecium* among vancomycin-resistant *E. faecium* prevalent in different German hospitals (2006: 53/302, 18%; 2007: 65/249, 26%; 2008: 95/298, 32%; 2009: 157/333, 52%; (Klare et al., 2010)). Preliminary findings direct to a similar trend in other European countries like Sweden (Soderblom et al., 2010; Fang et al., 2010). If this increased VanB-type prevalence is linked to a supposed reservoir of *vanB* among enterococcal or non-enterococcal intestinal colonizers (Stamper et al., 2007; Young et al., 2007; Graham et al., 2008; Usacheva et al., 2010; Bourdon et al., 2010; Werner et al., 2011c) or simply linked to an improved and better identification of low-level expressed VanB-type resistance (Pendle et al., 2008; Grabsch et al., 2008a; Grabsch et al., 2008b; Stamper et al., 2010) in relation to a reduced breakpoint as defined by EUCAST (EUCAST Clinical Breakpoint Table v. 1.1 2010-04-27)[6] remains to be elucidated in further studies.

6.2 Northern America

Canada and the USA illustrate two divergent scenarios concerning vancomycin resistance rates among enterococci. In Canada resistance rates are persistently low (Karlowsky et al., 1999; Zhanel et al., 2000; Nichol et al., 2006; Zhanel et al., 2008a; Zhanel et al., 2010b). Results of a recent CANWARD study performed in 2008 among 10 participating Canadian hospitals revealed 3.1% VRE among 320 clinical enterococcal isolates (Zhanel et al., 2010b). All 10 VRE were *vanA*-type *E. faecium*. VRE prevalence among Canadian ICU patients is low as well; VRE accounted for <1% (n= 17/ 4133) of all isolates and 6.7% (n= 17/255) of enterococcal isolates, majority of them (88%) possessed *vanA* (Zhanel et al., 2008b). Despite the low prevalence of the more common vancomycin resistance genotypes, a number of new and still rare vancomycin resistance genotypes of the *vanD*, *vanE*, *vanG* and *vanL* classes were identified in Canadian enterococci (Boyd et al., 2000; Van Caeseele et al., 2001; Boyd et al., 2002; Boyd et al., 2004; Boyd et al., 2006a; Boyd et al., 2008).

In contrast to the situation in Canada, vancomycin resistance among clinical enterococci from US medical centres is highly prevalent. It is mainly encoded by *vanA*-type resistance widely prevalent among hospital-associated clonal types of *E. faecium* (Karlowsky et al., 2004; Nichol et al., 2006). The rapid increase in vancomycin resistance among the *E. faecium* population in US hospitals in general and the intensive care setting especially after its first appearance within a 10 years' time span is a dramatic example of a fast growing resistance problem that nowadays neither can be controlled nor prevented or reversed. The obvious coincidence of a number of unfortunate circumstances and factors from either side, the health care setting (e. g., delayed compliance with infection control and prevention strategies; permission of oral vancomycin use) and the bacteria themselves (e. g., rapid spread of hospital-associated epidemic clones; vancomycin resistance genes in a stable and transferable genetic background) may have led to such a scenario (Martone 1998; Nichol et al., 2006). The Surveillance Network (TSN) collects data on blood culture isolates from patients from 268 US hospitals. Data for 2002 revealed in 67% vancomycin resistance among altogether 1.285 *E. faecium* isolates whereas the same resistance characteristics still remained

[6] http://www.eucast.org/fileadmin/src/media/PDFs/EUCAST_files/Disk_test_documents/EUCAST_breakpoints_v1.1.pdf

rare with <5% among *E. faecalis* isolates (Karlowsky et al., 2004). Results of other studies revealed similar rates (Nichol et al., 2006; Deshpande et al., 2007). The overall situation is even impaired during the last years showing a rise in the total number of hospitalisations due to VRE infections (Ramsey and Zilberberg 2009). The Nationwide Inpatient Sample available through the Healthcare Costs and Utilization Project Website showed increased incidence of VRE infections from 3.2 to 6.5 between 2003 and 2006. An increased use of vancomycin to treat increasing numbers of MRSA and *Clostridium difficile* infections was one of the major drivers.

6.3 Latin America

In Latin America, prevalence of VRE is generally considered to be low with rates <5% among enterococci in general and before 2005 (Quinones Perez 2006); however, reliable data based on comprehensive studies or data sets were missing. Results of a recent SENTRY study revealed a recognizable change of vancomycin resistance rates among clinical enterococcal isolates from participating Latin American countries/hospitals increasing from 5 to 15.5% within 6 years (between 2003 and 2008). The most significant increase was demonstrated for Brazil with VRE rates rising from 7 to 31% (Sader et al., 2009). Considering that the majority of enterococcal isolates is *E. faecalis* which mainly remained susceptible to vancomycin, the increase of vancomycin resistance among *E. faecium* isolates seems even more dramatic based on the numbers specified. A molecular characterization of prospectively collected 732 enterococcal isolates from 2006 to 2008 from 32 hospitals in Colombia, Ecuador, Peru and Venezuela revealed vancomycin resistance in 6% of all isolates (Panesso et al., 2010). Considering only isolates of *E. faecium* (n= 111) prevalence of vancomycin resistance ranged from 24 to 48%; however, sample size per country was quite limited and a sampling bias cannot be excluded. Nevertheless, all vancomycin-resistant *E. faecium* were of the *vanA* genotype and represented hospital-associated strain types as determined by MLST (ST17, ST18, ST203, ST280 and others). Tn*5382*-*vanB2* encoded VanB type resistance was demonstrated to be linked to two epidemic clones; a ST201 *E. faecalis* and a ST64 *E. faecium* disseminated among 9 and 15 Chilean hospitals, respectively (Lopez et al., 2009).

6.4 Asia, Australia and New Zealand

VanB-type resistance is only highly prevalent in certain parts of the world, for instance, in Australia (Christiansen et al., 2004; Pearman 2006; Worth et al., 2008; Pendle et al., 2008; Johnson et al., 2010) or Singapore (Koh et al., 2006; Koh et al., 2009) where *vanB*-type vancomycin resistance among clinical *E. faecium* is more prevalent than the *vanA*-type. The reason(s) for this remain unknown and are not linked to a supposed larger reservoir of the *vanB* cluster in commensal intestinal colonizers (Padiglione et al., 2000), rates of which were similar in Australian, US-American and European studies (Stamper et al., 2007; Graham et al., 2008; Grabsch et al., 2008b; Bourdon et al., 2010; Werner et al., 2011c). A larger reservoir of *vanB*-type resistance in isolates from commercial animal farming associated with an avoparcin use is unlikely; avoparcin use was ceased in Australia in 2000 and Singapore has no significant agriculture at all thus excluding a distinct animal *vanB*-type VRE reservoir (see chapter 7). However, community carriage linked to a consumption of imported and contaminated food cannot be excluded. Studies performed in New Zealand described a supposed dissemination of *vanA*-type resistance among *E. faecalis* strains rather then *E. faecium* in a background of generally low level of vancomycin resistance (Manson et al., 2003a; Manson et al., 2003b). VRE epidemiology in other Australasian countries reflects a similar scenario as in Europe or Northern America with *vanA*-type resistance highly prevalent among *E. faecium*. Several studies performed during outbreaks in Taiwanese hospitals revealed a preferred prevalence of (hospital-associated) *vanA*-type vancomycin-resistant *E. faecium* strains (Hsieh et al., 2009; Hsieh et al., 2010). In South-Korean hospitals (and outside hospitals) *vanA*-genotype (VanB phenotype) *E. faecium* were widely prevalent (Ko et al., 2005; Shin et al., 2006; Park et al., 2008). Recent reports from China revealed also a preferred prevalence of *vanA*-type vancomycin resistance among clinical VRE (Zheng et al., 2007a; Zheng et al., 2007b; Zhu et al., 2009).

7. Vancomycin resistance among enterococci from farm animals, feedstuff and non-hospitalized humans and the environment

Surveillance of antimicrobial resistance among enterococci as commensal colonizers of food-producing animals became prominent during the early and mid 1990ies. At this time scientific and public awareness arose due to the argument that use of antimicrobial growth promoters, focused on the glycopeptide avoparcin, added to the feed of food animals in sub-inhibitory concentrations is capable of selecting antibiotic-resistant bacteria; here glycopeptide/vancomycin-resistant enterococci. Large studies were initiated when higher numbers of VRE were suspiciously found in environmental samples without any known reservoir in or link to use of glycopeptides in human medicine (Klare et al., 1993; Torres et al., 1994). Soon after, avoparcin, another glycopeptide class antibiotic used in animal husbandry as a feed additive (growth promoter) was identified to select VRE in the animal setting (Bates et al., 1994; Klare et al., 1995a; Klare et al., 1995b; Bates 1997). Consequently, meat samples from commercially raised animals were highly contaminated with VRE including samples of pork, beef, chicken and turkey (Klare et al., 1995a; Klare et al., 1995b; Schouten et al., 1997; Klein et al., 1998; Simonsen et al., 1998; Kruse et al., 1999). Samples from organic or private farms of smaller sizes that did not use avoparcin or feed additives at all were free of VRE (Klare et al., 1995b; Klare and Witte 1998). Following the food chain, VRE reached humans and were capable of colonizing the intestines of healthy people; in contrast, a small study in vegetarians showed no detectable VRE counts (Schouten et al., 1997; Van Den Bogaard et al., 1997; Stobberingh et al., 1999). Similar studies were performed all over Europe and data have already been reviewed in previous papers and book chapters and are thus not discussed in greater details here (Woodford et al., 1998; Klare and Witte 1998; Aarestrup et al., 2000b; Bonten et al., 2001; Klare et al., 2003). In countries within the EU, avoparcin was abandoned in Norway and Denmark in 1995, Germany 1996 and in the remaining EU countries in 1997. Studies performed in some European countries soon after identified a reduced prevalence of VRE, their numbers dropped qualitatively and quantitatively in samples from commercial animal farms, food samples and following the food chain in humans of the general population (Klare et al., 1999). However, studies from Denmark and Norway showed that other antimicrobial growth promoters may lead to a co-selection phenomenon and reduced VRE numbers were only documentable when other growth promoters like macrolides (spiramycin, tylosin) were also banned. The reason was a genetic linkage of both resistance determinants *erm*(B) and *vanA* on similar plasmids (Aarestrup 2000; Borgen et al., 2002). Based on the precautionary principle the European

Commission postponed the further use of four antimicrobial growth promoters with a supposed link (same antibiotic class) to antibiotics used in human medicine in 1998. This decision was confirmed in 2003 specifying the phasing out of all antimicrobial growth promoters within the EU [Regulation (EC) No. 1831/2003 on additives for use in animal nutrition]. However, VRE counts did not drop to zero. Studies in animal farms performed several years after the ban of several growth promoters including avoparcin revealed a permanent reservoir of VRE (Borgen et al., 2000; Borgen et al., 2001; Ghidan et al., 2008). Recent studies performed in Swedish animal farms still highlighted a considerable reservoir of VRE (Nilsson et al., 2009b). Sweden banned avoparcin and other growth promoters already in 1986 and VRE prevalence among the clinical setting as well as the general population was and still is very low but somehow widely found in sewage (Sahlstrom et al., 2009). Phenotypic and genotypic characterization of the sewage VRE identified for the majority of them (a) species *E. faecium* and (b) the *vanB*-type. PFGE analysis revealed different strains prevalent over the study period. This finding is especially noticeable since a few years later rates of VanB-type *E. faecium* increased in certain Swedish hospitals (Soderblom et al., 2010; Fang et al., 2010).

Outside Europe similar scenarios of VRE epidemiology were described. In Korea, VRE were still prevalent in livestock samples four years after banning avoparcin (Lim et al., 2006). VRE were isolated from 17% of the chicken samples (n= 57 strains from 342 meat samples) and 2% of the pig samples (4 from 214 fecal samples) whereas no VRE were isolated from 110 bovine samples. All the 61 VRE isolates were *van*A-type *E. faecium.* A study performed in Japan three years after the ban of avoparcin (1997) did not identify any VRE among 515 fresh faecal samples from 178 beef cattle, 179 pig and 158 broiler chicken farms representing all 47 Japanese prefectures (Kojima et al., 2010) whereas in 1996, one year before the ban, 3% (8/263) of enterococci tested were vancomycin-resistant (Yoshimura et al., 1998). However, in these two studies it was only screened for enterococci in general and subsequently resistances were determined. So it cannot be ruled out that samples contained VRE but at lower numbers then statistically recognizable with the described non-selective screening strategy. Avoparcin use was banned in Taiwan in 2000. A nationwide surveillance was initiated to study VRE prevalence on chicken farms from 2000 to 2003 (Lauderdale et al., 2007). VRE were still identified, but counts dropped in a quantitative manner, only 8.8% (n= 7/80) of the chicken farms surveyed harboured VRE in 2003 compared with 25% (15/60) in 2000. Interestingly, majority were vancomycin-resistant *E. faecalis* (see below). This reflects a somehow different VRE epidemiology than in the rest of the world; similar to Australia where *vanB*-type *E. faecium* and *vanA*-type *E. faecalis* predominate (Worth et al., 2008; Johnson et al., 2010). In Australia, the general scenario appears to be different; a larger reservoir of VRE outside the clinical setting could not be identified despite an ongoing high use of avoparcin. For instance, prevalence rates of VRE in the general population were extremely low (0,2%), the two identified VRE among 1085 community specimens were *vanB*-type *E. faecium* (Padiglione et al., 2000).

In the US, avoparcin has never been used as a feed additive, a reservoir for VRE outside the clinical setting could not be identified when screening samples from various animal farms, meat, environmental sources and stool samples from healthy people during this time (Coque et al., 1996; McDonald et al., 1997; Martone 1998). However, situation changed the last years and vancomycin resistance was prevalent among 6 of 55 pig samples investigated in 2008 (Donabedian et al., 2010).

8. Localization and spread of *vanA*- and *vanB*-type resistance

Vancomycin resistance in animal, human commensal and environmental sources is mostly encoded by *vanA*-type resistance clusters and its reservoir is in isolates of *E. faecium*; thus it reflects the same situation as in the clinical setting in most parts of the world. Exchange of resistant strains among different ecosystems is less probable due to the supposed ecovar association, especially among hospital-associated *E. faecium* strains (see chapter 5), although dissemination across host barriers of vancomycin- and multi-resistant enterococci was described anecdotally, especially for the less strongly host-adapted *E. faecalis* strains (Manson et al., 2003a; Manson et al., 2003b; Manson et al., 2004; Agerso et al., 2008; Larsen et al., 2010; Hammerum et al., 2010; Freitas et al., 2011a). Vancomycin resistance among enterococci most probably spreads via a dissemination of mobile genetic elements of variants of the *vanA*-type element Tn*1546* mostly located on mobilizable or conjugative plasmids (Sletvold et al., 2007; Novais et al., 2008; Sletvold et al., 2008; Freitas et al., 2009; Rosvoll et al., 2009; Sletvold et al., 2010; Laverde Gomez et al., 2011; Werner et al., 2011b; Freitas et al., 2011b). In vitro transfer of *vanA* plasmids has been determined in a number of studies (Werner et al., 1997; van den Braak et al., 1998; Werner et al., 2010b) and transfer in vivo in digestive tracts of animals and human volunteers was also shown (Moubareck et al., 2003; Lester et al., 2006; Lester and Hammerum 2010). Transfer rates under natural conditions may be higher than determined in vitro (Dahl et al., 2007).

Molecular studies revealed a tremendous number of deletions, insertions, and modifications of the original Tn*1546*-like structure in different not epidemiologically linked VRE leading to a wide diversity of various Tn*1546* subtypes (van den Braak et al., 1998; Willems et al., 1999; Huh et al., 2004; Werner et al., 2006; Lim et al., 2006; Yoo et al., 2006). Despite its high diversity, identical cluster types were identified among clinical human and animal commensal and environmental strains suggesting a common reservoir and exchange of its mobile elements via conjugative plasmids or as part of larger mobile genomic islands in European, Asian and Australian studies (van den Braak et al., 1998; Jensen et al., 1998; Willems et al., 1999; Werner et al., 2006; Jung et al., 2007). Garcia-Migura and co-workers identified a hot spot for integration of Tn*1546*-like elements and it could be speculated if this integration site is more prevalent among plasmids and is the reason for the preferred prevalence of *vanA* clusters on specific plasmids (Garcia-Migura et al., 2008). Results of a recent study about horizontal transferability of *vanA* plasmids among enterococci, other lactic acid bacteria and bifidobacteria revealed a preferred transfer into and a possible host restriction within the species *E. faecium* (Werner et al., 2010b). In contrast, *vanB*-type elements preferably integrate into the chromosome, but are mobile as part of integrative and conjugative elements ICE (Paulsen et al., 2003; Hegstad et al., 2010). Occasionally *vanB* resides on (transferable) plasmids (Rice et al., 1998; Zheng et al., 2009); as noticed recently associated with larger VanB-type VRE outbreaks (Sivertsen et al., 2011; Bjorkeng et al., 2011). Many surveillance studies failed to recognize a considerable reservoir of *vanB* among enterococcal colonizers in animals and humans, whereas recent real-time based studies targeting *vanB* or improved methods of detection revealed a considerable reservoir among intestinal colonizers, maybe also non-enterococcal bacteria (see above). In general, the supposed low expression of vancomycin resistance among *vanB* strains may have lead to an underestimation of its general prevalence, since in many screening studies comparably high vancomycin concentrations were used to select VRE (Poole et al., 2005; Hershberger et al., 2005). Rates of clinical *vanB*-type VRE are increasing, at least in some European countries during last years (Johnson et al., 2010; Soderblom et al., 2010; Bourdon et al., 2011) and a link to a supposed reservoir outside the clinical setting, for instance, among mammal intestinal colonizers is discussed also in areas where *vanB*-type vancomycin resistance is more prevalent (Christiansen et al., 2004; Johnson et al., 2010).

9. Genereal conclusion

Vancomycin resistance in enterococci has established as an important health care problem worldwide. Eight genotypes of acquired vancomycin resistance in enterococci are known. The *vanA*-type resistance encoded by transposon Tn*1546* and Tn*1546*-derived elements is the most prevalent resistance determinant followed by *vanB*-type clusters which are mainly part of integrative and conjugative elements (ICE) mostly residing within the chromosome. The main *van* genotype reservoir is in *E. faecium*. Prevalence of VRE among the clinical setting varies in different parts of the world. Their increased incidence is linked to characteristic predisposing factors in affected patients but also to the bacteria themselves. The latter concerns a preferred spread of hospital-associated strain types among health care settings. These strains differ from commensal strains by their core genomes (different MLST types and clonal complexes) and an additional genomic content including specific (resistance) plasmids. However, countries and institutions having similar pre-conditions may experience different developments and changes in VRE prevalence are multifactorial and cannot be simply addressed to or predicted from specific factors and circumstances. VRE and their resistance determinants are still prevalent among commercial animal husbandry despite the glycopeptide avoparcin and other antimicrobial substances were banned for growth promotion in many parts of the world. Their role to feed the (vancomycin) resistance gene pool of hospital-associated strain types remains to be elucidated in further studies.

10. References

Aarestrup, F.M., 2000. Characterization of glycopeptide-resistant enterococcus faecium (GRE) from broilers and pigs in Denmark: genetic evidence that persistence of GRE in pig herds is associated with coselection by resistance to macrolides. J. Clin. Microbiol. 38, 2774-2777.

Aarestrup, F.M., Agerso, Y., Gerner-Smidt, P., Madsen, M., Jensen, L.B., 2000a. Comparison of antimicrobial resistance phenotypes and resistance genes in Enterococcus faecalis and Enterococcus faecium from humans in the community, broilers, and pigs in Denmark. Diagn. Microbiol. Infect. Dis. 37, 127-137.

Aarestrup, F.M., Bager, F., Andersen, J.S., 2000b. Association between the use of avilamycin for growth promotion and the occurrence of resistance among Enterococcus faecium from broilers: epidemiological study and changes over time. Microb. Drug Resist. 6, 71-75.

Abadia Patino, L., Christiansen, K., Bell, J., Courvalin, P., Perichon, B., 2004. VanE-type vancomycin-resistant Enterococcus faecalis clinical isolates from Australia. Antimicrob. Agents Chemother. 48, 4882-4885.

Abadia Patino, L., Courvalin, P., Perichon, B., 2002. vanE gene cluster of vancomycin-resistant Enterococcus faecalis BM4405. J. Bacteriol. 184, 6457-6464.

Agerso, Y., Lester, C.H., Porsbo, L.J., Orsted, I., Emborg, H.D., Olsen, K.E., Jensen, L.B., Heuer, O.E., Frimodt-Moller, N., Aarestrup, F.M., Hammerum, A.M., 2008. Vancomycin-resistant Enterococcus faecalis isolates from a Danish patient and two healthy human volunteers are possibly related to isolates from imported turkey meat. J. Antimicrob. Chemother. 62, 844-845.

Agerso, Y., Pedersen, A.G., Aarestrup, F.M., 2006. Identification of Tn5397-like and Tn916-like transposons and diversity of the tetracycline resistance gene tet(M) in enterococci from humans, pigs and poultry. J. Antimicrob. Chemother. 57, 832-839.

Arias, C.A., Courvalin, P., Reynolds, P.E., 2000. vanC cluster of vancomycin-resistant Enterococcus gallinarum BM4174. Antimicrob. Agents Chemother. 44, 1660-1666.

Arias, C.A., Martin-Martinez, M., Blundell, T.L., Arthur, M., Courvalin, P., Reynolds, P.E., 1999. Characterization and modelling of VanT: a novel, membrane-bound, serine racemase from vancomycin-resistant Enterococcus gallinarum BM4174. Mol. Microbiol. 31, 1653-1664.

Arias, C.A., Murray, B.E., 2008. Emergence and management of drug-resistant enterococcal infections. Expert. Rev. Anti. Infect. Ther. 6, 637-655.

Arsene, S., Leclercq, R., 2007. Role of a qnr-like gene in the intrinsic resistance of Enterococcus faecalis to fluoroquinolones. Antimicrob. Agents Chemother. 51, 3254-3258.

Arthur, M., Depardieu, F., Gerbaud, G., Galimand, M., Leclercq, R., Courvalin, P., 1997. The VanS sensor negatively controls VanR-mediated transcriptional activation of glycopeptide resistance genes of Tn1546 and related elements in the absence of induction. J. Bacteriol. 179, 97-106.

Arthur, M., Molinas, C., Depardieu, F., Courvalin, P., 1993. Characterization of Tn1546, a Tn3-related transposon conferring glycopeptide resistance by synthesis of depsipeptide peptidoglycan precursors in Enterococcus faecium BM4147. J. Bacteriol. 175, 117-127.

Arthur, M., Quintiliani, R., Jr., 2001. Regulation of VanA- and VanB-type glycopeptide resistance in enterococci. Antimicrob. Agents Chemother. 45, 375-381.

Ballard, S.A., Grabsch, E.A., Johnson, P.D., Grayson, M.L., 2005a. Comparison of three PCR primer sets for identification of vanB gene carriage in feces and correlation with carriage of vancomycin-resistant enterococci: interference by vanB-containing anaerobic bacilli. Antimicrob. Agents Chemother. 49, 77-81.

Ballard, S.A., Pertile, K.K., Lim, M., Johnson, P.D., Grayson, M.L., 2005b. Molecular characterization of vanB elements in naturally occurring gut anaerobes. Antimicrob. Agents Chemother. 49, 1688-1694.

Baptista, M., Rodrigues, P., Depardieu, F., Courvalin, P., Arthur, M., 1999. Single-cell analysis of glycopeptide resistance gene expression in teicoplanin-resistant mutants of a VanB-type Enterococcus faecalis. Mol. Microbiol. 32, 17-28.

Batchelor, M., Zhou, D., Cooper, M.A., Abell, C., Rayment, T., 2010. Vancomycin dimer formation between analogues of bacterial peptidoglycan surfaces probed by force spectroscopy. Org. Biomol. Chem. 8, 1142-1148.

Bates, J., 1997. Epidemiology of vancomycin-resistant enterococci in the community and the relevance of farm animals to human infection. J. Hosp. Infect. 37, 89-101.

Bates, J., Jordens, J.Z., Griffiths, D.T., 1994. Farm animals as a putative reservoir for vancomycin-resistant enterococcal infection in man. J. Antimicrob. Chemother. 34, 507-514.

Bischoff, K., Jacob, J., 1996. [The sat4 streptothricin acetyltransferase gene of Campylobacter coli: its distribution in the environment and use as epidemiological marker]. Zentralbl. Hyg. Umweltmed. 198, 241-257.

Bjorkeng, E., Rasmussen, G., Sundsfjord, A., Sjoberg, L., Hegstad, K., Soderquist, B., 2011. Clustering of polyclonal VanB-type vancomycin-resistant Enterococcus faecium in a low-endemic area was associated with CC17-genogroup strains harbouring transferable vanB2-Tn5382 and pRUM-like repA containing plasmids with axe-txe plasmid addiction systems. APMIS 119, 247-258.

Boguslawska, J., Zycka-Krzesinska, J., Wilcks, A., Bardowski, J., 2009. Intra- and interspecies conjugal transfer of Tn916-like elements from Lactococcus lactis in vitro and in vivo. Appl. Environ. Microbiol. 75, 6352-6360.

Bonora, M.G., Ligozzi, M., Luzzani, A., Solbiati, M., Stepan, E., Fontana, R., 2006. Emergence of linezolid resistance in Enterococcus faecium not dependent on linezolid treatment. Eur. J. Clin. Microbiol. Infect. Dis. 25, 197-198.

Bonora, M.G., Olioso, D., Lo, C.G., Fontana, R., 2007. Phylogenetic analysis of vancomycin-resistant Enterococcus faecium genotypes associated with outbreaks or sporadic infections in Italy. Microb. Drug Resist. 13, 171-177.

Bonten, M.J., Slaughter, S., Ambergen, A.W., Hayden, M.K., van, V.J., Nathan, C., Weinstein, R.A., 1998. The role of "colonization pressure" in the spread of vancomycin-resistant enterococci: an important infection control variable. Arch. Intern. Med. 158, 1127-1132.

Bonten, M.J., Willems, R., Weinstein, R.A., 2001. Vancomycin-resistant enterococci: why are they here, and where do they come from? The Lancet Infectious Diseases 1, 314-325.

Borgen, K., Simonsen, G.S., Sundsfjord, A., Wasteson, Y., Olsvik, O., Kruse, H., 2000. Continuing high prevalence of VanA-type vancomycin-resistant enterococci on Norwegian poultry farms three years after avoparcin was banned. J. Appl. Microbiol. 89, 478-485.

Borgen, K., Sorum, M., Wasteson, Y., Kruse, H., 2001. VanA-type vancomycin-resistant enterococci (VRE) remain prevalent in poultry carcasses 3 years after avoparcin was banned. Int. J. Food Microbiol. 64, 89-94.

Borgen, K., Sorum, M., Wasteson, Y., Kruse, H., Oppegaard, H., 2002. Genetic linkage between erm(B) and vanA in Enterococcus hirae of poultry origin. Microb. Drug Resist. 8, 363-368.

Borgmann, S., Schulte, B., Wolz, C., Gruber, H., Werner, G., Goerke, C., Klare, I., Beyser, K., Heeg, P., Autenrieth, I.B., 2007. Discrimination between epidemic and non-epidemic glycopeptide-resistant E. faecium in a post-outbreak situation. J. Hosp. Infect. 67, 49-55.

Boumghar-Bourtchai, L., Dhalluin, A., Malbruny, B., Galopin, S., Leclercq, R., 2009. Influence of recombination on development of mutational resistance to linezolid in Enterococcus faecalis JH2-2. Antimicrob. Agents Chemother. AAC-

Bourdon, N., Berenger, R., Lepoultier, R., Mouet, A., Lesteven, C., Borgey, F., Fines-Guyon, M., Leclercq, R., Cattoir, V., 2010. Rapid detection of vancomycin-resistant enterococci from rectal swabs by the Cepheid Xpert vanA/vanB assay. Diagn. Microbiol. Infect. Dis. 67, 291-293.

Bourdon, N., Fines-Guyon, M., Thiolet, J.M., Maugat, S., Coignard, B., Leclercq, R., Cattoir, V., 2011. Changing trends in vancomycin-resistant enterococci in French hospitals, 2001-08. J. Antimicrob. Chemother. 66, 713-721.

Bourgeois-Nicolaos, N., Massias, L., Couson, B., Butel, M.J., Andremont, A., Doucet-Populaire, F., 2007. Dose dependence of emergence of resistance to linezolid in Enterococcus faecalis in vivo. J Infect Dis 195, 1480-1488.

Boyd, D.A., Cabral, T., Van, C.P., Wylie, J., Mulvey, M.R., 2002. Molecular characterization of the vanE gene cluster in vancomycin-resistant Enterococcus faecalis N00-410 isolated in Canada. Antimicrob. Agents Chemother. 46, 1977-1979.

Boyd, D.A., Conly, J., Dedier, H., Peters, G., Robertson, L., Slater, E., Mulvey, M.R., 2000. Molecular characterization of the vanD gene cluster and a novel insertion element in a vancomycin-resistant enterococcus isolated in Canada. J. Clin. Microbiol. 38, 2392-2394.

Boyd, D.A., Du, T., Hizon, R., Kaplen, B., Murphy, T., Tyler, S., Brown, S., Jamieson, F., Weiss, K., Mulvey, M.R., 2006a. VanG-type vancomycin-resistant Enterococcus faecalis strains isolated in Canada. Antimicrob. Agents Chemother. 50, 2217-2221.

Boyd, D.A., Kibsey, P., Roscoe, D., Mulvey, M.R., 2004. Enterococcus faecium N03-0072 carries a new VanD-type vancomycin resistance determinant: characterization of the VanD5 operon. J. Antimicrob. Chemother. 54, 680-683.

Boyd, D.A., Miller, M.A., Mulvey, M.R., 2006b. Enterococcus gallinarum N04-0414 harbors a VanD-type vancomycin resistance operon and does not contain a D-alanine:D-alanine 2 (ddl2) gene. Antimicrob. Agents Chemother. 50, 1067-1070.

Boyd, D.A., Willey, B.M., Fawcett, D., Gillani, N., Mulvey, M.R., 2008. Molecular characterization of Enterococcus faecalis N06-0364 with low-level vancomycin resistance harboring a novel D-Ala-D-Ser gene cluster, vanL. Antimicrob. Agents Chemother. 52, 2667-2672.

Canton, R., Ruiz-Garbajosa, P., Chaves, R.L., Johnson, A.P., 2010. A potential role for daptomycin in enterococcal infections: what is the evidence? J. Antimicrob. Chemother. 65, 1126-1136.

Carias, L.L., Rudin, S.D., Donskey, C.J., Rice, L.B., 1998. Genetic linkage and cotransfer of a novel, vanB-containing transposon (Tn5382) and a low-affinity penicillin-binding protein 5 gene in a clinical vancomycin-resistant Enterococcus faecium isolate. J. Bacteriol. 180, 4426-4434.

Casadewall, B., Courvalin, P., 1999. Characterization of the vanD Glycopeptide Resistance Gene Cluster from Enterococcus faecium BM4339. J. Bacteriol. 181, 3644-3648.

Casetta, A., Hoi, A.B., de, C.G., Horaud, T., 1998. Diversity of structures carrying the high-level gentamicin resistance gene (aac6-aph2) in Enterococcus faecalis strains isolated in France. Antimicrob. Agents Chemother. 42, 2889-2892.

Cetinkaya, Y., Falk, P., Mayhall, C.G., 2000. Vancomycin-resistant enterococci. Clin. Microbiol. Rev. 13, 686-707.

Chang, S., Sievert, D.M., Hageman, J.C., Boulton, M.L., Tenover, F.C., Downes, F.P., Shah, S., Rudrik, J.T., Pupp, G.R., Brown, W.J., Cardo, D., Fridkin, S.K., the Vancomycin-Resistant Staphylococcus aureus Investigative Team, 2003. Infection with vancomycin-resistant Staphylococcus aureus containing the vanA resistance gene. N Engl J Med 348, 1342-1347.

Christiansen, K.J., Tibbett, P.A., Beresford, W., Pearman, J.W., Lee, R.C., Coombs, G.W., Kay, I.D., O'Brien, F.G., Palladino, S., Douglas, C.R., Montgomery, P.D., Orrell, T., Peterson, A.M., Kosaras, F.P., Flexman, J.P., Heath, C.H., McCullough, C.A., 2004. Eradication of a large outbreak of a single strain of vanB vancomycin-resistant

Enterococcus faecium at a major Australian teaching hospital. Infect. Control Hosp. Epidemiol. 25, 384-390.

Clark, N.C., Weigel, L.M., Patel, J.B., Tenover, F.C., 2005. Comparison of Tn1546-like elements in vancomycin-resistant Staphylococcus aureus isolates from Michigan and Pennsylvania. Antimicrob. Agents Chemother. 49, 470-472.

Coque, T.M., Tomayko, J.F., Ricke, S.C., Okhyusen, P.C., Murray, B.E., 1996. Vancomycin-resistant enterococci from nosocomial, community, and animal sources in the United States. Antimicrob. Agents Chemother. 40, 2605-2609.

Courvalin, P., 2005. Genetics of glycopeptide resistance in gram-positive pathogens. Int. J. Med. Microbiol. 294, 479-486.

Courvalin, P., 2006. Vancomycin resistance in gram-positive cocci. Clin. Infect. Dis. 42 Suppl 1, S25-S34.

Cui, L., Lian, J.Q., Neoh, H.M., Reyes, E., Hiramatsu, K., 2005. DNA microarray-based identification of genes associated with glycopeptide resistance in Staphylococcus aureus. Antimicrob. Agents Chemother. 49, 3404-3413.

Dahl, K.H., Mater, D.D., Flores, M.J., Johnsen, P.J., Midtvedt, T., Corthier, G., Sundsfjord, A., 2007. Transfer of plasmid and chromosomal glycopeptide resistance determinants occurs more readily in the digestive tract of mice than in vitro and exconjugants can persist stably in vivo in the absence of glycopeptide selection. J. Antimicrob. Chemother. 59, 478-486.

Dahl, K.H., Rokenes, T.P., Lundblad, E.W., Sundsfjord, A., 2003. Nonconjugative transposition of the vanB-containing Tn5382-like element in Enterococcus faecium. Antimicrob. Agents Chemother. 47, 786-789.

Dahl, K.H., Sundsfjord, A., 2003. Transferable vanB2 Tn5382-containing elements in fecal streptococcal strains from veal calves. Antimicrob. Agents Chemother. 47, 2579-2583.

David, V., Bozdogan, B., Mainardi, J.L., Legrand, R., Gutmann, L., Leclercq, R., 2004. Mechanism of intrinsic resistance to vancomycin in Clostridium innocuum NCIB 10674. J. Bacteriol. 186, 3415-3422.

de Vries, L.E., Christensen, H., Skov, R.L., Aarestrup, F.M., Agerso, Y., 2009. Diversity of the tetracycline resistance gene tet(M) and identification of Tn916- and Tn5801-like (Tn6014) transposons in Staphylococcus aureus from humans and animals. J. Antimicrob. Chemother. 64, 490-500.

Deghorain, M., Goffin, P., Fontaine, L., Mainardi, J.L., Daniel, R., Errington, J., Hallet, B., Hols, P., 2007. Selectivity for D-lactate incorporation into the peptidoglycan precursors of Lactobacillus plantarum: role of Aad, a VanX-like D-alanyl-D-alanine dipeptidase. J. Bacteriol. 189, 4332-4337.

Depardieu, F., Bonora, M.G., Reynolds, P.E., Courvalin, P., 2003a. The vanG glycopeptide resistance operon from Enterococcus faecalis revisited. Mol. Microbiol. 50, 931-948.

Depardieu, F., Foucault, M.L., Bell, J., Dubouix, A., Guibert, M., Lavigne, J.P., Levast, M., Courvalin, P., 2009. New combinations of mutations in VanD-Type vancomycin-resistant Enterococcus faecium, Enterococcus faecalis, and Enterococcus avium strains. Antimicrob. Agents Chemother. 53, 1952-1963.

Depardieu, F., Reynolds, P.E., Courvalin, P., 2003b. VanD-type vancomycin-resistant Enterococcus faecium 10/96A. Antimicrob. Agents Chemother. 47, 7-18.

Depardieu, F., Kolbert, M., Pruul, H., Bell, J., Courvalin, P., 2004. vanD-Type vancomycin-resistant Enterococcus faecium and Enterococcus faecalis. Antimicrob. Agents Chemother. 48, 3892-3904.

Deplano, A., Denis, O., Nonhoff, C., Rost, F., Byl, B., Jacobs, F., Vankerckhoven, V., Goossens, H., Struelens, M.J., 2007. Outbreak of hospital-adapted clonal complex-17 vancomycin-resistant Enterococcus faecium strain in a haematology unit: role of rapid typing for early control. J. Antimicrob. Chemother. 60, 849-854.

Derbise, A., Aubert, S., El, S.N., 1997. Mapping the regions carrying the three contiguous antibiotic resistance genes aadE, sat4, and aphA-3 in the genomes of staphylococci. Antimicrob. Agents Chemother. 41, 1024-1032.

Derbise, A., Dyke, K.G., El Solh, N., 1996. Characterization of a Staphylococcus aureus transposon, Tn5405, located within Tn5404 and carrying the aminoglycoside resistance genes, aphA-3 and aadE. Plasmid 35, 174-188.

Deshpande, L.M., Fritsche, T.R., Moet, G.J., Biedenbach, D.J., Jones, R.N., 2007. Antimicrobial resistance and molecular epidemiology of vancomycin-resistant enterococci from North America and Europe: a report from the SENTRY antimicrobial surveillance program. Diagn. Microbiol. Infect. Dis. 58, 163-170.

Domingo, M.C., Huletsky, A., Boissinot, M., Bernard, K.A., Picard, F.J., Bergeron, M.G., 2008. Ruminococcus gauvreauii sp. nov., a glycopeptide-resistant species isolated from a human faecal specimen. Int. J. Syst. Evol. Microbiol. 58, 1393-1397.

Domingo, M.C., Huletsky, A., Giroux, R., Boissinot, K., Picard, F.J., Lebel, P., Ferraro, M.J., Bergeron, M.G., 2005. High prevalence of glycopeptide resistance genes vanB, vanD, and vanG not associated with enterococci in human fecal flora. Antimicrob. Agents Chemother. 49, 4784-4786.

Domingo, M.C., Huletsky, A., Giroux, R., Picard, F.J., Bergeron, M.G., 2007. vanD and vanG-Like gene clusters in a Ruminococcus species isolated from human bowel flora. Antimicrob. Agents Chemother. 51, 4111-4117.

Donabedian, S.M., Perri, M.B., Abdujamilova, N., Gordoncillo, M.J., Naqvi, A., Reyes, K.C., Zervos, M.J., Bartlett, P., 2010. Characterization of vancomycin-resistant Enterococcus faecium isolated from swine in three Michigan counties. J. Clin. Microbiol.

Donskey, C.J., 2004. The role of the intestinal tract as a reservoir and source for transmission of nosocomial pathogens. Clin. Infect. Dis. 39, 219-226.

Dutta, I., Reynolds, P.E., 2002. Biochemical and genetic characterization of the vanC-2 vancomycin resistance gene cluster of Enterococcus casseliflavus ATCC 25788. Antimicrob. Agents Chemother. 46, 3125-3132.

EARSS, 2009. EARSS Annual report 2008. EARSS Annual report 2008 10, 1-180.

Facklam, R.R., Carvalho, M.d.G.S., Teixeira, L.M., 2002. History, taxonomy, biochemical characteristics, and antibiotic susceptibility testing of enterococci. In: Gilmore, M.S. (Eds), The enterococci: Pathogenesis, molecular biology, and antibiotic resistance. ASM Press, Washington, D.C., pp. 1-54.

Fang, H., Nord, C.E., Ullberg, M., 2010. Screening for vancomycin-resistant enterococci: results of a survey in Stockholm. APMIS 118, 413-417.

Fines, M., Perichon, B., Reynolds, P., Sahm, D.F., Courvalin, P., 1999. VanE, a new type of acquired glycopeptide resistance in Enterococcus faecalis BM4405. Antimicrob. Agents Chemother. 43, 2161-2164.

Finks, J., Wells, E., Dyke, T.L., Husain, N., Plizga, L., Heddurshetti, R., Wilkins, M., Rudrik, J., Hageman, J., Patel, J., Miller, C., 2009. Vancomycin-resistant Staphylococcus aureus, Michigan, USA, 2007. Emerg. Infect. Dis. 15, 943-945.

Fischer, A., Yang, S.J., Bayer, A.S., Vaezzadeh, A.R., Herzig, S., Stenz, L., Girard, M., Sakoulas, G., Scherl, A., Yeaman, M.R., Proctor, R.A., Schrenzel, J., Francois, P., 2011. Daptomycin resistance mechanisms in clinically derived Staphylococcus aureus strains assessed by a combined transcriptomics and proteomics approach. J. Antimicrob. Chemother. 66, 1696-1711.

Foglia, G., Del, G.M., Vignaroli, C., Bagnarelli, P., Varaldo, P.E., Pantosti, A., Biavasco, F., 2003. Molecular analysis of Tn1546-like elements mediating high-level vancomycin resistance in Enterococcus gallinarum. J. Antimicrob. Chemother. 52, 772-775.

Foucault, M.L., Courvalin, P., Grillot-Courvalin, C., 2009. Fitness cost of VanA-type vancomycin resistance in methicillin-resistant Staphylococcus aureus. Antimicrob. Agents Chemother. 53, 2354-2359.

Foucault, M.L., Depardieu, F., Courvalin, P., Grillot-Courvalin, C., 2010. Inducible expression eliminates the fitness cost of vancomycin resistance in enterococci. Proc. Natl. Acad. Sci. U. S. A 107, 16964-16969.

Fraimow, H., Knob, C., Herrero, I.A., Patel, R., 2005. Putative VanRS-like two-component regulatory system associated with the inducible glycopeptide resistance cluster of Paenibacillus popilliae. Antimicrob. Agents Chemother. 49, 2625-2633.

Freitas, A.R., Coque, T.M., Novais, C., Hammerum, A.M., Lester, C.H., Zervos, M.J., Donabedian, S., Jensen, L.B., Francia, M.V., Baquero, F., Peixe, L., 2011b. Human and swine hosts share vancomycin-resistant Enterococcus faecium CC17 and CC5 and Enterococcus faecalis CC2 clonal clusters harboring Tn1546 on indistinguishable plasmids. J. Clin. Microbiol. 49, 925-931.

Freitas, A.R., Coque, T.M., Novais, C., Hammerum, A.M., Lester, C.H., Zervos, M.J., Donabedian, S., Jensen, L.B., Francia, M.V., Baquero, F., Peixe, L., 2011a. Human and swine hosts share vancomycin-resistant Enterococcus faecium CC17 and CC5 and Enterococcus faecalis CC2 clonal clusters harboring Tn1546 on indistinguishable plasmids. J. Clin. Microbiol. 49, 925-931.

Freitas, A.R., Novais, C., Ruiz-Garbajosa, P., Coque, T.M., Peixe, L., 2009. Clonal expansion within clonal complex 2 and spread of vancomycin-resistant plasmids among different genetic lineages of Enterococcus faecalis from Portugal. J. Antimicrob. Chemother. 63, 1104-1111.

Galloway-Pena, J.R., Nallapareddy, S.R., Arias, C.A., Eliopoulos, G.M., Murray, B.E., 2009. Analysis of clonality and antibiotic resistance among early clinical isolates of Enterococcus faecium in the United States. J. Infect. Dis. 15, 1566-1573.

Galloway-Pena, J.R., Rice, L.B., Murray, B.E., 2011. Analysis of PBP5 of early U.S. isolates of Enterococcus faecium: Sequence variation alone does not explain increasing ampicillin resistance over time. Antimicrob. Agents Chemother. 55, 3272-3277.

Garcia-Migura, L., Hasman, H., Svendsen, C., Jensen, L.B., 2008. Relevance of hot spots in the evolution and transmission of Tn1546 in glycopeptide-resistant Enterococcus faecium (GREF) from broiler origin. J. Antimicrob. Chemother. 62, 681-687.

Garcia-Migura, L., Liebana, E., Jensen, L.B., 2007. Transposon characterization of vancomycin-resistant Enterococcus faecium (VREF) and dissemination of resistance associated with transferable plasmids. J. Antimicrob. Chemother. 60, 263-268.

Gfeller, K.Y., Roth, M., Meile, L., Teuber, M., 2003. Sequence and genetic organization of the 19.3-kb erythromycin- and dalfopristin-resistance plasmid pLME300 from Lactobacillus fermentum ROT1. Plasmid 50, 190-201.

Ghidan, A., Kaszanyitzky, E.J., Dobay, O., Nagy, K., Amyes, S.G., Rozgonyi, F., 2008. Distribution and genetic relatedness of vancomycin-resistant enterococci (VRE) isolated from healthy slaughtered chickens in Hungary from 2001 to 2004. Acta Vet. Hung. 56, 13-25.

Goffin, P., Deghorain, M., Mainardi, J.L., Tytgat, I., Champomier-Verges, M.C., Kleerebezem, M., Hols, P., 2005. Lactate racemization as a rescue pathway for supplying D-lactate to the cell wall biosynthesis machinery in Lactobacillus plantarum. J. Bacteriol. 187, 6750-6761.

Grabsch, E.A., Chua, K., Xie, S., Byrne, J., Ballard, S.A., Ward, P.B., Grayson, M.L., 2008a. Improved detection of vanB2-containing Enterococcus faecium with vancomycin susceptibility by Etest using oxgall supplementation. J. Clin. Microbiol. 46, 1961-1964.

Grabsch, E.A., Ghaly-Derias, S., Gao, W., Howden, B.P., 2008b. Comparative study of selective chromogenic (chromID VRE) and bile esculin agars for isolation and identification of vanB-containing vancomycin-resistant enterococci from feces and rectal swabs. J. Clin. Microbiol. 46, 4034-4036.

Graham, M., Ballard, S.A., Grabsch, E.A., Johnson, P.D.R., Grayson, M.L., 2008. High rates of fecal carriage of nonenterococcal vanB in both children and adults. Antimicrob. Agents Chemother. 52, 1195-1197.

Guardabassi, L., Christensen, H., Hasman, H., Dalsgaard, A., 2004. Members of the genera Paenibacillus and Rhodococcus harbor genes homologous to enterococcal glycopeptide resistance genes vanA and vanB. Antimicrob. Agents Chemother. 48, 4915-4918.

Guardabassi, L., Agerso, Y., 2006. Genes homologous to glycopeptide resistance vanA are widespread in soil microbial communities. FEMS Microbiology Letters 259, 221-225.

Guardabassi, L., Perichon, B., van Heijenoort, J., Blanot, D., Courvalin, P., 2005. Glycopeptide resistance vanA operons in Paenibacillus strains isolated from soil. Antimicrob. Agents Chemother. 49, 4227-4233.

Haenni, M., Saras, E., Chatre, P., Meunier, D., Martin, S., Lepage, G., Menard, M.F., Lebreton, P., Rambaud, T., Madec, J.Y., 2009. vanA in Enterococcus faecium, Enterococcus faecalis, and Enterococcus casseliflavus detected in French cattle. Foodborne. Pathog. Dis. 6, 1107-1111.

Hallgren, A., Saeedi, B., Nilsson, M., Monstein, H.J., Isaksson, B., Hanberger, H., Nilsson, L.E., 2003. Genetic relatedness among Enterococcus faecalis with transposon-mediated high-level gentamicin resistance in Swedish intensive care units. J. Antimicrob. Chemother. 52, 162-167.

Hammerum, A.M., Lester, C.H., Heuer, O.E., 2010. Antimicrobial-resistant enterococci in animals and meat: a human health hazard? Foodborne. Pathog. Dis. 7, 1137-1146.

Hegstad, K., Mikalsen, T., Coque, T.M., Werner, G., Sundsfjord, A., 2010. Mobile genetic elements and their contribution to the emergence of antimicrobial resistant Enterococcus faecalis and Enterococus faecium. Clin. Microbiol. Infect. 16, 541-554.

Heikens, E., van Schaik, W., Leavis, H.L., Bonten, M.J.M., Willems, R.J.L., 2008. Identification of a novel genomic island specific to hospital-acquired clonal complex 17 Enterococcus faecium isolates. Appl. Environ. Microbiol. 74, 7094-7097.

Hendrickx, A.P., Willems, R.J., Bonten, M.J., van, S.W., 2009. LPxTG surface proteins of enterococci. Trends Microbiol. 17, 423-430.

Hendrickx, A.P.A., Bonten, M.J.M., van Luit-Asbroek, M., Schapendonk, C.M.E., Kragten, A.H.M., Willems, R.J.L., 2008. Expression of two distinct types of pili by a hospital-acquired Enterococcus faecium isolate. Microbiology 154, 3212-3223.

Hendrickx, A.P.A., Van Wamel, W.J.B., Posthuma, G., Bonten, M.J.M., Willems, R.J.L., 2007. Five genes encoding surface exposed LPXTG proteins are enriched in hospital-adapted Enterococcus faecium Clonal Complex-17 isolates. J. Bacteriol. 189, 8321-8332.

Hershberger, E., Oprea, S.F., Donabedian, S.M., Perri, M., Bozigar, P., Bartlett, P., Zervos, M.J., 2005. Epidemiology of antimicrobial resistance in enterococci of animal origin. J. Antimicrob. Chemother. 55, 127-130.

Hooper, D.C., 2002. Fluoroquinolone resistance among Gram-positive cocci. The Lancet Infectious Diseases 2, 530-538.

Horinouchi, S., Weisblum, B., 1980. Posttranscriptional modification of mRNA conformation: mechanism that regulates erythromycin-induced resistance. Proc. Natl. Acad. Sci. U. S. A 77, 7079-7083.

Horodniceanu, T., Bougueleret, L., El-Solh, N., Bieth, G., Delbos, F., 1979. High-level, plasmid-borne resistance to gentamicin in Streptococcus faecalis subsp. zymogenes. Antimicrob. Agents Chemother. 16, 686-689.

Howden, B.P., Davies, J.K., Johnson, P.D., Stinear, T.P., Grayson, M.L., 2010. Reduced vancomycin susceptibility in Staphylococcus aureus, including vancomycin-intermediate and heterogeneous vancomycin-intermediate strains: resistance mechanisms, laboratory detection, and clinical implications. Clin. Microbiol. Rev. 23, 99-139.

Hsieh, Y.C., Lee, W.S., Ou, T.Y., Hsueh, P.R., 2010. Clonal spread of CC17 vancomycin-resistant Enterococcus faecium with multilocus sequence type 78 (ST78) and a novel ST444 in Taiwan. Eur. J. Clin. Microbiol. Infect. Dis. 29, 25-30.

Hsieh, Y.C., Ou, T.Y., Teng, S.O., Lee, W.C., Lin, Y.C., Wang, J.T., Chang, S.C., Lee, W.S., 2009. Vancomycin-resistant enterococci in a tertiary teaching hospital in Taiwan. J. Microbiol. Immunol. Infect. 42, 63-68.

Huh, J.Y., Lee, W.G., Lee, K., Shin, W.S., Yoo, J.H., 2004. Distribution of insertion sequences associated with Tn1546-like elements among Enterococcus faecium isolates from patients in Korea. J. Clin. Microbiol. 42, 1897-1902.

Jackson, C.R., Fedorka-Cray, P.J., Barrett, J.B., Ladely, S.R., 2004. Genetic relatedness of high-level aminoglycoside-resistant enterococci isolated from poultry carcasses. Avian Dis. 48, 100-107.

Jackson, C.R., Fedorka-Cray, P.J., Barrett, J.B., Ladely, S.R., 2005. High-level aminoglycoside resistant enterococci isolated from swine. Epidemiol. Infect. 133, 367-371.

Jacob, J., Evers, S., Bischoff, K., Carlier, C., Courvalin, P., 1994. Characterization of the sat4 gene encoding a streptothricin acetyltransferase in Campylobacter coli BE/G4. FEMS Microbiol. Lett. 120, 13-17.

Jacoby, G.A., 2005. Mechanisms of resistance to quinolones. Clin. Infect. Dis. 41 Suppl 2, S120-S126.

Jasni, A.S., Mullany, P., Hussain, H., Roberts, A.P., 2010. Demonstration of conjugative transposon (Tn5397)-mediated horizontal gene transfer between Clostridium difficile and Enterococcus faecalis. Antimicrob. Agents Chemother. 54, 4924-4926.

Jensen, L.B., Ahrens, P., Dons, L., Jones, R.N., Hammerum, A.M., Aarestrup, F.M., 1998. Molecular analysis of Tn1546 in Enterococcus faecium isolated from animals and humans. J. Clin. Microbiol. 36, 437-442.

Johnson, P.D., Ballard, S.A., Grabsch, E.A., Stinear, T.P., Seemann, T., Young, H.L., Grayson, M.L., Howden, B.P., 2010. A sustained hospital outbreak of vancomycin-resistant Enterococcus faecium bacteremia due to emergence of vanB E. faecium sequence type 203. J. Infect. Dis. 202, 1278-1286.

Jones, R.N., Deshpande, L.M., 2004. Are Enterococcus faecalis strains with vat(E) in poultry a reservoir for human streptogramin resistance? vat(E) occurrence in human enterococcal bloodstream infections in North America (SENTRY Antimicrobial Surveillance Program, 2002). Antimicrob. Agents Chemother. 48, 360-361.

Jung, W.K., Lim, J.Y., Kwon, N.H., Kim, J.M., Hong, S.K., Koo, H.C., Kim, S.H., Park, Y.H., 2007. Vancomycin-resistant enterococci from animal sources in Korea. Int. J. Food Microbiol. 113, 102-107.

Jung, Y.H., Shin, E.S., Kim, O., Yoo, J.S., Lee, K.M., Yoo, J.I., Chung, G.T., Lee, Y.S., 2010. Characterization of two newly identified genes, vgaD and vatG, conferring resistance to streptogramin A in Enterococcus faecium. Antimicrob. Agents Chemother. 54, 4744-4749.

JUREEN, R., MOHN, S.C., Harthug, S., HAARR, L., LANGELAND, N., 2004. Role of penicillin-binding protein 5 C-terminal amino acid substitutions in conferring ampicillin resistance in Norwegian clinical strains of Enterococcus faecium. APMIS 112, 291-298.

Karlowsky, J.A., Jones, M.E., Draghi, D.C., Thornsberry, C., Sahm, D.F., Volturo, G.A., 2004. Prevalence and antimicrobial susceptibilities of bacteria isolated from blood cultures of hospitalized patients in the United States in 2002. Ann. Clin. Microbiol. Antimicrob. 3, 7-

Karlowsky, J.A., Zhanel, G.G., Hoban, D.J., 1999. Vancomycin-resistant enterococci (VRE) colonization of high-risk patients in tertiary care Canadian hospitals. Canadian VRE Surveillance Group. Diagn. Microbiol. Infect. Dis. 35, 1-7.

Kawalec, M., Gniadkowski, M., Kedzierska, J., Skotnicki, A., Fiett, J., Hryniewicz, W., 2001b. Selection of a teicoplanin-resistant Enterococcus faecium mutant during an outbreak caused by vancomycin-resistant enterococci with the vanB phenotype. J. Clin. Microbiol. 39, 4274-4282.

Kawalec, M., Gniadkowski, M., Kedzierska, J., Skotnicki, A., Fiett, J., Hryniewicz, W., 2001a. Selection of a teicoplanin-resistant Enterococcus faecium mutant during an outbreak caused by vancomycin-resistant enterococci with the vanB phenotype. J. Clin. Microbiol. 39, 4274-4282.

Kawalec, M., Kedzierska, J., Gajda, A., Sadowy, E., Wegrzyn, J., Naser, S., Skotnicki, A.B., Gniadkowski, M., Hryniewicz, W., 2007. Hospital outbreak of vancomycin-resistant enterococci caused by a single clone of Enterococcus raffinosus and several clones of Enterococcus faecium. Clinical Microbiology and Infection 13, 893-901.

Kerr, I.D., Reynolds, E.D., Cove, J.H., 2005. ABC proteins and antibiotic drug resistance: is it all about transport? Biochem. Soc. Trans. 33, 1000-1002.

Klare, I., Badstubner, D., Konstabel, C., Bohme, G., Claus, H., Witte, W., 1999. Decreased incidence of VanA-type vancomycin-resistant enterococci isolated from poultry meat and from fecal samples of humans in the community after discontinuation of avoparcin usage in animal husbandry. Microb. Drug Resist. 5, 45-52.

Klare, I., Heier, H., Claus, H., Bohme, G., Marin, S., Seltmann, G., Hakenbeck, R., Antanassova, V., Witte, W., 1995a. Enterococcus faecium strains with vanA-mediated high-level glycopeptide resistance isolated from animal foodstuffs and fecal samples of humans in the community. Microb. Drug Resist. 1, 265-272.

Klare, I., Heier, H., Claus, H., Reissbrodt, R., Witte, W., 1995b. vanA-mediated high-level glycopeptide resistance in Enterococcus faecium from animal husbandry. FEMS Microbiol. Lett. 125, 165-171.

Klare, I., Heier, H., Claus, H., Witte, W., 1993. Environmental strains of Enterococcus faecium with inducible high-level resistance to glycopeptides. FEMS Microbiol. Lett. 106, 23-29.

Klare, I., Konstabel, C., Badstübner, D., Werner, G., Witte, W., 2003. Occurrence and spread of antibiotic resistances in Enterococcus faecium. Int. J. Food Microbiol. 88, 269-290.

Klare, I., Konstabel, C., Mueller-Bertling, S., Werner, G., Strommenger, B., Kettlitz, C., Borgmann, S., Schulte, B., Jonas, D., Serr, A., Fahr, A., Eigner, U., Witte, W., 2005. Spread of ampicillin/vancomycin-resistant Enterococcus faecium of the epidemic-virulent clonal complex-17 carrying the genes esp and hyl in German hospitals. European Journal of Clinical Microbiology & Infectious Diseases 24, 815-825.

Klare, I., Werner, G., Witte, W., 2010. Enterococci with vancomycin resistance from German hospitals in 2008/2009 (German). Epidemiologisches Bulletin 2010, 427-437.

Klare, I., Witte, W., 1998. VRE: animal reservoirs and food. In: Brun-Buisson, C., Eliopoulos, G.M., Leclercq, R. (Eds), Bacterial resistance to glycopeptides. Flammarion Médecine-Sciences, Paris, pp. 83-93.

Klein, G., Pack, A., Reuter, G., 1998. Antibiotic resistance patterns of enterococci and occurrence of vancomycin-resistant enterococci in raw minced beef and pork in Germany. Appl. Environ. Microbiol. 64, 1825-1830.

Ko, K.S., Baek, J.Y., Lee, J.Y., Oh, W.S., Peck, K.R., Lee, N., Lee, W.G., Lee, K., Song, J.H., 2005. Molecular characterization of vancomycin-resistant Enterococcus faecium isolates from Korea. J. Clin. Microbiol. 43, 2303-2306.

Koh, T.H., Hsu, L.Y., Chiu, L.L., Lin, R.V.T.P., 2006. Emergence of epidemic clones of vancomycin-resistant Enterococcus faecium in Singapore. Journal of Hospital Infection 63, 234-236.

Koh, T.H., Low, B.S., Leo, N., Hsu, L.Y., Lin, R.T., Krishnan, P., Chan, D., Nadarajah, M., Toh, S.L., Ong, K.H., 2009. Molecular epidemiology of vancomycin-resistant enterococci in Singapore. Pathology 41, 676-680.

Kojima, A., Morioka, A., Kijima, M., Ishihara, K., Asai, T., Fujisawa, T., Tamura, Y., Takahashi, T., 2010. Classification and antimicrobial susceptibilities of enterococcus species isolated from apparently healthy food-producing animals in Japan. Zoonoses. Public Health 57, 137-141.

Kruse, H., Johansen, B.K., Rorvik, L.M., Schaller, G., 1999. The use of avoparcin as a growth promoter and the occurrence of vancomycin-resistant Enterococcus species in Norwegian poultry and swine production. Microb. Drug Resist. 5, 135-139.

Kuzin, A.P., Sun, T., Jorczak-Baillass, J., Healy, V.L., Walsh, C.T., Knox, J.R., 2000. Enzymes of vancomycin resistance: the structure of D-alanine-D-lactate ligase of naturally resistant Leuconostoc mesenteroides. Structure. 8, 463-470.

Kwong, S.M., Lim, R., Lebard, R.J., Skurray, R.A., Firth, N., 2008. Analysis of the pSK1 replicon, a prototype from the staphylococcal multiresistance plasmid family. Microbiology 154, 3084-3094.

Larsen, J., Schonheyder, H.C., Lester, C.H., Olsen, S.S., Porsbo, L.J., Garcia-Migura, L., Jensen, L.B., Bisgaard, M., Hammerum, A.M., 2010. Porcine-origin gentamicin-resistant Enterococcus faecalis in Humans, Denmark. Emerg. Infect. Dis. 16, 682-684.

Lauderdale, T.L., Shiau, Y.R., Wang, H.Y., Lai, J.F., Huang, I.W., Chen, P.C., Chen, H.Y., Lai, S.S., Liu, Y.F., Ho, M., 2007. Effect of banning vancomycin analogue avoparcin on vancomycin-resistant enterococci in chicken farms in Taiwan. Environmental Microbiology 9, 819-823.

Launay, A., Ballard, S.A., Johnson, P.D.R., Grayson, M.L., Lambert, T., 2006. Transfer of vancomycin resistance transposon Tn1549 from Clostridium symbiosum to Enterococcus spp. in the gut of gnotobiotic mice. Antimicrob. Agents Chemother. 50, 1054-1062.

Laverde Gomez, J.A., van, S.W., Freitas, A.R., Coque, T.M., Weaver, K.E., Francia, M.V., Witte, W., Werner, G., 2010. A multiresistance megaplasmid pLG1 bearing a hyl(Efm) genomic island in hospital Enterococcus faecium isolates. Int. J. Med. Microbiol.

Laverde Gomez, J.A., van, S.W., Freitas, A.R., Coque, T.M., Weaver, K.E., Francia, M.V., Witte, W., Werner, G., 2011. A multiresistance megaplasmid pLG1 bearing a hylEfm genomic island in hospital Enterococcus faecium isolates. Int. J. Med. Microbiol. 301, 165-175.

Leavis, H.L., Willems, R.J., van Wamel, W.J., Schuren, F.H., Caspers, M.P., Bonten, M.J., 2007. Insertion sequence-driven diversification creates a globally dispersed emerging multiresistant subspecies of E. faecium. PLoS. Pathog. 3, e7-75.

Leavis, H.L., Willems, R.J.L., Top, J., Bonten, M.J.M., 2006. High-Level ciprofloxacin resistance from point mutations in gyrA and parC confined to global hospital-adapted clonal lineage CC17 of Enterococcus faecium. J. Clin. Microbiol. 44, 1059-1064.

Leclercq, R., Derlot, E., Duval, J., Courvalin, P., 1988. Plasmid-mediated resistance to vancomycin and teicoplanin in Enterococcus faecium. N. Engl. J. Med. 319, 157-161.

Leclercq, R., Derlot, E., Weber, M., Duval, J., Courvalin, P., 1989. Transferable vancomycin and teicoplanin resistance in Enterococcus faecium. Antimicrob. Agents Chemother. 33, 10-15.

Lee, S.Y., Park, K.G., Lee, G.D., Park, J.J., Park, Y.J., 2010. Comparison of Seeplex VRE detection kit with ChromID VRE agar for detection of vancomycin-resistant enterococci in rectal swab specimens. Ann. Clin. Lab Sci. 40, 163-166.

Lester, C.H., Hammerum, A.M., 2010. Transfer of vanA from an Enterococcus faecium isolate of chicken origin to a CC17 E. faecium isolate in the intestine of cephalosporin-treated mice. J. Antimicrob. Chemother. 65, 1534-1536.

Lester, C.H., Olsen, S.S., Schonheyder, H.C., Hansen, D.S., Tvede, M., Holm, A., Arpi, M., Friis-Moller, A., Jensen, K.T., Kemp, M., Hammerum, A.M., 2009. Typing of vancomycin-resistant enterococci obtained from patients at Danish hospitals and detection of a genomic island specific to CC17 Enterococcus faecium. Int. J. Antimicrob. Agents 35, 312-314.

Lester, C.H., Sandvang, D., Olsen, S.S., Schonheyder, H.C., Jarlov, J.O., Bangsborg, J., Hansen, D.S., Jensen, T.G., Frimodt-Moller, N., Hammerum, A.M., 2008. Emergence of ampicillin-resistant Enterococcus faecium in Danish hospitals. J. Antimicrob. Chemother. 62, 1203-1206.

Lester, C.H., Frimodt-Moller, N., Sorensen, T.L., Monnet, D.L., Hammerum, A.M., 2006. In vivo transfer of the vanA resistance gene from an Enterococcus faecium isolate of animal origin to an E. faecium isolate of human origin in the intestines of human volunteers. Antimicrob. Agents Chemother. 50, 596-599.

Lim, S.K., Kim, T.S., Lee, H.S., Nam, H.M., Joo, Y.S., Koh, H.B., 2006. Persistence of vanA-type Enterococcus faecium in Korean livestock after ban on avoparcin. Microbial Drug Resistance 12, 136-139.

Lobritz, M., Hutton-Thomas, R., Marshall, S., Rice, L.B., 2003. Recombination proficiency influences frequency and locus of mutational resistance to linezolid in Enterococcus faecalis. Antimicrob. Agents Chemother. 47, 3318-3320.

Lopez, M., Hormazabal, J.C., Maldonado, A., Saavedra, G., Baquero, F., Silva, J., Torres, C., Del, C.R., 2009. Clonal dissemination of Enterococcus faecalis ST201 and Enterococcus faecium CC17-ST64 containing Tn5382-vanB2 among 16 hospitals in Chile. Clin. Microbiol. Infect. 15, 586-588.

Mahbub, A.M., Kobayashi, N., Ishino, M., Sumi, A., Kobayashi, K., Uehara, N., Watanabe, N., 2005. Detection of a novel aph(2") allele (aph[2"]-Ie) conferring high-level gentamicin resistance and a spectinomycin resistance gene ant(9)-Ia (aad 9) in clinical isolates of enterococci. Microb. Drug Resist. 11, 239-247.

Mak, A., Miller, M.A., Chong, G., Monczak, Y., 2009. Comparison of PCR and culture for screening of vancomycin-resistant Enterococci: highly disparate results for vanA and vanB. J. Clin. Microbiol. 47, 4136-4137.

Mammina, C., Di Noto, A.M., Costa, A., Nastasi, A., 2005. VanB-VanC1 Enterococcus gallinarum, Italy. Emerg. Infect. Dis. 11, 1491-1492.

Manson, J.M., Keis, S., Smith, J.M., Cook, G.M., 2003a. Characterization of a vancomycin-resistant Enterococcus faecalis (VREF) isolate from a dog with mastitis: further evidence of a clonal lineage of VREF in New Zealand. J. Clin. Microbiol. 41, 3331-3333.

Manson, J.M., Smith, J.M., Cook, G.M., 2004. Persistence of vancomycin-resistant enterococci in New Zealand broilers after discontinuation of avoparcin use. Appl. Environ. Microbiol. 70, 5764-5768.

Manson, J.M., Keis, S., Smith, J.M.B., Cook, G.M., 2003b. A clonal lineage of VanA-type Enterococcus faecalis predominates in vancomycin-resistant enterococci isolated in New Zealand. Antimicrob. Agents Chemother. 47, 204-210.

Marner, E.S., Wolk, D.M., Carr, J., Hewitt, C., Dominguez, L.L., Kovacs, T., Johnson, D.R., Hayden, R.T., 2011. Diagnostic accuracy of the Cepheid GeneXpert vanA/vanB assay ver. 1.0 to detect the vanA and vanB vancomycin resistance genes in Enterococcus from perianal specimens. Diagn. Microbiol. Infect. Dis. 69, 382-389.

Marshall, C.G., Broadhead, G., Leskiw, B.K., Wright, G.D., 1997. D-Ala-D-Ala ligases from glycopeptide antibiotic-producing organisms are highly homologous to the enterococcal vancomycin-resistance ligases VanA and VanB. Proc. Natl. Acad. Sci. U. S. A 94, 6480-6483.

Marshall, C.G., Lessard, I.A., Park, I., Wright, G.D., 1998. Glycopeptide antibiotic resistance genes in glycopeptide-producing organisms. Antimicrob. Agents Chemother. 42, 2215-2220.

Marshall, S.H., Donskey, C.J., Hutton-Thomas, R., Salata, R.A., Rice, L.B., 2002. Gene dosage and linezolid resistance in Enterococcus faecium and Enterococcus faecalis. Antimicrob. Agents Chemother. 46, 3334-3336.

Martel, A., Devriese, L.A., Decostere, A., Haesebrouck, F., 2003. Presence of macrolide resistance genes in streptococci and enterococci isolated from pigs and pork carcasses. Int. J. Food Microbiol. 84, 27-32.

Martone, W.J., 1998. Spread of vancomycin-resistant enterococci: why did it happen in the United States? Infect. Control Hosp. Epidemiol. 19, 539-545.

McBride, S.M., Fischetti, V.A., Leblanc, D.J., Moellering, R.C., Jr., Gilmore, M.S., 2007. Genetic diversity among Enterococcus faecalis. PLoS. ONE. 2, e582-

McDonald, L.C., Kuehnert, M.J., Tenover, F.C., Jarvis, W.R., 1997. Vancomycin-resistant enterococci outside the health-care setting: prevalence, sources, and public health implications. Emerg. Infect. Dis. 3, 311-317.

McKessar, S.J., Berry, A.M., Bell, J.M., Turnidge, J.D., Paton, J.C., 2000. Genetic characterization of vanG, a novel vancomycin resistance locus of Enterococcus faecalis. Antimicrob. Agents Chemother. 44, 3224-3228.

Mevius, D., Devriese, L., Butaye, P., Vandamme, P., Verschure, M., Veldman, K., 1998. Isolation of glycopeptide resistant Streptococcus gallolyticus strains with vanA, vanB, and both vanA and vanB genotypes from faecal samples of veal calves in The Netherlands. J. Antimicrob. Chemother. 42, 275-276.

Meziane-Cherif, D., Saul, F.A., Moubareck, C., Weber, P., Haouz, A., Courvalin, P., Perichon, B., 2010. Molecular basis of vancomycin dependence in VanA-type Staphylococcus aureus VRSA-9. J. Bacteriol. 192, 5465-5471.

Min, Y.H., Kwon, A.R., Yoon, J.M., Yoon, E.J., Shim, M.J., Choi, E.C., 2008. Molecular analysis of constitutive mutations in ermB and ermA selected in vitro from inducibly MLSB-resistant enterococci. Arch. Pharm. Res. 31, 377-380.

Moore, I.F., Hughes, D.W., Wright, G.D., 2005. Tigecycline is modified by the flavin-dependent monooxygenase TetX. Biochemistry 44, 11829-11835.

Morris-Downes, M., Smyth, E.G., Moore, J., Thomas, T., Fitzpatrick, F., Walsh, J., Caffrey, V., Morris, A., Foley, S., Humphreys, H., 2010. Surveillance and endemic vancomycin-resistant enterococci: some success in control is possible. J. Hosp. Infect. 75, 228-233.

Moubareck, C., Bourgeois, N., Courvalin, P., Doucet-Populaire, F., 2003. Multiple antibiotic resistance gene transfer from animal to human enterococci in the digestive tract of gnotobiotic mice. Antimicrob. Agents Chemother. 47, 2993-2996.

Moubareck, C., Meziane-Cherif, D., Courvalin, P., Perichon, B., 2009. VanA-type Staphylococcus aureus strain VRSA-7 is partially dependent on vancomycin for growth. Antimicrob. Agents Chemother. 53, 3657-3663.

Murray, B.E., 1990. The life and times of the Enterococcus. Clin. Microbiol. Rev. 3, 46-65.

Murray, B.E., 2000. Vancomycin-resistant enterococcal infections. N. Engl. J. Med. 342, 710-721.

Nallapareddy, S.R., Singh, K.V., Okhuysen, P.C., Murray, B.E., 2008. A functional collagen adhesin gene, acm, in clinical isolates of Enterococcus faecium correlates with the recent success of this emerging nosocomial pathogen. Infect. Immun. 76, 4110-4119.

Nallapareddy, S.R., Wenxiang, H., Weinstock, G.M., Murray, B.E., 2005. Molecular characterization of a widespread, pathogenic, and antibiotic resistance-receptive Enterococcus faecalis lineage and dissemination of its putative pathogenicity island. J. Bacteriol. 187, 5709-5718.

Nannini, E., Murray, B.E., Arias, C.A., 2010. Resistance or decreased susceptibility to glycopeptides, daptomycin, and linezolid in methicillin-resistant Staphylococcus aureus. Curr. Opin. Pharmacol. 10, 516-521.

Naser, S.M., Vancanneyt, M., Hoste, B., Snauwaert, C., Vandemeulebroecke, K., Swings, J., 2006b. Reclassification of Enterococcus flavescens Pompei et al. 1992 as a later synonym of Enterococcus casseliflavus (ex Vaughan et al. 1979) Collins et al. 1984 and Enterococcus saccharominimus Vancanneyt et al. 2004 as a later synonym of Enterococcus italicus Fortina et al. 2004. Int. J. Syst. Evol. Microbiol. 56, 413-416.

Naser, S.M., Vancanneyt, M., Hoste, B., Snauwaert, C., Vandemeulebroecke, K., Swings, J., 2006a. Reclassification of Enterococcus flavescens Pompei et al. 1992 as a later synonym of Enterococcus casseliflavus (ex Vaughan et al. 1979) Collins et al. 1984 and Enterococcus saccharominimus Vancanneyt et al. 2004 as a later synonym of Enterococcus italicus Fortina et al. 2004. Int. J. Syst. Evol. Microbiol. 56, 413-416.

Neves, F.P., Ribeiro, R.L., Duarte, R.S., Teixeira, L.M., Merquior, V.L., 2009. Emergence of the vanA genotype among Enterococcus gallinarum isolates colonising the intestinal tract of patients in a university hospital in Rio de Janeiro, Brazil. Int. J. Antimicrob. Agents 33, 211-215.

Nichol, K.A., Sill, M., Laing, N.M., Johnson, J.L., Hoban, D.J., Zhanel, G.G., 2006. Molecular epidemiology of urinary tract isolates of vancomycin-resistant Enterococcus faecium from North America. International Journal of Antimicrobial Agents 27, 392-396.

Nilsson, O., Greko, C., Bengtsson, B., 2009a. Environmental contamination by vancomycin resistant enterococci (VRE) in Swedish broiler production. Acta Vet. Scand. 51, 49-

Nilsson, O., Greko, C., Top, J., Franklin, A., Bengtsson, B., 2009b. Spread without known selective pressure of a vancomycin-resistant clone of Enterococcus faecium among broilers. J. Antimicrob. Chemother. 63, 868-872.

Noble, W.C., Virani, Z., Cree, R.G., 1992. Co-transfer of vancomycin and other resistance genes from Enterococcus faecalis NCTC 12201 to Staphylococcus aureus. FEMS Microbiol. Lett. 72, 195-198.

Novais, C., Freitas, A.R., Sousa, J.C., Baquero, F., Coque, T.M., Peixe, L.V., 2008. Diversity of Tn1546 and its role in the dissemination of vancomycin-resistant enterococci in Portugal. Antimicrob. Agents Chemother. 52, 1001-1008.

Novick, R.P., Murphy, E., 1985. MLS-resistance determinants in Staphylococcus aureus and their molecular evolution. J. Antimicrob. Chemother. 16 Suppl A, 101-110.

Onodera, Y., Okuda, J., Tanaka, M., Sato, K., 2002. Inhibitory activities of quinolones against DNA gyrase and topoisomerase IV of Enterococcus faecalis. Antimicrob. Agents Chemother. 46, 1800-1804.

Oteo, J., Cuevas, O., Navarro, C., Aracil, B., Campos, J., on behalf of the Spanish Group of 'The European Antimicrobial Resistance Surveillance System' (EARSS), 2007. Trends in antimicrobial resistance in 3469 enterococci isolated from blood (EARSS experience 2001-06, Spain): increasing ampicillin resistance in Enterococcus faecium. J. Antimicrob. Chemother. 59, 1044-1045.

Oyamada, Y., Ito, H., Fujimoto, K., Asada, R., Niga, T., Okamoto, R., Inoue, M., Yamagishi, J.i., 2006a. Combination of known and unknown mechanisms confers high-level resistance to fluoroquinolones in Enterococcus faecium. J Med Microbiol 55, 729-736.

Oyamada, Y., Ito, H., Inoue, M., Yamagishi, J.i., 2006b. Topoisomerase mutations and efflux are associated with fluoroquinolone resistance in Enterococcus faecalis. J Med Microbiol 55, 1395-1401.

Padiglione, A.A., Grabsch, E.A., Olden, D., Hellard, M., Sinclair, M.I., Fairley, C.K., Grayson, M.L., 2000. Fecal colonization with vancomycin-resistant enterococci in Australia. Emerg. Infect. Dis. 6, 534-536.

Pai, M.P., Rodvold, K.A., Schreckenberger, P.C., Gonzales, R.D., Petrolatti, J.M., Quinn, J.P., 2002. Risk factors associated with the development of infection with linezolid- and vancomycin-resistant Enterococcus faecium. Clin. Infect. Dis. 35, 1269-1272.

Palmer, K.L., Carniol, K., Manson, J.M., Heiman, D., Shea, T., Young, S., Zeng, Q., Gevers, D., Feldgarden, M., Birren, B., Gilmore, M.S., 2010. High-quality draft genome sequences of 28 Enterococcus sp. isolates. J. Bacteriol. 192, 2469-2470.

Panesso, D., badia-Patino, L., Vanegas, N., Reynolds, P.E., Courvalin, P., Arias, C.A., 2005. Transcriptional analysis of the vanC cluster from Enterococcus gallinarum strains with constitutive and inducible vancomycin resistance. Antimicrob. Agents Chemother. 49, 1060-1066.

Panesso, D., Reyes, J., Rincon, S., Diaz, L., Galloway-Pena, J., Zurita, J., Carrillo, C., Merentes, A., Guzman, M., Adachi, J.A., Murray, B.E., Arias, C.A., 2010. Molecular epidemiology of vancomycin-resistant Enterococcus faecium: a prospective, multicenter study in South American hospitals. J. Clin. Microbiol. 48, 1562-1569.

Park, I.J., Lee, W.G., Lim, Y.A., Cho, S.R., 2007. Genetic rearrangements of Tn1546-like elements in vancomycin-resistant Enterococcus faecium isolates collected from hospitalized patients over a seven-year period. J. Clin. Microbiol. 45, 3903-3908.

Park, I.J., Lee, W.G., Shin, J.H., Lee, K.W., Woo, G.J., 2008. VanB phenotype-vanA genotype Enterococcus faecium with heterogeneous expression of teicoplanin resistance. J. Clin. Microbiol. 46, 3091-3093.

Patel, R., 2000. Enterococcal-type glycopeptide resistance genes in non-enterococcal organisms. FEMS Microbiol. Lett. 185, 1-7.

Patel, R., Piper, K., Cockerill, F.R., III, Steckelberg, J.M., Yousten, A.A., 2000. The biopesticide Paenibacillus popilliae has a vancomycin resistance gene cluster homologous to the enterococcal VanA vancomycin resistance gene cluster. Antimicrob. Agents Chemother. 44, 705-709.

Paulsen, I.T., Banerjei, L., Myers, G.S., Nelson, K.E., Seshadri, R., Read, T.D., Fouts, D.E., Eisen, J.A., Gill, S.R., Heidelberg, J.F., Tettelin, H., Dodson, R.J., Umayam, L., Brinkac, L., Beanan, M., Daugherty, S., DeBoy, R.T., Durkin, S., Kolonay, J., Madupu, R., Nelson, W., Vamathevan, J., Tran, B., Upton, J., Hansen, T., Shetty, J., Khouri, H., Utterback, T., Radune, D., Ketchum, K.A., Dougherty, B.A., Fraser, C.M., 2003. Role of mobile DNA in the evolution of vancomycin-resistant Enterococcus faecalis. Science 299, 2071-2074.

Pearman, J.W., 2006. 2004 Lowbury Lecture: the Western Australian experience with vancomycin-resistant enterococci - from disaster to ongoing control. Journal of Hospital Infection 63, 14-26.

Pendle, S., Jelfs, P., Olma, T., Su, Y., Gilroy, N., Gilbert, G.L., 2008. Difficulties in detection and identification of Enterococcus faecium with low-level inducible resistance to vancomycin, during a hospital outbreak. Clin. Microbiol. Infect. 14, 853-857.

Perichon, B., Courvalin, P., 2004. Heterologous expression of the enterococcal vanA operon in methicillin-resistant Staphylococcus aureus. Antimicrob. Agents Chemother. 48, 4281-4285.

Perichon, B., Courvalin, P., 2006. Synergism between beta-lactams and glycopeptides against VanA-type Methicillin-Resistant Staphylococcus aureus and heterologous expression of the vanA operon. Antimicrob. Agents Chemother. 50, 3622-3630.

Poole, T.L., Hume, M.E., Campbell, L.D., Scott, H.M., Alali, W.Q., Harvey, R.B., 2005. Vancomycin-resistant Enterococcus faecium strains isolated from community wastewater from a semiclosed agri-food system in Texas. Antimicrob. Agents Chemother. 49, 4382-4385.

Poyart, C., Pierre, C., Quesne, G., Pron, B., Berche, P., Trieu-Cuot, P., 1997. Emergence of vancomycin resistance in the genus Streptococcus: characterization of a vanB transferable determinant in Streptococcus bovis. Antimicrob. Agents Chemother. 41, 24-29.

Prystowsky, J., Siddiqui, F., Chosay, J., Shinabarger, D.L., Millichap, J., Peterson, L.R., Noskin, G.A., 2001. Resistance to linezolid: characterization of mutations in rRNA and comparison of their occurrences in vancomycin-resistant enterococci. Antimicrob. Agents Chemother. 45, 2154-2156.

Qi, C., Zheng, X., Obias, A., Scheetz, M.H., Malczynski, M., Warren, J.R., 2006. Comparison of testing methods for detection of decreased linezolid susceptibility due to G2576T mutation of the 23S rRNA gene in Enterococcus faecium and Enterococcus faecalis. J. Clin. Microbiol. 44, 1098-1100.

Quinones Perez, D., 2006. Epidemiology of antimicrobial resistance in Enterococcus spp. from Cuba and other Latin American countries. In: Kobayashi, N. (Eds), Drug resistance of enterococci: Epidemiology and molecular mechanisms. Research Signpost, Kerala, India, pp. 1-20.

Rahim, S., Pillai, S.K., Gold, H.S., Venkataraman, L., Inglima, K., Press, R.A., 2003. Linezolid-resistant, vancomycin-resistant Enterococcus faecium infection in patients without prior exposure to linezolid. Clin. Infect. Dis. 36, E146-E148.

Ramsey, A.M., Zilberberg, M.D., 2009. Secular trends of hospitalization with vancomycin-resistant enterococcus infection in the United States, 2000-2006. Infect. Control Hosp. Epidemiol. 30, 184-186.

Reynolds, E., Cove, J.H., 2005. Enhanced resistance to erythromycin is conferred by the enterococcal msrC determinant in Staphylococcus aureus. J. Antimicrob. Chemother. 55, 260-264.

Reynolds, E., Ross, J.I., Cove, J.H., 2003. Msr(A) and related macrolide/streptogramin resistance determinants: incomplete transporters? Int. J. Antimicrob. Agents 22, 228-236.

Reynolds, P.E., Arias, C.A., Courvalin, P., 1999. Gene vanXYC encodes D,D -dipeptidase (VanX) and D,D-carboxypeptidase (VanY) activities in vancomycin-resistant Enterococcus gallinarum BM4174. Mol. Microbiol. 34, 341-349.

Reynolds, P.E., Courvalin, P., 2005. Vancomycin resistance in enterococci due to synthesis of precursors terminating in D-alanyl-D-serine. Antimicrob. Agents Chemother. 49, 21-25.

Rice, L.B., 2006. Antimicrobial resistance in gram-positive bacteria. Am. J. Infect. Control 34, S11-S19.

Rice, L.B., Carias, L.L., Donskey, C.L., Rudin, S.D., 1998. Transferable, plasmid-mediated vanB-type glycopeptide resistance in Enterococcus faecium. Antimicrob. Agents Chemother. 42, 963-964.

Rice, L.B., Carias, L.L., Marshall, S., Rudin, S.D., Hutton-Thomas, R., 2005. Tn5386, a novel Tn916-like mobile element in Enterococcus faecium D344R that interacts with Tn916 to yield a large genomic deletion. J. Bacteriol. 187, 6668-6677.

Rice, L.B., Carias, L.L., Marshall, S.H., Hutton-Thomas, R., Rudin, S., 2007. Characterization of Tn5386, a Tn916-related mobile element. Plasmid 58, 61-67.

Rice, L.B., Carias, L.L., Rudin, S., Hutton, R., Marshall, S., Hassan, M., Josseaume, N., Dubost, L., Marie, A., Arthur, M., 2009. Role of class A penicillin-binding proteins in the expression of beta-lactam resistance in Enterococcus faecium. J. Bacteriol. 191, 3649-3656.

Rice, L.B., Carias, L.L., Rudin, S., Hutton, R.A., Marshall, S., 2010. Multiple copies of functional, Tet(M)-encoding Tn916-like elements in a clinical Enterococcus faecium isolate. Plasmid

Rice, L.B., Bellais, S., Carias, L.L., Hutton-Thomas, R., Bonomo, R.A., Caspers, P., Page, M.G.P., Gutmann, L., 2004. Impact of specific pbp5 mutations on expression of {beta}-lactam resistance in Enterococcus faecium. Antimicrob. Agents Chemother. 48, 3028-3032.

Roberts, A.P., Johanesen, P.A., Lyras, D., Mullany, P., Rood, J.I., 2001. Comparison of Tn5397 from Clostridium difficile, Tn916 from Enterococcus faecalis and the CW459tet(M) element from Clostridium perfringens shows that they have similar conjugation regions but different insertion and excision modules. Microbiology 147, 1243-1251.

Roberts, A.P., Mullany, P., 2009. A modular master on the move: the Tn916 family of mobile genetic elements. Trends Microbiol. 17, 251-258.

Roberts, A.P., Mullany, P., 2011. Tn916-like genetic elements: a diverse group of modular mobile elements conferring antibiotic resistance. FEMS Microbiol. Rev.

Roberts, M.C., 2005. Update on acquired tetracycline resistance genes. FEMS Microbiol. Lett. 245, 195-203.

Roberts, M.C., Sutcliffe, J., Courvalin, P., Jensen, L.B., Rood, J., Seppala, H., 1999. Nomenclature for macrolide and macrolide-lincosamide-streptogramin B resistance determinants. Antimicrob. Agents Chemother. 43, 2823-2830.

Rodriguez-Martinez, J.M., Velasco, C., Briales, A., Garcia, I., Conejo, M.C., Pascual, A., 2008. Qnr-like pentapeptide repeat proteins in gram-positive bacteria. J. Antimicrob. Chemother. 61, 1240-1243.

Rosato, A., Pierre, J., Billot-Klein, D., Buu-Hoi, A., Gutmann, L., 1995. Inducible and constitutive expression of resistance to glycopeptides and vancomycin dependence in glycopeptide-resistant Enterococcus avium. Antimicrob. Agents Chemother. 39, 830-833.

Rosato, A., Vicarini, H., Leclercq, R., 1999. Inducible or constitutive expression of resistance in clinical isolates of streptococci and enterococci cross-resistant to erythromycin and lincomycin. J. Antimicrob. Chemother. 43, 559-562.

Rosvoll, T.C.S., Pedersen, T., Sletvold, H., Johnsen, P.J., Sollid, J.E., Simonsen, G.S., Jensen, L.B., Nielsen, K.M., Sundsfjord, A., 2009. PCR-based plasmid typing in Enterococcus faecium strains reveals widely distributed pRE25-, pRUM-, pIP501-

and pHTbeta-related replicons associated with glycopeptide resistance and stabilizing toxin-antitoxin systems. FEMS Immunology and Medical Microbiology 58, 254-268.

Ruggero, K.A., Schroeder, L.K., Schreckenberger, P.C., Mankin, A.S., Quinn, J.P., 2003. Nosocomial superinfections due to linezolid-resistant Enterococcus faecalis: evidence for a gene dosage effect on linezolid MICs. Diagn. Microbiol. Infect. Dis. 47, 511-513.

Ruiz-Garbajosa, P., Bonten, M.J., Robinson, D.A., Top, J., Nallapareddy, S.R., Torres, C., Coque, T.M., Canton, R., Baquero, F., Murray, B.E., Del, C.R., Willems, R.J., 2006. Multilocus sequence typing scheme for Enterococcus faecalis reveals hospital-adapted genetic complexes in a background of high rates of recombination. J. Clin. Microbiol. 44, 2220-2228.

Sader, H.S., Moet, G.J., Jones, R.N., 2009. Antimicrobial resistance among Gram-positive bacteria isolated in Latin American hospitals. J. Chemother. 21, 611-620.

Saeedi, B., Hallgren, A., Isaksson, B., Jonasson, J., Nilsson, L.E., Hanberger, H., 2004. Genetic relatedness of Enterococcus faecalis isolates with high-level gentamicin resistance from patients with bacteraemia in the south east of Sweden 1994-2001. Scand. J. Infect. Dis. 36, 405-409.

Sahlstrom, L., Rehbinder, V., Albihn, A., Aspan, A., Bengtsson, B., 2009. Vancomycin resistant enterococci (VRE) in Swedish sewage sludge. Acta Vet. Scand. 51, 24-

Sahm, D.F., Kissinger, J., Gilmore, M.S., Murray, P.R., Mulder, R., Solliday, J., Clarke, B., 1989. In vitro susceptibility studies of vancomycin-resistant Enterococcus faecalis. Antimicrob. Agents Chemother. 33, 1588-1591.

San Millan, A., Depardieu, F., Godreuil, S., Courvalin, P., 2009a. VanB-type Enterococcus faecium clinical isolate successively inducibly resistant to, dependent on, and constitutively resistant to vancomycin. Antimicrob. Agents Chemother. 53, 1974-1982.

San Millan, A., Depardieu, F., Godreuil, S., Courvalin, P., 2009b. VanB-type Enterococcus faecium clinical isolate successively inducibly resistant to, dependent on, and constitutively resistant to vancomycin. Antimicrob. Agents Chemother. 53, 1974-1982.

Schmitz, F.J., Witte, W., Werner, G., Petridou, J., Fluit, A.C., Schwarz, S., 2001. Characterization of the translational attenuator of 20 methicillin-resistant, quinupristin/dalfopristin-resistant Staphylococcus aureus isolates with reduced susceptibility to glycopeptides. J. Antimicrob. Chemother. 48, 939-941.

Schouten, M.A., Voss, A., Hoogkamp-Korstanje, J.A., 1997. VRE and meat. Lancet 349, 1258-

Schwarz, F.V., Perreten, V., Teuber, M., 2001. Sequence of the 50-kb conjugative multiresistance plasmid pRE25 from Enterococcus faecalis RE25. Plasmid 46, 170-187.

Sebaihia, M., Wren, B.W., Mullany, P., Fairweather, N.F., Minton, N., Stabler, R., Thomson, N.R., Roberts, A.P., Cerdeno-Tarraga, A.M., Wang, H., Holden, M.T., Wright, A., Churcher, C., Quail, M.A., Baker, S., Bason, N., Brooks, K., Chillingworth, T., Cronin, A., Davis, P., Dowd, L., Fraser, A., Feltwell, T., Hance, Z., Holroyd, S., Jagels, K., Moule, S., Mungall, K., Price, C., Rabbinowitsch, E., Sharp, S., Simmonds, M., Stevens, K., Unwin, L., Whithead, S., Dupuy, B., Dougan, G., Barrell, B., Parkhill, J., 2006. The multidrug-resistant human pathogen Clostridium difficile has a highly mobile, mosaic genome. Nat. Genet. 38, 779-786.

Seedat, J., Zick, G., Klare, I., Konstabel, C., Weiler, N., Sahly, H., 2006. Rapid emergence of resistance to linezolid during linezolid therapy of an Enterococcus faecium infection. Antimicrob. Agents Chemother. 50, 4217-4219.

Shaw, J.H., Clewell, D.B., 1985. Complete nucleotide sequence of macrolide-lincosamide-streptogramin B-resistance transposon Tn917 in Streptococcus faecalis. J. Bacteriol. 164, 782-796.

Shin, E., Hong, H., Ike, Y., Lee, K., Park, Y.H., Cho, D.T., Lee, Y., 2006. VanB-vanA incongruent VRE isolated from animals and humans in 1999. J. Microbiol. 44, 453-456.

Shirano, M., Takakura, S., Yamamoto, M., Matsumura, Y., Matsushima, A., Nagao, M., Fujihara, N., Saito, T., Ito, Y., Iinuma, Y., Shimizu, T., Fujita, N., Ichiyama, S., 2010. Regional spread of vanA- or vanB-positive Enterococcus gallinarum in hospitals and long-term care facilities in Kyoto prefecture, Japan. Epidemiol. Infect. 1-7.

Sievert, D.M., Rudrik, J.T., Patel, J.B., McDonald, L.C., Wilkins, M.J., Hageman, J.C., 2008. Vancomycin-resistant Staphylococcus aureus in the United States, 2002-2006. Clin. Infect. Dis. 46, 668-674.

Sifaoui, F., Gutmann, L., 1997. Vancomycin dependence in a vanA-producing Enterococcus avium strain with a nonsense mutation in the natural D-Ala-D-Ala ligase gene. Antimicrob. Agents Chemother. 41, 1409-

Sillanpaa, J., Nallapareddy, S.R., Prakash, V.P., Qin, X., Hook, M., Weinstock, G.M., Murray, B.E., 2008. Identification and phenotypic characterization of a second collagen adhesin, Scm, and genome-based identification and analysis of 13 other predicted MSCRAMMs, including four distinct pilus loci, in Enterococcus faecium. Microbiology 154, 3199-3211.

Simjee, S., White, D.G., Wagner, D.D., Meng, J., Qaiyumi, S., Zhao, S., McDermott, P.F., 2002. Identification of vat(E) in Enterococcus faecalis isolates from retail poultry and its transferability to Enterococcus faecium. Antimicrob. Agents Chemother. 46, 3823-3828.

Simonsen, G.S., Haaheim, H., Dahl, K.H., Kruse, H., Lovseth, A., Olsvik, O., Sundsfjord, A., 1998. Transmission of VanA-type vancomycin-resistant enterococci and vanA resistance elements between chicken and humans at avoparcin-exposed farms. Microb. Drug Resist. 4, 313-318.

Sinclair, A., Arnold, C., Woodford, N., 2003. Rapid detection and estimation by pyrosequencing of 23S rRNA genes with a single nucleotide polymorphism conferring linezolid resistance in Enterococci. Antimicrob. Agents Chemother. 47, 3620-3622.

Singh, K.V., Malathum, K., Murray, B.E., 2001. Disruption of an Enterococcus faecium species-specific gene, a homologue of acquired macrolide resistance genes of staphylococci, is associated with an increase in macrolide susceptibility. Antimicrob. Agents Chemother. 45, 263-266.

Singh, K.V., Murray, B.E., 2005. Differences in the Enterococcus faecalis lsa locus that influence susceptibility to quinupristin-dalfopristin and clindamycin. Antimicrob. Agents Chemother. 49, 32-39.

Singh, K.V., Weinstock, G.M., Murray, B.E., 2002. An Enterococcus faecalis ABC homologue (Lsa) is required for the resistance of this species to clindamycin and quinupristin-dalfopristin. Antimicrob. Agents Chemother. 46, 1845-1850.

Sivertsen, A., Lundblad, E.W., Wisell, K.T., Liljequist, B., Billström, H., Ullberg, M., Heimer, D., Sjögren, I., Aasnaes, B., Sundsfjord, A., Hegstad, K., 2011. The widespread VRE outbreak in Swedish hospitals 2007-2009 was associated with clonal E. faecium CC17 genogroup strains harbouring several virulence traits and transferable vanB pRUM-like repA plasmids. Final Programme of the 21st ECCMID, Milano, May 7-10, 2011 Poster P924, 113-

Sletvold, H., Johnsen, P.J., Hamre, I., Simonsen, G.S., Sundsfjord, A., Nielsen, K.M., 2008. Complete sequence of Enterococcus faecium pVEF3 and the detection of an omega-epsilon-zeta toxin-antitoxin module and an ABC transporter. Plasmid 60, 75-85.

Sletvold, H., Johnsen, P.J., Simonsen, G.S., Aasnaes, B., Sundsfjord, A., Nielsen, K.M., 2007. Comparative DNA analysis of two vanA plasmids from Enterococcus faecium strains isolated from poultry and a poultry farmer in Norway. Antimicrob. Agents Chemother. 51, 736-739.

Sletvold, H., Johnsen, P.J., Wikmark, O.G., Simonsen, G.S., Sundsfjord, A., Nielsen, K.M., 2010. Tn1546 is part of a larger plasmid-encoded genetic unit horizontally disseminated among clonal Enterococcus faecium lineages. J. Antimicrob. Chemother. 65, 1894-1906.

Sng, L.H., Cornish, N., Knapp, C.C., Ludwig, M.D., Hall, G.S., Washington, J.A., 1998a. Antimicrobial susceptibility testing of a clinical isolate of vancomycin-dependent enterococcus using D-alanine-D-alanine as a growth supplement. Am. J. Clin. Pathol. 109, 399-403.

Sng, L.H., Cornish, N., Knapp, C.C., Ludwig, M.D., Hall, G.S., Washington, J.A., 1998b. Antimicrobial susceptibility testing of a clinical isolate of vancomycin-dependent enterococcus using D-alanine-D-alanine as a growth supplement. Am. J. Clin. Pathol. 109, 399-403.

Soderblom, T., Aspevall, O., Erntell, M., Hedin, G., Heimer, D., Hokeberg, I., Kidd-Ljunggren, K., Melhus, A., Olsson-Liljequist, B., Sjogren, I., Smedjegard, J., Struwe, J., Sylvan, S., Tegmark-Wisell, K., Thore, M., 2010. Alarming spread of vancomycin resistant enterococci in Sweden since 2007. Euro. Surveill 15, pii: 19620.

Sorum, M., Johnsen, P.J., Aasnes, B., Rosvoll, T., Kruse, H., Sundsfjord, A., Simonsen, G.S., 2006. Prevalence, persistence, and molecular characterization of glycopeptide-resistant enterococci in Norwegian poultry and poultry farmers 3 to 8 years after the ban on avoparcin. Appl. Environ. Microbiol. 72, 516-521.

Stamper, P.D., Shulder, S., Bekalo, P., Manandhar, D., Ross, T.L., Speser, S., Kingery, J., Carroll, K.C., 2010. Evaluation of BBL CHROMagar VanRE for detection of vancomycin-resistant Enterococci in rectal swab specimens. J. Clin. Microbiol. 48, 4294-4297.

Stamper, P.D., Cai, M., Lema, C., Eskey, K., Carroll, K.C., 2007. Comparison of the BD GeneOhm VanR Assay to culture for identification of vancomycin-resistant enterococci in rectal and stool specimens. J. Clin. Microbiol. 45, 3360-3365.

Stinear, T.P., Olden, D.C., Johnson, P.D., Davies, J.K., Grayson, M.L., 2001. Enterococcal vanB resistance locus in anaerobic bacteria in human faeces. The Lancet 357, 855-856.

Stobberingh, E., van Den, B.A., London, N., Driessen, C., Top, J., Willems, R., 1999. Enterococci with glycopeptide resistance in turkeys, turkey farmers, turkey slaughterers, and (sub)urban residents in the south of The Netherlands: evidence for transmission of vancomycin resistance from animals to humans? Antimicrob. Agents Chemother. 43, 2215-2221.

Straus, S.K., Hancock, R.E., 2006a. Mode of action of the new antibiotic for Gram-positive pathogens daptomycin: comparison with cationic antimicrobial peptides and lipopeptides. Biochim. Biophys. Acta 1758, 1215-1223.

Straus, S.K., Hancock, R.E., 2006b. Mode of action of the new antibiotic for Gram-positive pathogens daptomycin: comparison with cationic antimicrobial peptides and lipopeptides. Biochim. Biophys. Acta 1758, 1215-1223.

Tanimoto, K., Nomura, T., Maruyama, H., Tomita, H., Shibata, N., Arakawa, Y., Ike, Y., 2006. First VanD-Type vancomycin-resistant Enterococcus raffinosus isolate. Antimicrob. Agents Chemother. 50, 3966-3967.

Tenover, F.C., McDonald, L.C., 2005. Vancomycin-resistant staphylococci and enterococci: epidemiology and control. Curr. Opin. Infect. Dis. 18, 300-305.

Teuber, M., Schwarz, F., Perreten, V., 2003. Molecular structure and evolution of the conjugative multiresistance plasmid pRE25 of Enterococcus faecalis isolated from a raw-fermented sausage. International Journal of Food Microbiology 88, 325-329.

Thal, L.A., Silverman, J., Donabedian, S., Zervos, M.J., 1997. The effect of Tn916 insertions on contour-clamped homogeneous electrophoresis patterns of Enterococcus faecalis. J. Clin. Microbiol. 35, 969-972.

Toh, S.M., Xiong, L., Arias, C.A., Villegas, M.V., Lolans, K., Quinn, J., Mankin, A.S., 2007. Acquisition of a natural resistance gene renders a clinical strain of methicillin-resistant Staphylococcus aureus resistant to the synthetic antibiotic linezolid. Molecular Microbiology 64, 1506-1514.

Top, J., Willems, R., Blok, H., de Regt, M., Jalink, K., Troelstra, A., Goorhuis, B., Bonten, M., 2007. Ecological replacement of Enterococcus faecalis by multiresistant clonal complex 17 Enterococcus faecium. Clinical Microbiology and Infection 13, 316-319.

Top, J., Willems, R., Bonten, M., 2008a. Emergence of CC17 Enterococcus faecium: from commensal to hospital-adapted pathogen. FEMS Immunol. Med. Microbiol. 52, 297-308.

Top, J., Willems, R., van, d., V, Asbroek, M., Bonten, M., 2008b. Emergence of clonal complex 17 Enterococcus faecium in The Netherlands. J. Clin. Microbiol. 46, 214-219.

Torres, C., Reguera, J.A., Sanmartin, M.J., Perez-Diaz, J.C., Baquero, F., 1994. vanA-mediated vancomycin-resistant Enterococcus spp. in sewage. J. Antimicrob. Chemother. 33, 553-561.

Tsvetkova, K., Marvaud, J.C., Lambert, T., 2010. Analysis of the mobilization functions of the vancomycin resistance transposon Tn1549, a member of a new family of conjugative elements. J. Bacteriol. 192, 702-713.

Usacheva, E.A., Ginocchio, C.C., Morgan, M., Maglanoc, G., Mehta, M.S., Tremblay, S., Karchmer, T.B., Peterson, L.R., 2010. Prospective, multicenter evaluation of the BD GeneOhm VanR assay for direct, rapid detection of vancomycin-resistant Enterococcus species in perianal and rectal specimens. Am. J. Clin. Pathol. 134, 219-226.

Valdezate, S., Labayru, C., Navarro, A., Mantecon, M.A., Ortega, M., Coque, T.M., Garcia, M., Saez-Nieto, J.A., 2009. Large clonal outbreak of multidrug-resistant CC17 ST17 Enterococcus faecium containing Tn5382 in a Spanish hospital. J. Antimicrob. Chemother. 63, 17-20.

Van Caeseele, P., Giercke, S., Wylie, J., Boyd, D., Mulvey, M., Amin, S., Ofner-Agostini, M., 2001. Identification of the first vancomycin-resistant Enterococcus faecalis harbouring vanE in Canada. Can. Commun. Dis. Rep. 27, 101-104.

Van Den Bogaard, A.E., Mertens, P., London, N.H., Stobberingh, E.E., 1997. High prevalence of colonization with vancomycin- and pristinamycin-resistant enterococci in healthy humans and pigs in The Netherlands: is the addition of antibiotics to animal feeds to blame? J. Antimicrob. Chemother. 40, 454-456.

van den Braak, N., van Belkum, A., van Keulen, M., Vliegenthart, J., Verbrugh, H.A., Endtz, H.P., 1998. Molecular characterization of vancomycin-resistant enterococci from hospitalized patients and poultry products in The Netherlands. J. Clin. Microbiol. 36, 1927-1932.

van Schaik, W., Top, J., Riley, D.R., Boekhorst, J., Vrijenhoek, J.E.P.V., Schapendonk, C.M.E., Hendrickx, A.P.A., Nijman, I.J., Bonten, M.J.M., Tettelin, H., Willems, R.J.L., 2010. Pyrosequencing-based comparative genome analysis of the nosocomial pathogen Enterococcus faecium and identification of a large transferable pathogenicity island. BMC Genomics 11, 239-

van Schaik, W., Willems, R.J., 2010. Genome-based insights into the evolution of enterococci. Clin. Microbiol. Infect.

Weaver, K.E., Kwong, S.M., Firth, N., Francia, M.V., 2009. The RepA_N replicons of Gram-positive bacteria: a family of broadly distributed but narrow host range plasmids. Plasmid 61, 94-109.

Weber, P., Meziane-Cherif, D., Haouz, A., Saul, F.A., Courvalin, P., 2009. Crystallization and preliminary X-ray analysis of a D-Ala:D-Ser ligase associated with VanG-type vancomycin resistance. Acta Crystallogr. Sect. F. Struct. Biol. Cryst. Commun. 65, 1024-1026.

Weigel, L.M., Clewell, D.B., Gill, S.R., Clark, N.C., McDougal, L.K., Flannagan, S.E., Kolonay, J.F., Shetty, J., Killgore, G.E., Tenover, F.C., 2003. Genetic analysis of a high-level vancomycin-resistant isolate of Staphylococcus aureus. Science 302, 1569-1571.

Werckenthin, C., Schwarz, S., 2000. Molecular analysis of the translational attenuator of a constitutively expressed erm(A) gene from Staphylococcus intermedius. J. Antimicrob. Chemother. 46, 785-788.

Werckenthin, C., Schwarz, S., Westh, H., 1999. Structural alterations in the translational attenuator of constitutively expressed ermC genes. Antimicrob. Agents Chemother. 43, 1681-1685.

Werner, G., 2011. Surveillance of antimicrobial resistance among Enterococcus faecium and Enterococcus faecalis isolated from human (clinical/commensal), food animal, meat and environmental samples. In: Semedo-Lemsaddek, T., Barreto-Crespo, M.T., Tenreiro, R. (Eds), Enterococcus and safety. Nova Science Publishers Inc., Hauppage, N.Y., pp. [in press]-.

Werner, G., Bartel, M., Wellinghausen, N., Essig, A., Klare, I., Witte, W., Poppert, S., 2007a. Detection of mutations conferring resistance to linezolid in Enterococcus spp. by fluorescence in situ hybridization. J. Clin. Microbiol. 45, 3421-3423.

Werner, G., Coque, T.M., Hammerum, A.M., Hope, R., Hryniewicz, W., Johnson, A., Klare, I., Kristinsson, K.G., Leclercq, R., Lester, C.H., Lillie, M., Novais, C., Olsson-Liljequist, B., Peixe, L.V., Sadowy, E., Simonsen, G.S., Top, J., Vuopio-Varkila, J., Willems, R.J., Witte, W., Woodford, N., 2008a. Emergence and spread of vancomycin resistance among enterococci in Europe. Euro. Surveill 13, pii: 19046-

Werner, G., Dahl, K.H., Willems, R.J., 2006. Composite elements encoding antibiotic resistance in Enterococcus faecium and Enterococcus faecalis. In: Kobayashi, N. (Eds), Drug Resistance in Enterococci: Epidemiology and Molecular Markers. Research Signpost, Fort P.O., Trivandrum, Kerala, pp. 157-208.

Werner, G., Fleige, C., Ewert, B., Laverde-Gomez, J.A., Klare, I., Witte, W., 2010a. High-level ciprofloxacin resistance among hospital-adapted Enterococcus faecium (CC17). Int. J. Antimicrob. Agents 35, 119-125.

Werner, G., Fleige, C., Geringer, U., van, S.W., Klare, I., Witte, W., 2011a. IS element IS16 as a molecular screening tool to identify hospital-associated strains of Enterococcus faecium. BMC. Infect. Dis. 11, 80-

Werner, G., Freitas, A.R., Coque, T.M., Sollid, J.E., Lester, C., Hammerum, A.M., Garcia-Migura, L., Jensen, L.B., Francia, M.V., Witte, W., Willems, R.J., Sundsfjord, A., 2010b. Host range of enterococcal vanA plasmids among Gram-positive intestinal bacteria. J. Antimicrob. Chemother.

Werner, G., Freitas, A.R., Coque, T.M., Sollid, J.E., Lester, C., Hammerum, A.M., Garcia-Migura, L., Jensen, L.B., Francia, M.V., Witte, W., Willems, R.J., Sundsfjord, A., 2011b. Host range of enterococcal vanA plasmids among Gram-positive intestinal bacteria. J. Antimicrob. Chemother. 66, 273-282.

Werner, G., Gfrörer, S., Fleige, C., Witte, W., Klare, I., 2008b. Tigecycline-resistant Enterococcus faecalis strain isolated from a German ICU patient. J. Antimicrob. Chemother. 61, 1182-1183.

Werner, G., Hildebrandt, B., Witte, W., 2001a. Aminoglycoside-streptothricin resistance gene cluster aadE-sat4-aphA-3 disseminated among multiresistant isolates of Enterococcus faecium. Antimicrob. Agents Chemother. 45, 3267-3269.

Werner, G., Hildebrandt, B., Witte, W., 2001b. The newly described msrC gene is not equally distributed among all isolates of Enterococcus faecium. Antimicrob. Agents Chemother. 45, 3672-3673.

Werner, G., Hildebrandt, B., Witte, W., 2003a. Linkage of erm(B) and aadE-sat4-aphA-3 in multiple-resistant Enterococcus faecium isolates of different ecological origins. Microb. Drug Resist. 9 Suppl 1, S9-16.

Werner, G., Klare, I., Heier, H., Hinz, K.H., Bohme, G., Wendt, M., Witte, W., 2000. Quinupristin/dalfopristin-resistant enterococci of the satA (vatD) and satG (vatE) genotypes from different ecological origins in Germany. Microb. Drug Resist. 6, 37-47.

Werner, G., Klare, I., Konstabel, C., Witte, W., 2007b. The current MLVA typing scheme for Enterococcus faecium does not discriminate enough to resolve epidemic-virulent, hospital-adapted clonal types. BMC Microbiology 7, 28-

Werner, G., Klare, I., Spencker, F.B., Witte, W., 2003b. Intra-hospital dissemination of quinupristin/dalfopristin- and vancomycin-resistant Enterococcus faecium in a paediatric ward of a German hospital. J. Antimicrob. Chemother. 52, 113-115.

Werner, G., Klare, I., Witte, W., 1997. Arrangement of the vanA gene cluster in enterococci of different ecological origin. FEMS Microbiol. Lett. 155, 55-61.

Werner, G., Klare, I., Witte, W., 2002. Molecular analysis of streptogramin resistance in enterococci. Int. J. Med. Microbiol. 292, 81-94.

Werner, G., Serr, A., Schütt, S., Schneider, C., Klare, I., Witte, W., Wendt, C., 2011c. Comparison of direct cultivation on a selective solid medium, polymerase chain reaction from an enrichment broth, and the BD GeneOhm™ VanR Assay for identification of vancomycin-resistant enterococci in screening specimens. Diagnostic Microbiology and Infectious Diseases 70, 512-521.

Werner, G., Strommenger, B., Witte, W., 2008c. Acquired vancomycin resistance in clinically relevant pathogens. Future Microbiology 3, 547-562.

Werner, G., Klare, I., Fleige, C., Witte, W., 2007c. Increasing rates of vancomycin resistance among Enterococcus faecium isolated from German hospitals between 2004 and 2006 are due to wide clonal dissemination of vancomycin-resistant enterococci and horizontal spread of vanA clusters. International Journal of Medical Microbiology 298, 515-527.

Werner, G., Strommenger, B., Klare, I., Witte, W., 2004. Molecular detection of linezolid resistance in Enterococcus faecium and Enterococcus faecalis by use of 5' nuclease real-time PCR compared to a modified classical approach. J. Clin. Microbiol. 42, 5327-5331.

Willems, R.J., Hanage, W.P., Bessen, D.E., Feil, E.J., 2011. Population biology of Gram-positive pathogens: high-risk clones for dissemination of antibiotic resistance. FEMS Microbiol. Rev.

Willems, R.J., Homan, W., Top, J., van Santen-Verheuvel, M., Tribe, D., Manzioros, X., Gaillard, C., Vandenbroucke-Grauls, C.M., Mascini, E.M., van, K.E., Van Embden, J.D., Bonten, M.J., 2001. Variant esp gene as a marker of a distinct genetic lineage of vancomycin-resistant Enterococcus faecium spreading in hospitals. Lancet 357, 853-855.

Willems, R.J., Top, J., van Den, B.N., van, B.A., Mevius, D.J., Hendriks, G., van Santen-Verheuvel, M., Van Embden, J.D., 1999. Molecular diversity and evolutionary relationships of Tn1546-like elements in enterococci from humans and animals. Antimicrob. Agents Chemother. 43, 483-491.

Willems, R.J., van Schaik W., 2009. Transition of Enterococcus faecium from commensal organism to nosocomial pathogen. Future. Microbiol. 4, 1125-1135.

Willems, R.J., Top, J., Smith, D.J., Roper, D.I., North, S.E., Woodford, N., 2003. Mutations in the DNA mismatch repair proteins MutS and MutL of oxazolidinone-resistant or -susceptible Enterococcus faecium. Antimicrob. Agents Chemother. 47, 3061-3066.

Willems, R.J., Bonten, M.J., 2007. Glycopeptide-resistant enterococci: deciphering virulence, resistance and epidemicity. Current Opinion in Infectious Diseases 20, 384-390.

Woodford, N., Adebiyi, A.M., Palepou, M.F., Cookson, B.D., 1998. Diversity of VanA glycopeptide resistance elements in enterococci from humans and nonhuman sources. Antimicrob. Agents Chemother. 42, 502-508.

Woodford, N., Johnson, A.P., Morrison, D., Hastings, J.G., Elliott, T.S., Worthington, A., Stephenson, J.R., Chin, A.T., Tolley, J.L., 1994. Vancomycin-dependent enterococci in the United Kingdom. J. Antimicrob. Chemother. 33, 1066-

Woodford, N., Reynolds, R., Turton, J., Scott, F., Sinclair, A., Williams, A., Livermore, D., 2003. Two widely disseminated strains of Enterococcus faecalis highly resistant to gentamicin and ciprofloxacin from bacteraemias in the UK and Ireland. J Antimicrob. Chemother. 52, 711-714.

Worth, L.J., Slavin, M.A., Vankerckhoven, V., Goossens, H., Grabsch, E.A., Thursky, K.A., 2008. Virulence determinants in vancomycin-resistant Enterococcus faecium vanB: clonal distribution, prevalence and significance of esp and hyl in Australian patients with haematological disorders. J. Hosp. Infect. 68, 137-144.

Xu, X., Lin, D., Yan, G., Ye, X., Wu, S., Guo, Y., Zhu, D., Hu, F., Zhang, Y., Wang, F., Jacoby, G.A., Wang, M., 2010. vanM, a new glycopeptide resistance gene cluster found in Enterococcus faecium. Antimicrob. Agents Chemother. 54, 4643-4647.

Yoo, S.J., Sung, H., Cho, Y.U., Kim, M.N., Pai, C.H., Kim, Y.S., 2006. Role of horizontal transfer of the transposon Tn1546 in the nosocomial spread of vanA vancomycin-resistant enterococci at a tertiary care hospital in Korea. Infect. Control Hosp. Epidemiol. 27, 1081-1087.

Yoshimura, H., Ishimaru, M., Endoh, Y.S., Suginaka, M., Yamatani, S., 1998. Isolation of glycopeptide-resistant enterococci from chicken in Japan. Antimicrob. Agents Chemother. 42, 3333-

Young, H.L., Ballard, S.A., Roffey, P., Grayson, M.L., 2007. Direct detection of vanB2 using the Roche LightCycler vanA/B detection assay to indicate vancomycin-resistant enterococcal carriage - sensitive but not specific. J. Antimicrob. Chemother. 59, 809-810.

Zarrilli, R., Tripodi, M.F., Di, P.A., Fortunato, R., Bagattini, M., Crispino, M., Florio, A., Triassi, M., Utili, R., 2005. Molecular epidemiology of high-level aminoglycoside-resistant enterococci isolated from patients in a university hospital in southern Italy. J. Antimicrob. Chemother. 56, 827-835.

Zhanel, G.G., Calic, D., Schweizer, F., Zelenitsky, S., Adam, H., Lagace-Wiens, P.R., Rubinstein, E., Gin, A.S., Hoban, D.J., Karlowsky, J.A., 2010a. New lipoglycopeptides: a comparative review of dalbavancin, oritavancin and telavancin. Drugs 70, 859-886.

Zhanel, G.G., DeCorby, M., Adam, H., Mulvey, M.R., McCracken, M., Lagace-Wiens, P., Nichol, K.A., Wierzbowski, A., Baudry, P.J., Tailor, F., Karlowsky, J.A., Walkty, A., Schweizer, F., Johnson, J., Hoban, D.J., 2010b. Prevalence of antimicrobial-resistant pathogens in Canadian hospitals: results of the Canadian Ward Surveillance Study (CANWARD 2008). Antimicrob. Agents Chemother. 54, 4684-4693.

Zhanel, G.G., DeCorby, M., Laing, N., Weshnoweski, B., Vashisht, R., Tailor, F., Nichol, K.A., Wierzbowski, A., Baudry, P.J., Karlowsky, J.A., Lagace-Wiens, P., Walkty, A., McCracken, M., Mulvey, M.R., Johnson, J., Hoban, D.J., 2008a. Antimicrobial-resistant pathogens in intensive care units in Canada: results of the Canadian National Intensive Care Unit (CAN-ICU) study, 2005-2006. Antimicrob. Agents Chemother. 52, 1430-1437.

Zhanel, G.G., DeCorby, M., Nichol, K.A., Baudry, P.J., Karlowsky, J.A., Lagace-Wiens, P.R., McCracken, M., Mulvey, M.R., Hoban, D.J., 2008b. Characterization of methicillin-resistant Staphylococcus aureus, vancomycin-resistant enterococci and extended-spectrum beta-lactamase-producing Escherichia coli in intensive care units in Canada: Results of the Canadian National Intensive Care Unit (CAN-ICU) study (2005-2006). Can. J. Infect. Dis. Med. Microbiol. 19, 243-249.

Zhanel, G.G., Harding, G.K., Rosser, S., Hoban, D.J., Karlowsky, J.A., Alfa, M., Kabani, A., Embil, J., Gin, A., Williams, T., Nicolle, L.E., 2000. Low prevalence of VRE gastrointestinal colonization of hospitalized patients in Manitoba tertiary care and community hospitals. Can. J. Infect. Dis. 11, 38-41.

Zheng, B., Tomita, H., Inoue, T., Ike, Y., 2009. Isolation of VanB-type Enterococcus faecalis strains from nosocomial infections: first report of the isolation and identification of the pheromone-responsive plasmids pMG2200, Encoding VanB-type vancomycin resistance and a Bac41-type bacteriocin, and pMG2201, encoding erythromycin resistance and cytolysin (Hly/Bac). Antimicrob. Agents Chemother. 53, 735-747.

Zheng, B., Tomita, H., Xiao, Y.H., Ike, Y., 2007a. The first molecular analysis of clinical isolates of VanA-type vancomycin-resistant Enterococcus faecium strains in mainland China. Lett. Appl. Microbiol. 45, 307-312.

Zheng, B., Tomita, H., Xiao, Y.H., Wang, S., Li, Y., Ike, Y., 2007b. Molecular characterization of vancomycin-resistant Enterococcus faecium isolates from mainland China. J. Clin. Microbiol. 45, 2813-2818.

Zhu, W., Clark, N.C., McDougal, L.K., Hageman, J., McDonald, L.C., Patel, J.B., 2008. Vancomycin-resistant Staphylococcus aureus isolates associated with incl8-like vanA plasmids in Michigan. Antimicrob. Agents Chemother. 52, 452-457.

Zhu, W., Murray, P.R., Huskins, W.C., Jernigan, J.A., McDonald, L.C., Clark, N.C., Anderson, K.F., McDougal, L.K., Hageman, J.C., Olsen-Rasmussen, M., Frace, M., Alangaden, G.J., Chenoweth, C., Zervos, M.J., Robinson-Dunn, B., Schreckenberger, P.C., Reller, L.B., Rudrik, J.T., Patel, J.B., 2010. Dissemination of an Enterococcus Incl8-like vanA plasmid, associated with vancomycin-resistant Staphylococcus aureus. Antimicrob. Agents Chemother.

Zhu, X., Zheng, B., Wang, S., Willems, R.J., Xue, F., Cao, X., Li, Y., Bo, S., Liu, J., 2009. Molecular characterisation of outbreak-related strains of vancomycin-resistant Enterococcus faecium from an intensive care unit in Beijing, China. J. Hosp. Infect. 72, 147-154.

Zirakzadeh, A., Patel, R., 2006. Vancomycin-resistant enterococci: colonization, infection, detection, and treatment. Mayo Clin. Proc. 81, 529-536.

Zirakzadeh, A., Patel, R., 2005. Epidemiology and mechanisms of glycopeptide reistance in enterococci. Current Opinion in Infectious Diseases 18, 507-512.

13

Single Cell Level Survey on Heterogenic Glycopeptide and β-Lactams Resistance

Tomasz Jarzembowski, Agnieszka Jóźwik,
Katarzyna Wiśniewska and Jacek Witkowski
*Medical University of Gdańsk,
Poland*

1. Introduction

Traditional microbiological methods, which involve the study of populations rather than individual cells, obscure heterogeneity of microorganisms. Now this phenomenon is widely reported and study of individual cells rather than populations seems to be highly reasonable. Differences between cells can be observed, especially in bacterial biofilm structure. In the case of wide variety of cells in the mixture, flow cytometry has proved to be a successful method in investigating varied populations of cells. This technique operates essentially by monitoring bacteria in suspension flowing, so that only one cell at a time passes by a sensor. The information acquired based on size and inner complexity of particles as well as fluorescence emission following previous staining can deliver great amount of information. This process also provides an immediate assessment of cells populations.

Although more than three decades ago flow cytometry has been applied to measure bacteria (Paau et al. 1977, Bailey et al. 1977), its use in microbiology is still underestimated and far from fully utilized. One of the reasons for that is that bacteria in comparison to mammalian cells are so much more difficult to work with in terms of their size and cell structure. Nevertheless with increasingly sensitive equipment, flow cytometry is finding its utility in dealing with highly heterogeneous bacterial populations.

The best known example of heterogeneity of bacteria is antibiotic resistance (Davey et al., 2003; Falagas et al., 2008). It is defined as resistance to antibiotics expressed by a subpopulation of cells within strains susceptible to antibiotics according to traditional in-vitro susceptibility testing. The heteroresistance has been observed in a range of microbes, including Staphylococcus aureus, coagulase-negative staphylococci, Acinetobacter baumannii , Mycobacterium tuberculosis, Streptococcus pneumoniae , Enterococcus faecium and Cryptococcus neoformans (Alvarez-Barrientos et al., 2000). Most observations on heteroresistance reported in the literature concern staphylococci resistant to methicillin, vancomycin, and/or inhibitors of teichoic acid synthesis (Finan at all., 2002). Recently, β-lactams heteroresistance of S. pneumoniae and vancomycin heteroresistance of enterococci have been also reported (Hasman et al., 2006; Nottasorn et al., 2005). The mechanism of β-lactams resistance is a change in the affinity of penicillin-binding proteins or overproduction of specific penicillin-binding proteins. Williamson et al. showed that at least five PBPs had been found in E. faecalis. Vancomycin resistance is usually determined by one of the two related gene clusters, vanA and vanB, that encode a dehydrogenase (VanH or VanHB) and ligase (VanA or VanB). Expression of VanA- and VanB-type resistance is regulated by the VanRS and VanRBSB two-component regulatory systems, respectively (Arthur et al., 1992; Evers and Courvalin, 1996).

As flow cytometry involves the study of single cells, it is an excellent method for studying heterogeneous populations. While analyzing many more cells than by conventional cytometry, rare cell types are more likely to be detected and the results are accessible to statistical analysis. The multiparametric nature of flow cytometric measurements is also an advantage. These include differences in cell size, DNA content or antigenic properties. Additionally, many supplementary modifications of flow cytometry are used. An example is the study of heterogenic vancomycin resistance with the use of reporter system for single-cell analysis of van gene expression. In the study, plasmid containing gene coding a green fluorescent protein was constructed for fluorescence-activated cell sorter (FACS) analysis (Cormack et al., 1996).

So far flow cytometry has been found useful in general microbiology with some clinical uses, as well as in its more specific branches such as environmental (Troussellier et al., 1999) or industrial microbiology (Gunasekera et al., 2000). First attempts to use flow cytometry for bacterial detection in body fluids are dated for the 80's when a test was developed enabling E. coli detection in blood samples (Mansour et al., 1985). The approach using flow cytometry has been continued and was reported later to be successful in bile, pleural fluid, ascites and cerebrospinal fluid (Takashi et al., 2000). Lately new tools based on flow cytometry have been developed, providing detection of significant bacteriuria as well as enumeration of bacterial particles, appearing to be an effective screening method (Hiroshi et al., 2006).

The emergence of multi-drug resistant microbial strains has emphasised the need for rapid detection method of antibiotic resistance and in this case as well flow cytometry appeared to be an extremely attractive tool.

Population analysis, among others, is the golden standard for the identification of hetero resistant vancomycin intermediate Staphylococcus aureus (hVISA) due to the fact that a proportion of MRSA found to harbor hVISA can be up to 8.3%. Moreover, for as yet unknown reasons, virtually all clinical E. faecalis isolates are tolerant to β-lactams and glycopeptides. Minimal inhibitory concentrations (MICs) of antimicrobials remain the same but the minimal bactericidal concentrations (MBCs) increase in tolerance.

Enterococcus faecalis usually plays a role in commensal flora in the human gastrointestinal tract. However, it can become a pathogen involved in various infections such as endocarditis, urinary tract infections, meningitis, sepsis and intraabdominal infections. It is also a leading cause of nosocomial infections, and the emergence of vancomycin- and multidrug-resistant E. faecalis in the clinical setting is of particular concern (Bizzini et al., 2009).

Here, the authors will present the analysis of heterogeneity of resistance studied by flow cytometry with use of fluorescent antibiotics binding bacterial cells and fluorescent probes targeting resistance genes. The proposal of vancomycin and methicilin heteroresistant strain model will be presented. With use of the model, results obtained for clinical E.faecalis and S.aureus strain are discussed.

2. Material and methods

The study was performed on reference and clinical strains listed in Tab 1. Fourteen MRSA strains were isolated from patients of various wards of the University Clinical Centre in Gdańsk and 12 Enterococcus faecalis from patients of Kościerzyna Medical Centre. The staphylococcal strains were isolated in the hospital laboratory during the period March 2008 to March 2009 and were sent to the Microbiology Department of the Medical University of Gdańsk for epidemiological typing. One isolate per patient was included in the study. Bacteria were cultured from swabs: wound (4 isolates), nose (2 isolates) and fluids: tracheostomy tube fluid (3 isolates), blood (1 isolate), abscess fluid (1 isolate), pus (1 isolate), bronchial fluid (1 isolate), urine (1 isolate). The data about clinical recognitions were not available. The isolates were cultured on sheep blood agar and were identified as *S.aureus* by colony morphology, a positive plasma coagulase reaction and by biochemical tests (API, bioMerieux, France). Resistance to methicillin was primary tested using disc diffusion method with cefoxitin disc (Clinical and Laboratory Standards Institute,2006) and then was confirmed by detection of *mec A* gene by the Polymerase Chain Reaction (PCR) as described previously (Barski et al., 1996). DNA of bacterial isolates was extracted according to the previous report (Barski et al., 1996). For further analyses, the isolates were subcultured on nutrient broth and stored with glycerol at - 70°C.

Spa typing and BURP analyses. The polymorphic X region of the protein A gene (*spa*) was amplified from the isolates by PCR with primers and according to procedure described by Kobayashi (1999). *Spa* types were determined by using Ridom Staph Type software, according to Harmsen et al (2003). The *spa* types were clustered into *spa*-CCs (clonal complexes) using the algorithm BURP - based upon repeat pattern (Rupptisch et al., 2006).

Phage typing was performed according to Blair and Williams (1961). Two sets of phages were used as follows: a basic set of 23 phages with additional phages 88,89,187 and an additional set of phages MR8, MR12, MR25, 30, 33, 38, M3, M5, 622, 56B supplied by the Central Public Health Laboratory in London for use on MRSA strains (Richardson et al., 1999). The phages were used in concentrations at routine test dilution (RTD) and 100xRTD. Reactions for phages were noted as described by Blair and Williams (1961). The phage type was defined by all the phages with strong reaction.

The susceptibility of the MRSA isolates to antimicrobial agents other than cefoxitin was determined by the disc diffusion method according to the guidelines (Clinical and Laboratory Standards Institute. 2006). The following drugs were used for test: erythromycin, clindamycin, ciprofloxacin, co-trimoxazole, tetracycline, gentamycin, vancomycin, teicoplanin, fusidic acid, rifampicin, linezolid, synercid, chloramphenicol. For isolates identified as resistant to erythromycin, but susceptible to clindamycin, D-test was performed to detect inducible clindamycin resistance. For vancomycin, additionally, the minimal inhibitory concentration (MIC) was determined by E-tests as described by the manufacturer (AB Biodisc, Sweden).

Enterococci were identified by esculin hydrolysis on Coccosel agar (bioMerieux). Species-level identification was based on rapid Strep ID (bioMerieux). Susceptibility testing was performed by following the current guidelines of the National Committee for Clinical Laboratory Standards (2002). Isolates were additionally tested for resistance to nitrofurantoin, gentamycin, amikacin, tobramycin, kanamycin, streptomycin ,neomycin, penicilin, meropenem, ampicillin, piperacilin and differentiated by antibiotic resistance pattern.

No.	Clinical source	Antibiotic resistance pattern	Phage group	Phage type	Spa type
SA1	Urine	Te C	III	42E/53/75/83A	010
SA1	Nose	E Cc Cip	III	54/75/83A	003
SA3	Nose	Sensitive	I/V	55/94/96	018
SA4	Tracheostomy tube fluid	E Cc Cip	III	47/54/75/83A	003
SA5	Blood	Cip Te C/	NT	-	008
SA6	Wound	Cip Te C/	III	53/83A	2065
SA7	Pus	E Cc Cip Sxt Te Rf C/Ge	NT	-	037
SA8	Bronchial fluid	E Cc Cip Te Ge	NT	-	008
SA9	Tracheostomy tube fluid	E Cc Cip Te Ge	III	47/54/75/83A	008
SA10	Tracheostomy tube fluid	E Cc Cip C	III	47/54/75/83A	151
SA11	Wound	E Cc Cip	II	55/71	003
SA1	Abscess	E Cc Cip	III	75/83A	003
SA2	Wound	E Cc Cip	III	83A	003
SA12	Wound	E Cc Cip	NT	-	002
SA	ATCC 25923		-	-	
SA	ATCC 29213		-	-	
E.F	wound	Te,FM, Rf, E,CC,An,NN,K,S	-	-	
E.F	Bronchial fluid	Te,Rf,E,CC,NN,K,N,Me,Am	-	-	
E.F	urine	FM,C,E,CC,Ge,An,NN,K,S,N	-	-	
E.F	urine	CC,An,NN,K,S,N,	-	-	
E.F	wound	FM,Cip,Ra,C,CC,An,NN,K,S,N	-	-	
E.F	wound	Te,FM,CC,Ge,NN,K,S,N	-	-	
E.F	faeces	Te,FM,C,CC,An,NN,K,S	-	-	
E.F	wound	Te,Rf,C,CC,An,NN,K,N,P,·	-	-	
E.F	faeces	Te,Cip,Ra,C,CC,NN,K,	-	-	
E.F	faeces	Te,Ra,CC,NN,	-	-	
E.F	faeces	Cip,Ra,C,CC,An,NN,K,S,N	-	-	
E.F	faeces	FM,Cip,Rf,C,CC,An,NN,K,N,P, Mem,Am,PIP	-	-	
E.F	ATTC 51299	Van-R	-	-	
E.F	ATTC 29212	Van-S	-	-	

S.A Staphylococcus aureus, E.F. Enterococcus faecalis, ICU- intensive care unit; DVA - dermatology, venerology, alergology department; E - erytromycin; Cc – clindamycin (/ -inducible resistance to macrolides); Cip -ciprofloxacin; Te - tetracycline; C - chloramphenicol; Rf – rifampicin; Sxt trimetoprim/ sulfamethoxazole; Ge – gentamicin NT - non- typable; ° - inhibition reaction with phages; Cc – clonal complex; MIC – minimal inhibitory concentration; Va –vancomycin; FM- Nitrofurantoin, , Ge-gentamycin, AN- Amikacin, NN –Tobramycin, K- Kanamycin, S-streptomycin , N- Neomycin, P-penicilin, MeM- Meropenem, AM- Ampicilin, PIP piperacilin

Table 1. List of strains used in the study.

For flow cytometry analysis, the isolates were grown overnight on Tryptic Soy Broth (TSB) at 37ºC and standardized to OD 1 (600 nm). The cells were then centrifuged 5 min at 2500 rpm, washed and suspended in 200 µl PBS buffer. The binding assay was carried out by adding solution of Bocillin @fl or vancomycin @fl respecitivelly to the cell suspension of each strain. The reaction mixtures were incubated for 30 min at 37ºC and centrifuged. The pellets were collected and washed three times in 1 ml of PBS. Fluorescence of particles was determined by a FACS Scan flow cytometer (Becton Dickinson, San Jose, CA, USA).

2.1 Optymalisation of bocillin@fl and vancomycin@fl binding

In the previous study the relation between fluorescence and amount of used bocillin@fl was described by equation below;

$$y = 4.469\ln(x) + 3.427,\ R^2 = 0.944 \tag{1}$$

Following these results (Jarzembowski et al., 2008) and similar results obtained during study of vancomycin @fl binding (Jarzembowski et al., 2009) we stained cells by addition of 1µg/ml vancomycin@fl. Because of inductive mechanism of vancomycin resistance , before staining strain was cultured in presence of 2ug/ml vancomycin (Sigma). The reaction mixtures were incubated for 45 min at 37ºC and again centrifuged. The pellets were collected and washed three times in 1 ml of PBS. Fluorescence of particles was determined with the use of FACS Scan flow cytometer (Becton Dickinson, San Jose, CA, USA). Results of induction of reference resistant strain are shown on Fig 1.

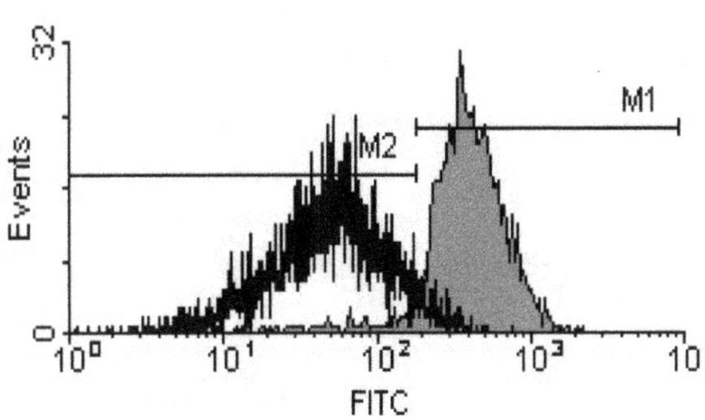

Fig. 1. Fluorescence (FL1) inducted (red) and uninducted (black) vancomycin resistant reference strain after staining with vancomycin@fl

To ensure cell nature of analysed particles we have excluded from procedure particles sized below 1µm based on value for size standard (Polysciences. Inc) and particles with low PI (propidium iodide) binding (Fig2).

2.2 Modeling of vancomycin heteroresistant strain

Mixture of the reference strains in proportion staring from 1.25 up to 50 % of resistant cells were composed to create model of heteroresistant strain. Cells binding and not binding vancomycin @fl were differentiated by markers consisting of 99.69 % of susceptible (M1) and 94% of resistant (M2) cells (Fig 3)

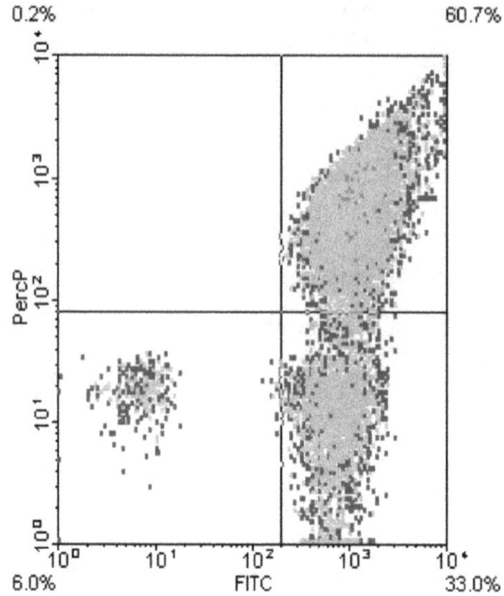

Fig. 2. Green (x axis) vancomycin@fl fluorescence and red (y axis) PI fluorescence reference susceptible strain. Only upper regions were included into further analysis.

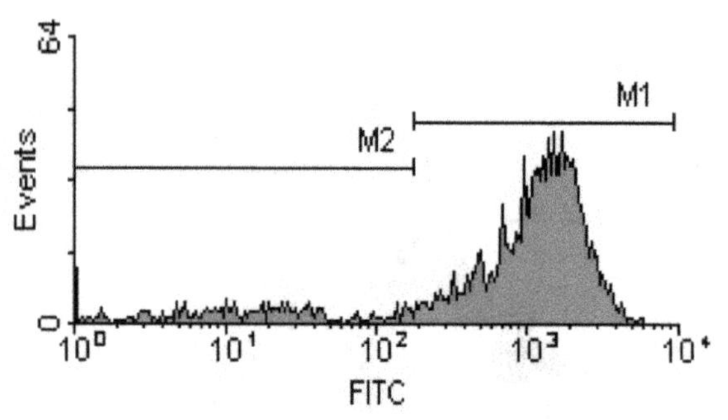

Fig. 3. Fluorescence (FL1) of mixed culture consisting of 25% resistant cells

2.3 Design and testing of DNA probes

Oligonucleotide probes were designed with the software package (Biosoft: Beacon Designer) and rRNA sequences were obtained from the Ribosomal Database Project (RDP) supplemented with newly deposited rRNA sequences from GenBank. As a positive control, Enfl84 probe (3'-ACGTGAGTTAACCTTTCTCC, Waar et al. 2005) targeting 16sRNA gene was used. Fluorescein-labelled oligonucleotides against selected specific target sequences (van genes) of *E. faecalis* were synthesized commercially (Metabion) and tested for specificity against the set of reference organisms. For hybridization, procedure described by Waar et al (2005) was adopted. Briefly, cell membrane was permeabilizated by incubation for 30 min at 37 °C in permeabilization buffer consisting of 1 mg lysozyme ml^{-1} (DNA Gdańsk). The cells were then centrifuged 5 min at 2500 rpm, washed and suspended in 200µl PBS buffer.

Subsequently, 200µl hybridization buffer containing FITC- labelled probe (1ng) was added. The probes were hybridizated at 50⁰C for 45 min.

3. Results and discussion

Heteroresistance, defined as a presence of subpopulations of resistant cells within susceptible majority was observed against β-lactams and glycopeptides. However, mechanism of actions of these groups of antibiotics is different.

The emergence of community acquired methicillin resistant Staphylococcus aureus (cMRSA) has renewed interest in the mechanisms of methicillin resistance (Okuma et al., 2002; Nunes et al., 2007). In contrast to vancomycin resistance, resistance to β-lactams (methicillin resistance) is constitutively mediated by a affinity change in penicillin-binding proteins (enzymes involved in cell wall synthesis). Because many genes are involved in cell wall biosynthesis, explanation of the nature of heterogeneous expression of methicillin resistance is very difficult (Markova et al., 2008). Since 2001, an increase in the number of MRSA strains with heteroresistance to oxacillin has been observed in the Netherlands. These strains can spread unnoticed, as their phenotypic heterogeneous resistance to beta-lactams affects the results of susceptibility testing (Wannet 2002). Coexistence of two subpopulations (susceptible and resistant) within a clinical isolate and expression of resistance only in a small number of cells leads to diagnostic problems in clinical laboratories (Markova et al., 2008). In methicillin-resistant Staphylococcus strain degree of heterogeneity is quite low: only 1 CFU of 10^4–10^7 CFU are phenotypically resistant (De Lencastre et al., 1993).

Invention of Bocillin@fl, commercially avaible fluorescent penicillin, significantly increased possibility of studying heteroresistance (Jarzembowski et al., 2010). Results of flow cytometry were found to be correlated with reference heteroresistant strain properties. Furthermore, use of fluorescent antibiotics in flow cytometry proved linear nature of heteroresistance (Fig.4.).

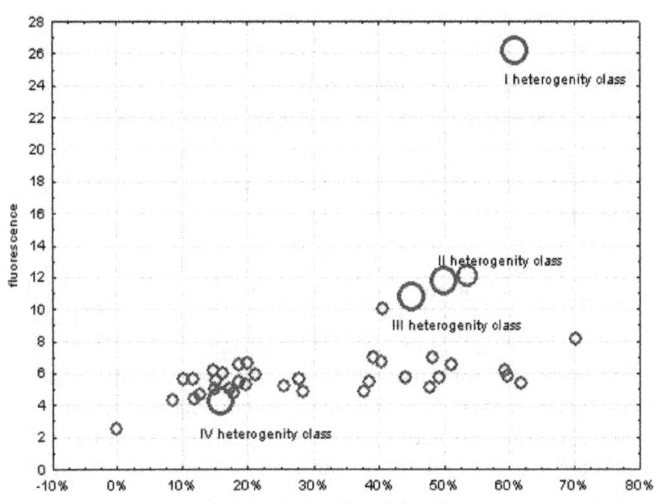

Fig. 4. Variance of bocillin @fl binding by medical isolates of S.aureus in relation to reference value

However, even in susceptible cell culture we always detect at least 1.47% antibiotic unbinding particles so it seems that the number of resistant cells in this method is overestimated.

Results of Markova et al study (2008) showed that also changes of cell structure can be involved in mechanism of heteroresistance. Both heteroresistant and methicillin susceptible strains (MSSA) may transform into cell wall-deficient form after exposure to sub tolerant conditions. The finding that methicillin sensitive strain and heteroresistant strain give rise to L-form colonial growth both on oxacillin-free and oxacillin-containing media appeared to be remarkable. It is known that the heterogeneous resistance phenotype of *mecA*-positive MRSA strains progresses to homogeneous resistance upon incubation with methicillin (Sakoulas et al., 2001). Study results of resistance demonstrate that differences reduction of antibiotic binding after preincubation can be proved with the use of flow cytometry (Fig.5).

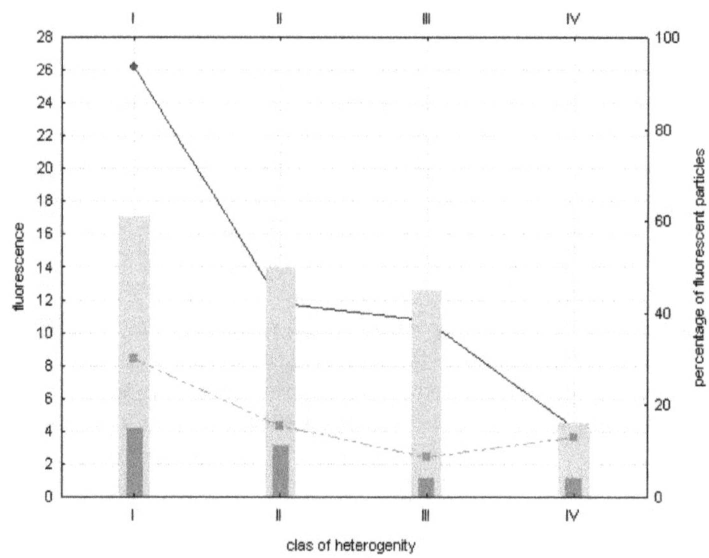

Fig. 5. Influence of incubation of heteroresistant strain with methicillin on Bocillin@fl binding

In contrast to MSSA and heteroresistant strains, homogenic MRSA strains did not convert to the cell wall-deficient forms (Markova et al., 2008).

Vancomycin resistance is an example of inductive reaction on presence of antibiotic. In presence of vancomycin high amount of cell wall precursor with low affinity to vancomycin (d-ala-d alla) is synthesized while native precursors are removed (Hasman et al., 2006). Because we aimed to detect resistant cells between susceptible majorities, the induction condition should be set to prevent inhibition of growth of susceptible strain. Thus, we set up inductive concentration below breakpoint value, at 0.016µg 0.8 µg, 2µg and 4µg/ml. The results showed optimal induction with final vancomycin concentration of 2µg/ml (data not shown). While there are no reference strains of different degree of vancomycin heteroresistance, model obtained by combination of resistant and susceptible strain was prepared. Vancomycin@fl binding by cells in this model is presented on fig 6. The high correlation between percentage of fluorescent particles and percentage of resistant cells can be seen. (Fig. 6)

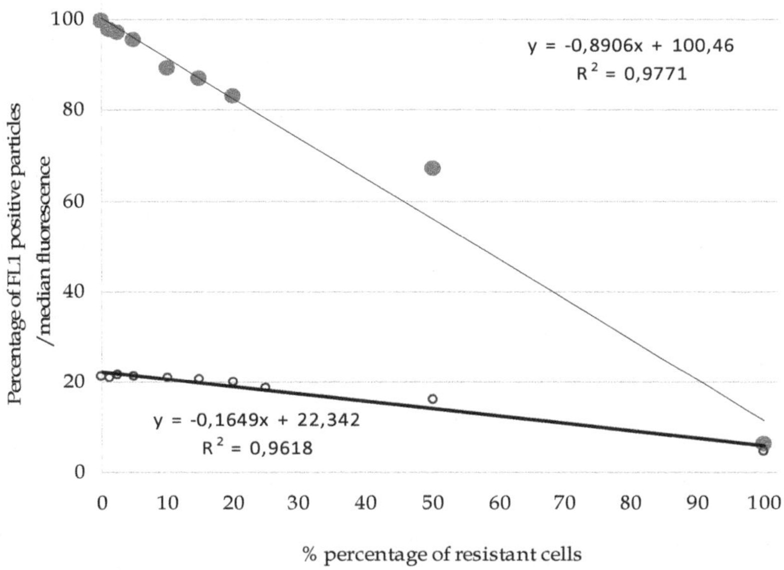

Fig. 6. Correlation between fluorescence (empty circles), FL1 positive particle (full circles) and percentage of resistant cells

The obtained model of vancomycin heteroresistance was then used for analysis of clinical strains. The percentage of stained particles ranged from 6.07% in resistant up to 99.66% in susceptible reference strains. Percentage in resistant unindicted strains was similar to the susceptible one (94.62 %). Reference strains showed also differences in fluorescence but they were not so significant (Tab. 3.) Similar, constant divergence was observed in the study of methicillin heteroresistance (Jarzembowski et al., 2010). Despite satisfactory differentiation of heteroresistance, the results showed some limitations of the method. Even in resistant strains some particles bind vancomycin@fl according to the chosen criteria. Among clinical strains, the percentage of unstained particles varies from 46.32 to 98.53 while median fluorescence varied from 547 to 1980.96. (Tab 2.). Generally, fluorescence of staphylococci was higher than fluorescence of enterococci

	percentage of FL1 positive particles	Median fluorescence	Mean fluorescence per particle
max in staphylococci	97.77	1980.96	37.01
max in enterococci	98.53	1684.85	27.26
Min in staphylococci	46.32	572.55	10.87
Min in enterococci	90.47	547.37	9.01
resistant reference strain	6.07	239.28	4.6
Susceptible reference strain	99.69	10009.04	21.2
Resistant uninducted strains	94.62	403.15	11.5

Table 2. Comparison of estimator values in groups of strains

In contrast to results of MIC based screening of vancomycin resistance, the results obtained in flow cytometry suggest heteroresistance of some strains (Fig. 7). It is obvious if we consider that presence of heteroresistant strains in US and Europe is quite high. Nunes et al. (2007) found a prevalence of 8.5 % (9/106) of glycopeptides-heteroresistant staphylococci isolated from bacteremia while others 7.4% (Frebourg et al., 1998).

None of the tested strains had a MIC value below 4µg/ml, so all of them should be considered as vancomycin susceptible. On the other hand, determination of MICs have shown good accuracy only to detect vancomycin intermediate Staphylococcus aureus (VISA) and fail in the detection of glycopeptides heteroresistant strains (Nunes et al., 2007). Heterogeneous phenotypes of clinical strains of *S. aureus* and CNS present MIC value below 4µg/ml (Nunes et al., 2007). That is why heteroresistance of the strains could be missed out in routine diagnostic.

The heteroresistance has been considered responsible for failure in the treatment. Unfortunately, there is no widely accepted method to detect heteroresistant strains. The lack of a standardized method makes it difficult to determine the clinical significance in the treatment of an infection with vancomycin. In the presence of vancomycin not only van genes change expression. There is some evidence that vancomycin influences biofilm formation, at least in S. epidermidis culture. Changes of cell surface structure and size seen in flow cytometry as SSC and FSC values were explained by the studied effect of the glycopeptide antibiotic on cell envelope properties and biofilm formation. SEM examination of cells grown in the presence of vancomycin revealed the presence of polymorphic form. Such changes in cell morphology could be the reason of extremely high fluorescence of some strains after staining with vancomycin@fl.

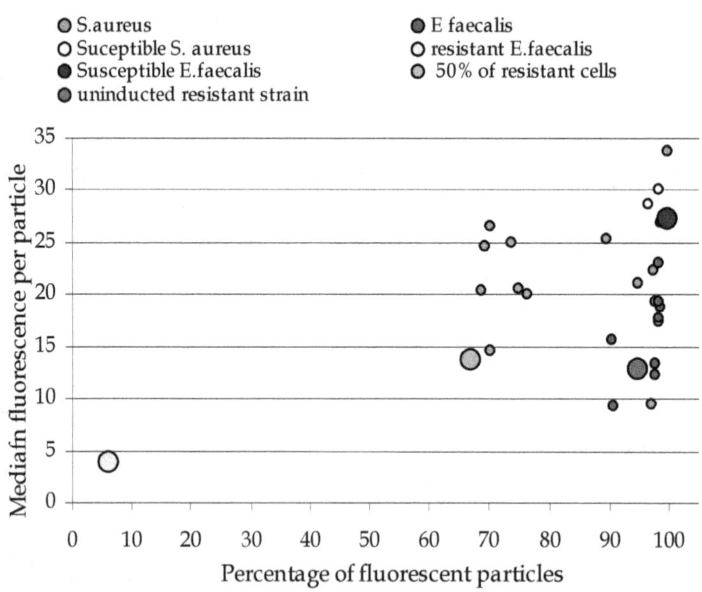

Fig. 7. Variance of vancomycin@fl binding by medical isolates of S.aureus and E. faecalis in relation to reference value

Both in study of vancomycin heteroresistance and study of methicillin resistance, median fluorescence per particle seems to be a very effective estimator (Fig. 1, 7). It is interesting to compare FCM results of "native 'methicillin heteroresistance (Fig. 4) and "artificial' model of vancomycin heteroresistance. Despite different resistance mechanism, changes of estimators are very similar. Both fluorescence and percentage of fluorescent particle decrease with amount of resistant cells (Fig. 7).

Detailed information about mechanism of heteroresistance can be explained by the study of resistance gene expression. At the first stage of our ongoing study we adopt protocol described by Warr (2005) to detect 16sRNA gene. In fact, Fig. 8 demonstrates successful detection of E. faecalis cells in flow cytometry. Furthermore, the protocol used determines the amount of cells in mixed culture.

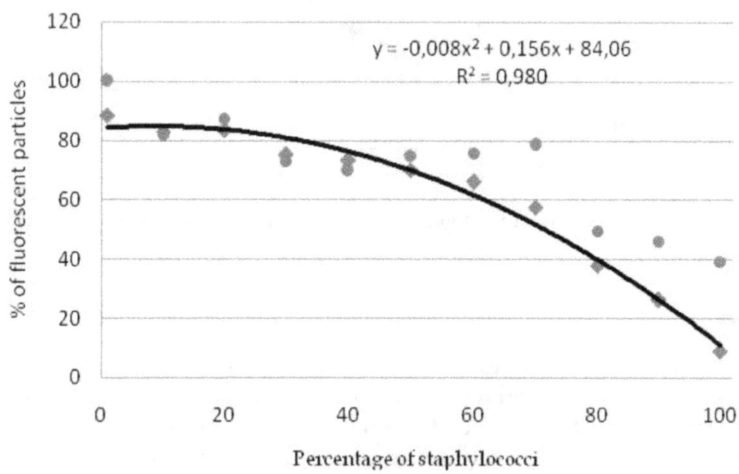

Fig. 8. Correlation between percentages of detectable particles in FLOW-FISH and proportion of E. faecalis cells in mixed culture stained by fluorescent 16sRNA probe

Detection of 16s RNA gene, which appeared to be successful in single cells, ranged between 10^4 and 10^5 ribosomes and, consequently, as many copies of 5S and 16Sand 23S-like rRNAs (Amman et al., 1990) making it was quite easy to get satisfactory signal. Despite the proven usefulness, serious limitations of FLOW- FISH technique in its sensitivity and resolution constitute an obstacle. It is believed that probes containing nucleic acid analogs with higher affinity for DNA and RNA may have the potential to reduce these problems (Kelly et al., 2009). An example of such probe is peptide nucleic acid (PNA), which binds to DNA and RNA with high affinity.

For our study, we decided to use another class of nucleic acid analogs in which the ribose sugar is constrained by a methylene bridge between 20-oxygen and 40-carbon, resulting in an N-type (3-endo) conformation , so called locked nucleic acids (LNAs) (Kelly et al., 2009).

LNA is able to hybridize with DNA and RNA according to Watson–Crick base-pairing rules and does so with unprecedented high affinity. As a result, LNAs have been shown to significantly improve the sensitivity and specificity.

This technique is expected to be particularly useful for the detection of lower mRNA transcript levels. In fact, preliminary results (Fig. 9) are promising. On the other hand, further studies are needed for validation of chosen approach.

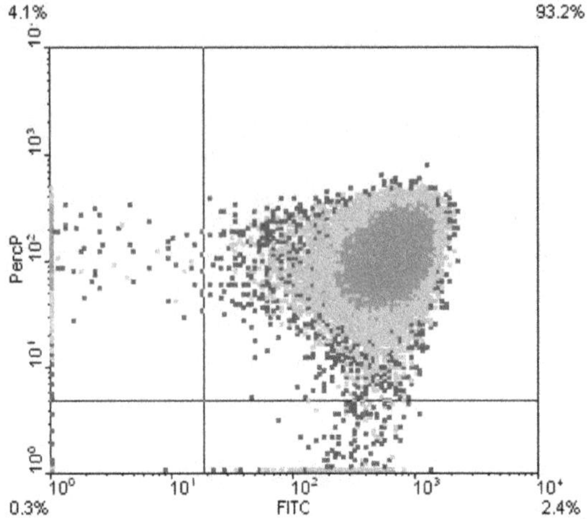

Fig. 9. Results of regulatory vancomycin gene detection with LNA probe (x axe- binding of probe, Y axe PI staining)

3. Conclusion

According to obtained results, fluorescent antibiotics are excellent tools both, for detection of resistance and studies of heteroresistance in flow cytometry. Model of vancomycin heteroresistance was successfully prepared and used in studies of clinical strains. Because it is believed that heteroresistance mechanism involves changes of cell structure, it is especially profitable in terms of antibiotic binding and changes in cell structure can be observed. However, overestimation of resistant cells in culture remain unsolved.

Preliminary results of FLOW-FISH are also promising. It seems, that use of LNA probes allows to express detection in single cells in culture. On the other hand, it is obvious that further studies are needed to evaluate the specifity ad sensitivity of this approach.

4. Acknowledgment

We thank Dr Agnieszka Daca and prof Ewa Bryl (Department of Physiopathology, Medical Unversity of Gdańsk) for their support of flow cytometry analysis of this study.

This study was supported by grants from: National Science CentreNN 401 597540

5. References

Amann, R., I.; Binder, B.; Olson, R., J.; Chisholm, S., W.; Devereux, R.; Stahl, D.,A.(1990)' Combination of 16S rRNA-Targeted Oligonucleotide Probes with Flow Cytometry for Analyzing Mixed Microbial Populations. Applied And Environmental Microbiology, 56, pp. 1919-1925

Alvarez-Barrientos, A.; Arroyo, J.; Canton, R.; Nombela, C.; Sanchez- Perez, M.(2000). Application of flow cytometry to clinical microbiology. Clin Microbiol Rev , 13, pp.167–195

Baptista, M.; Rodrigues, P.; Depardieu, F.; Courvalin, P.; Arthur, M.(1999) Single-cell analysis of glycopeptide resistance gene expression in teicoplanin-resistant mutants of a VanB-type Enterococcus faecalis. Molecular Microbiology , 32(1), pp.17±28

Barski, P.; Piechowicz, L.; Galiński, J.; Kur, J. (1996). Rapid assay for detection of methicillin-resistant *Staphylococcus aureus* using multiplex PCR. Molec. Cellul. Probs., 10, pp. 471–475

Bizzini, A.; Zhao, H.; Auffray, H., Hartke, A. The Enterococcus faecalis superoxide dismutase is essential for its tolerance to vancomycin and penicillin. Journal of Antimicrobial Chemotherapy, 64, pp. 1196–1202

Blair, J.E.; Williams, R.,E.,O. (1961). Phage typing of Staphylococci. Bull. World Health Organ, 24, pp. 771–784.

Cargill, S.; Upton, L. (2003). Low concentrations of vancomycin stimulate biofilm formation in some clinical isolates of Staphylococcus epidermidis. Curr. Issues Mol. Biol., 5, pp. 9-15.

Clinical and Laboratory Standards Institute. 2006. Performance standards for antimicrobial susceptibility testing; sixteenth informational supplement., Vol. 26, No. 3.

Davey, H.; Winson, M. (2003). Using Flow Cytometry to Quantify Microbial Heterogeneity Curr. Issues Mol. Biol., 5, pp. 9-15

De Lencastre, H.; Figueiredo, A.; Tomasz,. A. (1993). Genetic control of population structure in heterogeneous strains of methicillin resistant Staphylococcus aureus. Eur J Clin Microbiol Infect Dis , 12, pp. 13–18

Device , O.; Toshiro, S.; Akinobu, Gotoh.; Yutaka, K.; Satoru , Muto.; Hisamitsu, I.; Yukio, H.; Horie, S.(2006). Enumeration of Bacterial Cell Numbers and Detection of Significant Bacteriuria by Use of a New Flow Cytometry-Based Journal of Clinical Microbiology, pp. 3596–3599

Falagas, M., E.,; Makris, C., G., ; Dimopoulos, G.,; Matthaiou, D., K. (2008). Heteroresistance: a concern of increasing clinical significance? Clin Microbiol Infect , 14, pp 101–104

Fiebelkorn, K.,R.; Crawford, S.,A.; Mc Elmeel, M.,L.; Jorgensen, J.,H. et al. (2003). Practical disc diffusion method for detection of inducible clindamycin resistance in *Staphylococcus aureus* and coagulase- negative staphylococci. J. Clin. Microbiol., 41, pp. 4740-4744.

Finan, J., E.; Rosato, A.,E.; Dickinson, T.,M.; Ko, D.; Archer, G.,L. (2002). Conversion of oxacillin-resistant staphylococci from heterotypic to homotypic resistance expression. Antimicrob Agents Chemother, 46, pp. 24–30

Frebourg, N., B.; Nouet, D.; Lemée, L.; Martin , E; Lemeland, J.,F.(1998). Comparison of ATB staph, rapid ATB staph, Vitek, and E-test methods for detection of oxacillin heteroresistance in staphylococci possessing mecA. Clin Microbiol. , (Jan 1998) 36, (1) pp. 52-7..

Gazzola, S.; Cocconcelli, P., S. (2008). Vancomycin heteroresistance and biofilm formation in Staphylococcus epidermidis from food. Microbiology, 154, pp. 3224–3231

Gunasekera, T., S.; Attfield, P.,V.; Veal, D.,A.(2000). A flow cytometry method for rapid detection and enumeration of total bacteria in milk. Applied and Environmental Microbiology, 66, pp.1228-1232.

Hartman, B., J.; Tomasz, A. (1986). Expression of methicillin resistance in heterogeneous strains of Staphylococcus aureus. Antimicrob Agents Chemother, 29, pp. 85–92

Harmsen, D.; Claus, H.; Witte, W.; Rothganger, J.; Turnwald, D. et al., (2003). Typing of methicillin-resistant *Staphylococcus aureus* in a university hospital setting by using novel software for *spa* repeat determination and database management. J. Clin. Microbiol., 41, pp. 5442-5448.

Hasman, H.; Aarestrup, FM.; Dalsgaard, A.;Guardabassi, L. (2006) Heterologous expression of glycopeptide resistance vanHAX gene clusters from soil bacteria in Enterococcus faecalis Journal of Antimicrobial Chemotherapy 57, 648–653

Jarzembowski, T.; Wiśniewska, K.; Jóź wik, A.; Bryl, E.; Witkowski ,J. (2008). Flow cytometry as a rapid test for detection of penicillin resistance directly in bacterial cells in Enterococcus faecalis and Staphylococcus aureus. Curr Microbiol, 57, pp. 167–169

Jarzembowski, T.; Wiśniewska, K.; Jóź wik, A.; Witkowski ,J. (2009). Heterogeneity of Methicillin-Resistant Staphylococcus aureus Strains (MRSA) Characterized by Flow Cytometry, Curr Microbiol, 59, pp. 78–80

Jarzembowski, T.; Wiśniewska, K.; Jóź wik, A.; Witkowski ,J. (2010). Flow Cytometry Approach Study of Enterococcus faecalis Vancomycin Resistance by Detection of Vancomycin@FL Binding to the Bacterial Cells. Curr Microbiol , 61, pp. 407–410

Kelly, L.; Robertson, A.; Dzung, C., Thach, C.(2009). LNA flow–FISH: A flow cytometry–fluorescence in situ hybridization method to detect messenger RNA using locked nucleic acid probesAnalytical Biochemistry. 390, pp. 109–114

Kobayashi, N.; Urasawa, S.; Uehara, N.; Watanabe, N.(1999). Analysis of genomic diversity within the Xr-region of the protein A gene in clinical isolates of *Staphylococcus aureus*. Epidemiol. Infect., 122, pp. 241-249.

Mansour JD, Robson JA, Arndt CW, Schulte Detection of *Escherichia coli* in Blood Using Flow Cytometry. Cytometry, 6, pp. 186-190

Markova, N.; Haydoushka, I.; Michailova, L.; Ivanova, R.; Valcheva, V.; Jourdanova, M.; Popova, T.; Radoucheva, T. (2008). Cell wall deficiency and its effect on methicillin heteroresistance in *Staphylococcus aureus*.International Journal of Antimicrobial Agents , 31, pp. 255–260

National Committee for Clinical Laboratory Standards (2002). Methods for dilution antimicrobial susceptibility tests for bacteria that grow aerobically. 5th edn. Approved standard M7-A5. National Committee for Clinical Laboratory Standards, Wayne,PA

Nunes, A., P., F.; Schuenck, R., P.; Bastos, C., C.; Magnanini, M., M., F.; Long, J., B.; Iorio, N.; Netto dos Santos, K., R.(2007). Heterogeneous resistance to vancomycin and teicoplanin among *Staphylococcus* spp. isolated from bacteremia. Brazilian Journal of Infectious Diseases ,vol.11, no.3 (June 2007).

Nottasorn, P.; Gilat, L.; Heidi, B.; Thomson, R. (2005). Unstable vancomycin heteroresistance is common among clinical isolates of methiciliin-resistant Staphylococcus aureus Journal of clinical microbiology, Vol. 43, No. 5,(May 2005), pp. 2494-2496

Okuma, K.; Iwakawa , K.; Turnidge, J., D. et al (2002). Dissemination of new methicillin-resistant Staphylococcus aureus clones in the community. J Clin Microbiol, 40, pp. 4289-4294

Pe´richon, B., Courvalin, P.(2006). Synergism between _-Lactams and Glycopeptides against VanA-Type Methicillin-Resistant Staphylococcus aureus and Heterologousn Expression of the vanA Operon. Antimicrobial agents and chemotherapy, Vol. 50, No. 11 (Nov. 2006), pp. 3622-3630

Richardson, J.,F.; Rosdahl, V.,T.; van Leeuwen, W.,J.; Vickery, A.,M.; Vindel, A. et al. (1999).Phages for methicillin-resistant *Staphylococcus aureus*: an international trial. Epidemiol. Infect., 122, pp. 227-233.

Rupptisch, W.; Indra, A.; Stoger, A. et al. (2006). Classifying *spa* types in complexes improves interpretation of typing results for methicillin-resistant *Staphylococcus aureus*.J. Clin. Microbiol., 44, pp. 2442-2448.

Sakoulas, G.; Gold, H.,S.;Venkataraman, L.; Degirolami, P., C.; Eliopoulos, G., M. Qian, Q. (2001). Methicillin-Resistant *Staphylococcus Aureus*: Comparison Of Susceptibility Testing Methods And Analysis Of *Meca*-Positive Susceptible Strains. Journal Of Clinical Microbiology, 39, vol 11, pp. 3946-3951.

Saribas, S; Bagdatli, Y.(2004). Vancomycin tolerance in enterococci. Chemotherapy, 50, pp. 250-4.

Takashi, S.; Yoshitsugu, I.; Shunji, T.; Naoko, F.; Junya, I.; Yukio, H.; Satoshi, I.(2005). Feasibility of flow cytometry for the detection of bacteria from body fluid samples. J Infect Chemother, 11, pp. 220-225

Troussellier, M.; Courties, P.; Servais, P. (1999).Flow cytometric discrimination of bacterial populations in seawater based on SYTO 13 staining of nucleic acids. FEMS Microbiology Ecology, 29, pp. 319-330

Wannet, W., J. Spread of an MRSA clone with heteroresistance to oxacillin in the Netherlands. Euro Surveill. 2002;7(5):pii=367. Available online: http://www.eurosurveillance.org/ViewArticle.aspx?ArticleId=367

Wong, S.,S.,Y.; Ho, P.,L.; Woo, P.,C.,Y.; Yuen, K.,Y. (1999)Bacteremia caused by staphylococci with inducible vancomycin heteroresistance. Clin Infect Dis ,29, pp. 760-7.

Waar, K.; Degener, J.,E.; van Luyn, M., J.; Harmsen, H.,J.(2005) Fluorescent in situ hybridization with specific DNA probes offers adequate detection of Enterococcus faecalis and Enterococcus faecium in clinical samples. J Med Microbiol., 54, pp. 937-44.

Zhao, G.; Meier, T., I.; Kahl, S., D.; Gee, K., R.; Blaszczak, L.,C. (1999). Bocillin fl, a sensitive and commercially available reagent for detection of penicillin-binding proteins. Antimicrob Agents Chemother, 43, pp. 1124-1128

Zwirglmaier, K.; Ludwig, W.; Schleifer, K.,H.(2004). *R*ecognition of *in* dividual *g* enes in a single bacterial cell by fluorescence *in situ* hybridization - RING-FISH Molecular Microbiology , 51, vol 1, pp. 89-96

14

Clinically Relevant Antibiotic Resistance Mechanisms Can Enhance the *In Vivo* Fitness of *Neisseria gonorrhoeae*

Elizabeth A. Ohneck[1], Jonathan A. D'Ambrozio[2], Anjali N. Kunz[2], Ann E. Jerse[2] and William M. Shafer[3,4]
[1]*Emory University Laney Graduate School;*
[2]*Uniformed Services University of the Health Sciences;*
[3]*Emory University School of Medicine;*
[4]*Laboratories of Bacterial Pathogenesis, VA Medical Center (Atlanta, GA)*
USA

1. Introduction

In 2007 the Centers for Disease Control and Prevention placed *Neisseria gonorrhoeae* on the infamous "Super Bugs" list to highlight the high prevalence of strains resistant to relatively inexpensive antibiotics, such as penicillin, tetracycline and fluoroquinolones, previously used in therapy to treat gonorrhea (Shafer et al., 2010). This event was significant because the gonococcus, a strict human pathogen, causes > 95 million infections worldwide each year and since the mid-1940s mankind has relied on effective antibiotic therapy to treat infections and stop local spread of disease. Today, such therapy is threatened by antibiotic resistance. Specifically, the third generation cephalosporins, especially ceftriaxone, may be losing their effectiveness since some (albeit still rare) isolates in the Far East, most recently Japan, and Europe have displayed clinical resistance to currently used levels of ceftriaxone, and treatment failures have been reported (Ohnishi et al., 2011; Unemo et al., 2010). Concern has been raised that the spectrum of resistance expressed by some gonococcal strains may make standard antibiotic treatment for gonorrhea ineffective in the not too distant future (Dionne-Odom et al., 2011). Without new, effective antibiotics or novel combination therapies of existing antibiotics, the reproductive health of the world's sexually active population may be placed at risk due to such antibiotic resistant gonococci.

An important question regarding antibiotic resistance is whether a particular resistance mechanism has a fitness cost for the bacterium (Andersson & Levin, 1999; Andersson & Hughes, 2010), especially in the community where it competes with its antibiotic sensitive brethren. A fitness cost is typically experimentally measured as a deleterious change in bacterial growth rate in laboratory media or survival in experimental infection in the absence of antibiotic pressure. Fitness costs (or benefits) are best viewed during co-cultivation of isogenic strains that differ only in the resistance mechanism under study. For certain antibiotic resistance mechanisms, a significant fitness cost can be incurred. This general observation led to the idea that removal of the selective pressure imposed by the antibiotic in question would favor sensitive strains to predominate in the community and allow for the return of the antibiotic in question to treat the infection in question. By and large, this has proven not be the case (Andersson and Hughes, 2010). There are many reasons for this, including the unintentional selective pressure exerted by the widespread availability and use of antibiotics to treat bacterial infections in general, over-the-counter antimicrobials that confer selective pressure and provide cross-resistance (or decreased susceptibility) to the antibiotic in question, and host-derived antimicrobials that select for the particular resistance determinant. In addition to antimicrobial pressures, it has been repeatedly documented that compensatory, second site mutations can develop that reverse fitness costs while maintaining resistance (Schrag et al., 1997; Marcusson et al., 2009; Andersson and Hughes, 2010).

More recently, a new view has been taken regarding antibiotic resistance and fitness: some resistance systems actually provide the resistant strain with a fitness advantage over wild-type strains or can reverse a fitness burden imposed by a separate mutation that also participates in resistance to a particular antibiotic. Evidence for enhanced fitness of bacterial pathogens, in laboratory media or in experimental infection models, due to mutations or gene acquisition events that increase resistance to antibiotics has been provided for *Campylobacter jejuni* (Luo et al., 2005) and *Neisseria gonorrhoeae* (Warner et al., 2007, 2008). The idea that an antibiotic resistance mechanism could have negligible and even beneficial effects on fitness could help to explain, in part, why resistant strains persist in the community long after the antibiotic has been removed from the treatment regimen. For instance, gonococci expressing resistance to penicillin, tetracycline and/or fluoroquinolones have persisted in the community despite the removal of these antibiotics from the recommended gonorrhea treatment regimen for several years. Against this background, we herein review data and provide models as to how two mechanisms of antibiotic resistance expressed by *N. gonorrhoeae* can enhance fitness *in vivo*. The *in vivo* system employed in these studies is a female mouse model of lower genital tract infection that recapitulates many features of infection in human females, most notably the development of inflammation that occurs during cervicitis (Jerse, 1999; Packiam et al., 2010; Song et al., 2008). The two resistance mechanisms discussed below are multi-drug efflux by the MtrC-MtrD-MtrE pump (Hagman et al., 1995; Jerse et al., 2003) and quinolone resistance that develops due to point mutations in *gyrA* and *parC*. We discuss concepts regarding the evolution of antibiotic resistance expressed by gonococci in the context of how these resistance mechanisms may have endowed this strict human pathogen with a fitness advantage during infection.

2. Antimicrobial efflux and gonococcal fitness

The MtrC-MtrD-MtrE efflux pump of *N. gonorrhoeae* is a resistance-nodulation-division (RND) efflux pump family member that recognizes a diverse array of hydrophobic antimicrobial agents and exports these toxic compounds out of the gonococcal cell (Hagman et al., 1995). The *mtrCDE* operon is composed of three structural genes that encode the core proteins of the efflux pump: *mtrC*, which encodes a periplasmic membrane fusion protein; *mtrD*, encoding an energy-dependent inner membrane transporter; and *mtrE*, which encodes a TolC-like outer membrane channel protein (Delahay et al., 1997; Hagman et al., 1995; Hagman et al., 1997). In addition to these core efflux proteins, an accessory protein termed MtrF is required for high-level resistance to substrates of the pump and its gene (*mtrF*) is also located within the *mtr* locus (Figure 1) (Veal & Shafer, 2003).

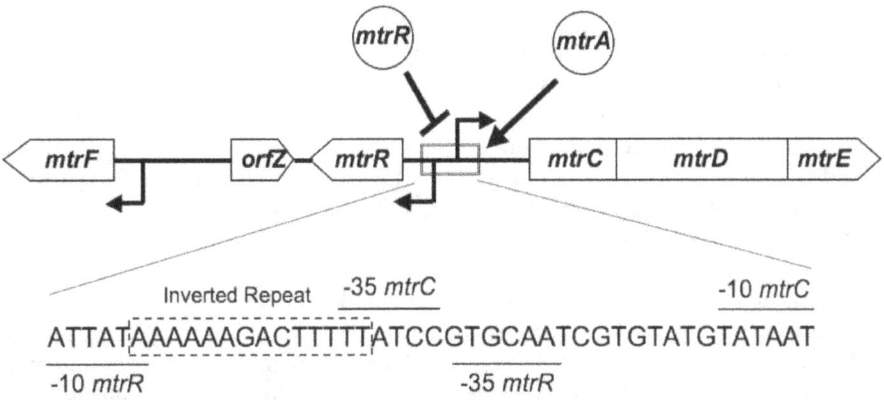

Fig. 1. **Organization of the *mtr* locus of *N. gonorrhoeae*.** Bent arrows mark the *mtrR*, *mtrF*, and *mtrCDE* promoters. *mtrR* and *mtrCDE* are divergently transcribed on opposite strands. Circles represent the transcriptional regulatory proteins MtrR and MtrA. The box represents the location of the expanded sequence. The *mtrR* and *mtrCDE* promoter elements are indicated in the expanded sequence; the dashed box marks the inverted repeat element of the *mtrR* promoter.

Transcription of the *mtrCDE* operon is negatively regulated by the TetR family transcriptional regulator, MtrR, which represses *mtrCDE* expression by the binding of two homodimers to pseudo-direct repeats within the *mtrCDE* promoter (Hoffman et al., 2005; Lucas et al., 1997). The *mtrR* gene is located 250 base pairs upstream of and is transcribed divergently from *mtrCDE* (Pan & Spratt, 1994). Additionally, transcription of *mtrCDE* may be induced in the presence of sub-lethal concentrations of nonionic, membrane-acting detergents through the action of an AraC/XylS family transcriptional activator, MtrA (Rouquette et al., 1999). Expression of *mtrF* is negatively regulated by both MtrR and the AraC family regulator MpeR (Folster and Shafer, 2005), as well as the availability of free iron (Mercante et al., 2012).

The MtrC-MtrD-MtrE efflux pump mediates resistance to structurally diverse hydrophobic antimicrobial agents, including ß-lactam antibiotics such as penicillin, macrolide antibiotics including erythromycin and azithromycin, dyes such as crystal violet, and detergents such as Triton X-100 and nonoxynol-9 (Hagman et al., 1995; Rouquette et al., 1999). Additionally, MtrC-MtrD-MtrE confers resistance to host antimicrobial compounds, including fatty acids, bile salts, progesterone, and the antimicrobial peptide LL-37 (Jerse et al., 2003; Morse et al., 1982; Shafer et al., 1995; Shafer et al., 1998). MtrC-MtrD-MtrE efflux pump-deficient mutants are highly attenuated in a female BALB/c mouse model of lower genital tract infection, even in the absence of pump substrate antibiotic treatment (Jerse et al., 2003). This attenuation is likely due to an increased susceptibility to host antimicrobial compounds, highlighting the importance of the *mtr* system in establishing gonococcal infection.

The production of efflux pumps is an energy-expensive process, and it might be hypothesized that high levels of MtrC-MtrD-MtrE production could stress the gonococcus, resulting in slower or defective growth, thereby conferring a fitness cost on strains with increased *mtrCDE* expression. In this respect, Eisenstein and Sparling noted that a mutant strain displaying the Mtr phenotype, now known to be due to a single base pair deletion in the inverted repeat in the *mtrR* promoter (Figure 1) that results in high-level antibiotic resistance through increased transcription of *mtrCDE* (Hagman & Shafer, 1995), had a slower growth rate *in vitro* (Eisenstein & Sparling, 1978). However, this same mutation confers a fitness advantage during competitive infection against wild-type strain FA19 in the female mouse model of infection in the absence of antibiotics (Warner et al., 2008) and is frequently found in clinical isolates (Shafer et al., 1995; Zarantonelli et al., 1999), particularly from men who have sex with men (Shafer et al., 1995; Xia et al., 2000). Additional mutations in the *mtrR* coding region and the *mtrR* promoter have been identified in clinical isolates that increase resistance to MtrC-MtrD-MtrE pump substrates as well as confer a survival advantage in the female mouse infection model (Table 1) (summarized in Warner et al., 2008). Mutations in the *mtrR* coding region, particularly those resulting in radical amino acid changes in the MtrR helix-turn-helix DNA binding domain, lead to low or intermediate levels of antimicrobial resistance that corresponds to a low to intermediate survival advantage during competitive infection in female mice (Warner et al., 2008). The single nucleotide deletion in the inverted repeat of the *mtrR* promoter and a recently identified mutation 120 base pairs upstream of the *mtrC* start codon (mtr_{120}) confer high-level resistance to pump substrates as well as a greater fitness advantage *in vivo* (Warner et al., 2008). These changes in fitness require an active efflux pump, as the effects were reversed in the regulatory mutant strains when the efflux pump system was genetically inactivated. Thus, it appears that the level of antibiotic resistance due to increased *mtrCDE* expression corresponds positively to the strength of the fitness advantage observed *in vivo*.

Genotype	CI at day 3
Single bp deletion in *mtrR* promoter	1000
mtr_{120} point mutation	1000
A39T change in DNA binding domain of MtrR	100
$mtrA::Km^R$	0.005
$mtrA::Km^R$ $mtrR_{1\text{-}53}$	100
$mtrA::Km^R$ $mtrR_{E202G}$	10
$mpeR::Km^R$	1

Table 1. Fitness of *mtr* regulatory mutants in mice compared to wild-type. CI: competitive index. Ratio of mutant to wild-type CFU (vaginal isolates) divided by mutant to wild-type CFU (inoculum).

Induction of *mtrCDE* expression by the activator MtrA is also important for gonococcal survival *in vivo*. Strains carrying a disrupted *mtrA* gene display a significant fitness disadvantage during competitive infection with wild-type strain FA19 in the female mouse model of infection (Warner et al., 2007). MtrA induction of *mtrCDE* expression occurs in the presence of nonionic detergents such as Triton X-100 (Rouquette et al., 1999). The presence of host antimicrobial factors that are pump substrates, such as fatty acids or CRAMP-38, the mouse homologue of the human cathelicidin LL-37, may have a similar effect. The decreased fitness of the *mtrA* mutants *in vivo* would therefore be attributed to failure of the gonococcus to respond to host defense factors due to inability to upregulate expression of the pump.

Interestingly, in a study by Warner et al., 2007, some *mtrA*-deficient strains developed mutations in the *mtrR* gene ($mtrR_{1\text{-}53}$ and $mtrR_{E202G}$) after inoculation into mice in the absence of antibiotics; these strains were recovered in high numbers and displayed increased antibiotic resistance as well as a fitness advantage during subsequent competitive infection against wild-type FA19 (Table 1). The development of compensatory mutations to overcome the cost of *mtrA* disruption highlights the importance of the MtrC-MtrD-MtrE efflux pump to gonococcal fitness *in vivo.*

The importance of the MtrC-MtrD-MtrE efflux pump *in vivo,* even in the absence of antibiotic treatment, suggests that this pump originally evolved as a mechanism to aid the gonococcus in escaping host defense mechanisms, rather than in response to the introduction of antibiotics to treat gonococcal infection. Increasing antibiotic use and the availability of the over-the-counter spermicide nonoxynol-9 may then have selected for pump mutants, such as those containing *mtrR* mutations frequently isolated from patients with gonococcal infection. These strains are not only able to resist antibiotic treatment, but also better able to resist host antimicrobial compounds, giving them a survival advantage *in vivo* and in the community (Xia et al., 2000). Thus, increased production of the MtrC-MtrD-MtrE efflux pump represents a mechanism of antibiotic resistance that imparts a fitness advantage upon the gonococcus, rather than a fitness cost. It is important to note that homologues of both the pump and its regulatory proteins exist in other Gram-negative bacteria. For example, the AcrA-AcrB-TolC efflux system of *Salmonella enterica* enhances the capacity of this pathogen to cause experimental infection in chickens (Webber et al., 2009). Lessons learned with the gonococcus regarding drug efflux and fitness may therefore have broader implications for how bacterial pathogens escape both classical antibiotics and host defense compounds.

3. Quinolone resistance and gonococcal fitness

The limited use of quinolones in the treatment of bacterial infections began after the 1962 discovery of nalidixic acid as a product of chloroquine synthesis. Subsequent development of fluoroquinolone derivatives amassed broad-spectrum appeal due to their effective targeting of many Gram-positive and Gram-negative pathogens (Emmerson, 2003). Continued development of this class of antibiotics was fueled by the concurrent progression of bacterial resistance to penicillin and tetracycline, including *N. gonorrhoeae* (Covino et al., 1990). By 1993, fluoroquinolones were recommended by the CDC as the first-line treatment option for uncomplicated gonococcal infections; however, within 10 years, over 80% of gonococcal isolates in the western Pacific region were ciprofloxacin resistant (Cip^R) (Tapsall, 2005; Trees et al., 2001). The eventual spread of quinolone resistant *N. gonorrhoeae* (QRNG) in the United States led to the removal of fluoroquinolones from the list of recommended first-line antibiotics for treatment of gonorrhea and related conditions by the CDC in 2007 (CDC, 2007).

Quinolones induce bacterial cell death by inhibiting the activity of the bacterial type IIA DNA topoisomerases DNA gyrase and topoisomerase IV (Emmerson, 2003; Hooper 1999). These enzymes are responsible for managing the topological state of genomic DNA and are necessary for resolving regions of topological stress that occur during critical cell processes such as DNA replication and the regulation of gene expression. DNA gyrase and topoisomerase IV are heterotetramers that bind to DNA and generate a double-stranded break in one region of the bound DNA duplex, which results results in a complex referred to as the G-segment. A second region of distant DNA duplex, referred to as the T-segment, passes through the G-segment and the cleaved substrate held in the G-segment is subsequently religated to complete a single round of topological adjustment (Bates et al., 2011; Chen and Lo 2003; Morais Cabral et al., 1997). Quinolones specifically target the G-segment of the enzyme-DNA complex. Presently, there is no universally accepted mechanism of how quinolones kill bacteria; however, mounting evidence suggests that two quinolone molecules stabilize the cleaved DNA duplex, resulting in the accumulation of lethal lesions within the genome of the cell (Laponogov et al., 2009).

Quinolone resistance in *N. gonorrhoeae* is due to point mutations in the quinolone resistance determining region (QRDR) of the A subunits of DNA gyrase (*gyrA*) and topoisomerase IV (*parC*) (Tanaka et al., 2000; Trees et al., 2001). Belland and colleagues were the first to delineate the genetic basis of quinolone resistance in *N. gonorrhoeae* in 1994. By analyzing ciprofloxacin resistant (Cip^R) mutants selected *in vitro*, these investigators showed Cip^R in *N. gonorrhoeae* is a two step process in which intermediate level ciprofloxacin resistance (Cip^I) occurs via point mutations in *gyrA* that encode amino acid substitutions at positions Ser91 and Asp95. Cip^I *gyrA* mutants then become Cip^R when point mutations occur in *parC* (Belland et al., 1994). This sequence of events is consistent with data from numerous molecular epidemiologic studies (Kam et al., 2003; Morris et al., 2009; Starnino et al., 2010; Tanaka, 1992; Trees et al., 2001; Vereshchagin et al., 2004). Analyses of clinical isolates have also provided insights into the nature of mutations directly associated with fluoroquinolone resistance in *N. gonorrhoeae*. Commonly isolated substitutions in the Ser91 position of the GyrA subunit include amino acids with bulky side chains (phenylalanine and tyrosine) and the hydrophobic leucine, while arginine is the most common substitution at position Asp95 (Kam et al., 2003; Morris et al., 2009; Ruiz et al., 2001; Starnino et al., 2010; Tanaka et al., 2000; Trees et al., 2001; Vereshchagin et al., 2004; Vernel-Paulillac et al., 2009). Double point mutations in *gyrA* that result in these amino acid substitutions are sufficient and also largely responsible for sterically hindering the intercalation of quinolone molecules (Xiong et al., 2011). The location specificity of *parC* mutations that lead to high level Cip^R appears to be less stringent than mutations in *gyrA*, with alterations at position 91 (the most common), 86, 87, or 88 identified among Cip^R isolates (Dewi et al., 2004; Morris et al., 2009; Tanaka et al., 2000; Trees et al., 2001) (Figure 2).

The impact of quinolone resistance mutations on microbial fitness has been studied in several bacterial species. Topoisomerase mutations often are associated with an *in vitro* fitness cost, although not all *gyrA* mutations or combinations of *gyrA* mutations or *gyrA, parC* mutations result in decreased growth *in vitro* (Bagel et al., 1999; Marcusson et al., 2009, Pope et al., 2008; Luo et al., 2005). Interestingly, in 2005 Zhang and colleagues showed *gyrA* mutations confer a fitness benefit to *C. jejuni in vivo* using a chicken intestinal colonization model (Luo et al., 2005). Based on this report and the wide prevalence of QRNG strains, we hypothesized that fluoroquinolone resistance mutations in *N. gonorrhoeae* may be accompanied by a transmission or survival advantage. To address the possibility that QRNG may be more fit *in vivo*, we constructed Cip^I and Cip^R mutants in *N. gonorrhoeae* strain FA19 that carry the commonly isolated *gyrA* (Ser91Phe and Asp95Asn) or *gyrA* (Ser91Phe and Asp95Asn) and *parC* (Asp86Asn) mutations, respectively, and measured their fitness relative to the Cip^S parent strain in the murine genital tract infection model. No *in vitro*

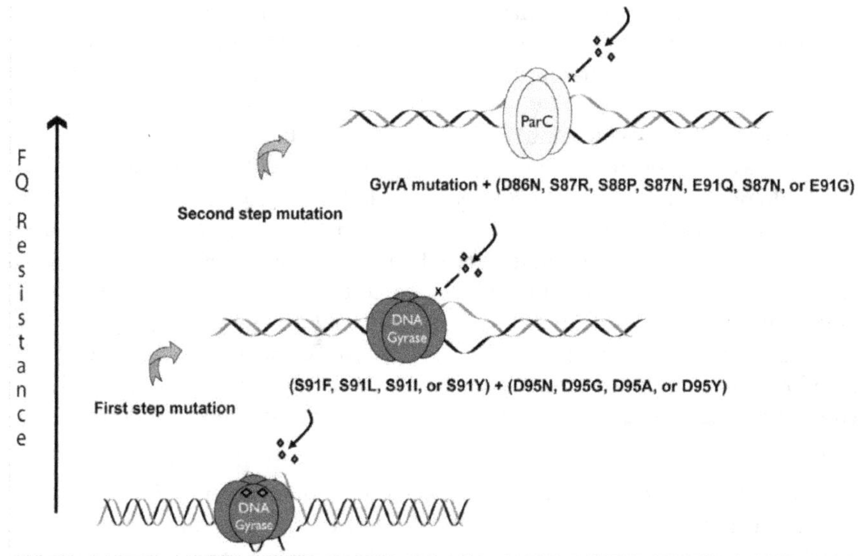

Fig. 2. **Evolution of quinolone resistance in *N. gonorrhoeae*.** Quinolone resistance in *N. gonorrhoeae* is a two-step process, beginning with point mutations in the QRDR of *gyrA*, which increase resistance to intermediate levels. Positions 91 and 95 are most often altered, with Ser91Phe and Asp95Asn the most common substitutions. Other substitutions have also been reported. High level resistance occurs upon mutation of the QRDR of *parC* mutation. *parC* mutations carried by Cip^R gonococci most often cause amino acid substations at position 91, 86, 87 or 88 (Kam et al., 2003; Ghanem et al., 2005; Morris et al., 2009; Ruiz 2001; Starnino et al., 2010; Tanaka et al., 2000; Trees et al., 2001; Vereshchagin et al., 2004; Vernel-Paulillac 2009).

fitness cost was associated with acquisition of the $gyrA_{91/95}$ mutations based on comparing the growth rates of the $gyrA_{91/95}$ mutant and the Cip^S wild-type strain, although a slight reduction (3-fold) in the recovery of the mutant was observed when co-cultured with the Cip^S wild-type strain (Table 2). Interestingly, however, the Cip^I $gyrA_{91/95}$ mutant exhibited a clear fitness advantage *in vivo* as evidenced by high competitive indices (CIs) over time and the isolation of only Cip^I bacteria from some mice on days 5 and 7 post-inoculation. In contrast, the Cip^R $gyrA_{91/95}$, $parC_{86}$ mutant grew significantly more slowly *in vitro* and exhibited reduced fitness *in vivo* relative to the wild-type Cip^S strain (Table 2) (Kunz et al., In Press).

Genotype	CI at day 3
$gyrA_{91/95}$	5-fold increase; 30-fold increase on day 5 compared to Cip^S wild-type strain
$gyrA_{91/95}$, $parC_{86}$	2-fold decrease compared to Cip^S wild-type strain
$gyrA_{91/95}$, *mtrR-79*	40-fold increase compared to Cip^S *mtr-56*mutant parent strain
$gyrA_{91/95}$, $parC_{86}$, *mtrR-79*	50-fold decrease compared to Cip^S *mtr-56* mutant parent strain

Table 2. Fitness of FQ-R mutations in mice compared to wild-type or *mtr* mutant Gc. CI: competitive index. Ratio of mutant to wild-type CFU (vaginal isolates) divided by mutant to wild-type CFU (inoculum).

As discussed, it is well established that *mtr* locus mutations increase gonococcal fitness in the mouse model, and we therefore wondered whether the fitness benefit conferred by $gyrA_{91/95}$ mutations would enhance the fitness advantage afforded by increased efflux of host substrates through the MtrC-MtrD-MtrE active efflux pump. Our alternative hypothesis was that increasing numbers of resistance mutations would impair growth to such an extent as to abrogate the fitness benefits associated with either resistance mutation. To test this hypothesis, we constructed $gyrA_{91/95}$ and $gyrA_{91/95}$, $parC_{86}$ mutants in an *mtr* mutant of strain FA19 that carries a commonly isolated *mtrR* promoter mutation (the single base pair deletion in the *mtrR* promoter termed hereafter as *mtrR-79*). The $gyrA_{91/95}$, *mtrR-79* mutant (Cip^{I}) showed no fitness difference compared to the *mtrR-79* mutant parent strain *in vitro*, but significantly out-competed the *mtrR-79* mutant during experimental murine infection. In contrast, the highly Cip^{R} $gyrA_{91/95}$, $parC_{86}$, *mtrR-79* mutant was severely attenuated both *in vitro* and *in vivo* relative to the $mtrR_{-56}$ mutant, with only $mtrR_{-56}$ mutant gonococci recovered from a majority of mice 5 days after inoculation (Table 2) (Kunz et al., In Press).

From these studies we conclude that the $gyrA_{91/95}$ mutation confers a fitness benefit to *N. gonorrhoeae* that is independent of the MtrC-MtrD-MtrE efflux pump system, but that an additional $parC_{86}$ mutation results in a net fitness cost. These data are intriguing and may help to explain the frequent isolation of Cip^{R} gonococci that also carry *mtrR* promoter or *mtrR* structural gene mutations, which has been interpreted by others as evidence that active efflux through the MtrC-MtrD-MtrE pump is another mechanism of fluoroquinolone resistance in *N. gonorrhoeae* (Dewi et al., 2004; Vereshchagin et al., 2004). The fact that we found no difference in the Cip MICs of the $gyrA_{91/95}$ versus $gyrA_{91/95}$, *MtrR-79* mutants or of $gyrA_{91/95}$, $parC_{86}$ versus $gyrA_{91/95}$, $parC_{86}$, *mtrR-79* mutants (Kunz et al., submitted), is strong genetic evidence that *mtr* mutations do not contribute to Cip^{R} in *N. gonorrhoeae*. Instead, the prevalence of Cip^{R} *mtr* strains may reflect increased microbial fitness conferred by these mutations.

It is important to remember that while mutations in both *gyrA* and *parC* led to reduced fitness in the mouse model, compensatory mutations may occur in nature that restore fitness while maintaining high level Cip^{R}. There is much evidence that fitness compensation can occur in bacteria without loss of antibiotic resistance (Balsalobre et al., 2011; Bjorkholm et al., 2001; Bjorkman et al., 1998; Giraud et al., 1999; Komp Lindgren et al., 2005; Marcussen et al., 2009; Nagaev et al., 2001). In support of this possibility for QRNG, we have observed that while Cip^{R} gonococci were outcompeted by Cip^{S} (wild-type) or Cip^{I} bacteria in a majority of mice tested, only Cip^{R} gonococci were recovered from some mice (10-17%) as infection progressed in each of several experiments (Figure 3). To further investigate this observation, we analyzed Cip^{R} bacteria isolated on day 5 in pure culture from a mouse inoculated with a mixture of Cip^{I} ($gyrA_{91/95}$, *mtrR-79*) and Cip^{R} ($gyrA_{91/95}$, $parC_{86}$, *mtrR-79*) mutants. Interestingly, these Cip^{R} bacteria grew better than the Cip ^{I} and Cip^{R} strains used to inoculate the mouse and the Cip^{S} *mtr* parent of the Cip^{I} and Cip^{R} strains. Unlike either of these strains, the *in vivo*-selected Cip^{R} mutant had a wild-type *mtr* locus and a *gyrA* allele that was predicted to encode a leucine instead of phenylalanine residue at position 91 (Phe91Leu) (Kunz et al., In Press). We conclude that one or more compensatory mutations occurred during infection that allowed highly Cip^{R} gonococci to out-compete Cip^{I} bacteria *in vivo*.

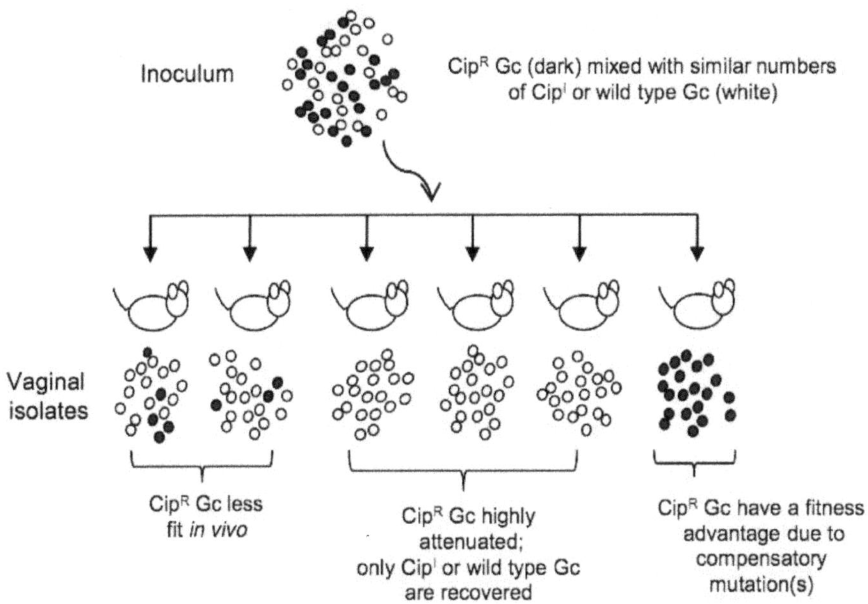

Fig. 3. **The fitness disadvantage of Cip^R gonococci can be overcome by selection for compensatory mutations**. Vaginal inoculation of estradiol-treated BALB/c mice with populations of Cip^S or Cip^I gonococci (white) mixed with similar numbers of Cip^R gonococci (black) results in the recovery of a higher proportion of Cip^S or Cip^I CFU, with some mice clearing the Cip^R bacteria. However, in 10-17% of mice tested, high numbers of only Cip^R CFU were recovered as infection progressed, most likely due to compensatory mutations (Kunz et al, In Press).

The basis for the reported *in vivo* fitness benefit shown by *gyrA* mutants in *N. gonorrhoeae* or *C. jejuni* (Luo et al., 2005) is not known. As topoisomerase mutations are accompanied by alterations in supercoiling (Bagel et al., 1999; Luo et al., 2005), changes in the expression of genes important for colonization, growth on mucosal surfaces, or evasion of host defenses are one possible explanation (Luo et al., 2005; Zhang et al., 2006). It is also possible that the *in vivo* fitness benefit exhibited by $gyrA_{91/95}$ mutants in *N. gonorrhoeae* is due to secondary mutations that were selected to compensate for alterations in GyrA as proposed by Marcusson *et al.* to explain the increased fitness of *gyrA* mutants of *E. coli* in a urinary tract infection model (Marcusson et al., 2009). The *E. coli* mutants tested in this study showed various degrees of fitness costs *in vitro*, however, and thus it is reasonable to assume that one or more compensatory mutations would be needed to promote fitness *in vivo*. In contrast, while *gyrA* mutations are associated with increased *in vivo* fitness in *C. jejuni* (Luo et al., 2005) and *N. gonorrhoeae* (Kunz et al., In Press), these mutations do not confer a significant growth cost *in vitro*; therefore, secondary mutations that restore growth may not be required for full fitness *in vivo*. Additionally, while not definitive evidence that *gyrA* mutations alone are responsible for the fitness we observe in the mouse model, we recently demonstrated that $gyrA_{91/95}$ mutations are accompanied by a pronounced fitness benefit in two other *N. gonorrhoeae* strains, and that this benefit was detected within one day of infection (Jonathan A. D'Ambrozio & Ann E. Jerse, unpublished observation).

Identification of the mechanism by which *gyrA* mutations enhance gonococcal fitness during experimental murine infection is important as it may reveal new and interesting facets of gonococcal pathogenesis. Additionally, our data suggest Cip^I strains may serve as a reservoir for Cip^R in *N. gonorrhoeae* since a single step mutation in *parC* is all that is then required for high-level resistance. We postulate the following scenario by which this may occur. First, low-levels of antibiotic pressure due to fluoroquinolone treatment for other infections or self-medication selects for Cip^I strains. Cip^I strains are then maintained within sexual networks, or even flourish, due to the fitness benefit conferred by the $gyrA_{91/95}$ mutations. Highly Cip^R strains would not flourish, possibly due to the more severe growth defect construed by mutation in $parC_{86}$ or the possibility that the $parC_{86}$ mutation or the combination of the $parC_{86}$, $gyrA_{91/95}$ mutations may have a negative impact on the expression of genes important for survival *in vivo*. However, some Cip^R gonococci will be selected due to compensatory mutations that restore fitness while maintaining high level Cip^R. Continued study of the frequency and nature of compensatory mutations that allow maintenance of high level Cip^R is important for understanding the spread of QRNG.

4. Conclusion

Antibiotic resistance expressed by many of the bacterial pathogens that infect humans represents one of the most important public health challenges for clinical medicine in the 21st century. During the early years of the antibiotic era of medicine (circa. 1945-1950) it became clear to physicians that antibiotic treatment failures were frequently the result of the infecting bacteria being resistant to the antibiotic being used; indeed, penicillinase-producing strains of *Staphylococcus aureus* were recognized and became wide-spread soon after penicillin was introduced as a therapeutic agent in 1943 (Bud, 2007). As the antibiotic era progressed and more antibiotics became available, disturbing reports of treatment failures became more prevalent. Fortunately, researchers trained in microbial physiology and bacterial genetics undertook studies to learn the mechanisms used by bacteria to resist a given antibiotic. These early investigators soon learned that while an antibiotic resistant strain had an advantage over a susceptible strain in the presence of the antibiotic in question, the resistance mechanism frequently came at a cost in the absence of the antibiotic. Thus, in the absence of the selective pressure brought by the antibiotic, the resistant strain frequently grew slower *in vitro* and in model systems of infection (cell culture or animals). However, for some resistance mechanisms, there was little if any cost when compared to a sensitive, but otherwise isogenic strain. The resulting dogma from this work was that antibiotic resistance in the absence of selective pressures could be costly for bacteria. In this case, removing the selective pressure would result in the evolution of more susceptible strains that would have an advantage in the community. By and large, this has not been the case (Anderson & Hughes, 2010).

Less clear, however, was whether in the absence of selective pressure, a resistant strain would have a fitness benefit during an infection over a sensitive counterpart. In this respect, the report of Luo *et al.* (2005) dealing with the increased fitness of a ciprofloxacin resistant strain of *C. jejuni* over a sensitive parent strain *in vivo* was a "game-changer" for antibiotic resistance researchers. Briefly, it forced us to consider the rather scary possibility that a mechanism of antibiotic resistance can actually enhance the ability of a pathogen to survive in the community. This possibility has a number of important implications for our understanding of bacterial pathogenesis and bacterial infections that should be considered. First, are there "antibiotic substitutes" *in vivo* that the resistance mechanism recognizes, allowing the resistant strain to out-compete the sensitive strain? Might these "host antibiotics" provide the selective pressure in the community? This is certainly likely for the fitness benefit imparted to those *N. gonorrhoeae* strains that over-express the Mtr efflux pump system. This pump, along with similar pumps produced by other Gram-negatives (Shafer et al., 2010), recognizes host antimicrobials (e.g., antimicrobial peptides) in addition to antibiotics such as beta-lactams and macrolides. In this context, efflux pump inhibitors (Lomovskaya & Bostian, 2006) may have clinical use as they would increase bacterial susceptibility to classical antibiotics as well as host antimicrobials. A second issue that requires further investigation is whether a resistance mechanism has secondary effects on the physiology of the resistant strain that results in an advantage during infection. This hypothesis may help to explain why $gyrA_{91/95}$ mutations can enhance the fitness of Cip^{I} strains of *N. gonorrhoeae*. Hopefully, ongoing transcriptional profiling studies that compare isogenic Cip^{I} and Cip^{S} strains will provide insights that will help us to understand fitness differences. A third point merits consideration: stable mutations that decrease bacterial susceptibility to a given antibiotic, but not to an extent that it pushes them across the MIC breakpoint, may be more advantageous for the bacteria than previously thought. In this respect, as emphasized throughout this text, mutations in *mtrR* or *gyrA* provide gonococci with a fitness advantage *in vivo*, but do not push them across the MIC breakpoint for either beta-lactams or quinolones, respectively. Importantly, both are necessary for clinically significant levels of resistance imparted by other mutations. Accordingly, strains bearing *mtrR* and/or *gyrA* mutations may not only be more fit during infection, but also more likely to subsequently develop clinical resistance to beta-lactams and quinolones than fully sensitive strains. This issue is of greater urgency now because the gonococcal strain that caused a ceftriaxone-resistant infection in Japan is an *mtrR* mutant (Ohnishi et al., 2011) even though the mutation by itself has little impact on the level of beta-lactam resistance (Veal & Shafer, 2003). Finally, if a resistance mutation enhances fitness and is stably maintained in a bacterial pathogen for years, it may be yet another reason why antibiotic re-cycling after extended absence from the treatment regimen may not be a viable option to combat the emergence and spread of antibiotic resistant bacteria.

We have used *N. gonorrhoeae* as a model human pathogen for studies on how bacterial fitness can be impacted by mechanisms of antibiotic resistance. Having been intimately associated with humans for thousands of years, it is of no surprise that the gonococcus has evolved novel ways to evade or resist the multitude of toxic agents that it encounters during infection. The continued emergence of strains expressing decreased susceptibility or even clinical resistance to frontline antibiotics used today (e.g., ceftriaxone) in therapy emphasizes the remarkable adaptive ability of this pathogen. The examples provided herein with the gonococcus emphasize that mechanisms of antibiotic resistance can enhance bacterial virulence, as defined by increased *in vivo* fitness. Understanding the processes that lead to increased fitness of the gonococcus (or any other pathogen) due to antibiotic resistance may result in novel strategies that could be used to inhibit bacterial replication *in vivo* directly or indirectly by enhancing the efficacy of the defensive systems of the host that operate locally.

5. Acknowledgments

This work was supported by the National Institute of Allergy and Infectious Diseases at the National Institute of Health [RO1 AI42053 and U19 AI31496 to A.E.J.; R37 AI21150 to

W.M.S.], and a USUHS training grant [C073-RT to A.N.K.]. W.M.S. was supported in part by a Senior Research Career Scientist Award from the VA Medical Research Service.

6. References

Andersson, D. & Levin, B. (1999) The Biological Cost of Antibiotic Resistance. *Current Opinion in Microbiology*, Vol. 2, No. 5, pp. 489 - 493, ISSN 1369-5274

Andersson, D. & Hughes, D. (2010) Antibiotic Resistance and Its Cost: Is It Possible to Reverse Resistance? *Nature Reviews Microbiology*, Vol. 8, No. 4, pp. 260 - 271, ISSN 1740 - 1526

Bagel, S., Hullen, V., Wiedemann, B. & Heisig, P. (1999) Impact of *gyrA* and *parC* Mutations on Quinolone Resistance, Doubling Time, and Supercoiling Degree in *Escherichia coli*. *Antimicrobial Agents and Chemotherapy*, Vol. 43, No. 4, pp. 868-875, ISSN 0066-4804

Balsalobre, L., Ferrandiz, J., de Alba, G. & de la Campa, A. (2011) Nonoptimal DNA Topoisomerases Allow Maintenance of Supercoiling Levels and Improve Fitness of *Streptococcus pneumoniae*. *Antimicrobial Agents and Chemotherapy*, Vol. 55, No. 3, pp. 1097-1105, ISSN 0066-4804

Bates, A., Berger, J. & Maxwell, A. (2011) The Ancestral Role of ATP Hydrolysis in Type II Topoisomerases: Prevention of DNA Double-Strand Breaks. *Nucleic Acids Research*, Vol. 39, No. 15, pp. 6327 - 6339, ISSN 0305-1048

Belland, R., Morrison, S., Ison, C. & Huang, W. (1994) *Neisseria gonorrhoeae* Acquires Mutations in Analogous Regions of *gyrA* and *parC* in Fluoroquinolone-Resistant Isolates. *Molecular Microbiology*, Vol. 14, No. 2, pp. 371-380, ISSN 0950-382X

Bjorkman J., Hughes, D. & Andersson, D. (1998) Virulence of Antibiotic-Resistant *Salmonella typhimurium*. *Proceedings of the National Acadamy of Science, USA*, Vol. 95, No. 7, pp. 3949-3953, ISSN 0027-8424

Bjorkholm, B., Sjolund, M., Falk, P., Berg, O., Engstrand, L. & Andersson, D. (2001) Mutation Frequency and Biological Cost of Antibiotic Resistance in *Helicobacter pylori*. *Proceedings of the National Acadamy of Science, USA*, Vol. 98, No. 25, pp. 146077-14612, ISSN 0027-8424

Bud, R. (2007) Fighting Resistance with Technology. In: *Penicillin: Triumph and Tragedy*, pp. 116 - 139, Oxford University Press, ISBN 978-0-19-925406-4, Oxford, UK

Centers for Disease Control and Prevention (CDC). (2007) Update to CDC's Sexually Transmitted Diseases Treatment Guidelines, 2006: Fluoroquinolones No Longer Recommended for Treatment of Gonococcal Infections. *Morbidity and Mortality Weekly Report*, Vol. 56, pp. 332-336

Chen, F.-J. & Lo, H.-J. (2003) Molecular Mechanisms of Fluoroquinolone Resistance. *Journal of Microbiology, Immunology, and Infection*, Vol. 36, No. 1, pp. 1-9, ISSN 1684-1182

Covino, J., Cummings, M., Smith, B., Benes, S., Draft, K. & McCormack, W. (1990) Comparison of Ofloxacin and Ceftriaxone in the Treatment of Uncomplicated Gonorrhea Caused by Penicillinase-Producing and Non-Penicillinase-Producing Strains. *Antimicrobial Agents and Chemotherapy*, Vol. 34, No. 1, pp. 148–149, ISSN 0066-4804

Delahay, R., Robertson, B., Balthazar, J., Shafer, W. & Ison, C. (1997) Involvement of the Gonococcal MtrE Protein in the Resistance of *Neisseria gonorrhoeae* to Toxic Hydrophobic Agents. *Microbiology*, Vol. 143, No. 7, pp. 2127 - 2133, ISSN 0002-1485

Dewi, B., Akira, S., Hayashi, H. & Ba-Thein, W. (2004) High Occurrence of Simultaneous Mutations in Target Enzymes and MtrRCDE Efflux System in Quinolone-Resistant

Neisseria gonorrhoeae. *Sexually Transmitted Diseases*, Vol. 31, No. 6, pp. 353-359, ISSN 0148-5717

Dionne-Odom, J., Tambe, P., Yee, E., Weinstock, H. & del Rio, C. (2011) Antimicrobial Resistant Gonorrhea in Atlanta: 1988 - 2006. *Sexually Transmitted Diseases*, Vol. 38, No. 12, pp. 780 - 782, ISNN 0148-5717

Eisenstein, B. & Sparling, P. (1978) Mutations to Increased Antibiotic Susceptibility in Naturally-Occurring Gonococci. *Nature*, Vol. 271, No. 5642, pp. 242 - 244, ISSN 0028-0836

Emmerson, A. M. (2003) The Quinolones: Decades of Development and Use. U.S. Patent 90001. *Journal of Antimicrobial Chemotherapy*, Vol. 51, Suppl1, pp. 13–20

Folster, J. & Shafer, W. (2005) Regulation of *mtrF* Expression in *Neisseria gonorrhoeae* and Its Role in High-Level Antimicrobial Resistance. *Journal of Bacteriology*, Vol. 187, N. 11, pp. 3713 - 3720, ISSN 0021-9193

Ghanem, K., Giles, J. & Zenilman, J. (2005) Fluoroquinolone-Resistant *Neisseria gonorrhoeae*: the Inevitable Epidemic. *Infectious Disease Clinics of North America*, Vol. 19, No. 2, pp. 351–365, ISSN 0891-5520

Giraud, E., Brisabois, A., Martel, J.-L. & Chaslus-Danclai, E. (1999) Comparative Studies of Mutations in Animal Isolates and Experimental *in vitro*- and *in vivo*-Selected Mutants of *Salmonella* spp. Suggest a Counterselection of Highly Fluoroquinolone-Resistant Strains in the Field. *Antimicrobial Agents and Chemotherapy*, Vol. 43, No. 9, pp. 2131-2137, ISSN 0066-4804

Hagman, K. & Shafer, W. (1995) Transcriptional Control of the *mtr* Efflux System of *Neisseria gonorrhoeae*. *Journal of Bacteriology*, Vol. 177, No. 14, pp. 4162 - 4165, ISSN 0021-9193

Hagman, K., Pan, W., Spratt, B., Balthazar, J., Judd, R. & Shafer, W. (1995) Resistance of *Neisseria gonorrhoeae* to Antimicrobial Hydrophobic Agents is Modulated by the *mtrRCDE* Efflux System. *Microbiology*, Vol. 141, No. 3, pp. 611 - 622, ISSN 0001-9400

Hagman, K., Lucas, C., Balthazar, J., Snyder, L., Nilles, M., Judd, R. & Shafer, W. (1997) The MtrD Protein of *Neisseria gonorrhoeae* is a Member of the Resistance/Nodulation/Division Protein Family Constituting Part of an Efflux System. *Microbiology*, Vol. 143, No. 7, pp. 2117 - 2125, ISSN 0002-1486

Hoffmann, K., Williams, D., Shafer, W. & Brennan, R. (2005) Characterization of the Multiple Transferable Resistance Repressor, MtrR from *Neisseria gonorrhoeae*. *Journal of Bacteriology*, Vol. 187, No 14, pp. 5008 - 5012, ISSN 0021-9193

Hooper, D. (1999) Mode of Action of Fluoroquinolones. *Drugs*, Vol. 58, Suppl 2, pp. 6–10, ISSN 0012-6667

Jerse, A. (1999) Experimental Gonococcal Genital Tract Infection and Opacity Protein Expression in Estradiol-Treated Mice. *Infection and Immunity* Vol. 67, No 11, pp. 5699-5708, ISSN 0019-9567

Jerse, A., Sharma, N., Simms, A., Crow, E., Snyder, L. & Shafer, W. (2003) A Gonococcal Efflux Pump System Enhances Bacterial Survival in a Female Mouse Model of Genital Tract Infection. *Infection and Immunity*, Vol. 71, No. 10, pp. 4476 - 5582, ISSN 0019-9567

Kam, K., Kam, S., Cheung, D., Tung, V., Au, W. & Cheung, M. (2003) Molecular Characterization of Quinolone-Resistant *Neisseria gonorrhoeae* in Hong Kong. *Antimicrobial Agents and Chemotherapy*, Vol 47, No. 1, pp. 436–439, ISSN 0066-4804

Komp Lindgren P., Marcusson, L., Sandvang, D., Frimodt-Moller, N. & Hughes, D. (2005) Biological Cost of Single and Multiple Norfloxacin Resistance Mutations in

Escherichia coli Implicated in Urinary Tract Infections. *Antimicrobial Agents and Chemotherapy*, Vol. 49, No. 6, pp. 2343-2351, ISSN 0066-4804

Kunz A., Begum, A., Wu, H., D'Ambrozio, J., Robinson, J., Shafer, W., Bash, M. & Jerse, A. (2012), Impact of Fluoroquinolone Resistance Mutations on Gonococcal Fitness and *in vivo* Selection for Compensatory Mutations. *Journal of Infectious Diseases* (In Press)

Laponogov, I., Sohi, M., Veselkov, D., Pan, X.-S., Sawhney, R., Thompson, A., McAuley, K., Fisher, L. & Sanderson, M. (2009) Structural Insight into the Quinolone-DNA Cleavage Complex of Type IIA Topoisomerases. *Nature Structural and Molecular Biology*, Vol. 16, No. 6, pp. 667–669, ISSN 1545-9993

Lomovskaya, O. & Bostian, K. (2006) Practical Applications and Feasibility of Efflux Pump Inhibitors in the Clinic—A Vision for Applied Use. *Biochemical Pharmacology*, Vol. 71, No. 7, pp. 910 - 918, ISSN 0006-2952

Lucas, C., Balthazar, J., Hagman, K. & Shafer, W. (1997) The MtrR Repressor Binds the DNA Sequence between the *mtrR* and *mtrC* Genes of *Neisseria gonorrhoeae*. *Journal of Bacteriology*, Vol. 179, No. 13, pp. 4123 - 4128, ISSN 0021-9193

Luo, N., Pereira, S., Sahin, O., Lin, J., Huang, S., Michel, L. & Zhang, Q. (2005) Enhanced *in vivo* Fitness of Fluoroquinolone-Resistant *Campylobacter jejuni* in the Absence of Antibiotic Selection Pressure. *Proceedings of the National Acadamy of Science, USA*, Vol. 102, No. 3, pp. 541-546, ISSN 0027-8424

Marcusson L., Frimodt-Moller, N. & Hughes, D. (2009) Interplay in the Selection of Fluoroquinolone Resistance and Bacterial Fitness. *PLoS Pathogens*, Vol. 5, No. 8, pp. e1000541, ISSN 1553-7366

Morais Cabral, J., Jackson, A., Smith, C., Shikotra, N., Maxwell, A. & Liddington, R. (1997) Crystal Structure of the Breakage-Reunion Domain of DNA Gyrase. *Nature*, Vol. 388, No. 6645, pp. 903–906, ISSN 0028-0836

Morris S., Moore, D., Hannah, P., Wang, S., Wolfe, J., Trees, D., Bolan, G. & Bauer, H. (2009) Strain Typing and Antimicrobial Resistance of Fluoroquinolone-Resistant *Neisseria gonorrhoeae* Causing a California Infection Outbreak. *Journal of Clinical Microbiology*, Vol. 47, No. 9, pp. 2944-2949, ISSN 0095-1137

Morse, S., Lysko, P., McFarland, L., Knapp, J., Sandstrom, E., Critchlow, C. & Holmes, K. (1982) Gonococcal Strains from Homosexual Men have Outer Membranes with Reduced Permeability to Hydrophobic Molecules. *Infection and Immunity*, Vol. 37, No. 2, pp. 432 - 438, ISSN 0019-9567

Mercante, A.D., Jackson, L., Johnson, P. J. T., Stringer, V. A., Dyer, D. W., & Shafer, W. M. (2012) MpeR Regulates the mtr Efflux Locus in *Neisseria gonorrhoeae* and Modulates Antimicrobial Resistance by an Iron-Responsive Mechanism. *Antimicrobial Agents and Chemotherapy*, Vol. 56, No. 3, pp. 1491 - 1501, ISSN 0066-4804.

Nagaev, I, Bjorkman, J., Andersson, D., & Hughes, D. (2001) Biological Cost and Compensatory Evolution in Fusidic Acid Resistant *Staphylococcus aureus*. *Molecular Microbiology*, Vol. 40, No. 2, pp. 443-449, ISSN 0950-382X

Ohnishi, M., Golparian, D., Shimuta, K., Saika, T., Hoshina, S., Iwasaku, K., Nakayama, S., Kitawaki, J. & Unemo, M. (2011) Is *Neisseria gonorrhoeae* Initiating a Future Era of Untreatable Gonorrhea?: Detailed Characterization of the First Strain with High-Level Resistance to Ceftriaxone. *Antimicrobial Agents and Chemotherapy*, Vol. 55, No. 7, pp. 3538 - 3545, ISSN 0066-4804

Packiam, M., Veit, S., Anderson, D., Ingalls, R. & Jerse, A. (2010) Mouse Strain-Dependent Differences in Susceptibility to *Neisseria gonorrhoeae* Infection and Induction of Innate Immune Responses. *Infection and Immunity*, Vol. 78, No. 1, pp. 433-440, ISSN 0019-9567

Pan, W. & Spratt, B. (1994) Regulation of the Permeability of the Gonococcal Cell Envelope by the *mtr* System. *Molecular Microbiology*, Vol. 11, No. 4, pp. 769 - 775, ISSN 0950-382X

Pope, C., Gillespie, S., Pratten, J. & McHugh, T. (2008) Fluoroquinolone-Resistant Mutants of *Burkholderia cepacia*. *Antimicrobial Agents and Chemotherapy*, Vol. 52, No. 3, pp. 1201-1203, ISSN 0066-4804

Rouquette, C., Harmon, J. & Shafer, W. (1999) Induction of the *mtrCDE*-Encoded Efflux Pump system of *Neisseria gonorrhoeae* Requires MtrA, an AraC-Like Protein. *Molecular Microbiology*, Vol. 33, No. 3, pp. 651 - 658, ISSN 1365-2958

Ruiz J., Jurado, A., Garcia-Méndez, E., Marco, F., Aguilar, L., Jiménez de Anta, M. & Vila, J. (2001) Frequency of Selection of Fluoroquinolone-Resistant Mutants of *Neisseria gonorrhoeae* Exposed to Gemifloxacin and Four Other Quinolones. *Journal of Antimicrobial Chemotherapy*, Vol. 48, No. 4, pp. 545-548, ISSN 0305-7453

Schrag, S., Perrot, V. & Levin, B. (1997) Adaptation to the Fitness Costs of Antibiotic Resistance in *Escherichia coli*. Proceedings of the Royal Society of Biological Sciences, Vol. 264, No. 1386, pp. 1287 - 1291, ISSN 0962-8452

Shafer, W., Balthazar, J., Hagman, K. & Morse, S. (1995) Missense Mutations that Alter the DNA-Binding Domain of the MtrR Protein Occur Frequently in Rectal Isolates of *Neisseria gonorrhoeae* that are Resistant to Fecal Lipids. *Microbiology*, Vol. 141, No. 4, pp. 907 - 911, ISSN 0001-9525

Shafer, W., Qu, X., Waring, A. & Lehrer, R. (1998) Modulation of *Neisseria gonorrhoeae* Susceptibility to Vertebrate Antibacterial Peptides due to a Member of the Resistance/Nodulation/Division Efflux Pump Family. *Proceedings of the National Academy of Science*, Vol. 95, No. 4, pp. 1829 - 1833, ISSN 0027-8424

Shafer, W., Folster, J. & Nicholas, R. (2010) Molecular Mechanisms of Antibiotic Resistance Expressed by the Pathogenic *Neisseria*. In: *Neisseria: Molecular Mechanisms of Pathogenesis*, Genco, C. & Wetzler, L. (Ed.), pp. 245 - 267, Caister Academic Press, ISBN 978-1-904455-51-6, Norfolk, UK

Song, W., Condron, S., Mocca, B., Veit, S., Hill, D., Abbas, A. & Jerse, A. (2008) Local and Humoral Immune Responses Against Primary and Repeat *Neisseria gonorrhoeae* Genital Tract Infections of 17ß-Estradiol-Treated Mice. *Vaccine*, Vol. 26, pp. 5741-5751, ISSN 0264-410X

Starnino, S., Conte, I., Matteelli, A., Galluppi, E., Cusini, M., Carlo, A., Delmonte, S. & Stefanelli, P. (2010) Trend of Ciprofloxacin Resistance in *Neisseria gonorrhoeae* Strains Isolated in Italy and Analysis of the Molecular Determinants. *Diagnostic Microbiology and Infectious Disease*, Vol. 67, No. 4, pp. 350–354, ISSN 0732-8893

Tanaka, M., Nakayama, H., Haraoka, M., Saika, T., Kobayashi, I., & Naito, S. (2000) Antimicrobial Resistance of *Neisseria gonorrhoeae* and High Prevalence of Ciprofloxacin-Resistant Isolates in Japan, 1993-1998. *Journal of Clinical Microbiology*, Vol. 38, No. 2, pp. 521-525, ISSN 0095-1137

Tapsall, J. W. (2005) Antibiotic Resistance in *Neisseria gonorrhoeae*. *Clinical Infectious Diseases*, Vol. 41, Suppl 4, pp. S263-8

Trees, D., Sandul, A., Neal, S., Higa, H., & Knapp, J. (2001) Molecular Epidemiology of *Neisseria gonorrhoeae* Exhibiting Decreased Susceptibility and Resistance to Ciprofloxacin in Hawaii, 1991-1999. *Sexually Transmitted Diseases*, Vol. 28, No. 6, pp. 309-14, ISSN 0148-5717

Unemo, M., Golparian, D., Syversen, G., Vestrheim, D. & Moi, H. (2010) Two Cases of Verified Clinical Failures Using Internationally Recommended First-Line Cefixime for Gonorrhoea Treatment, Norway, 2010. *Euro Surveillance*, Vol. 15, No. 47, ISSN 1025-496X

Veal, W. & Shafer, W. (2003) Identification of a Cell Envelope Protein (MtrF) Involved in Hydrophobic Antimicrobial Resistance in *Neisseria gonorrhoeae*. *Journal of Antimicrobial Chemotherapy*, Vol. 51, No. 1, pp. 27 - 37, ISSN 0305-7453

Vereshchagin V., Ilina, E., Malakhova, M., Zubkov, M., Sidorenko, S., Kuhanova, A. & Govorun, V. (2004) Fluoroquinolone-Resistant *Neisseria gonorrhoeae* Isolates from Russia: Molecular Mechanisms Implicated. *Journal of Antimicrobial Chemotherapy*, Vol. 53, No. 4, pp. 653-656, ISSN 0305-7453

Vernel-Pauillac F., Hogan, T., Tapsall, J. & Goarant, C. (2009) Quinolone Resistance in *Neisseria gonorrhoeae*: Rapid Genotyping of Quinolone Resistance-Determining Regions in *gyrA* and *parC* Gene by Melting Curve Analysis Predicts Susceptibility. *Antimicrobial Agents and Chemotherapy*, Vol. 53, No. 3, pp. 1264-1267, ISSN 0066-4804

Warner, D., Folster, J., Shafer, W. & Jerse, A. (2007) Regulation of the MtrC-MtrD-MtrE Efflux-Pump System Modulations the *in vivo* Fitness of *Neisseria gonorrhoeae*. *Journal of Infectious Diseases*, Vol. 196, No. 12, pp. 1804 - 1812, ISSN 0022-1899

Warner, D., Shafer, W. & Jerse, A. (2008) Clinically Relevant Mutations that Cause Derepression of the *Neisseria gonorrhoeae* MtrC-MtrD-MtrE Efflux Pump System Confer Different Levels of Antimicrobial Resistance and *in vivo* Fitness. *Molecular Microbiology*, Vol. 70, No. 2, pp. 462 - 478, ISSN 1365-2958

Webber, M., Baily, A., Blair, J., Morgan, E., Stevents, M., Hinton, J., Ivens, A., Wain, J. & Piddock, L. (2009) The Global Consequence of Disruption of the AcrAB-TolC Efflux Pump in *Salmonella enterica* Includes Reduced Expression of SPI-1 and Other Attributes Required to Infect the Host. *Journal of Bacteriology*, Vol. 191, No. 13, pp. 4276 - 4285, ISSN 0021-9193

Xia, M., Whittington, W., Shafer, W. & Holmes, K. (2000) Gonorrhea Among Men Who Have Sex with Men: Outbreak Caused by a Single Genotype of Erythromycin-Resistant *Neisseria gonorrhoeae* with a Single Base Pair Deletion in the *mtrR* Promoter Region. *Journal of Infectious Diseases*, Vol. 181, No. 6, pp. 2080 - 2082, ISSN 0022-1899

Xiong, X., Bromley, E., Oelschlaeger, P., Woolfson, D. & Spencer, J. (2011) Structural Insights into Quinolone AntibioticRresistance Mediated by Pentapeptide Repeat Proteins: Conserved Surface Loops Direct the Activity of a Qnr Protein from a Gram-Negative Bacterium. *Nucleic Acids Research*, Vol. 39, No. 9, pp. 3917–3927, ISSN 0305-1048

Zhang, Q., Sahin, O., McDermott, P. & Payot, S. (2006) Fitness of Antimicrobial-Resistant *Campylobacter* and *Salmonella*. *Microbes and Infection*, Vol. 8, No. 7, pp. 1972-1978, ISSN 1286-4579

Zarantonelli, L., Borthagaray, G., Lee, E. & Shafer, W. (1999) Decreased Azithromycin Susceptibility of *Neisseria gonorrhoeae* Due to *mtrR* Mutations. *Antimicrobial Agents and Chemotherapy*, Vol. 43, No. 10, pp. 2468 - 2472, ISSN 0066-4804

15

Mechanisms of Antibiotic Resistance in *Corynebacterium* spp. Causing Infections in People

Alina Olender
Department of Medical Microbiology, Medical University of Lublin
Poland

1. Introduction

In recent years we can observe an increasing number of publications describing different incidents of infections, where species of *Corynebacterium* are isolated as the etiological factor of infection (Anderson et al., 2008; Campanile et al., 2009; Chiner et al., 1999; Dela et al., 2008; Fernandez-Roblas et al., 2009; Funke et al., 1997a; Funke et al., 1997b; Lagrou et al., 1998; Otsuka et al., 2005; Ostuka et al., 2006; Williams et al., 1993). It is a large and very diverse group of microorganisms, in which *Corynebacterium diphtheriae* is the most important species, with the most important human-pathogenic significance (Gomes et al., 2009; Wagner et al., 2011; Wilson, 1995). Strains of this species produce a strong exotoxine and are responsible for causing diphtheria. Well-developed procedures for diagnosis of diphtheria and conducted large-scale vaccinations resulted in erradication of diphtheria in most countries. Beside the typical human-pathogenic *C. diphtheriae,* the genus *Corynebacterium* comprises more than 85 different species of pathogenic significance. This type includes species pathogenic for animals, e.g. *C. pseudotuberculosis* (Baird & Fontanie, 2007; Nieto et al., 2009), *C. kutscheri* (Amao et al., 2008; Suzuki et al., 1988), *C. canis* (Funke et al., 2009) and a very large group of species colonizing the skin and mucous membranes of man, which in favorable circumstances, may become the cause of serious infections in humans. These opportunistic organisms, e.g. *C. jeikeium* (Ifantidou et al., 2010; Pitcher et al., 1990; Rosato et al., 2001), *C. urealyticum* (Funke et al., 1997b; Garcia-Bravo et al. 1996; López-Medrano et al., 2008), *C. amycolatum* (Anderson et al., 2008; Dela et al., 2008; Funke et al., 1997b), *C. striatum* (Campanile et al., 2009; Funke et al., 1997b; Martinem-Martinez et al., 1995; Ostuka et al., 2006; Roberts et al., 1992), *C. pseudodiphtehriticum* (Chiner et al., 1999; Dorello et al., 2006; Freman et al., 1994; Olender & Niemcewicz, 2010), may cause infections of various course: mild, chronic and acute, as well as of invasive nature, life-threatening to a patient. The genus *Corynebacterium* includes also species unrelated to the human organism, e.g. *C. glutamicum,* producing L-glutamic acid and lysine, used in biotechnological processes on the industrial scale and in genetic studies (Katsumata et al., 1984; Serwold-Davis et al., 1987; Tauch et al., 1998; Wendisch et al., 2006; Valbuena et al., 2007, Yague Guirao et al., 2005).

Application of modern molecular biology techniques in genetic studies of unknown strains isolated from infections resulted in the detection and description of new species such as: *C. singulare* (Riegel etal., 1997), *C. auriscanis* (Collins et al., 1999), *C. resistens* (Otsuka et al. 2005),

C. imitans (Funke at al., 1997a), *C. sputi* (Yassin & Siering, 2008) and the reclassification of previously inaccurately determined ones, e.g.: *C. cystitidis, C. pilosum* (Takahashi et al., 1995).

In view of a widely conducted taxonomic research of species belonging to the genus *Corynebacterium*, the term "dyphteroids" has also been changed, which was used commonly for the opportunistic species, suggesting a direct relationship with *C. diphtheriae*. Nowadays taxonomists more and more replace it by a more universal name for this group of bacteria "coryneform" (Anderson et al., 2008; Balci et al., 2002; Funke et al., 1996; Funke et al., 1997b; Gomez-Garces et al., 2007; Lagrou et al., 1998; Ostuka et al., 2005), which seems fully justified.

Many opportunistic strains of the genus *Corynebacterium*, isolated from clinical materials, belong to species whose characteristics determining the pathogenic effect on the human body have not been thoroughly recognised and characterized yet. Therefore, the assessment of their role as pathogens is often very difficult. Undoubtedly, the common occurrence of coryneform on mucous membranes and the skin may cause doubts in interpretation of their contribution to infections, especially when the material is sampled from places non-sterile physiologically and there might be a suspicion of its contamination.

An increasing number of recognized and described incidents of infections and the observed increase in the number of publications on this topic is probably connected with the microbiological diagnostics currently carried out at a higher level and development of quick commercial tests for identification of species based on their biochemical properties. In reference to strains difficult to identify or requiring verification of uncertain biochemical determination, oftener methods of molecular biology are used, which has resulted in detection of new species and the reclassification of ones previously poorly assayed.

Infections caused by opportunistic *Corynebacterium spp.* generally refer to a group of people, who experience symptoms of immunodeficiency. The group of patients with a particular risk of infection includes primarily people with immunodeficiency due to disorders of bone marrow activity, the ongoing processes of cancer, post surgery or urological surgery, invasive diagnostic procedures and patients with AIDS. The risk of infection is increased by long-term hospitalization, antibiotic therapy, radiotherapy, treatment with cytostatics or steroids. A disturbing fact is occurrence of such infections in a group of people called "immunocompetent", in whom no symptoms of immunodeficiency were reported before (Chiner et al., 1999; Frejman et al., 1994).

The basis for treatment of infections caused by *Corynebacterium spp.* is taking up of an effective antibiotic therapy. For this group of microorganisms, until recently an obstacle in the evaluation of drug resistance was use of different criteria of interpretation that were recommended for other groups of microorganisms and determination of drug resistance with various methods, yet results presented by different authors have become the basis for information about occurrence of strains with high resistance to antibiotics among opportunistic *Corynebacterium spp.*, which indicate existence of different mechanisms of resistance in these strains.

The described multidrug-resistant strains of *C. jeikeium* (Rosato et al., 2001; Yagye Guirao et al., 2005) *C. amycolatum* (Yagye Guirao et al., 2005; Yoon et al., 2011), *C. striatum* (Campanile et al., 2009; Martinem-Martinez et al., 1995; Otsuka et al., 2006; Roberts et al., 1992) i *C. resistens* (Otsuka et al., 2005) confirm presence in *Corynebacterium spp.* of different mechanisms of resistance and genes, which may be differently located. Phenotypic tests of resistance to antibiotics have become the basis for search of the genes responsible for them and their transmission paths. They have also contributed to analyses and study of similarity in occurrence of resistance genes in other groups of microorganisms, often unrelated to the genus *Corynebacterium*, such as *Staphylococcus spp.* (Roberts et al., 1999), *Enterococcus* spp.(Power et al., 1995), *E. coli* (Deb & Noth,1999; Serwold-Davis et al., 1990; Serwold-Davis et al., 1987).

2. Mechanisms of resistance to antibiotics most commonly occurring in *Corynebacterium* spp.

The conducted study characterizing resistance to antibiotics isolated from clinical material of different species of the genus *Corynebacterium* (Anderson et al., 2008; Fernandez-Roblas et al., 2009; Funke et al., 1997a; Funke et al., 1997b; Garcia-Bravo et al., 1996; Gomez-Garceset al., 2007; Martinem-Martinez et al., 1995; Otsuka et al., 2006; Roberts et al., 1992, Troxler R et al., 2001, Weiss et al., 1996) draw attention to the most frequently occuring mechanisms of resistance to antibiotics in this group of microorganisms. The results show participation of extrachromosomal genetic elements in transmission of resistance genes in both pathogenic and potentially pathogenic - opportunistic and typically nonpathogenic ones, e.g. present in the soil or strains of *Corynebacterium spp.* (Kono et al., 1983; Vertes et al., 2005).

Antibiotic resistance genes in species of *Corynebacterium spp.* are often located on large plasmids, e.g. resistance to tetracycline, chloramphenicol, erythromycin and streptomycin on plasmid pTP10 in *C. xerosis* (Deb & Nath, 1999; Hodgson et al., 1990), but also on trensposons (Delal et al., 2008).

2.1 Resistance to macrolides, lincosamides and streptogramins B

The occurrence of simultaneous resistance to three groups of antibiotics: macrolides, lincosamides and streptogramins B, determined in short as MLSB, is characteristic mainly of staphylococci and streptococci. It is connected with occurrence of three different mechanisms of the effects of activity: modification of the ribosome binding site associated with methylation or mutation, the mechanism of active efflux of antibiotic from the cell and the least significant - enzymatic inactivation of the antibiotic. The first two MLSB resistance mechanisms are of the highest importance.

Methylation of the binding site causes conformational changes of the subunit 23S rRNA, which prevents binding of the antibiotic molecules in the peptidyltransferase center within the 50S ribosome subunit and leads to the blockade of the mRNA translation and inhibition of bacterial protein synthesis. In species of the genus *Corynebacterium* it is connected with presence of genes belonging to class *erm* (erythromycin ribosome methylation), encoding the rRNA methylase enzyme, which causes dimethylation of adenine present in the 23S rRNA (Arthur et al., 1990). The gene *erm* occurring in *Corynebacterium spp,* responsible for this mechanism of resistance has been classified as class X of genes *erm* (Roberts et al., 1999). Despite a high degree of homology between genes *ermX* isolated from different species of *Corynebacterium* (*C. diphtheriae, C. jeikeium and C. xerosis*), it has been found that they exhibit different locations. The gene *ermX* in *C. diphtheriae* was found within the 14.5-kbp plasmid pNG2 (Coyle et al., 1979), while the gene *ermX* in *C. xerosis* turned out to be located on transposon Tn5432, whose carrier is the 50-kbp plasmid pTP10 (Delal et al., 2008). In the strain *C. jeikeium* (Pitcher et al., 1990) and *C. striatum* (Roberts et al., 1992), the gene *ermX* was found on the chromosome, which has been confirmed also in other analysed strains of *C. jeikeium* (Rosato et al., 2001). Despite detection of different locations of genes *ermX* in certain strains of *C. jeikeium* and *C. xerosis,* it is assumed that its most typical location is primarily the transposon Tn*5432*. At the same time in other examined *Corynebacterium spp.*, in which the MLSB mechanism is not related to the location of genes *ermX* on transposon Tn*5432*, interesting results of research were obtained, indicating the possibility of reorganization of fragments of the transposon Tn*5432* and presence of all its components in the strain genome (Hall et al., 1999).

It is possible that mobile transpositional elements IS*1249* containing *ermX* may create new composite transposons containing other multidrug- resistant genes. This phenomenon is particularly disturbing since transposition of the insertional sequence IS*1249* is known for its capabilities to insert and transfer Tn*5432* from genomes of unrelated bacteria (Rosato et al., 2001).

Different results of studies suggesting different locations of the detected genes *ermX* referred to the species of *Corynebacterium,* which were isolated from strains coming from different geographical regions, which may explain such diversified locations in the genome. The strain of *C. diphthariae,* containing pNG2 and *C. striatum* came from patients from the north-western USA (Coyle et al., 1979; Hodgson et al., 1990; Roberts et al., 1992), *C. xerosis* from pTP10 from Japan (Tauch et al.1995), *C. jeikeium* from France (Rosato et al.2001) and *C. jeikeium* and *C. amycolatum* from Spain (Yague Guirao et al., 2005).

It is very likely that different locations of genes *ermX* may indicate the possibility of acquiring resistance genes by multidrug-resistant strains of *Corynebacterium spp.* from microorganisms colonizing the skin or mucous membranes. *ErmX* occurring in *C. diphtheriae* is contained in plasmid pNG2, similar to plasmids isolated from *Corynebacterium spp.* occurring on the skin (Serwold-Davis & Groman, 1986). The replicon 2.6-kb EcoRI-ClaI fragment (oriR) may be possessed by many microorganisms, including a popular commensal *E. coli* (Deb & Nath, 1999; Serwold-Davis et al., 1990; Serwold-Davis et al., 1987).

At the same time, as research indicates, the plasmid pNG2 seems an unlikely place of origin for genes *erm* occurring in *Corynebacterium spp.* More likely is transposon Tn*5432* associated with the chromosome, which may be mobile (Trauch et al., 1995). Tn*5432* was also found in the occuring on the skin strains of *Propionibacterium acnes, P. granulosum* and P. *avidum*, which suggests that multidrug –resistant strains of the genus *Corynebacterium* may be an important source in horizontal transfer of resistance genes to other human pathogens (Ross et al., 2002). Another source, from which strains may be derived or to which they may arrive, is bacterial flora occurring in animals. It may be confirmed by detection of gene *ermX* in the strain of *Corynebacterium spp.* isolated from pasteurized milk. It showed resistance to erythromycin and/or spiromycin (Perrin-Guyomard et al., 2005).

Beside gene *ermX*, in strains of *Corynebacterium* Group A with the MLSB mechanism of resistance, also gene *erm* class B has been found (Luna et al., 1999), which occurs in *Enterococcus spp.* and *Streptococcus spp.*, which may also suggest the participation of these microorganisms in spread of the MLSB mechanism in *Corynebacterium spp.*

The expression of the MLSB resistance may be constitutive or induced. In the case of the constitutive type of resistance, active mRNA, permitting synthesis of methylase, is created without an inducer, while the induced MLSB - inactive mRNA is synthesized, which is activated only under the influence of an inducer, which allows synthesis of the enzyme. Occurrence of the constitutive MLSB resistance mechanism is very popular in strains of *C. pseudodiphtheriticum,* present in mucous membranes of the upper respiratory tract in humans (Olender & Niemcewicz, 2010).

Formation of cross-resistance associated with the MLSB mechanism is also accompanied by the process of active efflux of antibiotic from the cell. In staphylococci they are transporters of the membrane protein nature (ETP - binding cassette), encoded by genes *msrA* (macrolide streptogramin resistance), carried on plasmids. These transporters act as a specific pump removing macrolides of 14 - and 15-membered lactone ring and streptogramins B from the bacterial cell. Macrolides of 16-membered lactose ring, lincosamides and telithromycin are not transported. In this case, this mechanism is referred to as MSB (Leclercq, 2002; Douthwaite &Champney, 2001)

It was found that presence of gene *msrA* is also associated with resistance to macrolides and streptogramins B in strains of *Corynebacterium spp.* (Ojo et al., 2006) and similarly with production of an active transport system of the antibiotic pumped out from the cell (macrolide efflux proteins). Gene *msrA* had been previously found only in *Staphylococcus spp.* (Roberts et al., 1999). It encodes the ATP relay needed by the cell to gain energy from hydrolysis ATP for active transport of erythromycin and streptogramin B, and enables synthesis of the ABC family of transporters, i.e. multiprotein systems to actively pump out the antibiotic from the cell.

In turn in reference to *S.pneumoniae, S. pyogenes, S. agalactiae* and other species of streptococci and enterococci, the efflux mechanism is associated with presence of the MCF transporters (macrolide-specific efflux) and refers only to macrolites with 14 - and 15-membered lactose rings. It does not apply to macrolites with a 16-membered lactose ring, ketolides, linkosamides and streptogramin B. It is associated with low levels of resistance to macrolides (Appelbaum, 2002).

Gene *mef,* causing active efflux of macrolides from the bacterial cell was also found in *Corynebacterium* group A, *C. jeikeium* and strains of *Corynebacterium spp.* (Luna et al., 1999).

2.2 Resistance to fluoroquinolones

In species of the genus *Corynebacterium,* resistance has been also observed to fluoroquinolones. It is associated with point mutations within the structural gene region of the gyrase subunit A, which is defined as the region determining resistance to quinolones (QRDR - quinolone resistance determining region).

Mutations are of the spontaneous nature, leading to changes in the amino acid sequences, on which depends the range of resistance to certain fluoroquinolones. The resulting level of resistance depends largely on the type of the amino acid that has been built-in as a result of mutation in place of the pre-existing one. Some of them cause a small loss of affinity and a slight decrease in sensitivity, other reduce potently the affinity and activity of fluoroquinolones. It is confirmed by studies of strains of *C. macginleyi,* in which resistance has been found to norfloxacin, ciprofloxacin and levofloxacin. By analyzing gene *gyraA* encoding the gyrase subunit A, a change of the amino acid in position 83 in the QRDR region was found (Serine to Arginine), which resulted in resistance in *C. macginleyi* to norfloxacin. A double mutation has been also found, leading to amino acid changes in positions 83 and 87, which conditioned resistance to all fluoroquinolones. It was observed that double mutations occurred in Ser-83 and Asp-87 in all strains of *C. macginleyi* with a high level of resistance (Eguchi et al., 2008).

Studies of the gene *gyr*A sequence were also conducted in strains of *C. striatum* and *C. amycolatum* (Sierra et al., 2005). A high resistance to quinolones in *C.amycolatum* resulted from a double mutation and amino acid changes in positions 87 and 97 or 87 and 88 (unusual location of mutation in *gyr*A). In the case of *C. striatum* mutations of amino acids in positions 87 and 91 occurred in *gyr*A, corresponding to resistance characterized by very high MIC values for ciprofloxacin and levofloxacin, while only moderately increased MIC values for moxifloxacin.

These studies showed various complex and intricate mechanisms of resistance to quinolones in the studied species of *Corynebacterium spp.* (Sierra et al., 2005), which depend on the number of mutations and the type of changed amino acids.

2.3 Resistance to tetracyclines

Phenotypic studies constituted the basis for detection of resistance to tetracycline in *Corynebacterium spp.* In the case of *C. striatum,* it was found in 97% of the tested strains (Martinem-Martinez, 1995). These observations were confirmed by detection of the gene *tet*M, responsible for resistance to all tetracyclines, which is due to the protective effect on the protein ribosome with the mass of about 72-72.5 kDa (Roberts et al., 1992).

In strains of *C. striatum* M82B resistance to tetracycline is associated with the region 50-kb R-plasmid pTP10. An analysis of the nucleotide sequence revealed two reading frames called *tet*A and *tet*B. For analysis of the *tet*AB genes function, their expression in *C. glutamicum* was used and thus it was confirmed that they are responsible for resistance to tetracycline, oxytetracycline, and at a low level to other derivatives, such as chlortetracycline, minocycline and doxycycline. At the same an increased MIC value for oxacycline was found in this strain. This effect is associated with participation of the *tet*AB genes that determine resistance of the transport nature. It creates a powerful mechanism of active transport (efflu) causing pumping out of drugs from the cell via specific transport protein localized in the cytoplasmic membrane (Tauch et al., 1999).

R-plasmid pTP10 found in *C. xerosis* also contains determinants of resistance to tetracycline with parallel resistance to other antibiotics, such as chloramphenicol, kanamycin and erythromycin (Kono et al., 1983; Tauch et al., 1995) whereas, in strains of *C. melassecola,* the species used to produce glutamate, the resistance gene to tetracycline was found on another mobile element - plasmid pAG1 (Deb & Nath, 1999).

2.4 Resistance to beta-lactam antibiotics

The common susceptibility to penicillin in toxic and nontoxic strains of *C. diphtheriae* made it one of the most frequently prescribed antibiotics in treatment of diphtheria (Wilson, 1995).

Despite this opinion, there have been cases observed in which it showed no efficacy. Phenotypic tests consisuted the basis (Von Hunostein et al., 2002), in which penicillin sensitivity of 24 nontoxic strains of *C. diphtheriae* biotype *gravis* was determined in the broth microdilution method and by Etests. The research conducted with two methods showed a high 98% consistency of results. MIC values for penicillin were in the range from 0.064 to 0.250 mg/l, with simultaneous very low values for erythromycin (MIC ≤ 0.016 mg/l), whereas MBC (Minimal Bactericidal Concentaration) - MBC50 and MBC90 for penicillin were respectively 2.0 and 8.0 mg/l and 17.0 and 24.0. In 71% of the tested strains the ratio MBC/MIC was ≥ 32. The results of the study indicated the insensitivity (tolerance) to penicillin, which was confirmed by a lack of a positive effect of treatment despite the MIC values indicating sensitivity of the tested strains to this antibiotic. Such an effect was also observed in the case of tolerance to amoxicillin in the strain *C. diphtheriae* isolated from the case of *endocarditis* (Dupon et al., 1995).

In other strains of *Corynebacterium spp.* a similar situation was found, i.e. creation of insensitivity to oxacillin with low MIC values. This effect was not associated with the existing mechanism of resistance to beta-lactam antibiotics, but with a very high phenotypic expression and activity of a pair of genes *tet*A and *tet*B present on the Tn3598-transposon Class II - 12kb, which determined resistance to tetracycline. The activity of these genes, which consists of powerful active pumping, resulted also in removal of a structurally different antibiotic, which was oxacillin (Tauch et al., 2000).

Based on the analysis of results of phenotypic and genotypic studies of different species of the genus *Corynebacterium* showing resistance to beta-laktam antibiotics, it can be concluded that both resistance mechanisms organisms occur in these microorganisms, i.e. production of beta-laktamases and modification of penicillin-binding proteins. It is confirmed by e.g. resistance to penicillin (MIC 90> 4 μg/ml) in strains of *C. jeikeium* and *C. urealyticum*, ampicillin (MIC90> 8 μg/ml) (Gomez-Garces et al., 2007), in *C. resistens* to penicillin, cefazolin, cefotiam, cefmetazol, cefepime (MIC> 64 μg/ml) and imipenem (MIC> 32 μg/ml) (Otsuka et al., 2005), in strains of *C. striatum* to penicillin, ampicillin (MIC90 = 16 μg/ml), cefazolin, cefotiam, cefotaxime, imipenem (MIC90> 32 μg/ml) (Otsuka et al., 2006). Just like in hospital strains of *C. urealyticum*, in which resistance to penicillin and cefotaxime was particularly high (MIC90> 512 μg/ml) (Garcia-Bravo et al., 1996).

It can be also confirmed by an analysis of the genome sequence of *C. glutamicum*, which showed presence of four genes encoding proteins PBP (Penicillin Binding Proteins) HMW (high-molecular-weight), i.e. PBP1a, PBP1b, PBP2a, PBP2b, two genes encoding PBP4, PBP4b (low-molecular-weight) and two probably encoding beta-laktamases (Valbuena et al., 2007).

2.5 Resistance to glycopeptides

An antibiotic recommended by many authors in the empirical treatment of invasive infections caused by species of the genus *Corynebacterium* is vancomycin. It is connected with the common sensitivity to this antibiotic of even multidug-resistant species, which pose the greatest problems in infections. It refers to such species as *C. jeikeium*, *C. resistant*, *C. amycolatum* and *C. striatum* (Wiliams et al., 1993). Unfortunately, still cases of isolated strains of *C. aquaticum* and *C. group B1* resistant to vancomycin have been reported.

Only single cases are described, in treatment of which other alternative antibiotics give very good results. An example might be a case of infection in a 44-year-old patient with *endocarditis* 4 months after a prosthetic mitral valve (Barnas et al., 1991). The strain of *Corynebacterium spp.* isolated from the blood turned out resistant to vancomycin and penicillin G, erythromycin, gentamicin and rifampicin. The use of imipenem and ciprofloxacin resulted in an effective cure of the infection.

In related species of Coryneform *Oerskovia turbata 892* and *Arcanobacterium* (former *Corynebacterium*) *haemolyticum 872,* resistance to vancomycin and teicoplanin was found of the constitutive nature. Presence of the VanA gene was detected, found on plasmids of 15 and 20 kb. In strains of *A. haemolyticum 872* the VanA gene sequence turned out the same as in vancomycin-resistant *Enterococcus faecium BM4147.* In the case of *O. turbata* 892 a change of sequence occurred in three points. Species *A. haemoliticum* and *O. turbata* show a natural sensitivity to vancomycin and teicoplanin, and resistance found in the tested strains resulted from presence of the VanA gene (Power et al., 1995). The resistance phenotype associated with presence of the VanA gene is characterized by a high degree of resistance to vancomycin and teicoplanin.

2.6 Resistance to chloramphenicol

Resistance genes to chloramphenicol were detected on plasmids - in the strain *Corynebacterium spp.* on the pXZ10145 plasmid - 5.3 kb and in *C. xerosis* on pTP10 - 45.0 kb (Deb & Nath, 1999). In *C. striatum* strain M82B (former *C. xerosis* M82B) (Tauch et al., 1998) chloramphenicol resistance gene cmx (chloramphenicol and exports) was detected as an integral part of the transposon Tn5564, which contains a complete copy of the insertion sequence IS1513. The *cmx* gene is responsible for encoding of a specific protein (transmembran chloramphenicol efflux protein), which inhibits the passage of the antibiotic into the cytoplasm, and gives the bacetrial cell resistance to chloramphenicol.

3. Problems with diagnostic of infection by coryneform

The increasing isolation of multidrug-resistant strains of the genus *Corynebacterium* from clinical materials draws attention to the emerging issues related to treatment of infections caused by this group of opportunistic bacteria. The problem is all the more important since the infections often concern diagnostically difficult cases, long-hospitalized patients, the chronically ill, often with an accompanying disease causing immunosuppression. The underrated contribution of coryneform in infections may lead to therapeutic errors. Their common occurrence on the mucous membranes and skin causes doubts about their recognition as the etiologic factor of the infection.

The next problem, that may determine the accuracy of microbiology result as well as confirmation of the presence of opportunistic *Corynebacterium spp.* in infection, is a choice of appropriate culture method - bacterial culture media, which composition supports the growth of different coryneforms species. It is applied mostly for lipophilic species, as *C. jeikeium, C. urealyticum.* It is very important to identify the isolated strains precisely, as this enables tracking multi drug-resistance in specific strains, their existence on specific areas and routes of transmission. These informations are specifically important for hospital areas, facilitating to make proper decision on limiting these types of infections.

Accurate microbiological diagnostics of infections caused by species of the genus *Corynebacterium*, identification of strains of the isolated species and determination of antibiotic susceptibility with methods enabling determination of the MIC values permit assessment of the existing and emerging mechanisms of drug resistance and result in making right decisions about the most appropriate antibiotic therapy for a given case. It is extremely important to apply correct interpretation criteria of the determined drug resistance for species of the genus *Corynebacterium*, specific for this group of microorganisms, based on the established and generally accepted recommendations (Clinical and Laboratory Standards Institute [CLSI], 2006; Łętowska & Olender, 2010). Application of methods of molecular biology and examination of resistance genes, their locations and transmission paths is a very important direction of research on monitoring of resistance mechanisms in coryneform and gives the ability to track and determine their role in transmission of genes also among other species.

4. Antibiotic therapy used in infections of *Corynebacterium spp.*

The basis for monitoring of the emerging multi-drug resistant strains for all bacteria, as well as species of the genus *Corynebacterium*, is conducting research characterizing their sensitivity to antibiotics, which is potentially useful in treating infections. Publication of such data is extremely important due to tips received about the most effective antibiotic therapy for a given group of microorganisms.

An analysis of sensistivity to antibiotics of a large group of strains of *C. urealyticum, C. amycolatum, C. jeikeium, C. coyleae, C. striatum, C. aurimucosum* and *C. afermentans* was conducted with assays using Etests (Fernandez-Roblas et al., 2009). The authors found that strains of all tested species were susceptible to glycopeptides, linezolid, chinupristin/dalphopristin and daptomycin, which was also confirmed in other studies (Funke et al., 1997a; Funke et al., 1997b).

The results obtained from research done in Italy, involving strains of *C. striatum* isolated from different infections, also indicated the need of analysis of drug resistance in *Corynebacterium*. Genetic studies of strains of *C. striatum* MDR (multidrug-resistant) revealed presence of a multidrug-resistant clone, whose strains isolated from cases of pneumonia, catheter related bacteremia and wound infections showed, despite resistance to other classes of antibiotics, susceptibility to glycopeptides, tigecyclin, chinupristyn/dalphopristin, daptomycin and linezolid (Campanile et al., 2009).

One of the most resistant species, which causes the biggest problems in hospitals and is frequently isolated from infections in hospitalized patients, is *C. jeikeium*. The study of 66 strains of *C. jeikeium* (Johnson et al. 2004) showed resistance to penicillin in all of them, in 94% resistance to erythromycin, and in 74% to tetracycline. Twenty-two strains of other examined species of the genus *Corynebacterium* had a significantly lower level of the resistant. But what is extremely important, all examined strains were susceptible to vancomycin (MIC = 0.5-4.0 mg/l), linezolid (MIC = 0.5-2.0 mg/l) and daptomycin (MIC ≤ 1mg/l) with the exception of two isolates of *C. auaticum,* whose MIC for daptomycin was 8 mg/l. At the same time effecacy of daptomycin was confirmed in the successfully applied combination with rifampicin in a patient with *endocarditis* caused by *C. amycolatum* (Dala et al., 2008) i *C. striatum* (Shah & Murillo, 2005).

Linezolid, as shown in published works, was also characterized by a very good action. High activity of linezolid was found in studies of 190 strains of coryneform (Gomez-Garces et al.,2007). It confirmed the possibility of equally successful application of this antibiotic in infections caused by Coryneform.

Diversity of antibiotic resistance in species of the genus *Corynebacterium* is strictly connected with the locations, in which the tested strains occur. As found in the conducted studies (Garcia-Bravo et al., 1996) strains of *C. urealyticum* coming from hospitalized patients show significantly higher resistance to antibiotics than those isolated from outpatients, from outside of the hospital environment. An analysis of frequency and duration of antibiotic therapy used in patients from both groups of respondents was conducted. It confirmed unequivocally that the hospital environment and more frequently used antibiotics in the hospitalized patients is conducive to occurence of multidrug-resistant strains, and the hospital environment in which such patients stay is the place from which strains of *C. urealyticum* came, causing infections in the hospitalized patients. At the same time considerably lower resistance to antibiotics of isolates coming from the outpatients indicates that the strains of *C.urealyticum* most likely are derived from microflora colonizing the skin of the examined outpatients.

A very disturbing fact is discovery of new multidrug-resistant species of the genus *Corynebacterium*, which suggests a progressive character of multidrug-resistance occurring in this group. It is confirmed by a description of a new multidrug-resistant species of *C. resistens* in 2005. It is lipophilic, with low fermentation properties (it ferments glucose), does not reduce nitrates, does not produce urease and pyrazinamidase. It is characterized by resistance to penicillin and cephalosporins (MIC > 64 μg/ml), imipenem (MIC > 32 μg/ml), aminoglycosides (MIC > 3 μg/ml 2), macrolides (MIC > 16 μg/ml), quinolones (MIC > 32 μg/ml) and sensitivity to teicoplanin (MIC ≤ 0.5 μg/ml) and vancomycin (MIC = 2 μg/ml) (Otsuka et al., 2005).

5. Conclusion

Presented by several authors results of their studies on antibiotics resistance show, that even though *Corynebacterium spp.* are the members of the normal flora, they are not universally susceptible to antibiotics, as could be expected. Opportunistic *Corynebacterium spp.*, until now considered as bacteria of low pathogenicity, may pose a diagnostic and therapeutic problems, as they are more and more commonly isolated from serious, life-threatening invasive infections. Observed in many cases multi drug-resistance may be connected with the possibility to acquire resistance genes by gene transfer within bacteria regarded as normal flora present in large number on a given body area (skin, mucous membranes). Drug resistance occurrence in opportunistic species is the result of antibiotics overuse. It is obvious that antibiotics used also influence on saprophytic bacteria. Resulting selection of resistant strains is commonly known and regarded as important process leading to multi drug-resistance. For these reasons, analysis of the process in opportunistic *Corynebacterium* is an important element in monitoring new multi drug-resistant strains derived from saprophytic flora, mostly in infections in patients from risk groups, under immunosuppression, hospitalized for long time. Studying mechanisms of drug resistance on the basis of phenotypic and genotypic expression is important for proper antibiotic therapies in infections caused by this group of microorganisms.

Studies on sensitivity to antibiotics of different multidrug-resistant species of the genus *Corynebacterium* indicate that the highest efficacy in treatment of infections is shown by glycopeptides, linezolid, daptomycin, tigecyclin and chinupristin/dalphopristin.

6. References

Adderson, E. E., Boudreaux, J. W. & Hayden, R. T. (2008). Infections caused by coryneform bacteria in pediatric oncology patients. *Pediatr Infect*. 27 (2): 136-141.

Amao, H., Moriguchi, N., Komukai, Y., Kawasami, H., Takahashi, S. & Sawada, T. (2008). Detection of *Corynebacterium kutscheri* in the feaces of subclinically infectied mice. *Lab Anim*. 42 (3): 376-382.

Appelbaum, P. C. (2002). Resistance among *Streptococcus pneumoniae*: Implications for drug selection. *Clin Infect Dis*. 34 (12): 1613-20.

Arthur, M., Nolinas, C., Mabilat, C. & Courvalin, P. (1990). Detection of erythromycin resistance by the Polymerase Chain Reaction using primers in conserved refion of *erm* rRNA methylase genes. *Antimicrob Agents Chemother*. 34 (10): 2024-26.

Baird, G. J., and Fontanie, M. C. (2007). *Corynebacterium pseudotuberculosis* and its role in ovine caseous lymphadenitis. *J Comp Pathol*. 137 (4): 179-210.

Balci, I., Esik, F., & Bayram, A. (2002). Coryneform bacteria isolated from blond cultures and their antibiotic susceptibilities. *J Intern Med Res*. 30 (4): 422-7.

Barnass, S., Holland, K. & Tabaqchali, S. K. (1991). Vancomycin-resistant *Corynebacterium species* causing prosthetic valve endocarditis successfully treated with imipenem and ciprofloxacin. *J Infect*. 22(2): 161-9.

Campanile, F., Carretto, E., Barbarini, D., Grigis, A., Falcone, M., Goglio, A., Venditti, M. & Stefani, S. E. (2009). Clonal multidrug - resistant *Corynebacterium striatum* strains, Italy. *Emerg Infect Dis*. 15(1): 75-78.

Chiner, E., Arriero, J. M., Signes-Costa, J., Marco, J., Corral, J., Gomez-Esparrago, A., Ortiz de la Tabla, V. & Martin, C. (1999). *Corynebacterium pseudodiphtheriticum* pneumonia in an immunocompetent patient. *Monaldi Arch Chest Dis*. 54 (4): 325-327.

Clinical and Laboratory Standards Institute. (2006). Method for antimicrobial dilution and disk susceptibility testing of infrequently isolated or fastidious bacteria. Approved standard M45-A. Wayne, PA. Clinical and Laboratory Standards Institute.

Collins, M. D., Hoyles, L., Lawson, P. A., Falsen, E., Robson, R. L. & Foster, G. (1999). Phenotypic and phylogenetic characterization of a new *Corynebacterium* species from dogs: description of *Corynebacterium auriscanis* sp.nov. *J Clin Microbiol*. 37(11): 3443-7.

Coyle, M. B., Minshew, B. H., Bland, J. A. & Hsu, P. C. (1979). Erythromycin and clindamycin resistance in *Corynebacterium diphtheriae* from skin lesion. *Antimicrob Agents Chemother*. 16 (4): 525-7.

Dalal, A., Urban, C. & Segal-Maurer, S. (2008). Endocarditis due *Corynebacterium amycolatum*. *J Med Microbiol*. 57 (10): 1299-1302.

Deb, J. K., and Nath, N. (1999). Plasmids of corynebacteria. *FEMS Microbiology Letters*. 175 (1): 11-20.

Dorella, F. A., Pacheco, L. G., Oliveira, S. C., Miyoshi, A. & Azevedo, V. (2006). *Corynebacterium pseudotuberculosis*: microbiology, biochemical properties, pathogenesis and molecular studies of virulence. *Vet Res*. 37 (2): 201-18.

Douthwaite, S., and Champney, W. S. (2001). Structures of ketolides and macrolides determine their mode of interaction with the ribosomal target site. *J Antimicrob Chemother.* 48 (Suppl T1): 1–8.

Dupon, C., Turner, L., Rouveix, E., Nicolas, M. H. & Dorra, M. (1995). Endocardite à *Corynebacterium diphtheriae* tolerant à l'amoxicillin. *Presse Med.* 24 (24): 1135.

Eguchi, H., Kuwahara, T., Miyamoto, T., Nakayama-Imaohji, H., Ichimura, M., Hayashi, T. & Shiota, H. (2008). High-level fluoroquinolone resistance in ophthalmic clinical isolates belonging to the species *Corynebacterium macginleyi. J Clin Microbiol.* 46 (2): 527-32.

Freeman, J. D., Smith, H. J., Haines, H. G. & Hellyar, A. G. (1994). Seven patients with respiratory infection due to *Corynebacterium pseudodiphtheriticum. Pathology.* 26 (3): 311-4.

Fernandez-Roblas, R., Adames, H., Martin-de-Hijas, N. Z., Garcia Almeida, D., Gadea, I. & Esteban, J. (2009). In vitro activity of tigecycline and 10 other antimicrobials against clinical isolates of the genus *Corynebacterium. Int J Antimicrob Agents.* 33 (5): 353-5.

Funke, G., Efstratiou, A., Kiklinska, D., Hutson, R., De Zoysa, A., Engler, K. H. & Collins, M. D. (1997a). *Corynebacterium imitans* sp.nov. isolated from patients with suspected diphtheria. *J Clin Microbiol.* 35 (8): 1978-83.

Funke, G., Englert, R., Frodl, R., Bernard, K. A. & Stenqer S. (2010). *Corynebacterium canis* sp. nov., isolated from a wound infection caused by a dog bite. *Int J Syst Evol Microbiol.* 60 (11): 2544-7.

Funke, G., Punter, V. & von Graevenitz, A. (1996). Antimicrobial susceptibility patterns of some recently established coryneform bacteria. *Antimicrob Agents Chemother.* 40 (12): 2874-8.

Funke, G., von Graevenitz, A., Clarridge III, J. E. & Bernard, K. A. (1997b). Clinical Microbiology of coryneform bacteria. *Clin Micrbiol Rev.*10 (1): 125-159.

Garcia-Bravo, M., Aguado, J. M., Morale, J. M. & Norwega, A. R. (1996). Influence of external factors in resistance of *Corynebacterium urealyticum* to antimicrobial agents. *Antimicrob. Agents Chemother.* 40 (2): 497-499

Gomes, D. L, Martins, C. A, Faria, L. M, Santos, L. S, Santos, C. S, Sabbadini, P. S, Souza, M. C, Alves, G. B, Rosa, A. C, Nagao, P. E, Pereira, G. A, Hirata, R. Jr, & Mattos-Guaraldi, A. L. (2009). *Corynebacterium diphtheriae* as an emerging pathogen in nephrostomy catheter-related infection: evaluation of traits associated with bacterial virulence. *J Med Microbiol.* 58 (11): 1419-27.

Gomez-Garces, J-L., Alos, J-I. & Tamayo, J. (2007). *In vitro* activity of linezolid and 12 other antimicrobials against coryneform bacteria, *Int J Antimicro Agents.* 29 (6): 688-692.

Hall, R. M., Collis, C. M., Kim, M. J., Partridge, S. R., Recchia, G. D. & Stokes, H. W. (1999). Mobile gene cassettes and integrons in evolution. *Ann N Y Acad Sci.* 18 (870): 68-80.

Hodgson, A.L., Krywult, J. & Radford, A. J. (1990). Nucleotide sequence of the erythromycin resistance gene from the *Corynebacterium* plasmid pNG2. *Nucleic Acods Res.* 18 (7): 1891.

Ifantidou, A. M, Diamantidis, M. D, Tseliki, G., Angelou, A. S., Christidou, P., Papa, A. & Pentilas, D. (2010). *Corynebacterium jeikeium* bacteremia in a hemodialyzed patient. *Int J Infect Dis.* 14 (3): 265-8.

Johnson, A. P., Mushtaq, S., Warner, M. & Livermore, D. M. (2004).Activity of daptomycin against multi-resistant Gram-positive bacteria including enterococci and *Staphylococcus aureus* resistant to linezolid. *Int J Antimicrob Agents.* 24 (4): 315-319.

Katsumata, R., Ozaki, A., Oka, T. & Furuya, A. (1984). Protoplast transformation of glutamate-producting bacteria with plazmid DNA. *J Bacteriol.* 159 (1): 306-311.

Kono, M., Sasatsu, M. & Aoki, T. (1983). R plasmids in *Corynebacterium xerosis* strains. *Antimicrob Agents Chemother.* 23 (3): 506-508.

Lagrou, J., Verhaegen, M., Janssens, G., Wauters, G. & Verbist, L. (1998). Prospective study of catalase-positive coryneform organisms in clinical specimens: identification, clinical relevance, and antibiotic susceptibility. *Diagn Microbiol Infect Dis.* 30 (1): 7-15.

Leclercq, R. (2002). Mechanisms of resistance to macrolides and lincosamides: nature of the resistance elements and their clinical implications. *Clin Infect Dis.* 34 (4): 482–92.

López-Medrano, F., García-Bravo, M., Morales, J. M., Andrés, A., San Juan, R., Lizasoain, M. & Aguado, J. M. (2008). Urinary tract infection due to *Corynebacterium urealyticum* in kidney transplant recipients: an underdiagnosed etiology for obstructive uropathy and graft dysfunction-results of a prospective cohort study. *Clin Infect Dis.* 46 (6): 825-30.

Luna, V.A., Coates, P., Eady, A., Cove, J. H., Nguyen, T. T. H. & Roberts, M. C. (1999). A variety of Gram-positive bacteria carry mobile mef genes. *J Antimicrob Chemother.* 44 (1): 19-25.

Łętowska, I. and Olender, A. (2010). Rekomendacje doboru testów do oznaczania wrażliwości bakterii na antybiotyki i chemioterapeutyki 2010. Oznaczanie wrażliwości pałeczek Gram-dodatnich z rodzaju *Corynebacterium* spp. Krajowy Ośrodek ds. Lekowrażliwości KORLD. www.korld.edu.pl

Martinez-Martinez, L., Suarez, A. I., Winstanley, J., Ortega, M. C. & Bernard, K. (1995). Phenotypic characteristics of 31 strains of *Corynebacterium striatum* isolated from clinical sample. *J Clin Microbiol.* 33 (9): 2458-2461.

Nieto, N. C, Foley, J. E, MacLachlan, N. J, Yuan, T. & Spier, S. J. (2009). Evaluation of hepatic disease in mice following intradermal inoculation with *Corynebacterium pseudotuberculosis. Am J Vet Res.* 70 (2): 257-62.

Ojo, K. K., Striplin, M. J., Ulep, C. C., Close, N. S., Zittle, J., Luis, H., Bernardo, M., Leitao, J. & Roberts, M. C. (2006). *Staphylococcus* efflux *msr*(A) gene characterized in *Streptococcus, Enterococcus, Corynebacterium,* and *Pseudomonas* isolates. *Antimicrob Agents Chemother.* 50 (3): 1089-1091.

Olender, A. and Niemcewicz, M. (2010). Macrolide, lincosamide, and streptogramin B-constitutive tract resistance in *Corynebacterium pseudodiphtheriticum* isolated from upper respiratory tract specimens. *Microb Drug Resist.* 16 (2): 119-22.

Otsuka, Y., Kawamura, Y., Koyama, T., Iihara, H., Ohkusu, K. & Azeki, T. (2005). *Corynebacterium resistens* sp.nov., a new multi-resistant coryneform bacterium isolated from human infection. *J Clin Microbiol.* 43 (8): 3713- 17.

Otsuka, Y., Ohkusu, K.,Kawamura, Y., Baba, S., Azeki, T. & Kiura, S. (2006). Emergence of multidrug-resistant *Corynebacterium striatum* as a nosocomial pathogen in long-term hospitalized patients with underlying diseases. *Diagn Microbiol Infect Dis.* 54 (2): 109-14.

Perrin-Guyomard, A., Soumet, C., Leclercq, R., Doucet-Populair, R. & Sanders, P. (2005). Antibiotic susceptibility of bacteria isolated from pasteurized milk and characterization of macrolide-lincosamide-streptogramin resistance genes. *J Food Prot.* 68 (2): 347-352.

Pitcher, D., Johnson, A., Allerberger, F., Woodford, N. & George, R. (1990). An investigation of nosocomial infection with *Corynebacterium jeikeium* in surgical patients using a ribosomal RNA gene probe. *Eur J Clin Microbiol Infect Dis.* 9 (9): 643-648.

Power, E. G., Abdullah, Y. H., Talsania, H. G., Spice, W., Aathithan, S. & French, G. L. (1995) VanA genes in vancomycin-resistant clinical isolates of *Oerskovia turbata* and *Arcanobacterium (Corynebacterium) haemolyticum. J Antimicrob Chemother.* 36 (4): 595-606.

Riegel, P., Ruimy, R., Renard, F. N. R., Freney, J., Prevost, G., Jehl, F., Christen, R. & Monteil, H. (1997). *Corynebacterium singulare* sp. nov., new species for urease-positive strains related to *Corynebacterium minutissimum. Int J Syst Bacteriol.* 36 (4): 1092-1096.

Roberts, M. C., Leonard, R. B., Briselden, A., Schoenknecht, F. D., & Coyle, M. B. (1992). Characterization of antibiotic-resistant *Corynebacterium striatum* strains. *J Antimicrob Chemother.* 30 (4): 463-474.

Roberts, M. C., Sutcliffe, J., Courvalin, P., Jensen, L. B., Rood, J. & Seppala, H. (1999). Nomenclature for macrolide and macrolide-lincosamide-streptogramin B resitance determinants. *Antimicrob Agents Chemother.* 43 (12): 2823-30.

Rosato, A. E., Lee, B. S. & Nash, K. A. (2001). Inducible macrolide resistance in *Corunebacterium jeikeium. Antimicrob Agents Chemother.* 45 (7): 1982-89.

Ross, J. I., Eady, A. A., Carnegle, E. & Cove, J. H. (2002). Detection of transposon Tn5432 - mediated macrolide- lincosamide-streptogramin B (MLSB) resistance in cutaneus propionibacterie from six European cities. *J Antimicrob Chemiother.* 49 (1): 165-168.

Serwold-Davis, T. M. and Groman, N. B. (1986). Mapping and cloning of *Corynebacterium diphtheriae* plasmid pNG2 and characterization of ist relatedness to plasmids from skin corynefrms. *Antimicrob Agents Chemother.* 30 (1): 69-72.

Serwold-Davis, T. M., Groman, N. B. & Kao, C. C. (1990). Localization of an orgin of replication in *Corynebacterium diphtheriae* broad host range plasmid pNG2 that also functions in Escherichia coli. *FEMS Microbiol Lett.* 54 (1-3): 119-23.

Serwold-Davis, T. M., Groman, N. & Rabin M. (1987). Transformaction of *Corynebacterium diphtheriae, Corynebacterium ulcerans, Corynebacterium glutamicum* and *Escherichia coli* with the *C.diphtheriae* plasmid pNG2. *Poc Natl Acad Sci USA.* 84 (14): 4964-68.

Shah, M. and Murillo, J. L. (2005). Successful treatment of *Corynebacterium striatum* endocarditis with daptomycin plus rifampin. *Ann Pharmacother.* 39 (10): 1741-4.

Sierra, J. M., Martinez-Martinez, L., Vazquez, F., Giralt, E. & Vila, J. (2005). Relationship between mutations in the *gyr*A gene and quinolone resistance in clinical isolates of *Corynebacterium striatum* and *Corynebacterium amycolatum, Antimicrob Agents Chemother.* 49 (5): 1714-9.

Suzuki, E., Mochida, K. & Nakagawa, M. (1988). Naturally occurring subclinical *Corynebacterium kutscheri* infection in laboratory rats: strain and age related antibody response. *Lab Anim Sci.* 38 (1): 42-5.

Takahashi, T., Tsuji, M., Kikuchi, N., Ishihara, C., Osanai, T., Kasai, N., Yanagawa, R. & Hiramune, T. (1995). Assignment of the bacterial agent of urinary calculus in young rats by the comparative sequence analysis of the 16s rRNA genes corynebacteria. *J Vet Sci.* 57 (3): 515-7.

Tauch, A., Kassing, F., Kalinowski, J. & Pühler, A. (1995). The *Corynebacterium xerosis* composite transposon Tn*5432* consists of two identical insertion sequences, designated IS*1249*, flanking the erythromycin resistance gene ermcx. *Plasmid.* 34 (2): 119-31.

Tauch, A., Kassing, F., Kalinowski, J. & Pühler, A. (1995). The erythromycin resistance gene of the *Corynebacterium xerosis* R-plasmid pTP10 also carrying chloramphenicol, kanamycin and tetracycline resistance is capable of transposition in *Corynebacterium glutamicum. Plasmid.* 33 (3): 168-79.

Tauch, A., Krieft, S., Kalinowski, J. & Pühler, A. (2000). The 51,409-bp R-plasmid pTP10 from the multiresistant clinical isolate *Corynebacterium striatum* M82B is composed of DNA segments initially identified in soil bacteria and in plant, animal, and human pathogens. *Mol Gen Genet.* 263 (1): 1-11.

Tauch, A., Krieft, S., Pühler, A. & Kalinowski, J. (1999). The *tetAB* of the *Corynebacterium striatum* R-lasmid pTP10 encode an ABC transporter and confer tetracycline, oxytetracycline and oxacillin resistance in *Corynebacterium glutamicum. FEMS Microbiol Lett.* 173 (1): 203-9.

Tauch, A., Zheng, Z., Pühler, A. & Kalinowski, J. (1998). *Corynebacterium striatum* chloramphenicol resistance transposon Tn5564: genetic organization and transposition in *Corynebacterium glutamicum. Plasmid.* 40 (2): 126-39.

Troxler, R., Funke, G., von Graevenitz, A. & Stock, I. (2001). Natural antibiotic susceptibility of recently established coryneform bacteria, *Eur J Clin Microbiol Infect Dis.* 20 (5): 315-23.

Wagner, K. S, White, J. M, Neal, S., Crowcroft, N. S, Kuprevičiene, N., Paberza, R., Lucenko, I., Jõks, U., Akbaş, E., Alexandrou-Athanassoulis, H., Detcheva, A., Vuopio, J., von Hunolstein, C., Murphy, P. G., Andrews, N., Members of the Diphtheria Surveillance Network & Efstratiou, A. (2011). Screening for *Corynebacterium diphtheriae* and *Corynebacterium ulcerans* in patients with upper respiratory tract infections 2007-2008: a multicentre European study. *Clin Microbiol Infect.* 17 (4): 519-25.

Weiss, K., Laverdiere, M. & Rivest, R. (1996). Comparison of antimicrobial susceptibilities of *Corynebacterium* species by broth microdilution and disc diffusion methods. *Antimicrob Agents Chemother.* 40 (4): 930-3.

Wendisch, V. F., Bott, M., Kalinowski, J., Oldiges, M. & Wiechert, W. (2006). Emerging *Corynebacterium glutamicum* systems biology, *J Biotechnol.* 124 (1): 74-92.

Williams, D. Y., Selepak, S. T., Gill, V. J. (1993). Identification of clinical isolates of nondiphterial *Corynebacterium* species and their antibiotic susceptibility patterns. *Diagn Microbiol Infect Dis.* 17 (1): 23-8.

Wilson, A. P. R. (1995). Treatment of infections caused by toxigenic and non-toxigenic strains of *Corynebacterium diphtheriae. J Antimicrob Chemother.* 35 (6): 717-20.

Valbuena, N., Letek, M., Ordonez, E., Atala, J., Daniel, R. A., Gil, J. A. & Mateos, L. M. (2007). Characterization of HMW-PBPs from the rod-shaped actinomecete *Corynebacterium glutamicum*: peptydoglycan synthesis in cells lacking actin-like cytoskeletal structures. *Mol Microbiol.* 66 (3): 643-57.

Vertes, A. A., Inui, M. & Yukawa, H. (2005). Manipulating Corynebacteria, from individual genes to chromosomes. *Appl Environ Microbiol.* 71 (12): 7633-42.

Von Hunolstein, C., Scopetti, F., Efstratiou, A. & Engler, K. (2002). Penicillin tolerance amongst non-toxigenic *Corynebacterium diphtheriae* isolated from cases of pharyngitis. *J. Antimicrob Chemother.* 50 (1): 125-8.

Yague Guirao, G., Mora Peris, B., Martinez-Toldos, M. C., Rodriguez Gonzalez, T., Valero Guillen, P.L. & Segovia Hernandez, M. (2005). Implication of *erm*X genes in macrolide- and telithromycin-resistance in *Corynebacterium jeikeium* and *Corynebacterium amycolatum. Rev Esp Quimioterap.* 18 (3): 136-242.

Yassin, A. F. and Siering, C. (2008). *Corynebacterium sputi* sp. nov., isolated from the sputum of the a patient with pneumonia. *Int J Syst Evol Microbiol.* 58 (12): 2876-9.

Yoon, S., Kim, H., Lee, Y. & Kim, S. (2011). Bacteremia caused by Corynebacterium amycolatum with a novel mutation in gyrA gene that confers high-level quinolone resistance. *Korean J Lab Med.* 31(1): 47-8.

16

The MarR Family of Transcriptional Regulators – A Structural Perspective

Thirumananseri Kumarevel
Biometal Science Laboratory, RIKEN Spring-8 Center, Harima Institute, Japan

1. Introduction

All living organisms have molecular systems that enable them to resist a variety of toxic substances and environmental stresses. Proteins belonging to the **M**ultiple **a**ntibiotic **r**esistance **R**egulators (MarR) family reportedly regulate the expression of proteins conferring resistance to multiple antibiotics, organic solvents, household disinfectants, oxidative stress agents and pathogenic factors (Alekshun & Levy, 1999a; Miller & Sulavik, 1996; Aravind et al., 2005). The *marR* gene was initially identified as a component of the negative regulator encoded by the *marRAB* locus in *Escherichia coli* (George & Levy, 1983a, b). Currently, a large number of MarR-like proteins (~12,000) can be found in bacterial and archaeal domains, and the physiological role of around 100 of them have been characterized. Members of the MarR family of transcriptional regulatory proteins form a homodimer to bind to their cognate double-stranded DNA (dsDNA). The protein-DNA interactions is regulated by specific phenolic (lipophilic) compounds, such as salicylate, ethidium, carbonyl cyanide m-chlorophenylhydrazone (CCCP) and benzoate. The MarR homologues contain a winged helix-turn-helix (wHtH) motif at the DNA binding site, and this motif is well known for DNA binding in eukaryotes, prokaryotes, archaea and viruses. In this chapter, we will discuss the identification, three-dimensional structure and interactions with ligand (drug)/DNA of MarR family proteins.

2. Identification and characterization of MarR family proteins

The MarR family of transcriptional regulators was first identified in multidrug resistant strains of *E. coli* K-12 (George & Levy, 1983a, b). This MarR protein plays a key role in regulating the multiple antibiotic resistance (*marRAB*) regulon, which is responsible for the mar phenotype manifesting as resistance to a variety of structurally and medicinally important antibiotics, including sodium salicylate, tetracycline, chloramphenicol, penicillins, β-lactams, puromycin, fluoroquinolones and organic solvents (Cohen et al., 1993a). The *marA* gene encodes a transcriptional regulatory protein MarA, which is a member of the AraC protein family. As an activator of the *marRAB* operon, MarA induces the expression of over 60 genes responsible for the mar phenotype, including the AcrAB-TolC multidrug efflux system (Alekshun & Levy, 1997; Okusu et al, 1996). The *in vivo* upregulation of *marRAB* expression and the mar phenotype have been experimentally shown to be activated by a wide range of antibiotics and phenolic compounds, such as 2,4-dinitrophenol, menadione, plumbagin and salicylate (Cohen etal., 1993b; Seoane & Levy, 1995).

Similar to MarR, MexR negatively regulates an operon in *Pseudomonas aeruginosa* that, when expressed, encodes a tri-partite multidrug efflux system that results in increased resistance to multiple antibiotics, including tetracycline, β-lactams, chloramphenicol, novobiocin, sulfonamides and fluoroquinolones (Li & Poole, 1999; Srikumar et al., 2000). Analysis of the open reading frame of *mepA* reveals that the gene is part of the *mepRAB* three gene cluster, which encodes MepR, a MarR family member. MepR binds to compounds like ethidium, DAPI and rhodamine 6G. Some members of the MarR family of DNA-binding proteins, such as hypothetical uricase regulator (HucR) and organic hydroperoxide resistance regulator (OhrR), mediate a cellular response to reactive oxidative stress (ROS) (Wilkinson & Grove, 2004; 2005). The *Deinococcus radiodurans* HucR was shown to repress its own expression as well as that of a uricase. This repression is alleviated both *in vivo* and *in vitro* upon binding uric acid, the substrate for uricase. As uric acid is a potent scavenger of reactive oxygen species, and *D. radiodurans* is known for its remarkable resistance to DNA-damaging agents, these observations indicate a novel oxidative stress response mechanism (Hooper et al., 1998; Kean et al., 2000; Ames et al., 1981). Similar to HucR, the OhrR protein of *Bacillus subtilis* also mediates a response to oxidative stress; however, for OhrR, it is oxidation of a lone cysteine residue by organic hydroperoxides that abrogates DNA binding (Fuangthong et al., 2001; Fuangthong & Helmann, 2002).

2.1 Crystal structure of MarR homologues

Recently, much structural information have become available for MarR homologues. The MarR proteins exist as homodimers in solution, and as mentioned above each monomer consists of a wHtH DNA binding motif. We have recently solved one of the MarR regulators, ST1710 in the absence (apo)/presence (complex) of salicylate and in the presence of the putative DNA promoter. The overall structure of ST1710 indicates that it belongs to the α/β family of proteins and resembles those of the MarR family of proteins. It consists of six α-helices and two β-strands, arranged in the order of α1-α2-α3-α4-β1-β2-α5-α6 in the primary structure. The asymmetric subunit contains one molecule of ST1710. Two monomers of ST1710 are related by a crystallographic 2-fold symmetry to form the dimer, and this is consistent with our gel-filtration analysis (Kumarevel et al., 2008) as well as with other MarR family proteins (Alekshun et al., 2001; Lim et al., 2002; Liu et al., 2001; Wu et al., 2003; Hong et al., 2005) (Fig. 1). The N- and C-terminal residues located at the helices of each monomer are closely intertwined and form a dimerization domain, which is stabilized by hydrophobic and hydrogen bonding interactions between the residues located within these regions. Apart from the dimerization domain, as observed in many DNA binding transcriptional regulators, the residues located within the α2-α3-α4-β1-β2 structure form the wHtH DNA binding motif (Alekshun et al., 2001; Hong et al., 2005; Bordelon et al., 2006; Newberry et al., 2007; Saridakis, et al., 2008). The residues involved in dimerization play a key role in maintaining the distance between the DNA recognition helices in the wHtH loops, which can ultimately affect the fidelity and strength of the protein-DNA interactions. Mutagenesis of the residues involved in the dimeric interface has been shown to cause low DNA binding affinity (Andresen et al., 2010). Furthermore, C-terminal deletion in MarR homologs decreases the ability to form dimers, which correlates with the attenuated DNA binding affinity and increased phenotypic resistance in *E. coli* (Linde et al., 2000).

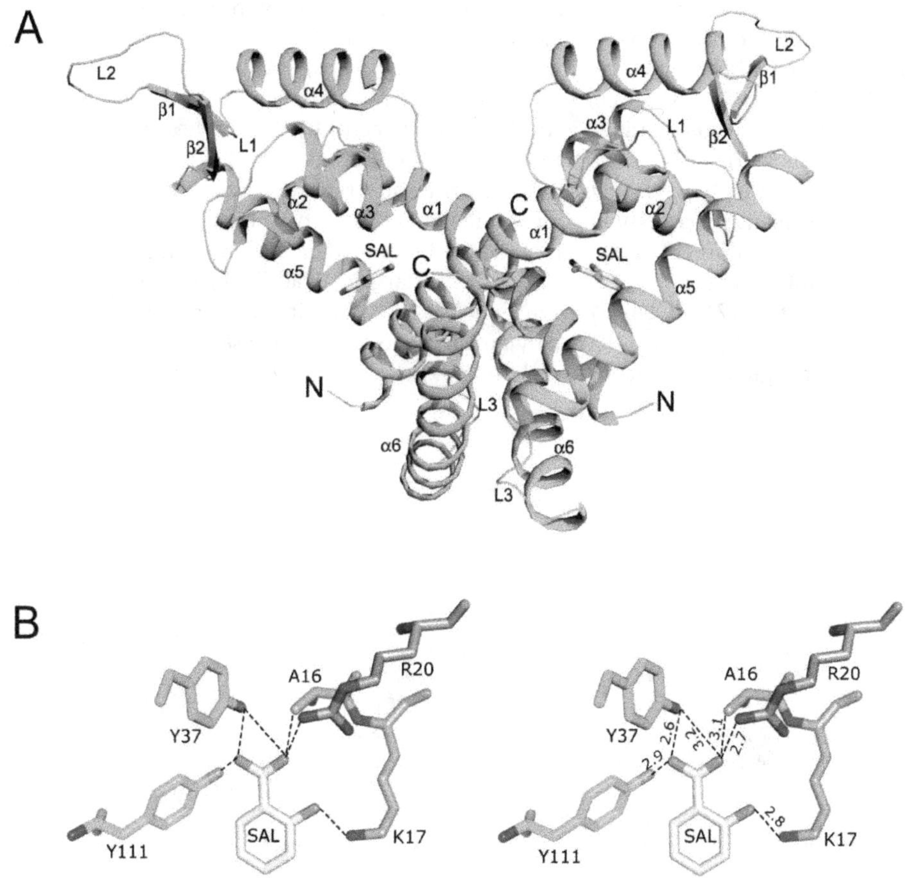

Fig. 1. Crystal structure of ST1710, a member of MarR family proteins. (A) A ribbon diagram of ST1710-salicylate complex dimer is shown. The secondary structure assignments and the N- /C-termini are labeled on the structure. (B) Close-up stereo view of salicylate binding site interactions with protein residues is shown. The hydrogen bonds are indicated by broken lines.

2.2 Structural comparison of MarR homologues

In a search for proteins with structural similarity to ST1710 protein within the known structures available in the Protein Data Bank (www.pdb.org) using the Dali program (Holm and Sander, 1996), we have identified many other protein structures within the MarR superfamily with good Z-scores. The highest ranked among those proteins is a Syla-like protein from *Enterococcus faecalis* (pdb id, 1lj9, Z-score=17.7, sequence identity=22%), which has been shown to up-regulate the expression of molecular chaperones, acid-resistance proteins and cytolysin, as well as to down-regulate several biosynthetic enzymes (Wu et al., 2003). The second highest ranked protein is a hypothetical regulator from *P. aeruginosa* (pdb ids, 2fbh, 2nnn, 2fbi), and the third one is OhrR from *B. subtilis*, an organic hydroperoxide-resistance regulator that controls the expression of the organic hydroperoxide resistance (*ohr*) gene by binding to *ohrA* promoter elements (Hong et al., 2005). Many proteins (1jgs, 1s3j, 2a61, 2nyx, 2hr3, 1xma, 3f3x, 2eth, 3nqd, 3nrv, 3bpv, 3bpx, 3s2w, 3deu, 3q5f, 3fm5, 3oop, 3cdh, 3cjn, 3e6m, 3k0l, 3bro, 3eco, 3jw4, 3bj6, 3g3z, 1lnw, 3bja, 3qww, 3kp6, 3bdd, 1z91, 2pex, 2bv6, 3hrm, 1ub9) were identified with Z-scores between 10-16. All of these proteins adopt a similar topology (rmsd between 1 to 4 Å), despite the low (~15-25%) sequence identities between them, and these sequence dissimilarities are reflected throughout the secondary structural elements (Figs. 2, 3). In addition, the high flexibility of the DNA binding domains displayed in the different crystals provides indirect evidence of the ability of this wHtH motif to adapt in order to recognize various DNA targets. In addition, a sequence homology search against ST1710 (Q96ZY1 from *Sulfolobus tokodaii*) in the non-redundant protein database using fasta revealed that many archaeal species have conserved motifs resembling MarR family regulatory sequences, including *Sulfolobus acidocaldarius*, *Sulfolobus solfataricus*,

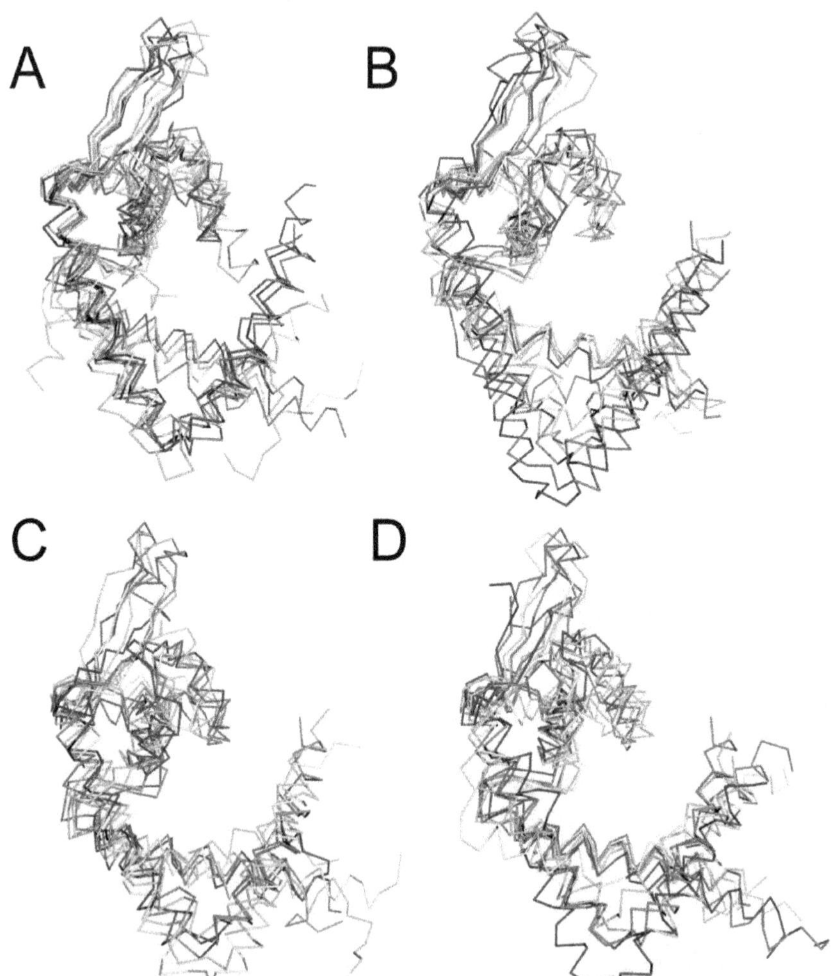

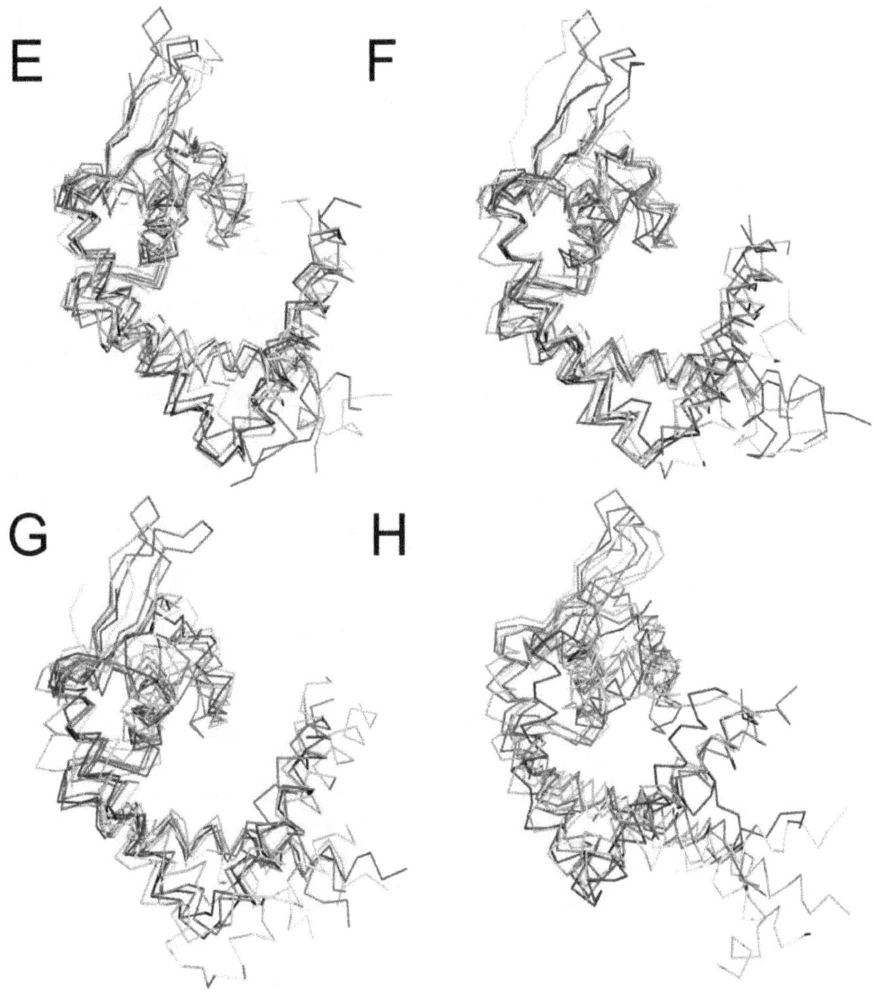

Fig. 2. Three-dimensional structural comparison of ST1710. Superposition of ST1710 with related MarR family proteins. (A) ST1710, 1JGS, 1LJ9, 1LNW, 1S3J, 1UB9 and 1XMA are colored in red, green, blue, yellow, majenta, cyan and orange, respectively. (B) ST1710, 1Z91, 2A61, 2BV6, 2ETH and 2FBH are colored in red, green blue, yellow, majenta and cyan, respectively. (C) ST1710, 2FBI, 2FNP, 2HR3, 2NNN and 2NYX are colored in red, green blue, yellow, majenta and cyan, respectively. (D) ST1710, 2PEX, 2QWW, 3BDD, 3BJ6 and 3BJA are colored in red, green blue, yellow, majenta and cyan, respectively. (E) ST1710, 3BPV, 3BPX, 3BRO, 3CDH and 3CJN are colored in red, green blue, yellow, majenta and cyan, respectively. (F) ST1710, 3DEU, 3E6M, 3ECO, 3F3X and 3FM5 are colored in red, green blue, yellow, majenta and cyan, respectively. (G) ST1710, 3G3Z, 3HRM, 3JW4, 3KOL and 3KP6 are colored in red, green blue, yellow, majenta and cyan, respectively. (H) ST1710, 3NQO, 3NRV, 3OOP, 3Q5F and 3S2W are colored in red, green blue, yellow, majenta and cyan, respectively.

A

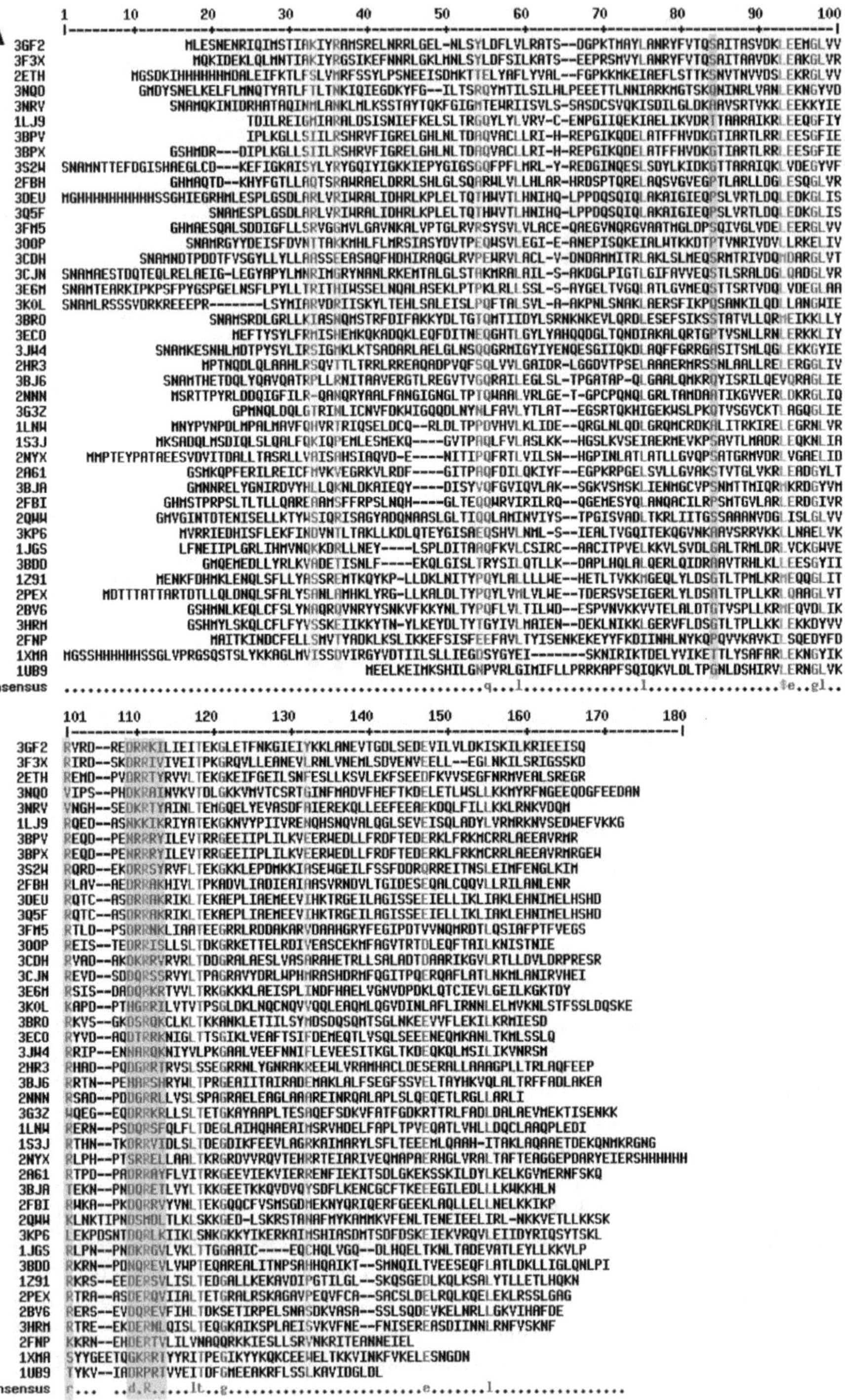
3GF2
3F3X
2ETH
3NQO
3NRV
1LJ9
3BPV
3BPX
3S2W
2FBH
3DEU
3Q5F
3FM5
3OOP
3CDH
3CJN
3E6M
3KOL
3BRO
3ECO
3JW4
2HR3
3BJ6
2NNN
3G3Z
1LNW
1S3J
2NYX
2A61
3BJA
2FBI
2QWW
3KP6
1JGS
3BDD
1Z91
2PEX
2BV6
3HRM
2FNP
1XMA
1UB9
Consensus

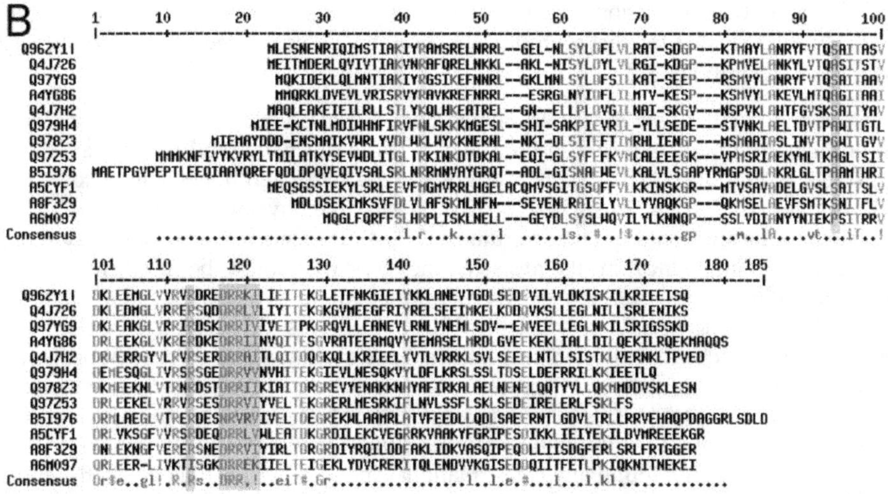

Fig. 3. Sequence alignment of ST1710 and its structurally and sequenctially related proteins from different species. (A) Structurally related proteins to ST1710, based on the Dali Zscore. (B) Sequentially related proteins from the non-reduntant sequence database. The highly redundant proteins are removed. The ligand and DNA binding residues are highlighted with yellow and green shades, respectively.

Metallosphaera sedula, Thermoplasma acidophilum, Thermoplasma volcanium, Streptomyces sviceus, Pelotomaculum thermopropionicum, Thermotoga lettingae, Clostridium beijerinckii and others. Among these, the amino acid sequence of ST1710 displays about 50% identity to the *S. acidocaldarius* (Chen et al., 2005) (17) and *S. solfataricus* (She et al., 2001) sequences, 41% identity to the M. sedula sequence (Copeland et al., 2006) and approximately 30-40% identity to others (Fig. 3).

2.1.1 Interactions between MarR homologues and ligands

MarR homologues are known to bind a variety of lipophilic compounds, including salicylate, ethidium and CCCP (Table 1). These bound molecules control interaction between protein-DNA molecules. Sodium salicylate is a well-known example of a compound that can inhibit MarR activity both *in vitro* and *in vivo* at millimolar concentrations (Alekshun and Levy, 1999b). Three different MarR proteins have been solved with the salicylate ligand, including ST1710 from *S. tokodaii*, MarR from *E. coli* and MTH313 from *Methanobacterium thermoautotrophicum*. Among these, ST1710 is the only MarR homologue solved in the apo form, complexed with salicylate ligand and complexed with a putative promoter DNA (Kumarevel et al., 2009). One salicylate ligand is identified and located at the interface between the helical dimerization and wHtH DNA-binding domains in ST1710 (Fig. 1A&B), and the bound salicylate ligand shows many interactions with the surrounding protein residues. In particular, the O2′ of salicylate is bonded to the side chain oxygens of Tyr37 and Tyr111. In addition, the side chain oxygen of Tyr37 is also bonded to the O1′ of the salicylate ligand molecule. The ligand oxygen O1′ is hydrogen bonded to the amino group (NH2) of residue Arg20, while the O2 of the ligand molecule is hydrogen bonded to the side chain nitrogen of

Lys17. The latter two interactions are from the symmetrically related molecule. Notably, all of the ST1710 residues that interact with the ligand are highly conserved among closely related species (>40% identity) (Fig. 3).

In contrast to ST1710, *E. coli* MarR was solved with two salicylate molecules per dimer, and both of them are highly exposed to the solvent. These salicylate binding sites are also not comparable to that of ST1710. The bound salicylate is hydrogen bonded with some of the MarR residues (Ala70, Thr72, Arg77, Arg86); however, the physiological relevance of either salicylate binding site could not be determined (Fig. 4). It seems that salicylate may stabilize the crystal packing, since in its absence, the crystals cannot be used for structure determination in the case of *E. coli* MarR (Alekshun et al., 2001). Analyses of another MarR homolog from *M. thermoautotrophicum* MTH313, which was also solved in the free (apo) form and complexed with salicylate, revealed a large asymmetrical conformational change that is mediated by the binding of sodium salicylate to two distinct locations in the dimer (Saridakis et al., 2008) (Fig. 4). The bound salicylate has two direct and one water mediated interactions with MTH313. Although the ligand binding sites in ST1710 and MTH313 are comparable, we have not found any conformational changes in ST1710 between the apo and ligand bound complexes, as observed in MTH313.

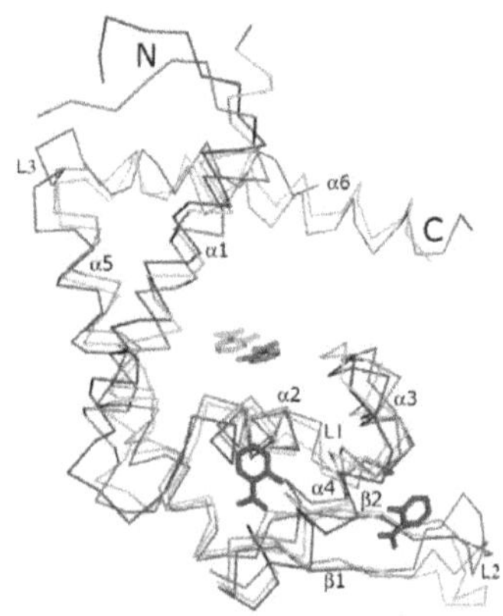

Fig. 4. Salicylate binding analysis in MarR homologues. Superposition of the ST1710-salicylate complex with other known MarR family of protein crystallized in the presence of salicylate. The ST1710, *E. coli* MarR and *M. thermoautotrophicum* MTH313 are shown in green, blue and red, respectively.

Meanwhile, eight salicylate molecules are bound to *Staphylococcus epidermidis* of TcaR (Chang et al., 2010). Among these eight molecules, two are bound similarly to that with MTH313, while the other two were observed in the more shallow binding pocket in each monomer. The remaining ligands are highly exposed to the solvent. TcaR has also been crystallized with four different antibiotics (ampicillin, kanamycin, methicillin and penicillin), revealing their interactions with the protein (Chang et al., 2010). The available biochemical and biophysical results suggest that the MarR regulators modulate the DNA binding affinity in the presence of ligands or drug molecules. However, more ligand bound complexes are required to generalize the binding pocket properties as well as to understand how these MarR regulators allosterically change their conformation in the presence of vaious drugs/ligands to mediate the protein-DNA interactions.

Protein	Organism	Footprint (DNA)	K_d (nM)	Ligand	K_d	Reference
ST1710	*Sulfolobus tokodaii*	30	200 ~ 1500	Salicylate, Ethidium Bromide, CCCP	~2-25 μM	Kumarevel et al., 2008 & 2009 Yu et al., 2009
MepR	*Staphylococcus aureus*	27,44	6.3	Ethidium, DAPI, Rhodamine 6G	~3-63 μM	Kumaraswami et al., 2009
MarR	*Escherichia coli*	21	1	Salicylate, Plumbagin, 2,4-dinitrophenol, menadione	0.5 – 1 mM	Martin & Rosner 1995; Cohen et al., 1993b; Seoane & levy, 1995; Alekshun & Levy 1999b; Alekshun et al, 2001
EmrR	*Escherichia coli*	42	-	Salicylate, Caronyl cyanide m-chlorophenylhydrozone, 2,4,-dinitrophenol, ethidium bromide	1.3 -11.1 μM	Xiong et al. 2000; Brooun et al., 1999
MexR	*Pseudomonos aeruginosa*	28	-	β-lactamin		Evans et al., 2001.
CbaR	*Comamonas testosteroni*	22	-	3-chlorobenzoate, protocatechuate		Providenti & Wyndham, 2001
CinR	*Butyrivibro fibrisolvens*	-	-	Cinnamic acid sugar esters		Dalrymple & Swadling, 1997
HpaR	*Escherichia coli*	27	-	4-hydroxyphenyl-acetic acid, 3-hydroxyphenyl acetic acid, 3,4-hydroxyphenyl acetic acid		Galan et al., 2003
ExpG	*Sinorhizobium meliloti*	21	0.58-1.3			Bartels et al, 2003; Baumgarth et al., 2005
PecS	*Erwinia chrysanthemi*	45	4-200			Reverchon et al., 2002; Rouanet et al., 2004
SlyA	*Salmonella typhimurium*	25	-			Stapleton et al., 2002
OhrR	*Xanthomonas campestris*	44	-	Tert-butyl hydroperoxide, cumene hydroperoxide		Mongkolsuk et al., 2002
OhrR	*Bacillus subtilis*	42	5	Tert-butyl hydroperoxide, cumene hydroperoxide		Fuangthong et al., 2001; Fuangthong & Helmann, 2002; Panamanee et al., 2002
HucR	*Deinococcus radiodurans*	21	0.29	Uric acid, Salicylate	11.6 μM	Wilkinson & Grove, 2004; 2005

Table 1. DNA and ligand binding data for MarR homologues.

2.1.1 Interactions between MarR proteins and DNA

It is well-known that members of the MarR family of regulatory proteins bind to their cognate double-stranded DNA by their winged HtH motif (Alekshun et al., 2001; Hong et al., 2005; Kumarevel et al., 2009). Footprinting analyses suggested that different MarR regulators recognize promoters of different lengths with different affinities (Table 1). In an earlier study, we have used the *OhrR* promoter sequence as a search model to identify the putative promoter DNA sequence for ST1710 from the *S. tokodaii* genomic sequence (Kumarevel et al., 1998). We have also shown the binding constant for DNA to be around 15 μM using gel mobility shift assays. Yu et al. (2009) subsequently showed by fluorescence spectroscopy that the affinity of the same DNA promoter we identified is increased significantly with increasing temperature. The affinity was shown to be approximately double from 10°C (K_d = 618 ± 34 nM) to 30°C (K_d = 334 ± 15 nM) and from 30°C to 50°C (K_d = 189 ± 9 nM). We later crystallized ST1710 along with two different DNA promoters (30-mer and 26-mer) and revealed the protein-DNA interactions and mode of binding as summarized below (Kumarevel et al., 2009).

The overall structure of the ST1710-DNA complex is shown in Fig. 5A & B. The bound DNA adopts a B-form right-handed structure, passing over the protein molecule by only contacting at the winged HtH loop regions. The wHtH domains recognize the promoter DNA (TAACAAT) (15-21) region, consistent with the -10 region of the OhrR-*ohrA* operator complex. The 4 and 3 bases at the 5′ and 3′-ends are highly disordered and hence not modeled. Of the bound 46 nucleotides, only 22 nucleotides were found to be involved in 36 contacts with six protein molecules. The critical protein-DNA contacts observed in this complex are as follows: Ser65 - Thy5′; Arg84 - G13′ and Ade17; Arg89 - Thy14′; Arg90 - Cyt18; Asp88 – Cyt18 (two salt bridge contacts); Lys91 - Ade19; Ile91 - Ade20. The observed salt bridge may be important in fixing the conformation of residue Arg90 in order to make contact with the nucleic acid base, Cyt18. Thus, the following residues Ser65, Arg84, Asp88, Arg89, Arg90, Lys91 and Ile92 interact with the bound promoter DNA. As further clarification of these protein-DNA interactions, our analysis of three mutant proteins (Arg89Ala, Arg90Ala, Lys91Ala) at the DNA binding loop region in gel mobility shift assays clearly support that these positively charged residues are important for DNA binding (Kumarevel et al., 2009). The DNA-binding residues in ST1710 are highly conserved among the closely related proteins Fig. (3). The winged loop region connecting the strands β1 and β2 apparently plays a major role in modulating their conformation for binding to the DNA molecule, and this mode of recognition is anticipated for the proteins closely related to ST1710 as well as those in the family of MarR regulators.

In our earlier report, we noticed only a small difference at the loop region connecting strands β1 and β2 in the protein conformers crystallized in two different space groups, but the overall structures are otherwise identical (Kumarevel et al., 2008). Similarly, we have not observe any conformational changes in comparisons of the ST1710-salicylate complex and native structure crystallized under the same conditions, and the subunits in the dimer are identical. In contrast to these observations, a significant conformational change has been observed between subunits (A, B chains) in the ST1710-DNA complex, although the overall structural topology remains identical. Specifically, the C-terminal helix and the winged HtH motif region show displacement relative to the other. The DNA binding motif is elevated

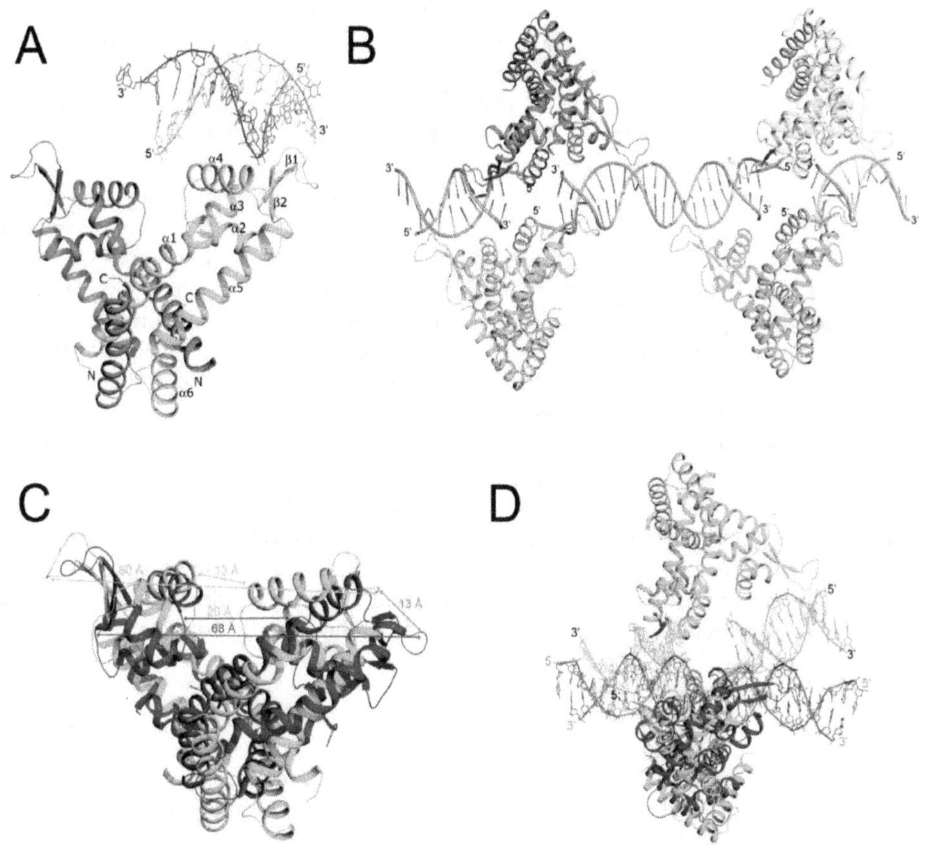

Fig. 5. Structure of ST1710-DNA complex and it's structural comparison with OhrR-*OhrA* complex. (A) ST1710-DNA complex observed in the aymmetric unit. The secondary structural assignments, N-/C- termini ends are labeled in one of the dimeric monomers. The complexed nucleic acids are shown as stick representations. (B) Part of the packing diagram. The 5′- and 3′- ends of each nucleotide chain is labeled. (C, D) Superposition of the OhrR-*OhrA* complex on the ST1710-DNA complex is shown without (A) and with nucleic acids (B). The protein and nucleic acids are shown in St1710-DNA complex are in cyan and green; while those in OhrR-*OhrA* complex are shown in blue and red, respectively.

compared to the other chain, while the C-terminal helix α6 is lower down. It is noteworthy to mention that the distances between the wHtH domains in the dimer are reduced by ~10 Å for the ST1710-DNA complex, compared to the native and salicylate complexes. These observed conformational changes are required in order to facilitate the DNA-binding and thus would explain the conformational flexibility of MarR homologues.

Another member of the MarR family of regulators that has been solved in complex with a promoter sequence is the *B. subtilis* OhrR. The OhrR was crystallized in the presence of a 29-mer duplex containing the -10 region of the cognate DNA. In the OhrR-*OhrA* complex, the wHtH motif contacts the DNA promoter sequence with substantial widening and deepening of the major groove that results from insertion of the recognition helix (α4) of the wHtH motif. The wHtH and recognition helices make many contacts with the DNA directly or mediated through water. The wHtH domain is important for the DNA interaction as evidenced by several mutagenic analyses, which show that the positively charged residues (Arg94) located at the terminals are important for the DNA contacts in *E. coli* MarR. In the OhrR-*ohrA* complex, the distance between wHtH loops is around 67 Å, and the distance between the recognition helices (α4) is about 20 Å, although the wings of the subunits are translocated about 16 Å compared to the structure of reduced OhrR (Hong et al., 2005) (Fig. 5C). In an attempt to clarify the binding mechanism of MarR regulators, a comparative analysis of our ST1710-DNA complex with the OhrR-*ohrA* complex (Fig. 5C & D) was performed, which revealed large conformational changes between these two complexes. Interestingly, we also observed unique conformational changes in the mode of DNA recognition. In contrast to the OhrR-*OhrA* complex, the bound promoter DNA passed over the wHTH motif without deepening the structure through the 2-fold axis in the ST1710-DNA complex. Despite their differences, it is interesting to note that the protein contacting residues are highly conserved between these two proteins and among the MarR family of regulators. This unexpected mode of DNA-binding in ST1710 is caused by one of the subunits translocated around 13 Å towards the 2-fold axis, reducing the distance between the recognition helix of the subunits to 13 Å. Thus, the mode of DNA binding observed in the OhrR-*ohrA* operator complex would be impossible for that of ST1710. Such unique conformational changes observed in these complexes explain how the MarR homolog regulators can modulate the DNA-binding affinity based on the cognate promoter or ligand molecules.

3. Conclusion

The MarR family of regulatory proteins in bacteria and archaea regulate a variety of biological functions, including those associated with the development of antibiotic resistance, a growing global health problem. Based on the existing crystal structures, it seems that members of the MarR family of proteins adopt similar topology, despite variations in sequence similarities among them. We have solved the crystal structure of ST1710 in three different forms (apo-form, ST1710-salicylate and ST1710-DNA complex) and demonstrated the functional importance of the ligand binding and DNA binding residues. The ligand or drug binding to the MarR regulators may regulate their promoter binding abilities as evidenced with MarR, ST1710 and MTH313. Furthermore, the promoter DNA is also recognized by the protein in a unique fashion as observed in OhrR-*OhrA* and ST1710-DNA complexes. Taken altogether, the current evidence describe the MarR regulators containing wHTH motifs as being prone to binding DNA through their positively charged residues located in their loops, and the mode of DNA binding depends on the subunit organization as observed in the MarR family of proteins (ST1710, OhrR). Through further structural and functional studies on MarR-DNA binding, we will be better poised to develop new drugs to specifically target those interactions that confer drug resistance to pathogenic organisms.

4. Acknowledgment

The author would like to thank Dr. T. Ishikawa for his moral support and encouragement.

5. References

Alekshun, M.M. & Levy, S.B. (1999a). Regulation of chromosomally mediated multiple antibiotic resistance: the mar regulon. *Antimicrob. Agents Chemother.* 41, 2067-2075.

Alekshun, M.N. & Levy, S.B. (1999b). Alteration of the repressor activity of MarR, the negative regulator of the *Escherichia coli marRAB* locus, by multiple chemicals *in vitro. J. Bacteriol.* 181, 4669-4672.

Alekshun, M.N.; Levy, S.B.; Mealy, T.R.; Seaton, B.A. & Head, J.F. (2001). The crystal structureof MarR, a regulator of multiple antibiotic resistance, at 2.3 Å resolution. *Natue Struct. Biol.* 8, 710-714.

Ames, B.N.; Cathcart, R.; Schwiers, E. & Hochstein, P. (1981). Uric acid provides an antioxidant defense in humans against oxidant- and radical-caused aging and cancer: a hypothesis. *Proc. Natl. Acad. Sci. USA* 78, 6858–6862.

Alekshun, M.N. & Levy, S.B. (1997). Regulation of chromosomally mediated multiple antibiotic resistance:the *mar* operons. *Antimicob Agents Chemother.* 41, 2067-2075.

Andresen, C.; Jalal, S.; Aili, D.; Wang, Y.; Islam, S.; Jarl, A.; Liedberg, B.; Wretlind, B.; Martensson, L.G. & Sunnerhagen, M. (2010). Critical biophyscial properties in the *Pseudomonas aeruginosa* efflux gene regulator MexR are targeted by mutations conferring multidrug resistance. *Protein Sci.* 19, 680-692.

Aravind, L.; Anantharaman, V.; Balaji, S.; Mohan Babu, M. & Iyer, L.M. (2005). The many faces of the helix-turn-helix domain: transcription regulation and beyond. *FEMS Microbiol. Rev.* 29, 231-262.

Bartels, F.W.; Baumgarth, B.; Anselmetti, D.; Ros, R. & Becker, A. (2003). Specific binding of the regulatory protein ExpG to promoter regions of the galactoglucan biosynthesis gene cluster of *Sinorhizobium meliloti* –a combined molecular biology and force spectroscopy investigation. *J. Struct. Biol.* 143, 145-152.

Baumgarth, B.; Bartels, F.W.; Anselmetti, D.; Becker, A. & Ros, R. (2005). Detailed studies of the binding mechanism of the *Sinorhizobium meliloti* transcriptional activator ExpG to DNA. *Microbiology* 151, 259-268.

Bordelon, T.; Wilkinson, S.P.; Grove, A. & Newcomer, M.E. (2006). The crystal structure of the transcriptional regulator HucR from *Deinococcus radiodurans* reveals a repressor preconfigured for DNA binding. *J. Mol. Biol.* 360, 168-177.

Brooun, A.; Tomashek, J.J. & Lewis, K. (1999). Purification and ligand binding of EmrR, a regulator of a multidrug transporter. *J. Bacteriol.* 181, 5131-5133.

Chang, Y.M.; Jeng, W.Y.; Ko, T.P.; Yeh, Y.J.; Chen, C.K. & Wang, A.H. (2010). Strutural study of TcaR and ist complexes with multiple antibiotics from *Staphylococcus epidermidis. Proc. Natl. Acad. Sci. USA.* 107, 8617-8622.

Chen, L.; Bruegger K.; Skovgaard, M.; Redder P.; She, Q.; Torarinsson, E.; Greve, B.; Awayez, M.; Zibat, A.; Klenk, H.P. & Garrett, R.A. (2005). The genome of *Sulfolobus acidocaldarius*, a model organism of the *Crenarchaeota. J. Bacteriol.* 187, 4992-4999.

Cohen, S.P.; Hachler, H. & Levy, S.B. (1993a). Genetic and functional analysis of the multiple antibiotic resistance (mar) locus in *Escherichia coli. J. Bacteriol.* 175, 1484-1492.

Cohen , S.P.; Levy, S.B.; Foulds, J. & Rosner, J.L. (1993b). Salicylate induction of antibiotic resistance in *Escherichia coli*: activation of the *mar* operon and a *mar* independent pathway. *J. Bacteriol.* 175, 7856-7862.

Copeland, A.; Lucas, S.; Lapidus, A.; Barry, K.; Glavina, del Rio, T.; Dalin, E.; Tice, H.; Bruce, D.; Pitluck, S. & Richardson, P. (2006). Sequencing of the draft genome and assembly of *Metallosphaera sedula* DSM 5348. Submitted (NOV-2006) to the EMBL/GenBank/DDBJ databases.

Dalrymple, B.P. & Swadling, Y. (1997). Expression of a *Butyrivibrio fibrisolvens* E14 gene (*cin*B) encoding an enzye with cinnamoyl ester hydrolase activity is negatively regulated by the product of an adjacent gene (*cin*R). *Microbiology* 143, 103-1210.

Evans, K.; Adewoye, L. & Poole, K. (2001). MexR repressor of the *mexAB-oprM* multidrug efflux operon of *Pseudomonas aeruginosa*: identification of MexR binding sites in the *mexA-mexR* intergenic region. *J. Bateriol.* 183, 807-812.

Fuangthong, M.; Atichartpongkul, S.; Mongkolsuk, S. & Helmann, J. D. (2001). OhrR is a repressor of *ohrA*, a key organic hydroperoxide resistance determinant in *Bacillus subtilis*. *J. Bacteriol.* 183, 4134-4141.

Fuangthong, M. & Helmann, J. D. (2002). The OhrR repressor senses organic hydroperoxide resistances by reversibile formation of a cycteine-sulfenic acid derivative. *Proc. Natl. Acad. Sci. USA* 99, 6690-6695.

Galan, B.; Kolb, A.; Sanz, J.M.; Garcia, J.L. & Prieto, M.A. (2003). Molecular determinants of the *hpa* regulatory system of *Escherichia coli*: the Hpa repressor. *Nucleic Acids Res.* 31, 6598-6609.

George, A.M. & Levy, S.B. (1983a). Amplifiable resistance to the tetracycline, chloramphenicol, and other antibiotics in *Escherichia coli*: Involvement of a nonplasmid -determined efflux of tetracycline. *J. Bacteriol.* 155, 531-540.

George, A.M. & Levy, S.B. (1983b). Gene in the major cotransduction gap of the *Escherichia coli* K-12 linkage map required for the expression of chromosomal resistance to tetracycline and other antibiotics. *J. Bacteriol.* 155, 541-548.

Holm, L. & Sander, C. (1996). A review of the use of protein structure comparison in protein classification and function identification. *Science* 273, 595-602.

Hong, M.; Fuangthong, M.; Helmann, J. D. & Brennan, R. G. (2005). Structure of an OhrR-ohrR operator complex reveals the DNA binding mechanism oft he MarR family. *Mol. Cell.* 20, 131-141.

Hooper, D.C.; Spitsin, S.; Kean, R.B.; Champion, J.M.; Dickson, G.M.; Chaudhry, I. & Koprowski, H. (1998). Uric acid, a natural scavenger of peroxynitrite, in experimental allergic encephalomyelitis and multiple sclerosis. *Proc. Natl Acad. Sci. USA* 95, 675–680.

Kean, R.B.; Spitsin, S.V.; Mikheeva, T.; Scott, G.S. & Hooper, D.C. (2000). The peroxynitrite scavenger uric acid prevents inflammatory cell invasion into the central nervous system in experimental allergic encephalomyelitis through maintenance of blood-central nervous system barrier integrity. *J. Immunol.* 165, 6511–6518.

Kumaraswami, M.; Schuman, J.T.; Seo, S. M.; Kaatz, G.W. & Brennan, R.G. (2009). Structural and biochemical characterization of MepR, a multidrug binding transcription regulator oft he *Staphylococcus aureus* multidrug efflux pump MepA. *Nucleic Acids Res.* 37, 1211-1224.

Kumarevel, T.S.; Tanaka, T.; Nishio, M.; Gopinath, S.C.B.; Takio, K.; Shinkai, A.; Kumar, P.K.R. & Yokoyama, S. (2008). Crystal structure oft he MarR family regulatory protein, ST1710, from *Sulfolobus tokodaii* strain 7. *J. Struct. Biol.* 16, 9-17.

Kumarevel, T.S.; Tanaka, T.; Umehara, T. & Yokoyama, S. (2009). ST1710-DNA complex crystal structure reveals the DNA binding mechanism oft he MarR family of regulators. Nucleic Acids Res. 37, 4723-47-35.

Li, X.Z. & Poole, K. (1999). Organic solvent tolerant mutants of *Pseudomonas aeruginosa* display multiple antibiotic resistance. *Can. J. Microbiol.* 45, 18-22.

Linde, H.J.; Notka, F.; Metz, F.; Kochanowski, B.; Heisig, P. & Lehn, N. (2000). In vivo increase in resistance to ciprofloxacin in *Escherichia coli* associated with deletion oft he C-terminal part of MarR. *Antimicrob.Agents Chemother.* 44, 1865-1868.

Yu, L.; Fang, J. & Wie, Y. (2009). Characterization oft he ligand and DNA binding properties of a putative archaeal regulators, ST1710. *Biochemistry* 48, 2099-2108.

Martin, R.G. & Rosner, J.L. (1995). Binding of purified multiple antibiotic-resistance repressor protein (MarR) to *mar* operator sequences. *Proc. Natl. Acad. Sci. USA.* 92, 5456-5460.

Miller, P.F. & Sulavik, M.C. (1996). Overlaps and parallels in the regulation of intrinsic multiple-antibiotic resistance in *Escherichia coli. Mol. Microbiol.* 21, 441-448.

Mongkolsuk, S.; Panmanee, W.; Atichartpongkul, S.; Vattanaviboon, P.; Whangsuk, W.; Fuangthong, M.; Eiamphungporn, W.; Sukchawalit, R. & Utamapongchai, S. (2002). The repressor for an organic peroxide-inducible operon is unlikely regulated at multiple levels. *Mol. Microbiol.* 44, 793-802.

Newberry, K.J.; Fuangthong, M.; Panmanee, W.; Mongkolsuk, S. & Brennan, R.G. (2007). Structural mechanism of organic hydroperoxide induction oft he transcription regulator OhrR. *Mol. Cell* 28, 652-664.

Okusu, H.; Ma, D. & Nikaido, H. (1996). AcrAB efflux pump plays a major role in the anibiotic resistance phenotype of *Escherichia coli* multiple antibiotic resistance(mar) mutants. *J. Bacterial.* 178, 306-308.

Panmanee, W.; Vattanaviboon, P.; Eiamphungporn, W.; Whangsuk, W.; Sallabhan, R. & Mongkolsuk, S. (2002). OhrR, a trancription repressor that senses and responds to changes in organic peroxide levels in *Xanthomonas campestris* pv. Phaseoli. *Mol. microbiol.* 45, 1647-1654.

Providenti, M.A. & Wyndham, R.C. (2001). Identification and functional chracterization of cbaR, a MarR-like modulator oft he *cbaABC*-encoded chlorobenzoate catabolism pathway. *Appl. Environ. Microbiol.* 67, 3530-3541.

Reverchon, S.; Rouanet, C.; Expert, D. & Nasser, W. (2002). Characterization of indigoidine biosynthetic genes in *Erwinia chrysanthemi* and role of this blue pigment in pathogenicity. *J. Bacteriol.* 184, 654-665.

Rouanet, C.; Reverchon, S.; Rodionov, D.A. & Nasser, W. (2004). Definition of a consensus DNA-binding site for PecS, a global regulator of virulence gene expression in *Erwinia chrysanthemi* and identification of new members oft he PecS regulon. *J. Biol. Chem.* 279, 30158-30167.

Saridakis, V.; Shahinas, D.; Xu, X. & Christendat, D. (2008). Structural insight on the mechanism of regulation oft he MarR family of proteins: high-resolution crystal structure of a transcriptional repressor from *Methanobacterium thermoautotrophicum. J. Mol. Biol.* 377, 655-667.

Seoane, A.S. & Levy, S.B. (1995). Characterization of MarR, the repressor oft he multiple antibiotic resistance (mar) operon in *Escherichia coli. J. Bacteriol.* 177, 3414-3419.

She, Q.; Singh, R.K.; Confalonieri, F.; Zivanovic, Y.; Allard, G.; Awayez, M.J.; Chan-Weiher, C. C. Y.; Clausen, I.G.; Curtis, B.A.; et al. (2001). The complete genome oft he crenarchaeon *Sulfolobus solfataricus* P2. *Proc. Natl. Acad. Sci. U.S.A.* 98, 7835-7840.

Srikumar, R.; Pau, C.J. & Poole, K. (2000). Influence of mutants in the mexR repressor gene on expression oft he MexA-MexB-oprM multidrug efflux system in *Pseudomonas aeruginosa*. *J. Bacteriol.* 182, 1410-1414.

Stapleton, M.R.; Norte, V.A.; Read, R.C. & Green, J. (2002). Interaction of the *Salmonella typhimurium* transcription and virulrnce factor SlyA with target DNA and identification of members of the SlyA regulon. *J. Biol. Chem.* 277, 17630-17637.

Wilkinson, S.P. & Grove, A. (2004). HucR, a novel uric acid responsive member of the MarR family of transcriptional regulators from *Deinococcus radiodurans*. *J. Biol. Chem.* 279, 51442-51450.

Wilkinson, S.P. & Grove, A. (2005). Negative cooperativity of uric acid Binding to the transcriptional regulator HucR from *Deinococcus radiodurans*. *J. Mol. Biol.* 350, 617-630.

Wu, R.Y.; Zhang, R.G.; Zagnitko, O.; Dementieva, I.; Maltzev, N.; Watson, J. D.; Laskowski, R.; Gornicki, P. & Joachimiak, A. (2003). Crystal structure of *Enterococcus faecalis* Syla-like transcriptional factor. *J. Bio. Chem.* 278, 20240-20244.

Xiong, A.; Gottman, A.; Park, C.; Baetens, M.; Pandza, S. & Martin, A. (2000). The EMrR protein represses the *Escherichia coli emrRAB* multidrug resistance operon by directly binding to ist promoter region. *Antimicrob. Agents Chemother*, 44, 2905-2907.

17

Antibiotic Resistance Patterns in Faecal *E. coli*: A Longitudinal Cohort-Control Study of Hospitalized Horses

Mohamed O. Ahmed[1,3‡], Nicola J. Williams[2], Peter D. Clegg[2], Keith E. Baptiste[4] and Malcolm Bennett[3]

[1]Department of Microbiology and Parasitology, Faculty of Veterinary Medicine, Tripoli university, Tripoli
[2]Department of Comparative Molecular Medicine,
[3]Department of Animal and Population Health,
[2,3]School of Veterinary Science, University of Liverpool, Leahurst,
[4]Department of Large Animal Sciences, Faculty of Life Sciences, University of Copenhagen, Taastrup,
[1]Libya
[2,3]UK
[4]Denmark

1. Introduction

Cross-sectional prospective surveys are a useful method for studying the effects of antimicrobials on animals (Dunowska et al., 2006; Thomson et al., 2008; Bunner et al., 2007) . However, there is a paucity of these studies in horses compared to other animals (Coe et al., 2008).

Although antibiotic consumption has been a major contributor to the antibiotic resistance phenomenon (Bunner et al., 2007) various different factors have added to the development and dissemination of antimicrobial resistance. For example, population densities among humans have been identified as risk factors for development and spread of antimicrobial resistance (Bruinsma et al., 2005; Zhang et al., 2006). Hospitalization, in humans for instance, is also associated with an increase in antibiotic resistance in pathogenic bacteria, while others have found a lack of a significant effect on the prevalence of resistance in *E. coli* (Koterba et al., 1986; Gaynes et al., 1997). A study by Dunowska and colleagues (Dunowska et al., 2006) concluded that both antimicrobial administration and hospitalization were associated with the shedding of *E. coli* resistant strains from equine faecal samples.

Certain antimicrobial administration regimes have been shown to give rise to antibiotic resistant bacteria, which then comprise a reservoir of resistant bacteria when shed into the environment (Ahmed et al., 2010; Fofana et al., 2006; Diarrassouba et al., 2007; Pallecchi et al., 2007). Linked resistance genes encoded on mobile genetic elements, can also contribute to the spread of resistance genes (Srinivasan et al., 2007), with exposure to one antimicrobial agent leading to selection for resistance against other, or multiple, antimicrobial drugs (Braoudaki et al., 2007; Schnellmann et al., 2006; Weese et al., 2006). Such genes can be maintained after antibiotic treatment, has been stopped such that removing the selective pressure does not necessarily lead to the loss of resistance (Ahmed et al., 2010; Kaszanyitzky et al., 2007; Ghidan et al.,2008). Mobile genetic elements are widely reported cause of the spread of antibiotic resistance in both *E. coli* and *Salmonella* commensals in animals bred for human consumption (Roest et al., 2007). Therefore, *E. coli* and other enteric organisms are widely used as an indicator organism (Kaneene et al., 2007; Bruinsma et al., 2003).

The purpose of this investigation was to identify changes in antibiotic resistant *E. coli* in faeces of horses entering the Philip Leverhulme Equine Hospital (PLEH), at the University of Liverpool, UK on arrival, during hospitalization, and after discharge. The dynamics affecting the prevalence of antibiotic resistant *E. coli* were used in this study in order to examine potential risk factors.

2. Materials and methods

2.1 Study design

Faecal samples were collected from horses admitted to the Philip Leverhulme Equine Hospital (PLEH) at the University of Liverpool for more than seven days at the following time points: 1st, on arrival, before treatment began; 2nd, one day; 3rd, 2-3 days after treatment had started; 4th, immediately before discharge. Further faecal samples were collected by the horse's owners, 4-8 weeks after discharge (5th), and also 6 months after discharge (6th). Horses were divided into three groups as follows: GI+, horses with gastrointestinal conditions and under antibiotic therapy; Non-GI+, horses with non-gastrointestinal conditions and under antibiotic therapy; Non-GI-, horses with non-gastrointestinal conditions and no antibiotic therapy.

2.2 Sample collection

Faecal samples were taken from stalls randomly and chosen from the firm part of the faecal balls. In total, 2-3 grams were collected and taken straight to the laboratory.

2.3 Bacterial culture

Standard microbiological methods and biochemical tests were used to isolate and confirm each *E. coli* as fully described by Ahmed et al 2010. Three single *E. coli* colonies were chosen from each sample, confirmed by biochemical testing (e.g. API system) and subjected to further susceptibility tests thereafter.

2.4 Antibiotic susceptibility tests

Antibiotic susceptibility testing was performed according to the BSAC guidelines (Andrews, 2008). Briefly, antimicrobial drugs tested for included: - ampicillin; if the isolates show resistance to ampicillin then isolates were also tested against other two cephalosporins (cefotaxime (30 µg) and ceftazidime (30µg) for extended resistance to cephalosporines and referred as potential ESBL producers (ESBLs*) for ampicillin resistant isolates), apramycin, chloramphenicol (and also against florfenicol, if chloramphenicol resistant), nalidixic acid (and also against ciprofloxacin, if nalidixic acid resistant), tetracycline and trimethoprim. Further susceptibility tests were also performed for gentamicin, spectinomycin, streptomycin and sulphamexazole for all collected resistant isolates. Isolates were considered resistant if resistance to at least one antibiotic was shown and classified as multidrug resistant isolates (MDR) if resistant to four or more classes of antibiotics (Ahmed et al., 2010). Guidelines for determining florfenicol and apramycin resistance were as followed and determined by Ahmed et al., 2010.

2.5 Identification of antibiotic resistance genes in resistant E. coli isolates

DNA was extracted by boiling: a 5µl drop of each isolate was suspended in 0.5 ml sterile water and heated for 20 minutes at 100°C. PCR assays, previously applied by Ahmed et al 2010 were also used to detect genes commonly associated with ampicillin, chloramphenicol, tetracycline and trimethoprim resistance, were carried out using modified versions of published protocols: Pitout, 1998 (Pitout et al., 1998) for ampicillin resistant genes (*tem* & *shv* genes); Vassort-Bruneau, 1996 (Vassort-Bruneau et al., 1996) and Keyes et al.,2000 (Keyes et al., 2000) for chloramphenicol resistant genes (*catI, catII catIII* & *cmlA* genes); Ng, 2001 (Ng et al., 2001) for tetracycline resistant genes (*tetA, tetB, tetC, tetD, tet E* and *tetG* genes); Gibreel & Sköld, 1998 (Gibreel et al., 1998) and Lee, 2001 (Lee et al., 2001) for trimethoprim resistant genes (*dfr1, dfr9 dfr12, dfr13, dfrA14* & *dfr17* genes).

2.6 Statistical data analysis

Data were analysed using Minitab software, in order to determine the 95% binomial confidence intervals (95%CI) and chi-square test (X^2).

2.7 Conjugation assays

Mating experiments to determine if resistance could be transferred by conjugation were carried out using a nalidixic acid resistant *E. coli* K12 as the recipient (as performed by Ahmed et al., 2010). The method was as following: *E. coli* K12 was inoculated into 20ml nutrient broths (LabM) and incubated overnight at 37°C. Resistant *E. coli* strains (donor strains) were inoculated into separate 3ml nutrient broths and incubated overnight; 4 ml of recipient strain was then added to the donor strain and incubated at 37°C for one hour. Broths were then streaked onto agar plates containing nalidixic acid (30µg/ml) plus ampicillin (8µg/ml). Plates were incubated for 24 hours. Successful transconjugants were subcultured onto nutrient agar for susceptibility testing by disc diffusion as previously described. The resistance profiles of the transconjugants were compared to the resistance profile of the original strains. Gene profiles of the donor isolates, characterized by PCR, were described prior to the tranconjugation experiments

3. Results

3.1 Prevalence of antibiotic resistant (AR) *E. coli* isolate

In total, 15 horses were used for the study: GI+ (n=6 horses), non-GI+ (n=4 horses) and non-GI- (n=5 horses). Six samples were collected from each horse (n=90 in total). The distribution of antibiotic resistance is presented in Tables 1 and 2.

Cohort group	No. of horses	No. of samples collected	No. of samples positive for AR *E. coli* (%)	Distribution of resistant samples(out of possible 6) for each sampling time 1st	2nd	3rd	4th	5th	6th
GI +	6	36	21 (58%)	2	4	5	5	3	2
NON GI +	4	24	18 (75%)	3	4	4	4	3	0
NON GI –	5	30	16 (53%)	1	3	4	4	4	0

Table 1. The number of horses, faecal samples collected and faecal samples positive for at least one antibiotic resistant (AR) *E. coli* isolate

Source of samples	Samples collected	Positive samples	Distributing of samples containing *E. coli* resistant isolates to different antibiotics AMP	CEP	APR	CHL	FLO	NAL	CIP	TET	TRI	MDR
GI +	36	21	15	1	1	5	5	8	6	15	19	8
NON GI +	*24*	18	12	10	0	10	0	11	11	11	18	11
NON GI –	*30*	16	14	4	0	7	2	7	5	11	13	10

*Abbreviations: Ampicillin (AMP), Cephalosporins (CEP), Apramycin (APR), Chloramphenicol (CHL), Florfenicol (FLO), Nalidixic acid (NAL), Ciprofloxacin (CIP), Teracycline (TET), Trimethoprim (TRI), MDR (multidrug resistance i.e. resistance to four or more antimicrobials), *ESBLs* isolates show resistance to ampicillin then isolates were also tested against other two cephalosporins (cefotaxime (30 µg) and ceftazidime (30µg) for extended resistance to cephalosporines andreferred as potential ESBL producers (ESBLs*)

Table 2. Summary of horses, faecal samples, faecal samples containing resistant *E. coli,* and the number of faecal samples with *E. coli* resistant to each individual antibiotic

The proportion of samples with at least one *E. coli* isolate resistant to at least one antibiotic ranged from 53-75% but did not vary significantly between treatment groups (GI +, non-GI+, non GI-) (Table1). All three treatment groups also showed a similar change in prevalence of resistant isolates recovered over the duration of the study (Table1). Furthermore, there were no significant differences in the antibiotic resistance profiles of the isolates in each group (Table2). Therefore, data from the three groups were subsequently combined for the analysis of changing resistance over time. A definite pattern was observed in the prevalence of overall resistance, which increased from 40 +/-6 % at the first time point, immediately prior to admission, to 86 +/- 28 % during hospitalization (3rd time point), and decreased to 12 +/- 30 % after release (6th time point) (Figure1).

To compare the prevalence of resistant isolates before hospitalisation, immediately before discharge and 6 months after discharge (at 1st, 4th and 6th time points respectively), data was analysed by X^2 testing, analysing each individual antimicrobial as well as multidrug resistance. With the exception of ampicillin, isolates resistant to each antimicrobial drug and multidrug resistant isolates (MDR) (i.e. isolates resistant to ≥ 4 antibiotic classes), increased significantly during hospitalization and decreased after the horses had returned home (Table3). The numbers of isolates resistant to florfenicol were too low for statistical analysis.

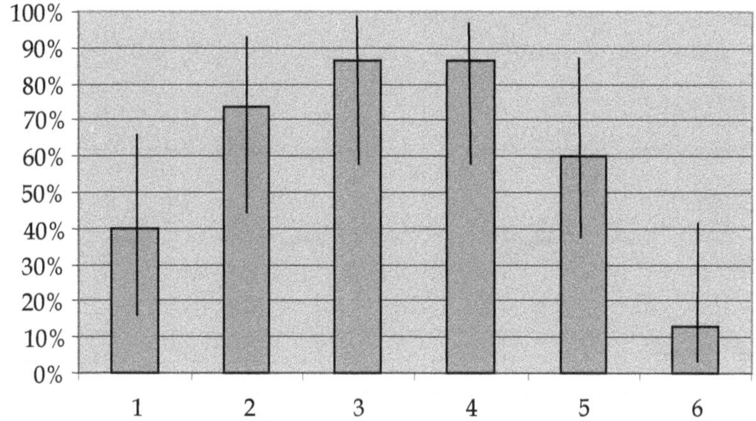

Fig. 1. Relationship between sampling time and the proportion of samples with ≥ one isolate resistant to at least one antibiotic (with 95% binomial CI); total from all three treatment groups GI+, non-GI+ and non-GI are combined (table1).

Prevalence of antibiotic resistance at sampling times	**Sampling times 1 & 4**		**Sampling times 4 & 6**	
	X^2	p	X^2	p
Resistant to at least one antibiotic	7.03	≤ 0.01	13.4	≤ 0.001
Amp	3.394	≥ 0.05	9.600	≤ 0.01
Cep	6.000	≤ 0.05	6.000	≤ 0.05
Chlo	6.136	≤ 0.05	9.130	≤ 0.01
Nal	7.500	≤ 0.01	7.500	≤ 0.01
Cip	7.500	≤ 0.01	7.500	≤ 0.01
Tet	15.000	≤ 0.001	11.627	≤ 0.001
Tri	10.995	≤ 0.001	13.393	≤ 0.001
MDR	10.909	≤ 0.001	10.109	≤ 0.001

Table 3. Two X^2 tests (2x2 analysis) to compare the effect of hospital admission and discharge on prevalence of resistance to particular antibiotic drugs.

3.2 Susceptibility testing of culture collection

In total, 138 *E. coli* isolates resistant to at least one antibiotic were collected. Of these, 71 (51.4%) were classified as MDR. Among these, two main distinctive MDR phenotypes (Ph_s) were found: Ph_s1;Amp,chlo,tet,tri,nal, comprising 93% of the MDR isolates, and mostly found among non-GI + samples; Ph_s2; Amp,chlo,tet,tri comprised 50% of the MDR isolates among the GI+ and the non-GI- samples. All the resistant isolates (n=138) were tested for susceptibility to further antibiotics. Overall, 38.5% were resistant to gentamicin, 71% to spectinomycin, 96% to streptomycin and 90% to sulphamexazole.

3.3 Molecular analysis of culture collection

PCRs revealed that *CatI [only](87%), tem(60.8%), tetA(60.8%, dfr17*(50.4%), *dfr1(38.5%)* were identified at higher prevalence among each positive collection of resistant isolates to each antibiotic (table4). MICs were also shown at higher values of ≥256 for most isolates to the selected drugs (table4).

Antibiotic	No. of Positive Sample	No. of Positive Isolates	MICs (ug/ml)	Resistance genes
Ampicillin	41	95	128 - >256	*tem (60.8%)* *shv (2%)*
Cephalosporines	15	34		
Chloramphenicol	22	51	256 - ≥256	*catI* (only) *(87%)*
Florfenicol	7	7		*catI (71%)*
Nalidixic acid	26	65		
Ciprofloxacin	22	64	4 - 16	
Tetracycline	37	89	64 - ≥256	*tetA (60.8%)* *tetB (19%)* *tetA&tetB(11.9%)*
Trimethoprim	50	127	>256	*dfr17* (50.4%) *dfr1 (38.5%)* *dfr12* (20%)

Table 4. Summary of antibiotic resistance, showing levels of resistance, MIC values and resistance gene prevalence in a total of 90 faecal samples and 138 isolates.

3.4 Conjugation experiments

Mating experiments were performed on selected isolates (n=73); those exhibiting nalidixic acid resistance were excluded 16 isolates (22% of the selected isolates & 11% of the overall culture collection) were able to transfer resistance by conjugation, and these were distributed across all cohort groups. Resistance profiles of the transconjugants, determined by susceptibility testing on the transconjugant, were identical to those of the donors (Table 5).

4. Discussion

Previous studies have given rise to conflicting conclusions as to whether or not hospitalization is associated with an increase in antibiotic resistance in bacteria (Bruinsma et al., 2003; Koterba et al., 1986). Factors other than the use of antimicrobial drugs could influence the maintenance and development of antibiotic resistance of enteric bacteria in the gastrointestinal tract (Dewulf et al., 2007). The use of antibiotics in animals is of concern (Mora et al., 2005) since resistant organisms might be excreted in the faeces of animals, following administration of antimicrobials, and contribute to the reservoir of resistant bacteria in the environment (Ahmed et al., 2010). Resistant bacteria could be selected or acquired in the hospital environment and may subsequently be disseminated to the horses' home environments.

No.	Origin	Resistance phenotype	Donor genes (previously identified by PCR)
1,	NON-GI-	AMP	*Tem*
2	NON-GI-	AMP	*Tem*
3	NON-GI-	MDR	*dfr1,dfr12,tetA,tem,catI*
4	NON-GI-	MDR	*dfr1,dfr12,tetA,tem*
5	NON-GI-	MDR	*dfr1,dfr12,tetA,tem,catI*
6	NON-GI-	MDR	*tem*
7	NON-GI-	MDR	*dfr1,dfr12,tetA,tem*
8	GI+	AMP	*tem*
9	GI+	AMP,TRI	*dfr(7-17)*
10	GI+	AMP,TRI	*not identified*
11	GI+	AMP	*tem*
12	GI+	AMP	*tem*
13	GI+	AMP	*tem*
14	GI+	AMP,TRI	*dfr1*
15	GI+	AMP,TRI	*tem*
16	NON-GI +	AMP	*tem*

Table 5. Characteristics of isolates showing of transferable resistance.

This study and in contrast with others found no obvious association between antibiotic treatment, or clinical condition, and resistance profiles in faecal *E. coli*. This may be due to the relatively small sample size, or because horses entering the PLEH are largely referral cases and likely to have received antibiotic therapy prior to admission.

However, overall resistance to most individual antibiotics, and the proportion of MDR isolates increased during hospitalization and thereafter decreased during convalescence in the home environment. Recent studies by Dunowska et al, on horses, concluded that both hospitalization and antimicrobial administration were associated with the shedding of antimicrobial resistance *E. coli* strains of faecal origin (Dunowska et al., 2006). An earlier study, from a university equine hospital, found that the rate of resistance amongst *E. coli* and *Klebsiella* was higher at day seven of hospitalization compared to day one (Koterba et al., 1986). This may be due to selection during hospitalization through antibiotic therapy, and also the ready availability of resistant isolates in the hospital environment. It would be interesting to undertake PFGE analysis of the *E. coli* over time to investigate whether resistance is due to infection with resistant strains or horizontal transmission of resistance to the existing gut flora.

Antimicrobials select for resistance (Tenover et al., 2006) but the restriction of antimicrobials does not necessarily reduce antimicrobial resistance (Hoyle et al., 2006). In our study, the prevalence of resistant *E. coli* dropped markedly after discharge from the hospital, which may suggest that both the increase and decrease in resistance are due to turnover of *E. coli* between the gut and the environment.

E. coli with simple and multiple antimicrobial resistance (MDR) has been widely documented (Fofana et al., 2006; Ahmed et al., 2010). Bacteria can acquire or develop resistance to antimicrobials in different ways, including acquisition of resistant genes. *E. coli* has been indicated as a possible reservoir for antimicrobial resistance genes and might play a role in the spreading of such determinants to other bacteria (Ahmed et al., 2010). The flora of healthy animals has also been implicated as a reservoir of antibiotic resistance genes (De Graef et al., 2004) and resistance transfer has been shown to occur between different animal species on farm premises (Hoyle et al., 2006). *E. coli* of animal origin with resistance to antibiotics and multiple antibiotics has been widely documented (Mora et al., 2005). The importance of farm animals in the spread of resistance to human populations is increased by worldwide reports of mobile genetic elements in animals raised for human consumption (Roest et al., 2007).

Our results for MICs and the genetic determination of resistance, suggest that, resistance was due to commonly reported genes causing such resistance in *E. coli* and other bacteria. It is interesting to note, that while some MDR transferred in the conjugation studies, many transconjugants were resistant to either ampicillin alone or ampicillin and trimethoprim (table 5). This suggests that both resistance profiles are encoded on mobile genetic elements. Horses in the GI+ and non-GI+ groups were the donors for most of the Amp and Amp/Trim transconjugants, and all the horses in both groups received therapy with cephalosporin drugs. It may, therefore be that these isolates represent either an endemic strain in the hospital, or an endemic plasmid moving rapidly between horses.

Multiple drug resistance phenotypes have been shown to be related to certain antibiotic drugs such as streptomycin and tetracycline (Mora et al., 2005). Also the resistance to a single antibiotic (i.e. tetracycline), in commensal *E. coli*, is linked to other antimicrobial resistances (e.g. ampicillin, trimethoprim and sulphonamides) (Dewulf et al., 2007). The *dfrA1, dfrA12, dfrA15* and *dfrA17* genes are documented to be carried on mobile genetic elements (i.e. integron classes), harboring resistance genes to at least three antimicrobials, and thus conferring multiple resistance (Ahmed et al., 2009). Other antibiotic resistances (i.e. ampicillin resistance) although found, were not strongly related to the presence of mobile genetic elements (Hoyle et al., 2005). Our PCR results in this study revealed similar observations within our collection of *E.coli* strains to other studies, although the conjugation results show that even isolates with single resistance (to ampicillin) transferred resistance (although not MDR). Thus, mobile genetic elements could also be responsible for single resistance and antimicrobial therapy might have resulted in such selection. The type of resistance and the identified genes (i.e. ampicillin resistance) could also be related to the type of antimicrobial therapy administered (e.g. cephalosporins). Such revelations, if proven by further studies, would mean that this kind of element may acquire further resistance genes in the future and help the dissemination and development of antibiotic resistance.

The importance of mobile gene pools in the spread of antibiotic resistance has been highlighted through comprehensive genomic analysis (Fricke et al., 2008). In our survey, a high proportion of the isolates tested in conjugation experiments were able to transfer resistance. *Dfr17* was the most prevalent trimethoprim resistance gene identified among the positive PCR isolates and *dfr1* was the second most prevalent. *tetA* was the most prevalent tetracycline resistant gene. This might indicate that the *dfr*17 and *tetA* resistant genes are more involved in the MDR mechanisms and most likely to be integrated within mobile genetic elements. The *tem* gene was also the most prevalent ampicillin resistant gene among the isolates and the *catI* gene was mostly found in MDR isolates. The *dfr17* is extensively reported to be involved in mobile genetic elements (Van et al., 2007). This, along with the conjugation results, suggests that these elements are present in the hospital environment or that they are already constituents of the horses' intestinal flora. The referral hospital deals with horses in the area and horses are likely to be referred more than once to this hospital, which might lead to increases in the dissemination of resistance phenotypes in horses. The similarity between MDR phenotypes among collected strains can be epidemiologically important and molecular characterization (i.e. PFGE) in future studies will enhance our understanding of the phenomena.

The florfenicol resistant isolates were positive by PCR (five out of seven were positive for *catI*) and the mechanisms of this resistance require further investigation. However florfenicol resistance has been documented in *E. coli* of animal origin (Singer et al., 2004) and it has been shown that *floR* genetic determinants and others (i.e. *cmlA, cat1, cat2*) were also largely related to florfenicol resistance (Li et al., 2007). Others have shown that *floR* mediated resistance to chloramphenicol and florfenicol is plasmid mediated and also carries resistance to other genes (Blickwede et al., 2007; Kehrenberg et al., 2008). Recent molecular analyses have suggested that florfenicol resistance is strongly due to horizontal rather than clonal dissemination (Kehrenberg et al., 2008). This correlates with our results, in that florfenicol resistance is entirely documented among MDR isolates (although not proven transconjugants by our experiments). The horses in this study had never been treated with these classes of drugs, implicating a mobile genetic system in the acquisition of resistance from other animals or the environment.

5. Conclusions

No association between therapy and resistance profile was found in this study. However, the prevalence of antimicrobial resistance, and of MDR strains, did increase during hospitalization and subsequently decreased upon release from hospital. Thus therapy and the general environment of the hospital do appear to select for resistance and resistant isolates may disseminate once horses have been discharged, leading to clinical and public health concerns.

6. Acknowledgements

Authors are grateful to all staff members at Philip Leverhulme Equine Hospital (PLEH) and the livery stables for their help and support throughout this work.

7. References

Ahmed, MO.; Clegg, P. D.; Williams, N. J.; Baptiste, K. E.; and Bennett, M.. (2010). Antimicrobial resistance in equine faecal Escherichia coli isolates from North West England. Ann.Clin.Microbiol.Antimicrob. 9:12.

Ahmed, AM.; Younis, EE.; Osman, SA.; Ishida, Y.; El-Khodery, SA.; Shimamoto, T. (2009). Genetic analysis of antimicrobial resistance in Escherichia coli isolated from diarrheic neonatal calves. *Vet Microbiol*, 136(3-4):397-402.

Andrews, JM. (2006). BSAC standardized disc susceptibility testing method (version 5). *J Antimicrob Chemother*, 58(3):511-529.

Blickwede, M.; Schwarz, S. (2004). Molecular analysis of florfenicol-resistant Escherichia coli isolates from pigs. *J Antimicrob Chemother*, 53(1):58-64.

Braoudaki, M.; Hilton, AC. (2004). Adaptive resistance to biocides in Salmonella enterica and Escherichia coli O157 and cross-resistance to antimicrobial agents. *J Clin Microbiol*, 42(1):73-78.

Bruinsma, N.; Filius, PM.; van den Bogaard, AE.; Nys, S.; Degener, J.; Endtz, HP.; Stobberingh, EE. (2003). Hospitalization, a risk factor for antibiotic-resistant Escherichia coli in the community? *J Antimicrob Chemother*, 51(4):1029-1032.

Bunner, CA.; Norby, B.; Bartlett, PC.; Erskine, RJ.; Downes, FP.; Kaneene, JB. (2007). Prevalence and pattern of antimicrobial susceptibility in Escherichia coli isolated from pigs reared under antimicrobial-free and conventional production methods. *J Am Vet Med Assoc*, 231(2):275-283.

Coe, PH.; Grooms, DL.; Metz, K.; Holland, RE. (2008). Changes in antibiotic susceptability of Escherichia coli isolated from steers exposed to antibiotics during the early feeding period. *Vet Ther*, 9(3):241-247.

De Graef, EM.; Decostere, S.; Devriese, LA.; Haesebrouck, F. (2004). Antibiotic resistance among fecal indicator bacteria from healthy individually owned and kennel dogs. *Microb Drug Resist*, 10(1):65-69.

Dewulf, J.; Catry, B.; Timmerman, T.; Opsomer, G.; de Kruif, A.; Maes, D. (2007). Tetracycline-resistance in lactose-positive enteric coliforms originating from Belgian fattening pigs: degree of resistance, multiple resistance and risk factors. *Prev Vet Med*, 78(3-4):339-351.

Diarrassouba, F.; Diarra, MS.; Bach, S.; Delaquis, P.; Pritchard, J.; Topp, E.; Skura, BJ. (2007). Antibiotic resistance and virulence genes in commensal Escherichia coli and Salmonella isolates from commercial broiler chicken farms. *J Food Prot*, 70(6):1316-1327.

Dunowska, M.; Morley, PS.; Traub-Dargatz, JL.; Hyatt, DR.; Dargatz, DA. (2006). Impact of hospitalization and antimicrobial drug administration on antimicrobial susceptibility patterns of commensal Escherichia coli isolated from the feces of horses. *J Am Vet Med Assoc*, 228(12):1909-1917.

Fofana, A.; Bada Alambedji, R.; Seydi, M.; Akakpo, AJ. (2006). Antibiotic resistance of Escherichia coli strains isolated from raw chicken meat in Senegal. *Dakar Med*, 51(3):145-150.

Fricke, WF.; Wright, MS.; Lindell, AH.; Harkins, DM.; Baker-Austin, C.; Ravel, J.; Stepanauskas, R. (2008). Insights into the environmental resistance gene pool from the genome sequence of the multidrug-resistant environmental isolate Escherichia coli SMS-3-5. *J Bacteriol*, 190(20):6779-6794.

Gaynes, R.; Monnet, D. (1997). The contribution of antibiotic use on the frequency of antibiotic resistance in hospitals. *Ciba Found Symp*, 207:47-56; discussion 56-60.

Ghidan, A.; Kaszanyitzky, EJ.; Dobay, O.; Nagy, K.; Amyes, SG.; Rozgonyi, F. (2008). Distribution and genetic relatedness of vancomycin-resistant enterococci (VRE) isolated from healthy slaughtered chickens in Hungary from 2001 to 2004. *Acta Vet Hung*, 56(1):13-25.

Gibreel, A.; Skold, O. (1998). High-level resistance to trimethoprim in clinical isolates of Campylobacter jejuni by acquisition of foreign genes (dfr1 and dfr9) expressing drug-insensitive dihydrofolate reductases. *Antimicrob Agents Chemother*, 42(12):3059-3064.

Hoyle, DV.; Davison, HC.; Knight, HI.; Yates, CM.; Dobay, O.; Gunn, GJ.; Amyes, SG.; Woolhouse, ME. (2006). Molecular characterisation of bovine faecal Escherichia coli shows persistence of defined ampicillin resistant strains and the presence of class 1 integrons on an organic beef farm. *Vet Microbiol*, 115(1-3):250-257.

Kaneene, JB.; Warnick, LD.; Bolin, CA.; Erskine, RJ.; May, K.; Miller, R. (2008). Changes in tetracycline susceptibility of enteric bacteria following switching to nonmedicated milk replacer for dairy calves. *J Clin Microbiol*, 46(6):1968-1977.

Kaszanyitzky, EJ.; Tenk, M.; Ghidan, A.; Fehervari, GY.; Papp, M. (2007). Antimicrobial susceptibility of enterococci strains isolated from slaughter animals on the data of Hungarian resistance monitoring system from 2001 to 2004. *Int J Food Microbiol*, 115(1):119-123.

Keyes, K.; Hudson, C.; Maurer, JJ.; Thayer, S.; White, DG.; Lee, MD. (2000). Detection of florfenicol resistance genes in Escherichia coli isolated from sick chickens. *Antimicrob Agents Chemother*, 44(2):421-424.

Kehrenberg, C.; Wallmann, J.; Schwarz, S. (2008) Molecular analysis of florfenicol-resistant Pasteurella multocida isolates in Germany. *J Antimicrob Chemother*, 62(5):951-955.

Koterba, A.; Torchia, J.; Silverthorne, C.; Ramphal, R.; Merritt, AM.; Manucy. (1986). Nosocomial infections and bacterial antibiotic resistance in a university equine hospital. *J Am Vet Med Assoc*, 189(2):185-191.

Lee, JC.; Oh, JY.; Cho, JW.; Park, JC.; Kim, JM.; Seol, SY.; Cho, DT. (2001) The prevalence of trimethoprim-resistance-conferring dihydrofolate reductase genes in urinary isolates of Escherichia coli in Korea. *J Antimicrob Chemother*, 47(5):599-604.

Li, XS.; Wang, GQ.; Du, XD.; Cui, BA.; Zhang, SM.; Shen, JZ. (2007). Antimicrobial susceptibility and molecular detection of chloramphenicol and florfenicol resistance among Escherichia coli isolates from diseased chickens. *J Vet Sci*, 8(3):243-247.

Mora, A.; Blanco, JE.; Blanco, M.; Alonso, MP.; Dhabi, G.; Echeita, A.; Gonzalez, EA.; Bernardez, MI.; Blanco, J. (2005). Antimicrobial resistance of Shiga toxin (verotoxin)-producing Escherichia coli O157:H7 and non-O157 strains isolated from humans, cattle, sheep and food in Spain. *Res Microbiol*, 156(7):793-806.

Ng, LK.; Martin, I.; Alfa, M.; Mulvey, M. (2001). Multiplex PCR for the detection of tetracycline resistant genes. *Mol Cell Probes*, 15(4):209-215.

Pallecchi, L.; Lucchetti, C.; Bartoloni, A.; Bartalesi, F.; Mantella, A.; Gamboa, H.; Carattoli, A.; Paradisi, F.; Rossolini, GM. (2007). Population structure and resistance genes in antibiotic-resistant bacteria from a remote community with minimal antibiotic exposure. *Antimicrob Agents Chemother*, 51(4):1179-1184.

Pitout, JD.; Thomson, KS.; Hanson, ND.; Ehrhardt, AF.; Moland, ES.; Sanders, CC. (1998). beta-Lactamases responsible for resistance to expanded-spectrum cephalosporins in Klebsiella pneumoniae, Escherichia coli, and Proteus mirabilis isolates recovered in South Africa. *Antimicrob Agents Chemother*, 42(6):1350-1354.

Roest, HI.; Liebana, E.; Wannet, W.; van Duynhoven, Y.; Veldman, KT.; Mevius, DJ. (2007). [Antibiotic resistance in Escherichia coli O157 isolated between 1998 and 2003 in The Netherlands]. *Tijdschr Diergeneeskd*, 132(24):954-958.

Singer, RS.; Patterson, SK.; Meier, AE.; Gibson, JK.; Lee, HL.; Maddox, CW. (2004). Relationship between phenotypic and genotypic florfenicol resistance in Escherichia coli. *Antimicrob Agents Chemother*, 48(10):4047-4049.

Schnellmann, C.; Gerber, V.; Rossano, A.; Jaquier, V.; Panchaud, Y.; Doherr, MG.; Thomann, A.; Straub, R.; Perreten, V. (2006). Presence of new mecA and mph(C) variants conferring antibiotic resistance in Staphylococcus spp. isolated from the skin of horses before and after clinic admission. *J Clin Microbiol*, 44(12):4444-4454.

Srinivasan, V.; Gillespie, BE.; Lewis, MJ.; Nguyen, LT.; Headrick, SI.; Schukken, YH.; Oliver, SP. (2007). Phenotypic and genotypic antimicrobial resistance patterns of Escherichia coli isolated from dairy cows with mastitis. *Vet Microbiol*, 124(3-4):319-328.

Tenover, FC. (2006). Mechanisms of antimicrobial resistance in bacteria. *Am J Med*, 119(6 Suppl 1):S3-10; discussion S62-70.

Thomson, K.; Rantala, M.; Hautala, M.; Pyorala, S.; Kaartinen, L. (2008). Cross-sectional prospective survey to study indication-based usage of antimicrobials in animals: results of use in cattle. *BMC Vet Res*, 4:15.

Van, TT.; Moutafis, G.; Tran, LT.; Coloe, PJ. (2007). Antibiotic resistance in food-borne bacterial contaminants in Vietnam. *Appl Environ Microbiol*, 73(24):7906-7911.

Vassort-Bruneau, C.; Lesage-Descauses, MC.; Martel, JL.; Lafont, JP.; Chaslus-Dancla, E. (1996). CAT III chloramphenicol resistance in Pasteurella haemolytica and Pasteurella multocida isolated from calves. *J Antimicrob Chemother*, 38(2):205-213.

Weese, JS.; Rousseau, J.; Willey, BM.; Archambault, M.; McGeer, A.; Low, DE. (2006). Methicillin-resistant Staphylococcus aureus in horses at a veterinary teaching hospital: frequency, characterization, and association with clinical disease. *J Vet Intern Med*, 20(1):182-186.

Zhang, R.; Eggleston, K.; Rotimi, V.; Zeckhauser, RJ. (2006). Antibiotic resistance as a global threat: evidence from China, Kuwait and the United States. *Global Health*, 2:6.

18

Clinical Impact of Extended-Spectrum β-Lactamase-Producing Bacteria

Yong Chong
Department of Blood and Marrow Transplantation, Hara-Sanshin Hospital, Fukuoka, Japan

1. Introduction

We have been forced to fight against the newly acquired antibiotic resistance of various bacteria. By the end of the 1970s, most *Escherichia coli* (*E. coli*) and *Klebsiella pneumoniae* (*K. pneumoniae*) strains contained plasmid-mediated, ampicillin-hydrolyzing β-lactamases, such as TEM-1, TEM-2, and SHV-1, and could be eliminated by the use of third-generation cephalosporins. [1] TEM-1 and TEM-2 were detected mainly in *E. coli*, and SHV-1 was mainly detected in *K. pneumoniae.* [2] The emergence of *K. pneumoniae* strains with a gene encoding β-lactamase that hydrolyzes the extended-spectrum cephalosporins was first reported by a study from Germany in 1983. [3] The gene encoding the new β-lactamase harbored a single-nucleotide mutation, as compared to the parental *bla*SHV-1 gene. In 1986, *K. pneumoniae* strains resistant to the third-generation cephalosporins were detected in France. [4] The resistance was attributed to a new β-lactamase gene, which was closely related to TEM-1 and TEM-2. These newly detected β-lactamases capable of hydrolyzing extended-spectrum β-lactam antibiotics were named extended-spectrum β-lactamases (ESBLs). [5] In 1989, the CTX-M type was reported as a new ESBL family member not belonging to either the TEM or SHV types. [6] Notably, the origin of CTX-M ESBLs is totally different from that of TEM or SHV ESBL. [7] Until the end of the 1990s, most of the ESBLs detected were either the TEM or SHV types and were usually associated with nosocomial outbreaks caused by *K. pneumoniae.* [1] In the new millennium, the worldwide spread of CTX-M-producing *E. coli* has been dramatic, and they are now considered to be the primary ESBL producers that are almost always associated with community-acquired infections. [8] ESBL-producing *E.coli* and *Klebsiella* spp. are now listed as one of the six drug-resistant pathogens for which few potentially effective drugs are available. [9] This chapter will outline the genetic aspects of TEM, SHV, and CTX-M ESBLs, including molecular epidemiology and mobile elements. In addition, we will also consider the impact of their genetic evolution on clinical aspects, including mode of infection and antibiotic resistance.

2. ESBL definition/classification

There is no exact definition of ESBLs. ESBLs are generally defined as β-lactamases that confer resistance to bacteria against the penicillins, the first-, second-, and third-generation cephalosporins, and to aztreonam by hydrolyzing these antibiotics, and are inhibited by β-lactamase inhibitors. [1] Most of ESBLs are classified as class A on the basis of the scheme devised by Ambler et al. [10] Class A ESBLs form a heterogeneous molecular group, which comprises β-lactamases sharing various identities, and consists of three major groups: the TEM, SHV, and CTX-M types. [7] TEM and SHV ESBLs genetically evolved from TEM-1, TEM-2, and SHV-1 progenitors (non-ESBLs), and CTX-M ESBLs developed independently from TEM and SHV ESBLs. Additional ESBL types, such as PER, VEB, and BES, are uncommon. [10] More than 130 TEM types and more than 50 SHV types are currently known. [10] The most common group of ESBLs not belonging to the TEM or SHV types is CTX-M, the name derives from the potent hydrolytic activity against cefotaxime. [1] More than 40 CTX-M types are now recognized and can be divided into five subgroups, CTX-M1, 2, 8, 9, and 25, according to their amino acid sequence similarities. [7]

3. Global epidemiology: dissemination of ESBLs

ESBLs were first detected in the first half of the 1980s in Europe, and they later disseminated worldwide. [1] Until the 1990s, the main producer of ESBLs was *K. pneumoniae* and nosocomial outbreaks caused by the organism were often reported. [1] The number of ESBL-producing *E. coli* isolates has been dramatically increasing during the 21st century. [11] A recent global surveillance database collected from Europe, North and South America, and Asia, showed that the detection frequencies for ESBL-producing *K. pneumoniae* and *E. coli* isolates were 7.5-44% and 2.2-13.5%, respectively. [12] The prevalence of ESBL-producing isolates increased to a greater degree, particularly in Asia than in other regions, and one study conducted in 2007 showed that the frequencies of ESBL-producing *K. pneumoniae* and *E. coli* isolates exceeded 30% in both bacterial populations. [13] A recent surveillance using samples collected from nine Asian countries showed ESBL producers accounted for 42.2% of *K. pneumoniae* isolates detected from patients with hospital-acquired pneumoniae. [14] Our data collected from one institution in Japan showed that the detection rate of the *E. coli* isolates increased first, followed by increased detection rates of the *K. pneumoniae* and *P. mirabilis* isolates. [15] (Figure1) These data suggest that *K. pneumoniae*, as well as *E. coli*, has been an important ESBL producer even in the last few years.

In the analysis of ESBL genotypes, TEM and SHV were predominantly observed until the 1990s, and it was most reported that SHV-producing *K. pneumoniae* strains showed clonal dissemination in hospitals. [1] Recent studies show that TEM and SHV types have been frequently detected up to the present day. Interestingly, in some cases, SHV has been found in isolates expressing other ESBL types, such as TEM and CTX-M. [16] Our study showed that multiple types of ESBLs, including TEM, SHV, and CTX-M, were most frequently detected in *K. pneumoniae* and *E. coli*. [15] (Table1) These findings suggest that the genetic mechanism underlying dissemination of ESBL genes has become more divergent and complicated. After the first half of the 2000s, it was often reported that the number of CTX-M ESBLs detected was on the rise, that the main carrier was *E. coli*, and that most of the CTX-M-producing *E. coli* strains were acquired in the community, not in hospitals. [11] The detection rate of CTX-M ESBLs has been dramatically rising, especially in the last 5 years. [17] The mechanism behind the spread of *bla*CTX-M genes differs from that observed in the case of *bla*TEM and *bla*SHV genes. *bla*TEM and *bla*SHV ESBL genes are associated with the dissemination of particular clones, known as an "epidemic" pattern; however, the mechanism by which *bla*CTX-M ESBL genes disseminate reflects the simultaneous spread of multiple specific clones, known as an "allodemic" pattern. [18] It has been indicated that various CTX-M-type ESBLs have spread

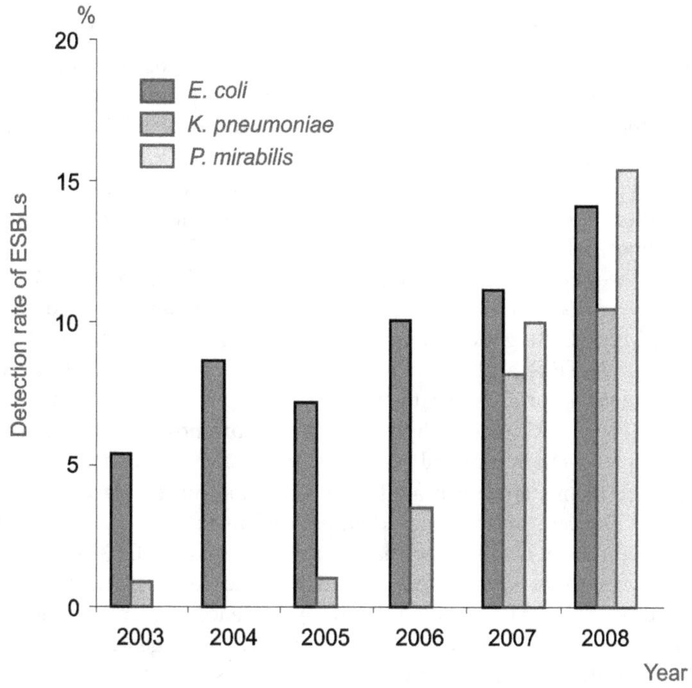

Fig. 1. Frequencies of ESBL-producing organisms at Hara-Sanshin Hospital in Fukuoka (Japan)

worldwide, and that specific CTX-M subgroups have been characterized in different geographic areas. [15,18,19] In contrast, CTX-M-15 ESBLs, which belong to the CTX-M-1 group, have been found worldwide. [18] Unlike in other countries, in the USA, ESBLs were rarely detected, until the first half of the 2000s; however, CTX-M ESBLs, specifically CTX-M-15, have frequently been encountered over the last 5 years. [20,21]

Year	Total no. of isolates	TEM/SHV	CTX-M	TEM/SHV+CTX-M
2003	11	0(0.0)	4 (36.4)	7(63.6)
2004	15	1(6.7)	5 (33.3)	9(60.0)
2005	15	0(0.0)	5(33.3)	10(66.7)
2006	20	0(0.0)	5 (25.0)	15(75.0)
2007	18	2(11.1)	7 (38.9)	9(50.0)
2008	25	5(20.0)	9(36.0)	11(44.0)
Total	104	8(7.7)	35(33.7)	61(58.6)

Table 1. Genotypes of ESBL-producing *Eschrichia coli* isolated from hospitalized patients

4. Genetic characteristics

Genes harboring ESBLs are associated with several specific genetic structures. A variety of mobile genetic elements, such as transposons, insertion sequences, and integrons, play important roles in the dissemination of ESBL genes. *bla*TEM-type ESBL genes are acquired by the mutation of plasmid-mediated, parent *bla*TEM-1 and *bla*TEM-2 genes, and the main producer of TEM-type ESBLs is *E. coli*; these genes occur within the earliest bacterial transposons identified. [2,22] *bla*SHV-type ESBL genes are the derivatives of chromosomal, parent *bla*SHV-1 genes, which occur mainly in *K. pneumoniae*,[23] and are likely acquired by the role of insertion sequences from chromosome to plasmid. [22] Notably, *bla*TEM-type and *bla*SHV-type ESBL genes located in the integron structures have never been identified. [22] The spread of *bla*CTX-M-type ESBL genes is associated with more complicated mobile elements, compared to that of *bla*TEM and *bla*SHV ESBL genes. *bla*CTX-M ESBL genes are not derivatives of *K. pneumoniae* or *E. coli* that contain original genes, as compared to *bla*TEM or *bla*SHV ESBL genes. *bla*CTX-M genes originate from the chromosomal β-lactamase genes of *Kluyvera* species, which are environmental bacteria found worldwide, and are captured mainly by insertion sequence elements translocated from chromosome to plasmid. [18] Original β-lactamase genes of *Kluyvera* species are identified in most CTX-M subgroups. [18] This differential origin might be involved in the characteristic spread of *bla*CTX-M ESBL genes, that is, an "allodemic" pattern of spread. All *bla*CTX-M genes are associated with insertion sequences. Well-studied, CTX-M-associated insertion sequence elements include IS*Ecp1* and IS*CR1*, which are involved in the mobilization of *bla*CTX-M genes by a transposition mechanism. [24,25,26] In addition, integron structures bearing insertion sequences and *bla*CTX-M genes can be linked to transposon elements, such as from the Tn*21* family, which has been intensively studied. Transposons of the Tn*21* family are disseminated worldwide in both environmental and clinical bacteria.[18,24] These highly efficient mobile genetic elements may have influenced the rapid and easy dissemination of *bla*CTX-M ESBL genes.

An antibiotic resistance plasmid itself is responsible for the efficiency of gene transfer, as well as the mobile genetic elements described above. It has been shown that ESBL gene-bearing plasmids can be transferred to different bacterial species by conjugation. [27,28] Previous studies have shown that *bla*TEM and *bla*SHV ESBL genes are associated with plasmids belonging to a few specific incompatibility (Inc) groups.[18] In contrast, *bla*CTX-M ESBL genes are carried by plasmids belonging to a variety of Inc groups including narrow- and broad-host-range types. [18,29] *bla*CTX-M-15 genes are located mainly on plasmids belonging to the IncF group. [29] Interestingly, a recent study has described the diversity of ESBL gene-bearing plasmids, including SHV types. [30] It was reported that a mosaic plasmid has been identified from a clonal CTX-M-producing *E. coli* isolate, suggesting genetic interactions among different plasmids. [31] In ESBL gene-bearing plasmids, the genetic diversity has been constantly increasing through the mechanism of gene transfer and gene shuffling.

5. Clinical impact

5.1 The mode of infection

5.1.1 Nosocomial infection

Up to the end of the 1990s, clinical infections caused by ESBL-producing bacteria were associated with nosocomial outbreaks, where the chief ESBL producer was *K. pneumoniae*, but not *E. coli.* In addition, the ESBL genotypes detected in the nosocomial setting were almost always TEM and SHV, but not CTX-M types. [1] SHV-producing *K. pneumoniae* strains were intensively examined in the analysis of clonal dissemination in hospitals. Clonally related SHV-4-producing *K. pneumoniae* isolates were shown to have spread to multiple hospitals within the specific region. [32] This phenomenon indicates that, at that time, the mode of spread for SHV-producing *K. pneumoniae* was the dissemination of particular clones, that is to say, an "epidemic" pattern. The number of nosocomial outbreaks caused by TEM- or SHV-producing *K. pneumoniae* strains have been decreased during this century; however, as observed in many studies, these organisms are frequently identified in many hospitals worldwide. Interestingly, the derivatives of TEM and SHV types have been reported to be more divergent in *K. pneumoniae* strains isolated in European hospitals. [16,33] Moreover, the new variants of *bla*SHV genes were detected from an Algerian hospital. [34]

5.1.2 Community-acquired infection

The mode of ESBL-related infection has dramatically changed since the 2000s. Community-acquired infections caused by ESBL-producing bacteria have been increasingly documented. [8] CTX-M-producing E. coli strains are chiefly responsible for community-acquired infections, which are related to an increase in the number of ESBL carriers in the general population. [11,35] One report describes a significant increase in the prevalence of ESBL carriers in a specific population from 2001 to 2006. [36] The interfamilial dissemination of ESBL-producing bacteria has also been suggested. [37] Notably, animals used as food and or pets are reported to carry CTX-M ESBLs, [38,39,40,41] and this finding may explain the dramatic spread of ESBLs in the community. The community-onset dissemination of ESBLs in both humans and animals may suggest that *bla*CTX-M ESBL genes detected in pathogenic bacteria are acquired from environmental bacteria. Branger et al showed that many CTX-M ESBLs were associated with the phylogenetic group D2 that lacked a virulence factor. [42, 43] The specific features may be related to the colonization and spread among the general population. The spread of ESBLs in the community is linked to the emergence of ESBL-related infections in outpatients, in whom urinary tract infections are most often reported along with bacteremia. [44,45, 46] One study has described the detection of CTX-M-producing *K. pneumoniae* in outpatients, [33] A nosocomial outbreak was caused by CTX-M-producing *K. pneumoniae* isolates from foods, suggesting the influx of ESBL-producing *K. pneumoniae* into a hospital. [47] These reports may account for the dissemination of CTX-M ESBL genes from *E. coli* to other bacteria in the community.

5.2 Antibiotic resistance

Antibiotic resistance is of utmost importance for the clinical impact of ESBL-producing bacteria. A meta-analysis showed increased mortality and delay in effective antibiotic use in ESBL-related bacteremia, [48] indicating the importance of constant surveillance for an antibiotic resistance pattern in organisms with ESBLs. ESBL-producing bacteria are resistant to almost all β-lactam antibiotics, except carbapenems, as indicated by their definition. In addition, most ESBL-producing bacteria, particularly those with the TEM, SHV, and CTX-M genotypes, exhibit co-resistance to aminoglycosides, tetracyclines, and sulfonamides. [18] Organisms with CTX-M genotypes, such as those with CTX-M-9, -14, and -15, are reported to be resistant to fluoroquinolones. [18] This additional resistance is induced by the main mechanism that *bla*CTX-M genes are directly linked to quinolone resistance genes, *qnr* genes. IS*CR1*, a mobile element for *bla*CTX-M genes, is associated with *qnr* genes, [26] indicating an effective transfer of quinolone resistance genes together with *bla*CTX-M genes. This genetic finding is interesting for clinical reasons. Selective pressure by the use of fluoroquinolones may induce the emergence of CTX-M ESBL-producing bacteria. As a consequence, the therapeutic options for infections caused by ESBL-producing bacteria may be more limited. Tigecycline has been shown to be microbiologically active against ESBL-producing *E. coli* and *K. pneumoniae,* [49,50] whereas, fosfomycin has been reported to be effective against urinary tract infections caused by ESBL-producing *E. coli.* [51,52]

6. Spread of CTX-M-15-producing ST131 *E. coli* clones

The dissemination of CTX-M-15 producing *E. coli* strains has become a major concern of research in antibiotic resistance. The first isolation of CTX-M-15-type ESBLs was reported in India in 2001. [53] CTX-M-15 is derived from CTX-M-3, belonging to the CTX-M-1 group, differing by one amino acid substitution. *bla*CTX-M-15 genes are transferred mainly by the IncF group plasmids, which are well adapted to *E. coli* and have acquired many antibiotic resistance genes. [54,55,56] Recently, Mnif et al reported that the IncF plasmids carrying *bla*CTX-M-15 genes contained many addiction systems, which could contribute to their maintenance in *E. coli* host strains. [57] The detection rate of the CTX-M-15 producing *E. coli* strains with multidrug resistance has been dramatically increasing worldwide since the 2000s. [56] This CTX-M-15-producing *E. coli* strain is often thought to be associated with ST131 clones. [56] Most of the CTX-M-15-producing *E. coli* strains isolated from three continents were O25:H4-ST131 clones that show highly similar PFGE profiles, suggesting a recent emergence of these clones. [58] The emergence of the CTX-M-15-producing ST131 *E. coli* clones is highly related to the recent dissemination of ESBLs in the USA. [59, 60] The worldwide spread of the multi-drug-resistant ST131 *E. coli* clones can be explained by the acquisition of IncFII plasmids harboring *bla*CTX-M-15 genes and many other antibiotic resistance genes. Interestingly, these ST131 *E. coli* clones belong to the highly virulent, phylogenetic group B2. [56] Over the past 5 years, CTX-M-15-producing ST131 *E. coli* clones have become an important causative agent for community-acquired ESBL infections, mainly urinary tract infections and bacteremia. [45]

7. Clinical impact on immunodeficient patients

The sufficient therapy for ESBL-related infections is important, especially in immunodeficient patients. One study has shown that approximately 13% of *E. coli*-related bacteremia cases detected in patients with cancer and neutropenia were caused by ESBLs, that CTX-M types were predominant among the ESBLs, and that the bacteremia induced by ESBL-producing *E. coli* strains was linked to inadequate empirical antibiotic therapy. [61] In our institution, the detection rate of ESBL-related bacteremia has been increasing in febrile neutropenic patients with hematological malignancies, and consequently, we have been forced to use carbapenems for the therapy. [62,63] In immunodeficient patients, such as those undergoing chemotherapy, serious ESBL-related infections may result in a poor prognosis owing to the failure of the initial therapy. Recently, M. D. Anderson Cancer Center has reported an interesting finding that pyomyositis was caused by ESBL-producing *E. coli* strains in neutropenic patients with hematological malignancies, and that the *E. coli* strains were ST131 clones belonging to phylogenetic group B2. [64] This notable finding implies that ESBL-producing ST131 *E. coli* clones cause fatal damage in the case of immunodeficient patients because of their high virulence.

8. Conclusions

The spread of ESBL-producing bacteria in the community has begun influencing outpatient therapy. Community-acquired bacteremia, due to ESBL-producing *E. coli* strains, is becoming a critical concern for outpatients, because inappropriate use of empirical antibiotics, such as cephalosporins and fluoroquinolones, has resulted in high mortality. [65,66] One study has shown that the resistance of CTX-M-15-producing ST131 *E. coli* strains isolated from the community to fosfomycin has increased. [67] In the near future, we may be forced to use carbapenems as the first choice for the empirical therapy of patients with community-acquired infections due to ESBL-producing bacteria. The identification of carbapenemase-producing *E coli* and *K. pneumoniae* strains has been frequently documented as evidence for additional β-lactamases-producing bacteria other than the ESBL-producing bacteria. [68] The study of NDM-1-type carbapenemase-producing *E coli* and *K. pneumoniae* is currently a topic of much interest in multidrug-resistant bacteria research. Notably, some of the NDM-1-type-producing *E coli* and *K. pneumoniae* strains express *bla*CTX-M-15 ESBL genes in a single isolate. [69,70,71] A worldwide surveillance recently showed that many NDM-1-producing bacteria detected carried additional ESBL genes. [72] The acquisition of efficient mobile elements has accelerated the transfer of various antibiotic resistance genes. Potentially, a "super bug," resistant to almost all licensed antibiotics, may emerge in the future. Constant and careful worldwide surveillance for multidrug-resistant bacteria is urgently warranted.

9. References

[1] Paterson DL, Bonomo RA. Extended-spectrum beta-lactamases: a clinical update. *Clin Microbiol Rev* 2005; 18: 657-86.

[2] Livermore DM. beta-Lactamases in laboratory and clinical resistance. *Clin Microbiol Rev* 1995; 8: 557-84.

[3] Knothe H, Shah P, Krcmery V, Antal M, Mitsuhashi S. Transferable resistance to cefotaxime, cefoxitin, cefamandole and cefuroxime in clinical isolates of Klebsiella pneumoniae and Serratia marcescens. *Infection* 1983; 11: 315-7.

[4] Brun-Buisson C, Legrand P, Philippon A, Montravers F, Ansquer M, Duval J. Transferable enzymatic resistance to third-generation cephalosporins during nosocomial outbreak of multiresistant Klebsiella pneumoniae. *Lancet* 1987; 2: 302-6.

[5] Philippon A, Labia R, Jacoby G. Extended-spectrum beta-lactamases. *Antimicrob Agents Chemother* 1989; 33: 1131-6.

[6] Bauernfeind A, Grimm H, Schweighart S. A new plasmidic cefotaximase in a clinical isolate of Escherichia coli. *Infection* 1990; 18: 294-8.

[7] Bonnet R. Growing group of extended-spectrum beta-lactamases: the CTX-M enzymes. *Antimicrob Agents Chemother* 2004; 48: 1-14.

[8] Pitout JD, Laupland KB. Extended-spectrum beta-lactamase-producing Enterobacteriaceae: an emerging public-health concern. *Lancet Infect Dis* 2008; 8: 159-66.

[9] Talbot GH, Bradley J, Edwards JE, Jr., Gilbert D, Scheld M, Bartlett JG. Bad bugs need drugs: an update on the development pipeline from the Antimicrobial Availability Task Force of the Infectious Diseases Society of America. *Clin Infect Dis* 2006; 42: 657-68.

[10] Jacoby GA, Munoz-Price LS. The new beta-lactamases. *N Engl J Med* 2005; 352: 380-91.

[11] Oteo J, Perez-Vazquez M, Campos J. Extended-spectrum [beta]-lactamase producing Escherichia coli: changing epidemiology and clinical impact. *Curr Opin Infect Dis* 2010; 23: 320-6.

[12] Reinert RR, Low DE, Rossi F, Zhang X, Wattal C, Dowzicky MJ. Antimicrobial susceptibility among organisms from the Asia/Pacific Rim, Europe and Latin and North America collected as part of TEST and the in vitro activity of tigecycline. *J Antimicrob Chemother* 2007; 60: 1018-29.

[13] Hawser SP, Bouchillon SK, Hoban DJ, Badal RE, Hsueh PR, Paterson DL. Emergence of high levels of extended-spectrum-beta-lactamase-producing gram-negative bacilli in the Asia-Pacific region: data from the Study for Monitoring Antimicrobial Resistance Trends (SMART) program, 2007. *Antimicrob Agents Chemother* 2009; 53: 3280-4.

[14] Lee MY, Ko KS, Kang CI, Chung DR, Peck KR, Song JH. High prevalence of CTX-M-15-producing Klebsiella pneumoniae isolates in Asian countries: diverse clones and clonal dissemination. *Int J Antimicrob Agents* 2011; 38: 160-3.

[15] Chong Y, Yakushiji H, Ito Y, Kamimura T. Clinical and molecular epidemiology of extended-spectrum beta-lactamase-producing Escherichia coli and Klebsiella pneumoniae in a long-term study from Japan. *Eur J Clin Microbiol Infect Dis* 2011; 30: 83-7.

[16] Canton R, Novais A, Valverde A, Machado E, Peixe L, Baquero F et al. Prevalence and spread of extended-spectrum beta-lactamase-producing Enterobacteriaceae in Europe. *Clin Microbiol Infect* 2008; 14 Suppl 1: 144-53.

[17] Rossolini GM, D'Andrea MM, Mugnaioli C. The spread of CTX-M-type extended-spectrum beta-lactamases. *Clin Microbiol Infect* 2008; 14 Suppl 1: 33-41.

[18] Canton R, Coque TM. The CTX-M beta-lactamase pandemic. *Curr Opin Microbiol* 2006; 9: 466-75.

[19] Suzuki S, Shibata N, Yamane K, Wachino J, Ito K, Arakawa Y. Change in the prevalence of extended-spectrum-beta-lactamase-producing Escherichia coli in Japan by clonal spread. *J Antimicrob Chemother* 2009; 63: 72-9.

[20] Lewis JS, 2nd, Herrera M, Wickes B, Patterson JE, Jorgensen JH. First report of the emergence of CTX-M-type extended-spectrum beta-lactamases (ESBLs) as the predominant ESBL isolated in a U.S. health care system. *Antimicrob Agents Chemother* 2007; 51: 4015-21.

[21] Sidjabat HE, Paterson DL, Adams-Haduch JM, Ewan L, Pasculle AW, Muto CA et al. Molecular epidemiology of CTX-M-producing Escherichia coli isolates at a tertiary medical center in western Pennsylvania. *Antimicrob Agents Chemother* 2009; 53: 4733-9.

[22] Poirel L, Naas T, Nordmann P. Genetic support of extended-spectrum beta-lactamases. *Clin Microbiol Infect* 2008; 14 Suppl 1: 75-81.

[23] Babini GS, Livermore DM. Are SHV beta-lactamases universal in Klebsiella pneumoniae? *Antimicrob Agents Chemother* 2000; 44: 2230.

[24] Novais A, Canton R, Valverde A, Machado E, Galan JC, Peixe L et al. Dissemination and persistence of blaCTX-M-9 are linked to class 1 integrons containing CR1 associated with defective transposon derivatives from Tn402 located in early antibiotic resistance plasmids of IncHI2, IncP1-alpha, and IncFI groups. *Antimicrob Agents Chemother* 2006; 50: 2741-50.

[25] Poirel L, Lartigue MF, Decousser JW, Nordmann P. ISEcp1B-mediated transposition of blaCTX-M in Escherichia coli. *Antimicrob Agents Chemother* 2005; 49: 447-50.

[26] Toleman MA, Bennett PM, Walsh TR. ISCR elements: novel gene-capturing systems of the 21st century? *Microbiol Mol Biol Rev* 2006; 70: 296-316.

[27] Palucha A, Mikiewicz B, Hryniewicz W, Gniadkowski M. Concurrent outbreaks of extended-spectrum beta-lactamase-producing organisms of the family Enterobacteriaceae in a Warsaw hospital. *J Antimicrob Chemother* 1999; 44: 489-99.

[28] Baraniak A, Fiett J, Sulikowska A, Hryniewicz W, Gniadkowski M. Countrywide spread of CTX-M-3 extended-spectrum beta-lactamase-producing microorganisms of the family Enterobacteriaceae in Poland. *Antimicrob Agents Chemother* 2002; 46: 151-9.

[29] Carattoli A. Resistance plasmid families in Enterobacteriaceae. *Antimicrob Agents Chemother* 2009; 53: 2227-38.

[30] Diestra K, Juan C, Curiao T, Moya B, Miro E, Oteo J et al. Characterization of plasmids encoding blaESBL and surrounding genes in Spanish clinical isolates of Escherichia coli and Klebsiella pneumoniae. *J Antimicrob Chemother* 2009; 63: 60-6.

[31] Lavollay M, Mamlouk K, Frank T, Akpabie A, Burghoffer B, Ben Redjeb S et al. Clonal dissemination of a CTX-M-15 beta-lactamase-producing Escherichia coli strain in the Paris area, Tunis, and Bangui. *Antimicrob Agents Chemother* 2006; 50: 2433-8.

[32] Yuan M, Aucken H, Hall LM, Pitt TL, Livermore DM. Epidemiological typing of klebsiellae with extended-spectrum beta-lactamases from European intensive care units. *J Antimicrob Chemother* 1998; 41: 527-39.

[33] Valverde A, Coque TM, Garcia-San Miguel L, Baquero F, Canton R. Complex molecular epidemiology of extended-spectrum beta-lactamases in Klebsiella pneumoniae: a long-term perspective from a single institution in Madrid. *J Antimicrob Chemother* 2008; 61: 64-72.

[34] Ramdani-Bouguessa N, Manageiro V, Jones-Dias D, Ferreira E, Tazir M, Canica M. Role of SHV {beta}-lactamase variants in resistance of clinical Klebsiella pneumoniae strains to {beta}-lactams in an Algerian hospital. *J Med Microbiol* 2011; 60: 983-7.

[35] Valverde A, Coque TM, Sanchez-Moreno MP, Rollan A, Baquero F, Canton R. Dramatic increase in prevalence of fecal carriage of extended-spectrum beta-lactamase-producing Enterobacteriaceae during nonoutbreak situations in Spain. *J Clin Microbiol* 2004; 42: 4769-75.

[36] Woerther PL, Angebault C, Lescat M, Ruppe E, Skurnik D, Mniai AE et al. Emergence and dissemination of extended-spectrum beta-lactamase-producing Escherichia coli in the community: lessons from the study of a remote and controlled population. *J Infect Dis* 2010; 202: 515-23.

[37] Rodriguez-Bano J, Lopez-Cerero L, Navarro MD, Diaz de Alba P, Pascual A. Faecal carriage of extended-spectrum beta-lactamase-producing Escherichia coli: prevalence, risk factors and molecular epidemiology. *J Antimicrob Chemother* 2008; 62: 1142-9.

[38] Kojima A, Ishii Y, Ishihara K, Esaki H, Asai T, Oda C et al. Extended-spectrum-beta-lactamase-producing Escherichia coli strains isolated from farm animals from 1999 to 2002: report from the Japanese Veterinary Antimicrobial Resistance Monitoring Program. *Antimicrob Agents Chemother* 2005; 49: 3533-7.

[39] Carattoli A, Lovari S, Franco A, Cordaro G, Di Matteo P, Battisti A. Extended-spectrum beta-lactamases in Escherichia coli isolated from dogs and cats in Rome, Italy, from 2001 to 2003. *Antimicrob Agents Chemother* 2005; 49: 833-5.

[40] Ho PL, Chow KH, Lai EL, Lo WU, Yeung MK, Chan J et al. Extensive dissemination of CTX-M-producing Escherichia coli with multidrug resistance to 'critically important' antibiotics among food animals in Hong Kong, 2008-10. *J Antimicrob Chemother* 2011; 66: 765-8.

[41] Leverstein-van Hall MA, Dierikx CM, Cohen Stuart J, Voets GM, van den Munckhof MP, van Essen-Zandbergen A et al. Dutch patients, retail chicken meat and poultry share the same ESBL genes, plasmids and strains. *Clin Microbiol Infect* 2011; 17: 873-80.

[42] Deschamps C, Clermont O, Hipeaux MC, Arlet G, Denamur E, Branger C. Multiple acquisitions of CTX-M plasmids in the rare D2 genotype of Escherichia coli provide evidence for convergent evolution. *Microbiology* 2009; 155: 1656-68.

[43] Branger C, Zamfir O, Geoffroy S, Laurans G, Arlet G, Thien HV et al. Genetic background of Escherichia coli and extended-spectrum beta-lactamase type. *Emerg Infect Dis* 2005; 11: 54-61.

[44] Ben-Ami R, Schwaber MJ, Navon-Venezia S, Schwartz D, Giladi M, Chmelnitsky I et al. Influx of extended-spectrum beta-lactamase-producing enterobacteriaceae into the hospital. *Clin Infect Dis* 2006; 42: 925-34.

[45] Pitout JD, Gregson DB, Campbell L, Laupland KB. Molecular characteristics of extended-spectrum-beta-lactamase-producing Escherichia coli isolates causing bacteremia in the Calgary Health Region from 2000 to 2007: emergence of clone ST131 as a cause of community-acquired infections. *Antimicrob Agents Chemother* 2009; 53: 2846-51.

[46] Meier S, Weber R, Zbinden R, Ruef C, Hasse B. Extended-spectrum beta-lactamase-producing Gram-negative pathogens in community-acquired urinary tract infections: an increasing challenge for antimicrobial therapy. *Infection* 2011.

[47] Calbo E, Freixas N, Xercavins M, Riera M, Nicolas C, Monistrol O et al. Foodborne nosocomial outbreak of SHV1 and CTX-M-15-producing Klebsiella pneumoniae: epidemiology and control. *Clin Infect Dis* 2011; 52: 743-9.

[48] Schwaber MJ, Carmeli Y. Mortality and delay in effective therapy associated with extended-spectrum beta-lactamase production in Enterobacteriaceae bacteraemia: a systematic review and meta-analysis. *J Antimicrob Chemother* 2007; 60: 913-20.

[49] Morosini MI, Garcia-Castillo M, Coque TM, Valverde A, Novais A, Loza E et al. Antibiotic coresistance in extended-spectrum-beta-lactamase-producing Enterobacteriaceae and in vitro activity of tigecycline. *Antimicrob Agents Chemother* 2006; 50: 2695-9.

[50] Kelesidis T, Karageorgopoulos DE, Kelesidis I, Falagas ME. Tigecycline for the treatment of multidrug-resistant Enterobacteriaceae: a systematic review of the evidence from microbiological and clinical studies. *J Antimicrob Chemother* 2008; 62: 895-904.

[51] Falagas ME, Kastoris AC, Kapaskelis AM, Karageorgopoulos DE. Fosfomycin for the treatment of multidrug-resistant, including extended-spectrum beta-lactamase producing, Enterobacteriaceae infections: a systematic review. *Lancet Infect Dis* 2010; 10: 43-50.

[52] Rodriguez-Bano J, Alcala JC, Cisneros JM, Grill F, Oliver A, Horcajada JP et al. Community infections caused by extended-spectrum beta-lactamase-producing Escherichia coli. *Arch Intern Med* 2008; 168: 1897-902.

[53] Karim A, Poirel L, Nagarajan S, Nordmann P. Plasmid-mediated extended-spectrum beta-lactamase (CTX-M-3 like) from India and gene association with insertion sequence ISEcp1. *FEMS Microbiol Lett* 2001; 201: 237-41.

[54] Boyd DA, Tyler S, Christianson S, McGeer A, Muller MP, Willey BM et al. Complete nucleotide sequence of a 92-kilobase plasmid harboring the CTX-M-15 extended-spectrum beta-lactamase involved in an outbreak in long-term-care facilities in Toronto, Canada. *Antimicrob Agents Chemother* 2004; 48: 3758-64.

[55] Marcade G, Deschamps C, Boyd A, Gautier V, Picard B, Branger C et al. Replicon typing of plasmids in Escherichia coli producing extended-spectrum beta-lactamases. *J Antimicrob Chemother* 2009; 63: 67-71.

[56] Peirano G, Pitout JD. Molecular epidemiology of Escherichia coli producing CTX-M beta-lactamases: the worldwide emergence of clone ST131 O25:H4. *Int J Antimicrob Agents* 2010; 35: 316-21.

[57] Mnif B, Vimont S, Boyd A, Bourit E, Picard B, Branger C et al. Molecular characterization of addiction systems of plasmids encoding extended-spectrum beta-lactamases in Escherichia coli. *J Antimicrob Chemother* 2010; 65: 1599-603.

[58] Nicolas-Chanoine MH, Blanco J, Leflon-Guibout V, Demarty R, Alonso MP, Canica MM et al. Intercontinental emergence of Escherichia coli clone O25:H4-ST131 producing CTX-M-15. *J Antimicrob Chemother* 2008; 61: 273-81.

[59] Peirano G, Costello M, Pitout JD. Molecular characteristics of extended-spectrum beta-lactamase-producing Escherichia coli from the Chicago area: high prevalence of ST131 producing CTX-M-15 in community hospitals. *Int J Antimicrob Agents* 2010; 36: 19-23.

[60] Johnson JR, Johnston B, Clabots C, Kuskowski MA, Castanheira M. Escherichia coli sequence type ST131 as the major cause of serious multidrug-resistant E. coli infections in the United States. *Clin Infect Dis* 2010; 51: 286-94.

[61] Gudiol C, Calatayud L, Garcia-Vidal C, Lora-Tamayo J, Cisnal M, Duarte R et al. Bacteraemia due to extended-spectrum beta-lactamase-producing Escherichia coli (ESBL-EC) in cancer patients: clinical features, risk factors, molecular epidemiology and outcome. *J Antimicrob Chemother* 2010; 65: 333-41.

[62] Chong Y, Yakushiji H, Ito Y, Kamimura T. Cefepime-resistant Gram-negative bacteremia in febrile neutropenic patients with hematological malignancies. *Int J Infect Dis* 2010; 14 Suppl 3: e171-5.

[63] Muratani T, Kobayashi T, Matsumoto T. Emergence and prevalence of beta-lactamase-producing Klebsiella pneumoniae resistant to cephems in Japan. *Int J Antimicrob Agents* 2006; 27: 491-9.

[64] Vigil KJ, Johnson JR, Johnston BD, Kontoyiannis DP, Mulanovich VE, Raad, II et al. Escherichia coli Pyomyositis: an emerging infectious disease among patients with hematologic malignancies. *Clin Infect Dis* 2010; 50: 374-80.

[65] Rodriguez-Bano J, Navarro MD, Romero L, Muniain MA, de Cueto M, Rios MJ et al. Bacteremia due to extended-spectrum beta -lactamase-producing Escherichia coli in the CTX-M era: a new clinical challenge. *Clin Infect Dis* 2006; 43: 1407-14.

[66] Rodriguez-Bano J, Picon E, Gijon P, Hernandez JR, Ruiz M, Pena C et al. Community-onset bacteremia due to extended-spectrum beta-lactamase-producing Escherichia coli: risk factors and prognosis. *Clin Infect Dis* 2010; 50: 40-8.

[67] Oteo J, Orden B, Bautista V, Cuevas O, Arroyo M, Martinez-Ruiz R et al. CTX-M-15-producing urinary Escherichia coli O25b-ST131-phylogroup B2 has acquired resistance to fosfomycin. *J Antimicrob Chemother* 2009; 64: 712-7.

[68] Bush K. Alarming beta-lactamase-mediated resistance in multidrug-resistant Enterobacteriaceae. *Curr Opin Microbiol* 2010; 13: 558-64.

[69] Poirel L, Al Maskari Z, Al Rashdi F, Bernabeu S, Nordmann P. NDM-1-producing Klebsiella pneumoniae isolated in the Sultanate of Oman. *J Antimicrob Chemother* 2010.

[70] Poirel L, Lagrutta E, Taylor P, Pham J, Nordmann P. Emergence of metallo-beta-lactamase NDM-1-producing multidrug-resistant Escherichia coli in Australia. *Antimicrob Agents Chemother* 2010; 54: 4914-6.

[71] Poirel L, Revathi G, Bernabeu S, Nordmann P. Detection of NDM-1-Producing Klebsiella pneumoniae in Kenya. *Antimicrob Agents Chemother* 2011; 55: 934-6.

[72] Lascols C, Hackel M, Marshall SH, Hujer AM, Bouchillon S, Badal R et al. Increasing prevalence and dissemination of NDM-1 metallo-{beta}-lactamase in India: data from the SMART study (2009). *J Antimicrob Chemother* 2011.

19

Occurrence, Antibiotic Resistance and Pathogenicity of Non-O1 *Vibrio cholerae* in Moroccan Aquatic Ecosystems: A Review

Khalid Oufdou and Nour-Eddine Mezrioui
Laboratory of Biology and Biotechnology of Microorganisms, Faculty of Sciences, Semlalia, Cadi Ayyad University, Morocco

1. Introduction

The problem of water scarcity is becoming more pronounced especially in countries with arid and semi-arid climates such as Morocco. Wastewaters discharge into different aquatic ecosystems (groundwater, sea water, river, lake water...), are draining different types of microorganisms and hazardous chemicals. The microbiological risk is not negligible, especially in areas where wastewater or other contaminated water, are reused for irrigation without preliminary treatment or for direct consumption by human and animals.

The emergence of bacteria resistant to antibiotics is common in areas where antibiotics are widely used, but the occurrence of antibiotic-resistant bacteria is also increasing in aquatic environments. Some pathogenic bacteria may occur naturally with the spread of resistance genes.

Vibrio cholerae is a natural inhabitant of the aquatic environment where water plays an important role in its transmission and epidemiology (WHO 1993; Chakraborty et al. 1997). This bacterium plays a role in ecological ecosystems and it is widely distributed in bays, estuaries, coastal water, reservoirs, rivers and possible water supplies for human consumption (Pathak et al., 1992; Caldini et al., 1997; Isaac-Marquez et al., 1998; Dumont et al., 2000).

The interest in examining the non-O1 serogroup of *V. cholerae* has been accentuated at an international level, given that some recent epidemic outbreaks in India and Bangladesh have been caused by non-O1 *V. cholerae* isolated in aquatic environment (Ramamurthy et al., 1993). Currently, it is recognized that non-O1 *V. cholerae* plays an important role as the causative agent of sporadic cases of cholera-like disease and isolated outbreaks linked to the consumption of contaminated water (Yamamoto et al., 1983; Chakraborty et al., 1997; Bag et al., 2008). Non-O1 *V. cholerae* has also been implicated in extra intestinal infections, including wounds, ear, sputum, urine and cerebrospinal fluid (WHO, 1993).

Resistance of *V. cholerae* to commonly used antimicrobials is increasing both in the farm animal and public health sectors and has emerged as a global problem.

This review present a synthesis of our research works on non-O1 *V. cholerae* since 1992, in comparison to faecal indicator bacteria, in some Moroccan aquatic ecosystems especially in wastewaters and groundwaters. We will discuss and compare our works with some other studies over the world.

2. Occurrence, pathogenicity of non-O1 *V. cholerae* in some Moroccan aquatic ecosystems

2.1 Occurrence and ecology of non-O1 *V. cholerae*

The use of untreated wastewater for agriculture irrigation poses serious health problems over the world. Several treatment systems of wastewater were developed to reduce the load of pollution. The stabilization pond system was tested in Marrakech region (Mezrioui et al., 1995; Mezrioui & Oufdou, 1996; Oufdou et al. 2004). It is composed of two oval ponds linked in series, each is of 2500 m^2 in area. The first pond is anaerobic (depth of water 2.3 m) and the second pond is facultative aerobic (depth : 1.5 m). The raw sewage flow to the system is maintained at 5.4 L/sec. The total hydraulic retention time was set at about 18 days with 10.5 days in the first pond and 7.5 days in the second pond.

Non-O1 *V. cholerae* was quantified using the most probale number (MPN) method using three tubes or flasks per inoculated volume and a series of 100, 10, 1 mL, and dilutions of water. They were inoculated into the three tubes with 3 stages: (i) enrichment by culture of 100, 10 or 1 mL of the sample from the series of three tubes of alkaline peptone water (1% peptone, 1% NaCl, pH 8.6) incubated at 37 °C for 18 h. (ii) Isolation was performed by culture of 0.1 mL taken from the surface in each enrichment tube or from one of its dilutions on thiosulfate-citrate-bile-sucrose agar (TCBS), incubated at 37 °C for 24 h. (iii) Identification of the colonies assumed to be those of non-O1 *V. cholerae* was carried out according to the methodology described by Lesne *et al.* (1991), Mezrioui and Oufdou (1996), Lamrani Alaoui et al. (2008) and Lamrani et al. (2010).

The seasonal abundance of non-O1 *V. cholerae* in wastewaters before and after treatment in stabilization ponds in an arid Mediterranean climate has been undertaken. A series of stations along the two stabilization ponds were sampled during two periods. The cold (or hot) period corresponds to months when the water temperature is below (or above) 22°C. This temperature was the average water temperature for the whole period of study (16 months).

Results showed that high abundances of non-O1 *V. cholerae* were noted during the hot months and low abundances during the cold months. In treated wastewaters, high abundances of non-O1 *V. cholerae* were recorded during hot period with an average abundance of $1.7x10^3$ MPN/mL. During cold periods, these densities were calculated to be $2.5x10^1$ MPN mL^{-1}. These seasonal dynamics were confirmed by the autocorrelation coefficient showing the cyclic nature of non-O1 *V. cholerae* abundances (Mezrioui et al., 1995).

In contrast, the spatial-temporal dynamics of faecal coliforms (FC) were the inverse of those of non-O1 *V. cholerae* abundances. Average FC abundances at the system's inflow point were $1.7x10^5$ cfu/mL, while at the seconf pond's outflow, they were $8.3x10^3$ cfu/mL.

The average seasonal variation of FC abundances at the second pond's outflow point was evaluated to 8.3x10^3 cfu/mL at the cold period and 1.8x10^3 cfu/mL at the hot period (Mezrioui & Oufdou, 1996). The inverse relationship between non-O1 *V. cholerae* and FC was more pronounced at the outflow point of the second pond (R^2= 0.68) than that of the first pond (R^2= 0.51).

As for removal efficiency, stabilization pond system of Marrakech led to 97.97% average overall reduction in FCs, whereas this system treatment is not efficient in removing non-O1 *V. cholerae* abundances (Mezrioui et al., 1995; Mezrioui & Oufdou, 1996).

We have also followed the dynamics of non-O1 *V. cholerae* in Marrakech groundwater (in supplying well waters) in comparison with other bacteria of sanitary interest. Sixteen wells covering two regions (Tensift and Jbilet) were studied. They are situated at the North of Marrakesh city (31°36′ N, 08°02′ W, Morocco) (Lamrani et al., 2010).

Detectable non-O1 *V. cholerae* was present in 81% of samples and the average abundances ranged from 0 to 11100 MPN/100 mL. Detectable *P. aeruginosa* was present in 88% of samples and its abundances ranged from 0 to 1670 cfu/100 mL. The total occurrence of FC and Faecal Streptococci (FS) during the period of study was 94% and their densities varied respectively from a minimum of 0 cfu/100 mL to a maximum of 10200 cfu/100 mL for FC and 6700 cfu/100 mL for FS. The annual average densities of non-O1 *V. cholerae* were 4903 MPN/100 mL in all samples. Whereas, the annual average densities of *P. aeruginosa*, FC and FS were respectively 206 cfu/100 mL, 1891 cfu/100 mL and 1246 cfu/100 mL (Lamrani et al., 2010).

Our results demonstrated that non-O1 *V. cholerae* and the other studied bacteria, occurred in the majority of the studied wells water. These wells serve as an important natural resource for drinking water, domestic water supply and recreation for rural and suburban populations. This fact could be responsible for potential health effects on populations using this groundwater. According to WHO standards, the studied wells are completely unsuitable for drinking water and other domestic uses.

The highest abundances of studied bacteria were detected at the wells located near malfunctioning septic systems or beside a high number of pollution sources such as infiltration of wastewater, septic tanks seepage, discharge leachates or human and animal faecal materials nearby the studied wells. Moreover, the majority of the studied wells are situated at 0 m to 400 m from pollution sources. These factors led to the contamination of the groundwater.

Based on the results of the present study, it is possible to conclude that groundwater can play an important role as a transmission vehicle of non-O1 *V. cholerae* and the other studied bacteria. Isaac-Marquez et al. (1998) considered that the presence of non-O1 *V. cholerae* in water supplies might be responsible for a proportion of diarrheic diseases among population of the city of Campeche and the rural locality of Becal (Mexico). Several reports have demonstrated that gastrointestinal and extra-intestinal infections caused by non-O1 *V. cholerae* are linked with contaminated water and other activities in aquatic environments, and this bacterium could therefore pose a problem for public health (WHO, 1993; Chakraborty et al., 1997).

Our findings (Lamrani et al. 2010) are in agreement with those reported by Nogueira *et al.* (2003) and Isaac-Marquez *et al.* (1998). These authors investigated water quality at sources and points of consumption of urban and rural communities. According to these authors, water distribution system, spring water and private wells samples had high coliforms positive and high percentages of non-O1 *V. cholerae.*

The comparison of non-O1 *V. cholerae* and FC abundances, using the Spearman correlation test, has showed that there is generally a positive relationship between these bacteria in the studied wells. FC can be used to detect the presence of non-O1 *V. cholerae* in Marrakesh groundwater. However, no significant relationship was observed between the presence of non-O1 *V. cholerae* and *P. aeruginosa* (Lamrani et al., 2010).

The ecological role of *V. cholerae* in environment implies a direct influence of environmental conditions and climate on the presence, persistence and abundance of bacteria in the aquatic ecosystem. To explain this difference of behavior of these bacteria, we have established the correlation of some of these factors with non-O1 *V. cholerae* abundances. We also tested some experimental studies on the effects of some environmental factors (temperature, pH, sunlight and algae) on survival of non-O1 *V. cholerae* compared to faecal indicator bacteria (Oufdou et al., 1998; Oufdou et al., 1999; Lamrani et al., 2009; Oufdou & Oudra, 2009).

The correlation of non-01 *V. cholerae* abundances in Marrakech stabilization ponds (Spearman correlation) was carried out. A positive and very significant correlation ($p<0.01$) between water temperature and pH was observed at the system's outflow point. At this point, Spearman coefficients values were respectively 0.91 and 0.76. In the system's inflow, an extremely significant correlation was observed only with temperature (Mezrioui et al., 1995).

The experimental effects of pH, temperature and sunlight were carried out. The strains of non-O1 *V. cholerae* and *E. coli* tested were isolated from the first pond of Marrakech stabilization pond. The survival of these bacteria was studied in experimental microcosms of 500mL flasks, each contained 200mL of filtered outflow water. Each microcosm was seeded separately with a standard inoculums (approximately 10^5 cfu/mL) prepared from a bacterial suspension (non-O1 *V. cholerae* or *E. coli*) in physiological water (0.9% NaCl).

The pH values tested (6.6, 7.3, 8 and 8.8) and the temperature values tested (8, 15, 23 and 30°C) corresponded to those measured at the stabilization ponds over the year.

The effect on bacterial survival was evaluated after calculation of the die-off coefficient *k* which is determined in accordance with the formula:

$$N_t = N_0 e^{-kt}$$

Where N_0 and N_t are respectively the initial bacterial number and the number of bacteria at time t. *k* is the die-off coefficients expressed in hourly terms (/h) (Crane and Moore, 1986).

The effect of pH on the behaviour of non-O1 *V. choleare* differed from the effect on *E. coli.* The greatest survival of non-O1 *V. cholerae* was at pH 8 (k = 0.0164/h) followed by the pH 8.8 (k= 0.0170/h). Whereas at the pH values of 6.6 and 7.3, the die-off coefficient were respectively 0.0197/h and 0.0195/h. The alkaline pH of 8.8 promoted survival of non-O1 *V. cholerae* (k=0.0170/h) and reduced that of *E. coli* (k=0.0232/h). At neutral pH (7.3), non-O1 *V. cholerae* did not survive as well (k= 0.0195/h) as *E. coli* (k=0.0124/h).

The minor variations in pH occurring in natural environments, making pH a relatively unimportant variable compared with other environmental factors, such as sunlight, temperature... However, in aquatic ecosystems such as stabilization ponds, phytoplanktonic blooms appears systematically and increase pH values (Oufdou et al., 2004; Oufdou & Oudra, 2008). The pH is a parameter that was used to improve the isolation of *V. cholerae* environmental samples by enrichment (using alkaline peptone water at pH 8.6) (Lipp et al., 2002).

Non-01 *V. cholerae* and *E. coli* survived longer at low temperatures. The survival of both bacteria was noticeably reduced at 23 and 30°C. This low survival rate of non-01 *V. cholerae* did not explain the high positive correlation between the non-01 *V. cholerae* abundances and temperature. Indeed, it would appear that the effect of temperature is a function of other factors such as nutrients. In microcosms such as flasks, where there is considerable confinement, nutrients are heavily depleted at 23 or 30°C, with a resultant decrease in bacterial survival. In the environments like wastewater, where there is no lack of nutrients, high temperatures lead to a multiplication of bacteria.

Solar radiation had a much greater effect on *E. coli* than it did on non-O1 *V. cholerae* (Mezrioui et al. 1995). This difference in bacterial survival as a result of sunlight factor could be explained by a difference in the bacterial's reaction to sunlight. Indeed, sunlight is absorber by a sensitizer that reacts with oxygen to form peroxides or hydroxyl radicals (Curtis et al., 1992). These authors indicated that damage to the membrane of an organism is ecologically important, since it makes the organism more sensitive to the effects of other factors such as the high pH values encountered in stabilization ponds. The obtained results by Mezrioui et al. (1995) showed that alkaline pH values inhibit the survival of *E. coli*, and its survival is thus less after exposure to sunlight. Non-O1 *V. cholerae*, on other hand, which survived better at pH 8 than at pH 7.3, is less sensitive to sunlight.

The effect of the cyanobacterium *Synechocystis* sp. on the survival of non-O1 *V. cholerae* was carried out (Oufdou et al., 1998 ; Oufdou et al., 2000). Blooms of this cyanobacterium occur during hot periods in wastewater stabilization ponds of Marrakech. Oufdou et al. (1998) have studied the effect of the picocyanobacterium Chroococcale: *Synechocystis* sp. on the behaviour of non-O1 *V. cholerae* in comparison to those of *E. coli* and *Salmonella* sp.. *Synechocystis* sp. was isolated from this ecosystem and cultivated in laboratory at controlled conditions of light and temperature.

Extracellular and intracellular products released by this microalga were tested on studied bacteria. Extracellular products obtained at the supernatant of algal culture in stationary phase, reduced *E. coli* and *Salmonella* sp. growth and stimulated non-O1 *V. cholerae* growth. Intracellular products obtained after lysing algal cells by ether, reduced *E. coli* and *Salmonella* sp. growth. The effect of products released by *Synechocystis* sp. was compared for axenic and non axenic strain alga. Obtained results showed that the presence of heterotrophic bacteria increased the reduction of *E. coli* and *Salmonella* sp. growth by extracellular and intracellular products of *Synechocystis* sp..

Blooms of this picocyanobacterium in Marrakech waste stabilization ponds, is among the important factors that affect the dynamics and survival of studied bacteria in this aquatic ecosystems which functions under a Mediterranean arid climate.

2.2 Pathogenicity of non-O1 *V. cholerae*

Several virulence factors such heat stable toxin (ST) (Arita et al., 1986), hemolysin (Yoh et al., 1986; Bag et al., 2008) and other cell-associated hemagglutinins (Banerjee et al., 1990) have been identified in non-O1 *V. cholerae.* Production of hemolysin and surface hemagglutinins of pathogenic bacteria, are important virulence determinants as they may serve as recognition and invasion molecules in cell-cell interaction affecting the host-pathogen relationship (Guhathakurta et al., 1999; Singh et al., 2001; Chatterjee et al., 2009). It has been demonstrated that non-O1 *V. cholerae* adheres and invades the epithelial cells of gut mucosa and starts its multiplication (Nishibuchi et al., 1983). This situation occurs only with expression of certain virulence factors as previously cited (Nishibuchi et al., 1983; O'Brien et al., 1984; Ichinose et al., 1987).

To characterize the virulence factors of the bacterial isolates in our study, hemolysis and hemagglutination with human erythrocytes were realized.

The hemagglutination and hemolytic activities of non-O1 *V. cholerae* strains isolated from wastewater and suburban and rural groundwater supplies of Marrakech region were carried out. Non-O1 *V. cholerae* strains isolated from Marrakech wastewater showed a hemagglutination rate of 55%. The distinction between the degrees of hemagglutination showed that 42.5% of non-O1 *V. cholerae* strains are able to agglutinate with a high level, red cells of human blood O group, while the percentage of strains showing hemagglutination reaction with low level is only 12.5%. As for the production of hemolysins, non-O1 *V. cholerae* strains showed 37.5% of β-hemolytic activity whereas no hemolytic activity α was noted.

In the groundwater, bacterial strains were found to be adhesive (hemagglutination), with percentages of 63.09%, 65.09%, 84.06% and 87.98% respectively for non-O1 *V. cholerae*, FS, FC and *P. aeruginosa.* Non-O1 *V. cholerae* strains had the highest percentage of hemolytic activities (production of hemolysin: α+β) (71.29%), in comparison to FS (20.71%), to FC (16.88%) and to *P. aeruginosa* strains (9.13%).

Analysis of a total of 1183 strains isolated from the studied wells, revealed that non-O1 *V. cholerae* had the highest β hemolytic activity (33.12%), while only 3.44% of FC and 4.44% of FS strains have this type of hemolysis. As for *P. aeruginosa,* β hemolytic activity was very low (1.44%). FC, FS and *P. aeruginosa* strains isolated from Marrakech groundwater expressed significantly lower hemolytic activity compared to non-O1 *V. cholerae* ($P < 0.05$, test of two proportions). Hemolysin of *V. cholerae* is suggested to be a virulence factor contributing towards pathogenesis (Nagamune et al., 1995). Guhathakurta et al. (1999) purified a bifunctional hemolysin-phospholipase C molecule from non-O1 *V. cholerae* (O139) showing enterotoxic activity, as shown by fluid accumulation in the ligated rabbit ileal loop and in the intestine of suckling mice (Pal et al., 1998).

The percentages of hemolytic isolates observed in this study are comparable to those reported by Begum et al. (2006). These authors found that 80% of the total non-O1 and non-O139 *V. cholerae* isolates were hemolysin positive. However, our results were lower than those obtained by Amaro et al. (1990). These authors showed that 97% of environmental non-O1 *V. cholerae* strains displayed hemolytic activity for human blood.

Adhesion to the intestinal mucosa represents the first step in the infectivity of bacterial pathogens such as *V. cholerae* (Booth and Finkelstein, 1986). This process is mediated by non-specific (mainly hydrophobic) and specific (binding of the bacterial adhesin with its receptor on the epithelial cell) interactions (Kabir and Ali, 1983). Agglutination of erythrocytes is among the most useful assays to test the attachment ability of potential pathogens.

Bacterial strains isolated from Marrakesh groundwater were found to be adhesive, with a range of hemagglutination activities varying from 63.09% for non-O1 *V. cholerae* to 65.09% for FS, 84.06% for FC and 87.98% for *P. aeruginosa.*

Among 317 strains of non-O1 *V. cholerae,* 60 strains (18.93%) were strongly adhesive (+2) and 140 (44.16%) were partially agglutinated (+1) to erythrocytes. On the other hand, 69.06% of FC strains and 62.02% of *P. aeruginosa* expressed complete agglutination (+2) capacity, and respectively 15% and 25.96% of them agglutinated partially (+1) to erythrocytes.

Our findings are in agreement with previous studies on hemagglutination distribution in *V. cholerae* (Amaro et al., 1990). These authors showed that 109 (78%) of the environmental non-Ol *V. cholerae* strains assayed, possessed agglutinating capacity.

Determination of several potential virulence factors in *Vibrio* spp. by Baffone et al. (2001) demonstrated that species were adhesive, with percentages ranging from 40% for *V. fluvialis* to 55-80% for *V. alginolyticus,* non-O1 *V. cholerae* and *V. parahaemolyticus.*

2.3 Antibiotic resistance of non-O1 *V. cholerae*

Among the 240 non-O1 *V. cholerae* strains isolated from Marrakech stabilization ponds, 89 (37.1%) isolates were resistant to at least one of 14 tested antibiotics (Mezrioui et al., 1995; Mezrioui & Oufdou, 1996). The levels of antibiotic resistance at the inflow and outflow points of the system were respectively 40 and 34% and were not significantly different. This antibiotic resistance level was lower than that obtained by Amaro et al. (1988). These authors showed that among 146 non-O1 *V. cholerae* strains isolated from the environment and tested for antibiotic resistance, 93% were resistant to at least one antibiotic.

It appears that in wastewater treated by Marrakech stabilization ponds treatment, non-O1 *V. cholerae* antibiotic resistance was not significantly modified. However, in the same treatment system, Hassani et al. (1992) have showed that the antibiotic resistance increased in 693 *E. coli* strains as they passed through the ponds. Levels of *E. coli* antibiotic resistance on the inflow and the outflow were 21% and 34% respectively.

Mezrioui & Oufdou (1996) have noted that non-O1 *V. cholerae* showed high resistance to ampicillin, amoxicillin and mezlocillin at all sampling points of Marrakech stabilisation pond system, followed by resistance to cefalexin, cefoperazone and amikacin.

Combined resistance to ampicillin and amoxicillin or to ampicillin and mezlocillin were the most frequently observed resistance pattern. Few isolates were resistant to cefalexin, cefoperazone or amikacin (less than 9%).

More importantly, some strains of non-O1 *V. cholerae* were found to be capable of receiving and stably maintaining plasmids conjugally transferred from *E. coli.* Antibiotic resistance can be transferred from non-O1 *V. cholerae* to other members of the *Enterobacteriaceae* family such as *E. coli* K12. Transfer frequencies in nutrient broth and filtered wastewater were respectively 3×10^{-5} and 2×10^{-8} (Mezrioui & Oufdou, 1996).

As for antibiotic resistance in groundwater of Marrakech-Tensift-Al Haouz region, antibiotic susceptibility testing revealed that the overall resistance (resistance to at least one antibiotic) of non-O1 *V. cholerae* strains was 79%, while it was 100% for *P. aeruginosa*, faecal coliforms (FC) and Faecal streptococci (FS) strains (Lamrani et al. 2010). 317, 208, 320 and 338 strains were respectively tested. The multiresistance level of non-O1 *V. cholerae* strains (69%) was significantly lower than that of FC and FS strains (95%), whereas 100% of *P. aeruginosa* strains were multiresistant. The monoresistance (resistance to one antibiotic) of non-O1 *V. cholerae* was 10% while it was 5% for FC and FS strains. Sixty six strains (21%) of non-O1 *V. cholerae* were susceptible to all antibiotics tested, while none of the isolates *P. aeruginosa*, FC and FS was susceptible to all antibiotics tested. Our results showed that among non-O1 *V. cholerae* strains resistance was most commonly observed towards sulfamethoxazole (75%), followed by streptomycin (62%) and cephalothin (60%) and trimethoprim (49%). A smaller proportion of these isolates were resistant to erythromycin (18%), kanamycin and polymyxin B (12%), cephotaxim (8%), gentamycin (7%) and tetracycline (2%). All the 317 non-O1 *V. cholerae* isolates were susceptible to chloramphenicol, nalidixic acid and novobiocin.

The obtained results showed correlation between bacteriological pollution and their antibiotic resistance and virulence.

The dominant multiresistant profiles noted for non-O1 *V. cholerae* were to seven antibiotics; of 220 strains resistant to at least two antibiotics, 53 strains (24.09%) were resistant to seven antibiotics. The maximal multiresistance was to ten antibiotics with two profiles: "Gm, Str, Km, Tpm, Smx, Amp, Amx, Cfl, Cfm, Ery" and "Gm, Str, Km, Tpm, Smx, Tc, Amp, Amx, Cfl, Cfm".

Of the antimicrobial resistant FC strains isolated, 80% were resistant to five or more antibiotics. The dominant multiresistant profile noted for FC was to eight antibiotics (11.6%). The maximal multiresistance was to fourteen antibiotics with two profiles: "Amp, Amx, Amx-clav, Cfl, Cfm, Cft, Chl, Gm, Na, PB, Smx, Str, Tc, Tpm" and "Amp, Amx, Amx-clav, Cfl, Cfm, Cft, Gm, Km, Na, PB, Smx, Str, Tc, Tpm".

3. Conclusion

Although the stabilization ponds showed considerable effectiveness in eliminating faecal coliforms, the system's final effluent contained not inconsiderable non-O1 *V. cholerae* concentrations. Their presence in treated wastewater limits their re-use in agriculture. The risks associated with the presence of non-O1 *V. cholerae* in effluent will be greater if these bacteria are multi-antibiotic resistant. The addition of a third maturation pond to Marrakech stabilization ponds may help in the reduction of bacteria.

The experimental studies on the effects of some environmental factors (temperature, pH, sunlight and the cyanobacterium; *Synechocystis*) on survival of both bacteria, showed that the alcaline pH (>8) seems to present a more bactericidal effect on FC than on non-O1 *V. cholerae*. Thus, the Cyanobacteria blooms, occurring periodically during summer in sewage stabilization ponds of Marrakech, will be considered as one of the major factors leading to high levels of non-O1 *V. cholerae* and low abundances of FC bacteria during the hot period.

Conjugative transfer of resistance genes occurred between non-01 *V. cholerae* strains and other bacteria such as *E. coli*. The high dissemination capacity for these R-factors plasmids can occur even when intergeneric transfer frequencies are relatively low.

Effluent discharged from stabilization ponds into receptor environment or re-used for irrigation purposes should be purified by more advanced methods prior to discharge in areas of greatest human impact and where antibiotic resistance could well prove to be a serious human problem in the future.

The bacteriological quality of groundwater in Marrakech region suggested that the studied wells water were heavily contaminated with FC, FS, *P. aeruginosa* and non-O1 *V. cholerae*. Their presence could have significant health risks for local population when it is used as a drinking water. According to WHO standards for drinking water, the studied well waters were unsuitable for the consumers. The characteristics of the environment of the prospected wells and their proximity from many sources of pollution as well as the lack of rigorous protection contributed to their contamination. In these wells water, the result of the interaction network underwent a high variability. This may be at the origin of a high ecological instability of the studied bacteria and physicochemical parameters. The need for guidelines to protect groundwater quality in Morocco is imperative.

Non-01 *V. cholerae* and the other studied bacteria isolated from Marrakesh groundwater are virulent since most of them are producers of hemolysins, hemagglutinins and are multiresistant to antibiotics. These bacteria may have important public health implications. Their role in several cases of gastro-enteric and systemic pathologies noted at the local population of Marrakech area (Jbilet and Tensift region) deserve greater interest and attention.

Urgent reactions are required to apply adequate solutions such as disinfection of groundwater, protection of the wells, public awareness. This study may be considered a typical example of what is happening in other cities in the developing world and it is estimated to assist local authorities in developing plans and actions to improve groundwater quality.

4. Acknowledgment

This work is partly financed by the ifs projects n°F/2826-2 and F/2826-3F.

5. References

Amaro, C., Aznar, R., Garay, E. & Alcaid, E. (1988). R plasmids in environmental *Vibrio cholerae* non-O1 strains. *Applied and Environmental Microbiology*, 54: 277 l-2776.

Amaro, C., Toranzo, A.E., Gonzalez, E.A., Blanco, J., Pujalte, M. J., Aznar, R. & Garay, E. (1990). Surface and Virulence Properties of Environmental *Vibrio cholerae* Non-O1 from Albufera Lake (Valencia, Spain). *Applied and Environmental Microbiology*, 56: 1140-1147.

Arita, M., Takeda, T., Honda, T. & Miwatani, T. (1986). Purification and characterization of *Vibrio cholerae* non-Ol heat-stable enterotoxin. *Infection and Immunity*, 52: 45-49.

Baffone, W., Citterio, B., Vittoria, E., Casaroli, A., Pianetti, A., Campana, R. & Bruscolini, F. (2001). Determination of several potential virulence factors in *Vibrio* spp. isolated from seawater. *Food Microbiology*, 18: 479-488.

Bag, P.K., Bhowmik, P., Hajra, T.K., Ramamurthy, T., Sarkar, P., Majumder, M., Chowdhury, G. & Das, S.C. (2008). Putative Virulence Traits and Pathogenicity of

Vibrio cholerae Non-O1, Non-O139 Isolates from Surface Waters in Kolkata, India. *Applied and Environmental Microbiology*, 74 (18): 5635-5644

Banerjee, K.K., Ghosh, A.N., Dutta-Roy, K., Pal, S.C. & Ghose, A.C. (1990). Purification and characterization of a novel hemagglutinin from *Vibrio cholerae. Infection and Immunity*, 58: 3698-3705.

Begum, K., Ahsan, C.R., Ansaruzzaman, M., Dutta, D.K., Ahmad, Q.S. & Talukder, K.A. (2006). Toxin(s), other than cholera toxin, produced by environmental non-O1 non-O139 *Vibrio cholerae. Cellular and Molecular Immunology*, 3: 115-121.

Booth, B.A. & Finkelstein, R.A. (1986). Presence of hemagglutinin/protease and other potential virulence factors in O1 and non-O1 *Vibrio cholerae. Journal of Infectious Diseases*, 154: 183-186.

Caldini, G., Neri, A., Cresti, S., Boddi, V., Rossolini, G.M. & Lanciotti, E. (1997). High Prevalence of *Vibrio cholerae* Non-O1 Carrying Heat-Stable-Enterotoxin-Encoding Genes among *Vibrio* Isolates from a Temperate-Climate River Basin of Central Italy. *Applied and Environmental Microbiology*, 63 (7): 2934-2939.

Chakraborty, S., Nair, G.B. & Shinoda, S. (1997). Pathogenic *Vibrios* in the natural aquatic environment. *Review of Environmental Health*, 12: 63-80.

Chatterjee, S., Ghosh, K., Raychoudhuri A., Basu, A., Rajendran K., et al. (2009). Incidence, virulence factors, and clonality among clinical strains of non-O1, non-O139 *Vibrio cholerae* isolates from hospitalized diarrheal patients in Kolkata, India. *Journal of Clinical Microbiology*, 47: 1087–1095.

Crane, S. R., Moore, J. A. (1986). Modeling enteric bacteria die off: a review. *Water, Air and Soil Pollution*, 27: 411-439.

Curtis T., Mara D., Silva S. (1992). The effect of sunlight on fecal coliforms in ponds: implications for research and design. *Water Science Technology*, 26: 1729-1738.

Dumont, S., Krovacek, K., Svenson, S.B., Pasquale, V., Baloda, S.B. & Figliuolod G. (2000). Prevalence and diversity of *Aeromonas* and *Vibrio* spp. in coastal waters of Southern Italy. *Comparative Immunology Microbiology and Infectious Diseases*, 23: 53-72.

Guhathakurta, B., Sasmal, D., Pal, S., Chakraborty, S., Nair, G.B. & Datta, A. (1999). Comparative analysis of cytotoxin, hemolysin, hemagglutinin and exocellular enzymes among clinical and environmental isolates of *Vibrio cholerae* O139 and non-O1, non-O139. *FEMS Microbiology Letters*, 179: 401-407.

Hassani, L., Imziln, B., Boussaid, A. & Gauthier, M.J. (1992). Seasonal incidences of and antibiotic resistance among *Aeromonas* species isolated from domestic wastewater before and after treatment in stabilization ponds. *Microbial Ecology*, 23: 227-237.

Ichinose, Y., Yamamoto, K. & Nakasone, N. (1987). Enterotoxicity of El Tor-like hemolysin of non-O1 *Vibrio cholerae. Infection and Immunity*, 55: 1090-1093.

Isaac-Marquez, A.P., Lezama-Davila, C.M., Eslava-Campos, C., Navarro-Ocana, A. & Cravioto-quintana, A. (1998). Serotype of *Vibrio cholerae* non-O1 isolated from water supplies for human consumption in Campeche, Mexico and their antibiotic resistance susceptibility pattern. *Memorias do Instituto Oswaldo Cruz, Rio de Janeiro*, 93: 17-21.

Kabir, S. & Ali, S. (1983). Characterization of surface properties of *Vibrio cholerae. Infection and Immunity*, 39: 1048-1058.

Lamrani Alaoui, H., Oufdou, K. & Mezrioui, N. (2008). Environmental pollutions impacts on the bacteriological and physicochemical quality of suburban and rural groundwater supplies in Marrakesh area (Morocco). *Journal of Environmental Monitoring and Assessment.* 145: 195-207.

Lamrani Alaoui, H., Oufdou, K. & Mezrioui, N. (2009). Rôle de la désinfection par rayonnement solaire ou par chloration dans l'amélioration de la qualité bactériologique des eaux de puits de la région de Marrakech. *Revue Electronique de Microbiologie Industrielle Sanitaire et Environnementale.* 03 (1) : 96-124.

Lamrani Alaoui, H., Oufdou, K. & Mezrioui, N. (2010). Determination of several potential virulence factors in non-O1 *Vibrio cholerae, Pseudomonas aeruginosa,* fecal coliforms and streptococci isolated from Marrakesh groundwater. *Water Science and Technology.* 61 (7) : 1895-1905.

Lesne, J., Baleux, B., Bousaid, A. & Hassani, L. (1991). Dynamics of non-O1 *Vibrio cholerae* in experimental sewage stabilization ponds under arid Mediterranean climate. *Water Science and Technology,* 22: 387-390.

Lipp, E.K., Huq, A. & Colwell, R.R. (2002). Effects of global climate on infectious disease: the cholera model. *Clinical Microbiology Reviews,* 15: 757–770.

Mezrioui, N., Oufdou, K. & Baleux, B. (1995). Dynamics of non-O1 *Vibrio cholerae* and fecal coliforms in experimental stabilization ponds in the arid region of Marrakesh, Morocco, and the effect of pH, temperature and sunlight on their experimental survival. *Canadian Journal of Microbiology,* 41: 489-498.

Mezrioui, N. & Oufdou, K. (1996). Abundance and antibiotic resistance of non-O1 *Vibrio cholerae* strains in domestic wastewater before and after treatment in stabilization ponds in an arid region (Marrakesh, Morocco). *FEMS Microbiology Ecology,* 21: 277-284.

Nagamune, K., Yamamoto, K. & Honda, T. (1995). Cloning and sequencing of a novel hemolysin gene of *Vibrio cholerae. FEMS Microbiology Letters,* 128: 265-269.

Nishibuchi, M., Seidler, R.J., Rollins, D.M. & Joseph, S.W. (1983). *Vibrio* factors cause rapid fluid accumulation in suckling mice. *Infection and Immunity,* 40: 1083-1091.

Nogueira G., Celso V.N., Maria C.B.T., Benécio A.A.F., Benedito P.D.F. (2003). Microbiological quality of drinking water of urban and rural communities. *Review Saùde Pùblica,* 37: 232-236

O'Brien, A.D., Chen, M.E., Holmes, R.K., Kaper, J. & Levine, M.M. (1984). Environmental and human isolates of *Vibrio cholerae* and *Vibrio parahaemolyticus* produce a *Shigella dysenteriae* 1 (Shiga)-like cytotoxin. *Lancet,* i: 77–78.

Oufdou, K. & Oudra, B. (2009). Substances bioactives élaborées par des cyanobactéries isolées de certains écosystèmes aquatiques marocains. *Afrique Science.* 05 (2): 260-279.

Oufdou, K. & Oudra, B. (2008). Impact des blooms à cyanobactéries sur certaines bactéries d'intérêt sanitaire dans le lac-réservoir Lalla Takerkoust (Marrakech, Maroc). *Bulletin de la Société d'Histoires Naturelles de Toulouse.* 144: 35-41.

Oufdou, K., Oudra, B. & Mezrioui, N. (2004). Interactions between bacteria and cyanobacteria in the stabilisation ponds of Marrakech (Morocco): Their role in purification of wastewater. *Proceeding of 3rd International training program TCTP' 2004 "Technologies on Waste Treatment and Environmental Pollution Control".* INRST-LEE / JICA : 67-74.

Oufdou, K., Mezrioui, N., Ait Melloul, A., Barakate, M. & Ait Alla, A. (1999). Effects of sunlight and *Synechocystis* sp. (picocyanobacterium) on the incidence of antibiotic resistance in wastewater enteric bacteria. *World Journal of Microbiology and Biotechnology*, 15 : 553-559.

Oufdou, K., Mezrioui, N., Oudra, B., Barakate, M., Loudiki, M. & Ait Alla, A. (2000). Relationships between bacteria and cyanobacteria in the Marrakech waste stabilisation ponds. *Water Science and Technology*, 42, N° 10-11 : 553-559.

Oufdou, K., Mezrioui, N., Oudra, B. & Ouhdouch, Y. (1998). Etude expérimentale de l'effet de *Synechocystis* sp. (picocyanobactérie) sur le comportement de certaines bactéries d'intérêt sanitaire. *International Journal of Limnology*, 34, (3): 259-268.

Pal, S., Datta, A., Nair, G.B. & Guhathakurta, B. (1998). Use of monoclonal antibodies to identify phospholipase C as the enterotoxic factor of the bifunctional hemolysin phospholipase C molecule of *Vibrio cholerae* O139. *Infection and Immunity*, 66: 3974-3977.

Pathak, S.P., Gautam, A.R., Garg, N. & Bhattacharjee, J.W. (1992). Ecology and toxigenicity of *Vibrio cholerae* non-O1 isolated from tropical river water. Journ*al of General Applied Microbiology*, 38: 253-262.

Ramamurthy, T., Garg, S., Sharma, R., Bhattacharya, S.K., Nair, G.B., Shimada, T., Takeda, T., Karasawa, T., Kurazano, H., Pal, A. & Takeda, Y. (1993). Emergence of novel strain of *Vibrio cholerae* with epidemic potential in southern and eastern India. *Lancet*, 341: 703–704.

Singh, D.V., Matte, M.H., Matte, G.R., Jiang, S., Sabeena, F., Shukla, B.N., Sanyal, S.C., Huq A. & Colwell, R.R. (2001). Molecular analysis of *Vibrio cholerae* O1, O139, non-O1, and non-O139 strains: clonal relationships between clinical and environmental isolates. *Applied and Environmental Microbiology*, 67 (2): 910 - 921.

WHO (1993). Epidemic diarrhea due to *Vibrio cholerae* non-O1. *Weekly Epidemiological Report*, 68: 141-142.

Yamamoto, K., Takeda, Y., Miwatani, T. & Craig, J.P. (1983). Purification and some properties of a non-O1 *Vibrio cholerae* enterotoxin that is identical to cholera enterotoxin. *Infection and Immunity*, 39: 1128-1135.

Yoh, M., Honda, T. & Miwatani, T. (1986). Purification and partial characterization of a *Vibrio hollisae* hemolysin that relates to the thermostable direct hemolysin of *Vibrio parahaemolyticus*. *Canadian Journal of Microbiology*, 32: 632-636.

20

Antimicrobial Resistance of Bacteria in Food

María Consuelo Vanegas Lopez
Universidad de los Andes,
Colombia

1. Introduction

Antibiotics are a major tool utilized by the healthcare industry to fight bacterial infections; however, bacteria are highly adaptable organisms, able develop resistance to antibiotics. Consequently, decades of antibiotic use, or rather misuse, have resulted in bacterial resistance to many modern antibiotics. This resistance can cause significant danger and suffering for many people with common bacterial infections, which were once easily treatable with this type of medication [1]. Antibiotics are widely used in human and veterinary medicine as well as in agriculture for the treatment of infections, to improve growth and for animal prophylaxis, which can generate a selection of multiresistant bacteria. However, is it not fully understood how widespread antibiotic resistant bacteria are in agricultural settings. The lack of such surveillance data is especially evident in dairy farm environments.

Over the past 6 decades, the introduction of new class or modifications of antimicrobial has been marched slowly but surely by the development of new bacterial resistance mechanisms. Since the first reports different estudies have demonstrated that increases in antimicrobial resistance among both pathogenic and commensal bacteria can be observed after introduction of antimicrobial[2]. Therefore in this chapter I will discuss some of the research which in which they reported the presence of antibiotic-resistant bacteria that are of importance in foods.

2. *Campylobacter*

Campylobacter was identified as a human diarrheal pathogen in 1973. *Campylobacter* is a major cause of disease in humans and poultry around the world and *Campylobacter* was, is the most frequently diagnosed bacterial cause for human gastroenteritis in the United States and throughout the world. Most cases of *Campylobacter* infections do not require antimicrobial treatment, being clinically mild and self-limiting [4]. Macrolides are considered the first choice drug for *C. jejuni* and *C. Coli* enteritis,erythromycin and ciprofloxacin are the drugs of choice for treatment of human campylobacteriosis and fluoroquinilones are also used. Contaminated food is the usual source of human infection; therefore, the presence of antimicrobial resistant strains in the food chain has raised concerns that the treatment of human infections will be compromised. Most disease in humans is associated with the consumption of contaminated poultry or cross-contamination with other foods [4]

This section provides a review of resistance prevalence in *C.jejuni* and *C.coli* from food. In this study, was investigated the prevalence of resistance to erythromycin and ciprofloxacin in *Campylobacter* isolates recovered from turkey carcasses at two processing plants. Ciprofloxacin and erythromycin resistance in *Campylobacter* recovered from processed turkey occurred more frequently among *C. coli* than *C. jejuni*. Molecular subtyping in this study provides further information about the relationships between antimicrobial-resistant *Campylobacter* at processing level [5]

The antimicrobial resistance profiles of *Campylobacter* isolates recovered from a series of samples of retail food (n = 374) and humans (n = 314) to eight antimicrobial compounds were investigated. High levels of resistance in isolates of *C.jejuni* were observed for ceftiofur (58%), ampicillin (25%) and nalidixic acid (17%) with lowest levels observed for streptomycin (7.9%) and chloramphenicol (8.3%). A total of 80% of isolates *of C. jejuni* were resistant to human ceftiofur, while 17% were resistant to ampicillin and nalidixic acid, 8.6% to streptomycin and 4.1% to chloramphenicol. Antimicrobial resistance of clinical relevance, such as erythromycin, ciprofloxacin and tetracycline were 6.7, 12 and 15% respectively for all food isolates and was similar to the corresponding prevalence of resistance observed in human isolates, where 6 , 4%, 12 and 13, respectively, were found to be resistant. Comparisons of strains of *C. jejuni* at each site showed a high degree of similarity although some regional variations exist. Comparison of the total populations of *C. jejuni* and *C. coli* showed minor differences, with *C. jejuni* strains resistant to ampicillin and ceftiofur. Patterns of multidrug resistance showed some profiles common to the human strains and clinical [6].

Antimicrobial resistance was evaluated in *Campylobacter* spp isolated of beef cattle in four commercial feedlots in Alberta (Canada). All calves were given chlortetracycline and oxytetracycline in food, and most animals (93%) were injected with long-acting oxytetracycline. A total of 1586 *Campylobacter* strains were isolated, these consist of *Campylobacter* coli (n = 154), *Campylobacter fetus* (n = 994), *Campylobacter jejuni* (n = 431), *Campylobacter hyointestinalis* (n = 4), and *Campylobacter lanienae* (n = 3) which were recovered and characterized [4]. Increases in the prevalence of strains resistant to tetracycline and doxycycline (56 to 89%) of *C. coli, C. fetus* and *C. jejuni* were observed [4]. Increased resistance to erythromycin was also found in strains of *C. coli* in the three episodes of isolation. Most isolates of *C. fetus* recovered were resistant to nalidixic acid and a relatively small number of multi-drug resistant strains were recovered. Widespread use of antimicrobial agents in meat production and possible horizontal transfer of mobile genetic elements with resistance determinants among bacteria *Campylobacter* and other taxa emphasized [4].

Campylobacter has become the leading cause of zoonotic enteric infections in developed and developing countries worlwide. Epidemiological and microbial studies show that poultry is the most important source for quinolone-susceptible and quinolone-resistant campylobacter infections in humans. Trend over time for macrolide resistance show stable low rates in most countries, and macrolides should remain the drugs class of choice for *C. jejuni* and *C. coli* enteritis. However, macrolide resitance is emerging in some countries and needs to be monitored.[7].

3. *Salmonella*

Salmonella spp. is widely distribuited in nature, colonizing a range of animal hosts. *Salmonella* entérica is recognized as one of the most common bacteria causes of food borne diarrheal illness worldwide. It had been estimated that annually there are about 1.3 billion cases of acute gastroenteritis due to nontyphoidal salmonelosis, resulting in 3 million deaths. In industrialized countries food animals are the main reservoir for human infections, the majority of which originate from contaminated meat products and eggs. It is very important the issue of antibiotic resistance of *Salmonella* spp, which has been investigated as its ecology and pathogenesis

Substantial effort has been made to disclose the genetic means by which *Salmonella* spp has evolved to resist antimicrobials. Acquired resistance arises by two ways: by mutations in chromosomally encoded genetic elements and by acquisition of exogenous mobile resistance genes by plasmids, integrons and transposons. Both mechanisms can led to rapid changes of a bacterial populations, horizontal genes transfer apppers to be most important in the evolutions of salmonella resistance.[8] In this section I summarize some examples which show the presence antimicrobial resistance *Salmonella* spp in food.

Burgos et al. isolated and identified enteric bacteria in the soil of dairy farms and found that enteric bacteria from dairy farm soil are resistant to multiple drugs and carriers of antibiotic resistance plasmids. This suggests that the surface layer of farm land plays an important role, as it is an environment that can be a reservoir for the development of bacterial resistance against antibiotics [3].

In another study undertaken in Alberta during 1996 and 1999, 209 strains of *Salmonella*, obtained from food animals were isolated and 17 antimicrobial drugs were tested and , 11.8% of strains were positive for resistance. These strains were commonly resistant to tetracycline (35.4%), streptomycin(32.5%), sulfamethoxazole (28.7%), ticarcillin (27.3%) and ampicillin (26.8%)[9]. *Salmonella* enterica serovar Heidelberg frequently causes foodborne illness in humans. The authors compared the prevalence of Salmonella serotype Heidelberg in a sampling of 20,295 meats, including chicken breast ,ground turkey, ground beef and pork ribs, collected between 2002 and 2006 a total of 298 Salmonella serovar Heidelberg isolates were recovered, representing 21.6% of all Salmonella serovars from retail meats. One hundred seventy-eight (59.7%) were from ground turkey, 110 (36.9%) were from chicken breast, and 10 (3.4%) were from pork chops; none was found in ground beef. One hundred ninety-eight isolates (66.4%) were resistant to at least one compound, and 49 (16.4%) were resistant to at least five compounds. Six strains (2.0%), all ground turkey, were resistant to at least nine antimicrobial agents. The greatest resistance in isolates from poultry was to tetracycline (39.9%), followed by streptomycin (37.8%), sulfamethoxazole (27.7%), gentamicin (25.7%), kanamycin (21.5%), ampicillin (19.8%), amoxicillin-clavulanate (10.4%) and ceftiofur (9.0%). These data indicate that *Salmonella* serovar Heidelberg is a common serovar in retail poultry meat and includes widespread clones of multidrug-resistant strains [10].

Recently, *Salmonella* Enterica *subsp. enterica* serovar *Saintpaul* has been increasingly observed in several countries, including Germany. However, the pathogenic potential and epidemiology of this serotype are not very well known. Fifty-five isolates of *S. turkey saintpaul* Germany and Turkey food products isolated from 2000 to 2007 were analyzed using an antimicrobial agent, organic solvents, and disinfectant susceptibility testing, detection of determinants of resistance, plasmid profiles, pulsed-field gel electrophoresis (PFGE) and hybridization experiments[11].The pattern of resistance was observed for ampicillin, amoxicillin-clavulanate, gentamicin, kanamycin, nalidixic acid, streptomycin, spectinomycin, and several third-generation cephalosporins (including ceftiofur and cefoxitin. This study revealed that a multiresistant S. saintpaul line Saintpaul is widespread in turkeys and turkey products in Germany.[11]

In Denmark, Skov, M et al, compared 8144 Salmonella isolates collected from meat imported or produced, as well as the Danish patients. Isolates from imported meat showed a higher rate of antimicrobial resistance, including resistance to multiple drugs, which were isolated from domestic beef. Isolates from humans showed resistance rates lower than those found in imported meat. These findings suggest that programs to control resistant *Salmonella spp.* are a worldwide problem [12]

A study in Vietnam shows that enteric bacteria in samples of raw foods contain a set of mobile genetic elements and the transfer of antibiotic resistance can easily occur between similar bacteria. This study was undertaken to examine the contamination rate and molecular characteristics of enteric bacteria isolated from a selection of food sources in Vietnam [16]. One hundred and eighty raw food samples were tested; 60.8% of the samples were from meat and 18.0% of samples of shellfish contaminated with *Salmonella* spp. More than 90% of all food sources contained *Escherichia coli.* The isolates were selected for antibiotic resistance against 15 antibiotics, and 50.5% of *Salmonella* isolates and 83.8% of isolates of *E. coli* were resistant to at least one antibiotic[13]. Isolates were screened for the presence of mobile genetic elements that confer resistance to antibiotics. Fifty-seven percent of *E. coli* and 13% of *Salmonella* isolates were found to contain integrons, and some isolates contained two integrons Plasmids were also detected in the 23 *Salmonella* isolates resistant to antibiotics and 33 isolates of *E. coli.* One hundred thirty-five *Salmonella* isolates and 76% of *E. coli* isolates contained plasmids of 95 kb, and some isolates contained two large plasmids. Conjugation experiments showed the successful transfer of all or part of the phenotypes of antibiotic resistance among isolates of *Salmonella* and *E. coli* contaminated food. The results show that enteric bacteria in raw food samples from Vietnam contain a set of mobile genetic elements and the transfer of antibiotic resistance can easily occur between similar bacteria[13]

Another study in Vietnam, was undertaken to examine the levels of *Salmonella* in samples of raw foods, including chicken, beef, pork and shellfish to determine their antibiotic resistance. A total of 180 samples were collected and analyzed, we obtained 91 isolates of *Salmonella.* Sixty-one percent of meat and 18% of shellfish samples were contaminated with *Salmonella spp.* The susceptibility of all isolates to a variety of antimicrobial agents was tested, and resistance to tetracycline, ampicillin / amoxicillin, nalidixic acid and streptomycin sulfafurazole was found in 40.7%, 22.0%, 18.7%, 16.5% and 14.3% of the isolates, respectively. Resistance to enrofloxacin, trimethoprim, chloramphenicol, kanamycin, and gentamicin was also detected (8.8 to 2.2%). About half (50.5%) of the *Salmonella* isolates were resistant to at least one of the antibiotics.[14]

4. *Escherichia coli*

E. coli is a bacterium, which very easily and frequently exchanges genetic information through horizontal gene transfer (e.g. by conjugation, transformation or transduction) with other related bacteria, such as other *E. coli* strains, *Salmonella, Shigella.* Therefore, *E. coli* strains may exhibit characteristics that have been acquired from a wide variety of sources.A recent review describes the population structure of commensal *E. coli*, the factors involved in the spread of different strains, how the bacteria can adapt to different niches, and how a commensal life style can evolve into a pathogenic one (Tenaillon et al., 2010). All humans and animals carry *E. coli* in their intestines as they are part of the normal gut flora and usually harmless. However, there are several types of *E. coli* strains that may cause gastrointestinalillness in humans. These strain types can be divided into several pathogroups These strain types can be divided into several pathogroups, resistant to ampicillin, amoxicillin/clavulanic acid,piperacillin/sulbactam, piperacillin/tazobactam, cefuroxime, etc.The strain carries plasmid-borne *bla*CTX-M-15 and a *bla*TEM-1 genes.An *E. coli* O104:H4 with a MLST ST678 was previously observed about 10 years ago in Germany in a Haemolytic Uremic Syndrome (HUS) case (Mellmann et al., 2008), the STEC O104:H4 outbreak strain shows an unusual combination of virulence factors of STEC and EAEC which has only been reported sporadically in humans before (Morabito et al., 1998) [16].

Another study analyzed the prevalence of *Escherichia coli* O157 in patients with diarrhea and surface water of some selected sources in Zaria (Nigeria), was evaluated of susceptibility to antibiotics and plasmid profiles of 184 isolates of *E. coli*, obtained from water samples of 228 and 112 diarrheal stool samples (collected from children <15 years) using standard methods. The most active antibiotics were gentamicin, chloramphenicol, and fluoroquinolones. Seventy-nine (42.9%) of 184 *E. coli* isolates were resistant to four or more antibiotics. The Multidrug Resistance (MDR) was higher among water isolates than clinical isolates. Of the 35 MDR isolates (20 of which were O157 strains), 22 (62.9%) harbored plasmids, all of which not less than 2.1 kb in size. Among the 20 strains of *E. coli* O157, only seven (35.0%) contained multiple plasmids. An *E. coli* O157 isolated from the aquatic system contains two plasmids resistant to seven drugs, including ampicillin, cefuroxime, ciprofloxacin, cotrimoxazole, nalidixic acid, nitrofurantoin and tetracycline. Loss of plasmids correlated with the loss of resistance to antibiotics (mutant) strains selected on tetracycline (50 mg / mL) in nutrient agar plates [17] .

The role of animal-based foods as vehicles for antibiotic-resistant bacteria has also been studied. One study on chickens fattening evaluated the incidence and distribution of antibiotic resistance in 197 commensal *Escherichia coli* strains. The effects of supplementation with antimicrobial agents approved bambermycin, penicillin, salinomycin and bacitracin or a combination of salinomycin more bacitracin. All isolates showed some degree of resistance to multiple antibiotics and resistance to tetracycline (68.5%), amoxicillin (61.4%), ceftiofur (51.3%), spectinomycin(47.2%), and sulfonamides (42%). These data demonstrate that the multidrug resistance of *E.coli* can be found in broilers, regardless of antimicrobial growth promoters used.

Water can also be an important vehicle for transmission of bacteria durability antibiotics, so I quote a study that was performed on wastewater from a plant to produce antibiotics which characterized the population of bacteria in surface waters of production plant of oxytetracycline (OTC). Found high levels of TBT in the wastewater (WW) and the antibiotic was still detectable at 20 Km (RWD), with undetectable levels in the water upstream (RWU). A total of 341 bacterial strains, most identified as Gammaproteobacteria. The most of the isolates (94.2% and 95.4% respectively WW and RWD) had tet (A) gene and it was the most common (67.0%), followed by tet (W), tet (C), tet (J), tet (L), tet (D), tet (y) and tet (K) (in the range between 21.0% and 40.6%). The authors propose that the strong selective pressure imposed by high concentrations of TBT contributes to the widespread dissemination of resistance genes and other genes of tetracycline resistance to antibiotics, possibly through mobile genetic elements[15]

5. *Enterococcus*

Enterococci colonize the gastrointestinal tract of the oral cavity and vaginal tract of humans and most animals [18]. The emergence of antimicrobial resistance represents the greatest threat to the treatment of human enterococcal infections. Enterococci are intrinsically resistant to a number of antimicrobial agents normally used to treat infections caused by grampositive bacteria. The enterococci have a remarkable ability to acquire new mechaninms of resistance and to transfer resistance determinans by way of conjugation [19]. In this section I focus in a review of antimicrobial resistant enterococci strains isolated from somefood.

From a medical point of view, the resistance of enterococci to vancomycin, teicoplanin and streptogramins is of special interest. In the case of vancomycin, there are identical types of groups of vanA of enterococci genes from fecal samples of animals, pet food, hospital patients, people in the community and water samples, these resistance genes may contaminate humans through the food chain [20]. Also, it was found that the most frequently isolated species are *Enterococcus faecium* (32.61%), followed by *E. faecalis* (21.74%), with high levels of resistance to streptomycin and gentamicin. These results confirm the presence of enterococci whitin the community having susceptibility profiles similar to those of strains found in hospital . [21].

A study at the Faculty of Pharmaceutical Sciences, University of Sao Paulo, Brazil, reported that 52.5% of the samples of raw and pasteurized milk, meat, cheese and vegetables were positive for enterococci; the most contaminated being the meat and the cheese. *E. faecium* was the predominant species, followed by E. faecalis, E. gallinarum and E.casseliflavus. Virulence genes were found and resistance to gentamicin, tetracycline and erythromycin in *E. faecalis* and three strains of *E. faecium* were resistant to vancomycin [22]. From the strains resistant to antibiotics, 72.4% of *E. faecalis* were able to form biofilm and 13.8% to adhere to Caco-2, which shows a virulent capacity of these types of enterococci [22].

The importance of ready-to-eat food (RTEF) and the Antibiotic Resistance (AR) gene flow has been assessed. RTEF are consumed frequently and may play a role in the acquisition of the determinants of AR in the human digestive tract. The study by Macovei et al, evaluated three RTEFs (chicken salad, a chicken burger and carrot cake) which were taken as samples from five fast food restaurants five times in the summer and 5 in the and winter. The overall concentrations of enterococci during the two seasons were similar (10^3 CFU / g), the most prevalent were *Enterococcus casseliflavus* (41.5% of isolates) and *Enterococcus hirae* (41.5%) in winter and *Enterococcus faecium* (36.8%), *E. casseliflavus* (27.6%) and *Enterococcus faecalis* (22.4%) in summer. In winter isolates were resistant mainly in to tetracycline (50.8%), ciprofloxacin (13.8%) and erythromycin (4.6%). In summer isolates were resistant mainly to tetracycline (22.8%), erythromycin (22.1%), and kanamycin (13.0%). The most common gene was *tet (M)* (35.4%) Genotyping of *E. faecalis* and *E. faecium* with pulsed-field gel electrophoresis revealed that the food contamination likely originated from various sources and is not clonal [23].

Another study from the southwestern United States, which characterized the profiles of antibiotic resistance of enterococci isolated from fresh produce harvested, found that of 185 Enterococci isolates, 97 (52%) were *Enterococcus faecium*, 38 (21%) were *Enterococcus faecalis*, and 50 (27%) were other Enterococcus species. Of clinical significance in humans is the fact that strains of *E. faecium* had a much higher prevalence of resistance to ciprofloxacin, tetracycline and nitrofurantoin than *E. faecalis*. 34% of the strains had multiple patterns of drug resistance, excluding intrinsic resistance. These data may help to elucidate the role of food in the transmission of antibiotic-resistant strains in human populations [24].

Additionally, one hundred and five VanA of the Glycopeptide-resistant enterococci (GRE) isolated from, human; animal, and food , were studied for genetic variability and molecular markers. The presence of indistinguishable *vanA* elements,mostly plasmid-borne, and virulence determinants in different species and PFGE-diverse populations suggested that all GRE might be potential reservoirs of resistance determinants and virulence traits transferable to human-adapted clusters. [25].

Research undertaken in Turkey has assessed vancomycin resistance and antibiotic resistance profiles of enterococci in different types of food purchased in local markets. Of a total of 200 samples, 50% had high levels of enterococci contamination, the greater resistance being found in samples of cream cheese. Only 4 strains were identified as resistant to vancomycin and identified as *E. faecalis*, from chicken. The results of this study emphasize the urgency of preventive measures to be taken to control antibiotic use on farms [26].

In addition, a study led by Martins et. al in Portugal whereby a total of 983 strains of enterococci were isolated from sewage sludge and effluent waste. These were tested against 10 different antibiotics. Multiresistance was found in 49.4% of the strains. Only 3.3% and 0.6% were resistant to ampicillin and vancomycin, respectively. However, observed 51.5% resistance to rifampicin, tetracycline 34.6%, 24.8% and 22.5% for erythromycin, nitrofurantoin. These results indicate that the use of antibiotics has created a large pool of resistance genes and the processes of wastewater treatment do not prevent the spread of resistant enterococci in the environment [27].

Different species of enterococci can frequently be isolated from environmental samples such as soil, water, plants or animal raw products.. In a study led by M.T. Tejedor Junco in 2009, isolated 78 strains of enterococci, from alfalfa (Medicago sativa) plant samples, drip irrigated with conventional water and a secondary effluent. *E. faecalis* (10.2%), *E. faecium* (2.6%), *E. hirae* (5.1%), *E. casseliflavus* (2.6%) and *E. mundtii* (79.5%) were isolated , In They found that all strains of enterococci, were susceptible to glycopeptides, penicillin and ampicillin. They did not detect strains with high level resistance to aminoglycosides. [28].

Additionally, the products supplied for feeding animals have been widely studied because they are potential vehicles for transmission of resistant bacteria. This has been demonstrated in a study conducted in 2006 in Portugal where 1137 enterococci strains and 163 *Escherichia coli* strains were recovered from 89 poultry feed samples, where 69.1% of enterococci isolates obtained from broiler feed were resistant to tetracycline and *E. coli* were resistant to ampicillin, tetracycline and streptomycin in 22.9%, 27.6% and 19.0% respectively. These data allow us to infer that the animal feed is a significant source of antibiotic resistant bacteria , thus leading to their introduction in the farm enviroment. The Poultry feed is at the start of the food safety chain, and might serve as a source of antimicrobial resistant bacteria present in poultry meat [29].

Some antibiotics had been used as growth promoters in Europe for several years, creating strains of resistant *E. faecium* .Resistant bacteria, have been isolated from samples of sewage, animal stools, meat products, samples from community and clinical samples from different European populations. Glycopeptide-resistant *E.faecium* (GREF), can be found in hospitals and outside them, and in the food chain by contaminated meat products.This suggests that the origin of these strains are other sources outside the hospital, probably for commercial ranching. Thus, to prevent the spread of antibiotic resistant strains such as enterococci, or transferable resistance genes, prudent use of antibiotics is necessary in human medicine and veterinary and in the animal husbandry [20].

There are no available studies about strains of enterococci resistant to antibiotics, isolated from Colombian food. Its been reported to a clinical level that the rate of vancomycin resistance in isolates of Enterococcus species by 2004 was about 7% in Brazil - Pan-American Health Organization (PAHO). In Colombia the problem is raised to similar levels and is a common source of nosocomial infections [1].

6. *Staphylococcus aureus*

S. aureus is one of the most important human and veterinary pathogens, and the epidemiology,pathology and antimicrobial resistance of this bacterium has been studied intensively in innumerable studies. *S. aureus* was one of the first bacteria in which the development of antimicrobial resistance (penicillin) was observed [2]. In human medicine, methicillin resistance is not only observed among *S. aureus,* but is also prevalent among other staphylococci as, *S. intermedius, S. epidermidis, S. hominis,*etc, have been isolated from animal sources in different studies and have been demostraded that they strains have mec A gene and are Methicillin resistan bacteria. [4]

In the United States, during 1992–2003, the number of health care–associated infections due to MRSA increased from 35.9% to 64.4% and in UK, death certificates increased by 39% [30]. In Colombia, the CA-MRSA (community-acquired, or community-associated *Staphylococcus aureus*) increased from 1% in 2001 to 5.4% in 2006 [31].

While environmental MRSA transmission has been investigated, transmission through food products has not received enough attention [32, 33]. However, Normmano et al. established the presence of *S.aureus* strains that harboured the mecA gene isolated from food samples such as bovine milk, mozzarella cheese, and pecorino cheese [33]. Other than information from that report the current prevalence of resistant bacteria in food matrices and levels of MRSA consumer exposure risks remain unknown.

Nowadays the assessment of the activity of an antibiotic is crucial to the successful outcome of antimicrobial therapy; however, the development of resistance both in human and animal bacterial pathogens has been associated with the extensive therapeutic use of antimicrobials or with their administration as growth promoters in meat production *[34, 35].*

In order to achieve the detection of sensitivity or resistance of *Staphylococcus aureus* strains, various techniques have been described, such as the employment of a cefoxitin 30 ug disc, using semiconfluent inoculums and overnight incubation at 35°C, resulting in a sensitivity of 100% and a specificity of 99%. In this way, disc diffusion remains the method of choice for routine screening for methicillin resistance, when the technical or economic capabilities are absent in the microbiological laboratories [36]

In addition, the most widely used molecular typing method for the study of local and global epidemiologies of MRSA is pulsed field gel electrophoresis (PFGE). This method has been used to identify MRSA clones that have a particular ability to cause major outbreaks [37, 38].

An unpublished study developed by the "Laboratorio de Ecología Microbiana y de Alimentos" (LEMA at the Universidad de los Andes), in Colombia genotyped the MRSA strain detecting *mecA* gene isolated from food samples circulating in Bogotá. Positive strains were genotyped for the identification of clonal groups using pulsed field electrophoresis (PFGE). 5 of the 149 strains were confirmed to have the *mecA* gene, indicating the presence of the SCC cassette. The electrophoretic pattern obtained by PFGE for these strains has revealed that 4 (80%) of the 5 strains belong to the Chilean clone, with 100% genetic similarity; this clone has been associated with 65% of infections associated with health care. This is the first evidence of the presence of MRSA in food in Colombia; nevertheless, this study is not published yet but is in the process of submission to publication[39].

Furthermore, a review of the resistance of gram-positive cocci in Colombia shows how our neighbors, Ecuador and Venezuela have a lower rate of resistance to that identified in our country at that time (25% vs. 47%) for coagulase-negative staphylococci-hospital in 2004 to the Pan American Health Organization (PAHO), where the frequency of *S. aureus* resistant to methicillin is much higher, with maximum values for Bogotá 60% and 70% for the 2001 to 2003 period. [40]. Reyes. J. et al, investigated the resistance profiles and mechanism of macrolide resistance in isolates of *Streptococcus pneumoniae* (1679), *Staphylococcus aureus* (348), coagulase-negative staphylococci (CoNS) (175), and *Enterococcus* spp. (123) from Colombian hospitals. The prevalence of macrolide resistance is low in Colombian pneumococci and high in MRSA (cMLS$_B$-type). [41].

7. Lactic acid bacteria (LAB)

For several decades, studies on the selection and spread of antibiotic resistance have focused mainly on clinically relevant species. However, recently several researchers have suggested that commensal bacteria such as lactic acid bacteria (LAB) may act as reservoirs of genes resistance to antibiotics similar to those found in human pathogens [42]. The main threat associated with these bacteria is that these resistance genes can be transferred to pathogenic bacteria [43].

Genes that confer resistance to tetracycline, erythromycin and vancomycin have been detected and characterized in *Lactococcus lactis,* enterococci and, recently, in lactobacilli isolated from fermented meat and milk products [1]. One example of the this resistance is the presented by lactobacilli, *pediococci* and *Leuconostoc spp.* which have been reported to have a high natural resistance to vancomycin, a property that is useful to separate them from other Gram-positive bacteria [44].

Thirty-one strains of *Lactobacillus delbrueckii* subsp. *bulgaricus* as components of yoghurt cultures showed intrinsic resistance towards mycostatin, nalidixic acid, neomycin, polymyxin B, trimethoprim, colimycin, sufamethoxazol and sulphonamides. Susceptibilities to cloxacillin, dihydrostreptomycin, doxcycline, furadantin, novobiocin, oleandomycin, oxacillin and streptomycin were prominent while kanamycin and streptomycin susceptibilities varied [45]. This has raised the discussion of new issues concerning the safety of probiotics in relation to the nature of the procurement and distribution of antimicrobial resistance genes [46].

Starter cultures of *Lactobacillus, Weissella* and *Bifidobacterium* of African and European origins were studied for their susceptibility to antimicrobials. Ouoba et al, evaluated and compared on its investigation to 24 antimicrobial, variations were observed and high levels of intrinsic resistence were found among the species studied. These authors confirmed the ability of *Lb. reuteri* from Africa to transfer by conjugation the gene erm(B), (resistance to erythromycin) to enterococci in vitro experiments [47]. Finally, they also identified a higher prevalence of phenotypic resistance to aminoglycosides in isolation from Europe. This is corroborated by recent publications in which they documented the transfer of macrolide resistance in Enterococcus from *Lactobacillus* in vivo [48] .

Pan L. et al, reported the presence of higher MICs (Minimal Inhibitory Concentration) in 14 of 202 strains of LAC, isolated from Chines fermented food. 14 strains reported the presence of multi-resistance and the presence of genes tet (M) and erm (B), mefA and aphA3 located on plasmids or chromosome. They found that lactic acid bacteria resistant to antibiotics are widespread among traditional Chinese fermented food and the incidence of this resistance was dependent on raw materials and manufacturing area of food; thus, the incidence of LAC resistance isolated during fermentation of sausages is much higher than that presented in the fermentation of vegetables. The results presented in these studies indicate the posssible role of LAC as f reservoirs for dissemination of antibiotic resistance in food and environment[49].

In Colombia there are some reports about antimicrobial resistance of bacterias responsible for human diseases, but its unkwon how frequent is the presence of these bacterias in food and its importance in human illness. The following are some comments about the problem of antimicrobial resistance in Colombia. Currently in Colombia, we have data based on antibiotic resistance of nosocomial strains, usually in intensive care units (ICU). This highlights the lack of a comprehensive study of this aspect in the Industrial and Food Process. Data record of 4008 set out the isolates from ICUs in 2003, 4,004 in 2004 and 4304 in 2005, where the most frequent were, in order: *S. aureus, E. coli, P. aeruginosa K. pneumoniae, A. baumannii* and *E. cloacae*. There was a statistically significant decrease in the number of isolates of *A. baumannii*. Salient issues that expose this study is the high resistance to ciprofloxacin (CIP) from *E. coli*, which is used as a marker, because once a gram-negative bacteria is resistant to this antibiotic it must be considered resistant to other quinolones.The resistance phenotype of this organism to third generation cephalosporins suggests the production of beta-lactamases of extended spectrum (ESBL) during the three year study. [50]. Of all the bacteria studied, *A. baumannii* showed the highest rates of multidrug resistance. Therefore, although there was a significant decrease in the number of isolates of this bacterium, in ICU this is a major concern. Among all prevalent in this study enterobacteria, *E. cloacae* could have the most ability to select resistance, including the carbapenems, to produce very high amounts of AmpC and close porins [50]. However, recent studies suggest that the prevalence of vancomycin resistance by the isolation of *Enterococcus faecium* found in South America is low (only 6%) compared to that presented in the United States [51]. Finally, according to the findings of this study, it is urgent to continue working with the national surveillance network of the resistance of both the hospital and those pathogens resistant organisms from food or water, in order to assist in the control of this public health problem of great importance [51].

8. References

[1] Mathur, S. and R. Singh, *Antibiotic resistance in food lactic acid bacteria--a review.* International Journal of Food Microbiology, 2005. 105(3): p. 281-295.

[2] Frank, A., *Antimicrobial Resistance In Bacteria of Animal Origin.* 2006, PP 160

[3] Burgos, J.M., B.A. Ellington, and M.F. Varela, *Presence of Multidrug-Resistant Enteric Bacteria in Dairy Farm Topsoil.* Journal of Dairy Science, 2005. 88(4): p. 1391-1398.

[4] Frank, A., *Antimicrobial Resistance In Bacteria of Animal Origin.* 2006 PP 269.

[5] Lutgen, E., et al., *Antimicrobial resistance profiling and molecular subtyping of Campylobacter spp. from processed turkey.* BMC Microbiology, 2009. 9(1): p. 203.

[6] Inglis, G.D., et al., *Temporal Prevalence of Antimicrobial Resistance in Campylobacter spp. from Beef Cattle in Alberta Feedlots.* Appl. Environ. Microbiol., 2006. 72(6): p. 4088-4095.

[7] Frank, A., *Antimicrobial Resistance In Bacteria of Animal Origin.* 2006 PP 284.

[8] Frank, A., *Antimicrobial Resistance In Bacteria of Animal Origin.* 2006 PP 293.

[9] Johnson J, A.R., and Lynn M. McMullen, *Antimicrobial resistance of selected Salmonella isolates from food animals and food in Alberta.* Can Vet J. , 2005. 46(2): p. 141-146.

[10] Zhao, S., et al., *Antimicrobial Resistance in Salmonella enterica Serovar Heidelberg Isolates from Retail Meats, Including Poultry, from 2002 to 2006.* Appl. Environ. Microbiol., 2008. 74(21): p. 6656-6662.

[11] Beutlich, J., et al., *A predominant Multidrug resistant Salmonella Saintpaul clonal line in German turkey and related food products.* Appl. Environ. Microbiol., 2010: p. AEM.02744-09.

[12] Skov, M., Andersen, J. , Aabo, S. , Ethelberg, S. , Aarestrup, F. , Sørensen, A. , Sørensen, G. , et al, *Antimicrobial Drug Resistance of Salmonella Isolates from Meat and Humans, Denmark.* Emerging Infectious Diseases, 2007. 13(4): p. 638-641.

[13] Van, T.T.H., et al., *Antibiotic Resistance in Food-Borne Bacterial Contaminants in Vietnam.* Appl. Environ. Microbiol., 2007. 73(24): p. 7906-7911.

[14] Van, T.T.H., et al., *Detection of Salmonella spp. in Retail Raw Food Samples from Vietnam and Characterization of Their Antibiotic Resistance.* Appl. Environ. Microbiol., 2007. 73(21): p. 6885-6890.

[15] Li, D., et al., *Antibiotic Resistance Characteristics of Environmental Bacteria from an Oxytetracycline Production Wastewater Treatment Plant and the Receiving River.* Appl. Environ. Microbiol., 2010. 76(11): p. 3444-3451.

[16] EFSA, *Urgent advice on the public health risk of Shiga-toxin producing Escherichia coli in fresh vegetables.* European Food Safety Authority, 2011. 9(6):2274.

[17] Vincent N. Chigor, V.J.U., 2 Stella I. Smith,3 Etinosa O. Igbinosa,1 and Anthony I. Okoh1, *Multidrug Resistance and Plasmid Patterns of Escherichia coli O157 and Other E.*

coli Isolated from Diarrhoeal Stools and Surface Waters from Some Selected Sources in Zaria, Nigeria. Int J Environ Res Public Health, 2010. 7(10): p. 3831-3841.

[18] B.D. Jett, M.M.H., M.S. Gilmore, *Virulence of enterococci.* Clin. Microbiol., 1994.

[19] Frank, A., *Antimicrobial Resistance In Bacteria of Animal Origin.* 2006 PP 319.

[20] Klare, I., et al., *Occurrence and spread of antibiotic resistances in Enterococcus faecium.* International Journal of Food Microbiology, 2003. 88(2-3): p. 269-290.

[21] Ronconi, *Detección de Enterococcus resistentes a altos niveles de aminoglucósidos y resistentes a glucopéptidos en Lactuca sativa (lechuga).* Enferm Infecc Microbiol Clin 2002. 20(8): p. 380-383.

[22] Gomes, B.C., et al., *Prevalence and characterization of Enterococcus spp. isolated from Brazilian foods.* Food Microbiology, 2008. 25(5): p. 668-675.

[23] Macovei, L. and L. Zurek, *Influx of Enterococci and Associated Antibiotic Resistance and Virulence Genes from Ready-To-Eat Food to the Human Digestive Tract.* Appl. Environ. Microbiol., 2007. 73(21): p. 6740-6747.

[24] Johnston, L.M. and L.-A. Jaykus, *Antimicrobial Resistance of Enterococcus Species Isolated from Produce.* Appl. Environ. Microbiol., 2004. 70(5): p. 3133-3137.

[25] Biavasco, F., et al., *VANA-TYPE ENTEROCOCCI FROM HUMANS, ANIMALS AND FOOD: species distribution, population structure, Tn1546-typing and location, and virulence determinants.* Appl. Environ. Microbiol., 2007: p. AEM.02239-06.

[26] Koluman, A., L.S. Akan, and F.P. Çakiroglu, *Occurrence and antimicrobial resistance of enterococci in retail foods.* Food Control, 2009. 20(3): p. 281-283.

[27] Martins da Costa, P., P. Vaz-Pires, and F. Bernardo, *Antimicrobial resistance in Enterococcus spp. isolated in inflow, effluent and sludge from municipal sewage water treatment plants.* Water Research, 2006. 40(8): p. 1735-1740.

[28] Tejedor J, G.M., Gómez L, Mendoza V, Grimón M, Palacios P, *Aislamiento, identificación y resistencia a antibióticos en cepas de Enterococcus aisladas de plantas de Medicago sativa regadas con agua convencional y depurada* Higiene y Sanidad Ambiental, 2009. 9: p. 418-421.

[29] da Costa, P.M., et al., *Antimicrobial resistance in Enterococcus spp. and Escherichia coli isolated from poultry feed and feed ingredients.* Veterinary Microbiology, 2007. 120(1-2): p. 122-131.

[30] Jarvis, W.R., *Prevention and control of methicillin-resistant Staphylococcus aureus: dealing with reality, resistance, and resistance to reality.* Clin Infect Dis, 2010. 50(2): p. 218-20.

[31] Manuel, G.-B., et al., *Epidemiology of meticillin-resistant Staphylococcus aureus (MRSA) in Latin America.* International journal of antimicrobial agents, 2009. 34(4): p. 304-308.

[32] Normanno, G., et al., *Coagulase-positive Staphylococci and Staphylococcus aureus in food products marketed in Italy.* International Journal of Food Microbiology, 2005. 98(1): p. 73-79.

[33] Normanno, G., et al., *Methicillin-resistant Staphylococcus aureus (MRSA) in foods of animal origin product in Italy.* Int J Food Microbiol, 2007. 117(2): p. 219-22.

[34] Normanno, G., et al., *Coagulase-positive Staphylococci and Staphylococcus aureus in food products marketed in Italy.* Int J Food Microbiol, 2005. 98(1): p. 73-9.

[35] Normanno, G., et al., *Occurrence, characterization and antimicrobial resistance of enterotoxigenic Staphylococcus aureus isolated from meat and dairy products.* Int J Food Microbiol, 2007. 115(3): p. 290-6.

[36] Skov, R., et al., *Evaluation of a cefoxitin 30 μg disc on Iso-Sensitest agar for detection of methicillin-resistant Staphylococcus aureus.* Journal of Antimicrobial Chemotherapy, 2003. 52(2): p. 204-207.

[37] Enright, M.C., et al., *Multilocus Sequence Typing for Characterization of Methicillin-Resistant and Methicillin-Susceptible Clones of Staphylococcus aureus.* J. Clin. Microbiol., 2000. 38(3): p. 1008-1015.

[38] Oliveira, D.C., A. Tomasz, and H. de Lencastre, *Secrets of success of a human pathogen: molecular evolution of pandemic clones of meticillin-resistant Staphylococcus aureus.* The Lancet Infectious Diseases, 2002. 2(3): p. 180-189.

[39] Rodriguez-Noriega, E., et al., *Evolution of methicillin-resistant Staphylococcus aureus clones in Latin America.* Int J Infect Dis, 2010. 14(7): p. e560-6.

[40] Espinosa, C., Cortés, J., Castillo, J. & Leal, A *Revisión sistemática de la resistencia antimicrobiana en cocos Gram positivos intrahospitalarios en Colombia.* Biomédica, 2011. 31: p. 27-34.

[41] Reyes, J., et al., *Characterization of macrolide resistance in Gram-positive cocci from Colombian hospitals: a countrywide surveillance.* International Journal of Infectious Diseases, 2007. 11(4): p. 329-336.

[42] Levy, S.B., Salyers, A.A. *Reservoirs of antibiotic resistance (ROAR) Network.* 2002 [cited 2011; Available from: http://www.healthsci.tufts.edu/apua/Roar/roarhome.htm.

[43] Perreten, V., et al., *Antibiotic resistance spread in food.* Nature, 1997. 389(6653): p. 801-802.

[44] Hamilton, M. and Shah, *Vancomycin susceptibility as an aid to the identification of lactobacilli.* Letters in Applied Microbiology, 1998. 26(2): p. 153-154.

[45] Sozzi, T.S., M *Antibiotic Resistances of Yogurt Starter Cultures Streptococcus thermophilus and Lactobacillus bulgaricus.* Applied and Environmental Microbiology, 1980. 40(862-865).

[46] Çataloluk, O. and B. Gogebakan, *Presence of drug resistance in intestinal lactobacilli of dairy and human origin in Turkey.* FEMS Microbiology Letters, 2004. 236(1): p. 7-12.

[47] Gevers, D., G. Huys, and J. Swings, *In vitro conjugal transfer of tetracycline resistance from Lactobacillus isolates to other Gram-positive bacteria.* FEMS Microbiology Letters, 2003. 225(1): p. 125-130.

[48] Ouoba, L.I.I., V. Lei, and L.B. Jensen, *Resistance of potential probiotic lactic acid bacteria and bifidobacteria of African and European origin to antimicrobials: Determination and transferability of the resistance genes to other bacteria.* International Journal of Food Microbiology, 2008. 121(2): p. 217-224.

[49] Pan, L., X. Hu, and X. Wang, *Assessment of antibiotic resistance of lactic acid bacteria in Chinese fermented foods.* Food Control, 2011. 22(8): p. 1316-1321.

[50] Briceño, D.F.C., Adriana; Valencia, Carlos; Torres, Julián Andrés; Pacheco, Robinson; Montealegre, María Camila; Ospina, Diego; Villegas, María Virginia, *Actualización*

de la resistencia a antimicrobianos de bacilos Gram negativos aislados en hospitales de nivel III de Colombia: años 2006, 2007 y 2008 Biomédica, 2010. 30(3): p. 371-381.

[51] Panesso, D., et al., *Molecular Epidemiology of Vancomycin-Resistant Enterococcus faecium: a Prospective, Multicenter Study in South American Hospitals.* J. Clin. Microbiol., 2010. 48(5): p. 1562-1569.

21

Antimicrobial Resistance Arising from Food-Animal Productions and Its Mitigation

Lingling Wang[1] and Zhongtang Yu[1,2,3,*]
Department of Animal Sciences[1],
Environmental Science Graduate Program[2],
Public Health Preparedness (PHP) Program[3],
The Ohio State University,
USA

1. Introduction

Antibiotics are routinely used in livestock production to treat and prevent diseases, or more often to promote growth of animals at sub-therapeutic doses. However, the huge amount of antibiotics used selects for resistant bacteria, resulting in development of antimicrobial resistance (AMR) mostly in intestinal microbiota of food animals. Therefore, animal manure constitutes the single largest reservoir of AMR. Although most of the AMR is carried by commensal bacteria, AMR genes can be transferred to pathogens of both animals and humans through horizontal gene transfer (HGT). Therefore, animal manure is a source of AMR contamination and poses a potential risk to human health. Because animal manure is the largest reservoir of AMR, management and treatment of animal manure provide an opportunity to contain and destruct AMR arising from food animal production. Several technologies are available for management and disposal of animal manure, including lagoon storage, intensive biological treatments, composting, and land application. These technologies differ in containing and reducing AMR as they create different physiochemical and biological conditions, which affect the survival of bacteria including antimicrobial-resistant bacteria. In this chapter, we discuss the development and occurrence of AMR arising from food animal production, as well as strategies and technologies to mitigate dissemination of AMR off farms to broad environment.

2. Use of antibiotics in food animal industry and development of antimicrobial resistance

In commercial food animal production, large quantities of antimicrobials are used to treat and prevent diseases and to promote animal growth (Prescott, 2008). In the latter case, antimicrobials are added to feed or drinking water at subtherapeutic levels. The Union of Concerned Scientists (UCS) reported that 11,200 metric tons of antimicrobials were used annually in the swine, poultry, and cattle industries for nontherapeutic purposes alone (Mellon *et al.*, 2001). In the United States and other countries as well, up to 50% of the

* Corresponding Author

antibiotics produced annually are used in food-animal production at therapeutic and subtherapeutic (for prophylaxis and growth promotion) levels (Barton, 2000; Teuber, 2001). Antimicrobials of almost all classes have been used in animal production. Some classes are primarily used for disease treatment or prevention, such as quinolones, lincosamides, and aminoglycosides, while others are used for both growth promotion and disease treatment/prevention, such as penicillins, macrolides, polypeptides, streptogramins, and tetracyclines. A survey by the American Health Institute (AHI, 2001) showed that among the antimicrobials used also in human medicine, tetracyclines leads the usage with an assumption of 3,239 tons per year followed by a combination of macrolides, lincosamides, polypeptides, streptogramins, and cephalosporins with an annual usage of 1,937 tons (Chee-Sanford *et al.*, 2009). Such usage of antimicrobials creates selective pressure for development of AMR.

Most of the bacteria carried by individual animals are within the intestinal tract, reaching a density of 10^{11} bacteria/g fecal content. In mammalian animals, bacteria account for about 50% of the feces. Most of the intestinal bacteria are commensal bacteria belonging to several hundred species (Andremont, 2003). Because antimicrobials were fed to animals for extended periods of time (weeks or months), intestinal bacteria are under persistent selective pressure to develop resistance to the antimicrobials used. As a result, AMR develops primarily in the intestinal tract and feces becomes the single largest reservoir of AMR arising from food animal production (Chee-Sanford *et al.*, 2009; Chen *et al.*, 2008). It is estimated that 180 million dry tons of livestock and poultry manure is generated annually in the US (Roe & Pillai, 2003). That can be translated into 90 dry tons of bacteria, many of which can be resistant to one or more antimicrobials. Although the majority of AMR present in animal manure is carried by commensal bacteria, the resistance genes can be transferred to bacteria pathogenic to animals and/or humans (Brody *et al.*, 2008; Witte, 2000). Figure 1 illustrates the dissemination of AMR to broad environments through vertical gene transfer (VGT) and horizontal gene transfer (HGT).

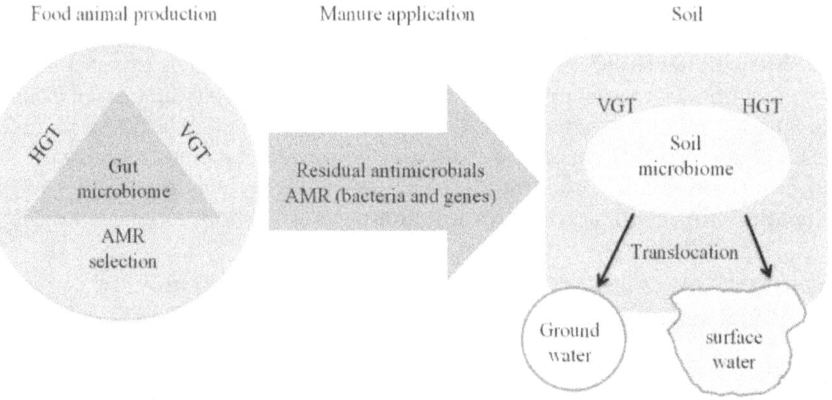

Fig. 1. Conceptualized view showing the possible fates of antimicrobial resistance (AMR) and residual antimicrobials after land application of animal manure (modified based on Chee-Sanford, *et al.*, 2009).

It has been well documented that bacteria resistant to antimicrobials abound in the intestinal tract and manure (Chen *et al.*, 2008). Antibiotic resistance was detected in *E. coli* isolated from animals soon after antibiotics were introduced to animal husbandry in the 1950s. Tetracycline-resistant *E. coli* was first found in chickens and pigs fed tetracycline in UK (Smith, 1967). With increasing use of various antimicrobials in food animals, AMR has been on the rise (Prescott, 2008). Numerous studies have been reported that examined the relationship between usage of antimicrobials and development of AMR in food animals. Although no precise quantitative relationship has been established, the accumulating body of data indicates a positive correlation between antimicrobial use and AMR development in food animals (Aarestrup *et al.*, 2008; Mathew *et al.*, 2007). As one example, in two farms where tylosin was used for growth promotion or treatment of diseases, 59% and 28%, respectively, of the *E. coli* isolates were resistant to tylosin, while only 2% of the *E. coli* isolated from an organic farm were resistant (Jackson *et al.*, 2004). In another study, as much as 71% of the *Enterococcus faecalis* isolated from swine manure was resistant to tetracycline (Haack & Andrews, 2000). These high levels of prevalence of AMR highlight the magnitude of AMR problem from animal manure.

The severity of AMR is also reflected by the wide occurrence of AMR to many drugs important to both animals and humans. Resistance has been seen to almost all kinds of veterinary antibiotics, including aminoglycoside, sulfadiazine, ampicillin, erythromycin, chloramphenicol, streptomycin, sulphonamide and tetracycline (Agustin *et al.*, 2005; Dubel *et al.*, 1982; Dunlop *et al.*, 1998; Hendriksen *et al.*, 2008; Hendriksen *et al.*, 2008; Lundin *et al.*, 2008). Additionally, AMR is distributed in many bacterial species. For example, resistance to tetracycline has been found in 26 different bacterial genera and in 60 species from swine manure (Stine *et al.*, 2007). Furthermore, with the wider use of antibiotics, multiple drug resistance often develops (Chen *et al.*, 2008; D'Lima *et al.*, 2007; Luangtongkum *et al.*, 2006). A study conducted in the 1980s on swine manure showed low levels of multiple drug resistance (Hanzawa *et al.*, 1984). However, there has been a rapid emergence of multiple drug resistance concomitant with widespread use of antimicrobials in both human medicine and animal husbandry in the past 10 to 15 years (Hawkey & Jones, 2009; Huang *et al.*, 2009).

Multiple drug resistance stems from clustering of multiple AMR genes together, primarily on mobile genetic elements. As a consequence, selection by one antibiotic drug can co-select multiple drug resistance. The selection of tetracycline resistance in beef cattle fed tylosin, a macrolide drug, (Chen *et al.*, 2008) attests this notion. Also, because multiple AMR genes are physically located on the same mobile genetic elements, multiple drug resistance can be readily transferred to other bacteria through HGT. Binh *et al* investigated the types of transferable plasmids that carry multiple AMR genes in piggery manure (Binh *et al.*, 2008) and found many of the 81 plasmids carry multiple AMR genes. Transposons and integrons were also found to carry multiple AMR genes (Barlow *et al.*, 2008; D'Lima *et al.*, 2007). This finding corroborates the potential risk posed from food animal production where antimicrobials are routinely used.

3. Impact of AMR in livestock manure on the development of AMR in environment

Animal manure from food animals is primarily applied to land either directly or after initial treatment or storage in on-farm animal facilities. Antimicrobial-resistant bacteria are, therefore, introduced to soil and disseminated to both soil and aquatic environments. Some studies have been carried out to determine the survival of manure bacteria after land application. Data from human pathogens, such as *Salmonella* and *Campylobacter*, *Yersinia enterocolitica* and *Escherichia coli* O157:H7, showed that their survival in water, soil and manure slurry varies dramatically, ranging from one day to longer than one year (Buswell *et al.*, 1998; Guo *et al.*, 2002; Santo Domingo *et al.*, 2000; Tauxe, 1997; Wang & Doyle, 1998). Although the survival of these manure bacteria remains to be determined, likely depending on the physiological and ecological features of the resistant bacteria, the resistance genes can be transferred to indigenous soil bacteria. AMR can then be further disseminated to other environments, such as groundwater and surface water through seepage and run off, respectively. Eventually, resistant bacteria can enter the food chain through crops grown on the affected land (Boehme *et al.*, 2004). There is a great interest in assessing the likelihood of AMR transfer from manure impacted soil to produce, especially ready-to-eat vegetables (Egea *et al.*, 2011; Rizek *et al.*, 2011).

The impact of AMR from animal manure to soil is also reflected at genetic level. Numerous studies have demonstrated the dissemination of AMR genes from manure to soil after land application. Although most of the manure bacteria may not survive long after manure application, the large number of manure bacteria and soil bacteria can create frequent HGT by which AMR genes are transferred to bacteria indigenous to soil (Sengeløv *et al.*, 2003). These researchers also detected increased levels of tetracycline resistance gene (*tet*) with increased application of pig manure slurry to soil. Our own data also demonstrated an increase in *tet* genes and erythromycin resistance genes (*erm*) in soil impacted by the use of antimicrobials in swine production (unpublished data).

Both surface water and groundwater can also be contaminated by AMR arising from food animal production. Groundwater downstream of a swine manure lagoon was found to contain a much higher level of *tet* genes than the groundwater upstream of the swine lagoon (Koike *et al.*, 2007). Seepage from the lagoon was responsible to the increase in *tet* genes in the groundwater. By the same token, AMR can be readily disseminated to groundwater and surface water following manure application to land and rainfall.

Significant portion (25-75%) of the antibiotic drugs consumed by food animals are excreted by the animal (Chee-Sanford *et al.*, 2009). The half-life of these excreted antimicrobials varies depending on the drugs concerned and the abiotic and biotic conditions that drugs come in contact. A few studies have found that some residual antimicrobials can persist in waste treatment systems and in the environment for long periods of time (Zilles *et al.*, 2005). It is not well understood to what extent the antimicrobials from animal manure can contribute to development of AMR in environment. However, some researchers showed that microbial populations in soil and water bodies could be affected by antimicrobial-containing manure (Campagnolo *et al.*, 2002; Kong *et al.*, 2006; Martinez, 2009).

Antimicrobial resistance is becoming an increasing health concern because antimicrobial-resistant commensal bacteria function as a huge resistance reservoir and can spread AMR to the environment and humans. Antimicrobial resistance can be transferred to human by bacteria that can survive in both animals and humans. And greater concerns come from the possibility of AMR transfer from bacteria of animal origin to those in humans. Additionally, the microbiomes present in water, soil, and crops should also be taken into consideration because the dynamics and population structure of their microbial communities can be affected by animal wastes. Although it remains to be determined if environmental AMR reservoir can serve as an intermediate between AMR genes between bacteria of animals and humans (Canton, 2009; Wright, 2010), some *in-vitro* studies did indicate possible exchange of

AMR genes between soil bacteria and bacterial of animal origin via broad host-range plasmids (Heuer & Smalla, 2007; Smalla *et al.*, 2000). Horizontal transfer of AMR genes can occur among bacteria that are not phylogenetically closely related, and such HGT aggravates the concern. In recent years, numerous studies have been reported on the emergence of multiple drug resistance and its linkage to the mobile genetic elements. Although no proof has been found of exchange of genes between environmental bacteria and human intestinal microbiota, the risk remains.

Cases of food contaminated with common pathogenic bacteria (e.g., *Campylobacter jejuni, E coli, Salmonella* and *Enterococcus faecium*) carrying resistant genes have been reported (Yan & Gilbert, 2004; Zhao *et al.*, 2003). The possible aftermath of AMR mediated via food chain could have two ramifications. First, the colonization of zoophilic resistant bacteria in human gut could compromise the therapeutic effect of treatment of human infections because most antibiotics either are used both in humans and animals or share the same resistance mechanism. Second, there is the risk of gene exchange between colonized exogenous resistant bacteria and bacteria indigenous to human intestines (Hammerum & Heuer, 2009; Luangtongkum *et al.*, 2009; Walsh & Fanning, 2008). Although it remains to be determined if colonization of pathogens of animal origin in human gut results in transfer of their resistant gene to human intestinal microbiome, the potential warrants careful examination in future studies.

Antimicrobial resistance arising from animals can also spread to humans by contact. Akwar *et al.* (Akwar *et al.*, 2007) indicated that occupational exposure of farmers to animals carrying resistant bacteria may constitute a source of AMR in humans. Ahmad *et al.* (Ahmad *et al.*, 2011) reported that insects, which can move freely over long distance, could acquire multi-drug (mainly tetracycline and erythromycin) resistant enterococci from swine manure and transfer them among animal production farms and from farms to food.

4. Mobile genetic elements and horizontal resistance gene transfer

Horizontal gene transfers (HGT), which is primarily mediated by mobile genetic elements, play an essential role in dissemination of AMR genes. Conjugative plasmids, transposons, integrons, phages, and insertion elements have all been implicated in horizontal resistance gene transfer (Barlow, 2009). Since *tet* genes were found on plasmids in the 1960s, most of the known AMR genes have been found residing on mobile genetic elements (Barlow *et al.*, 2008; Lawley *et al.*, 2000; Nandi *et al.*, 2004; Rice, 1998). By analyzing resistant strains isolated from a conventional swine farm, Stine *et al* (Stine *et al.*, 2007) found recombination of *tet* genes and multiple different *tet* genes carried in single bacterial isolates. HGT is primarily responsible for the development of multiple drug resistance (Hawkey & Jones, 2009).

It should be noted that HGT can occur between bacteria that belong to different species. As such, AMR genes can be transferred from manure bacteria to indigenous bacteria, which are adapted to the soil environment and amplify the AMR through proliferation (i.e. vertical gene transfer). Additionally, because transformation does not need a live donor, AMR released from dead bacteria can also contribute to HGT through natural transformation. Thus, AMR genes inside of dead bacteria or released from dead bacteria also constitute a portion of the AMR reservoir and should be included in risk assessment of AMR arising from animal production. Additionally, most bacteria in soil or manure are viable but not culturable. In the case of soil bacteria, as much as 99% may not be cultured (Torsvik *et al.*, 1990). Therefore, most AMR is carried by unculturable bacteria, and AMR present in both culturable and unculturable bacteria should be examined to account for the entire AMR reservoir.

5. Mitigation of AMR arising from animal production

Although antibiotics are widely thought to be the most successful drug in human medicine, risk of AMR to human health emerged from the early clinical practices (Gezon & Cryst, 1948; Rutherford *et al.*, 1946). As elaborated above, extensive use of antimicrobials in livestock production made AMR situation worse. The potential but great risk precipitated the ban, at first partially and now completely, of antimicrobials as growth promoters in Europe (Casewell *et al.*, 2003). The ban led to significant decrease in AMR though not completely eliminated AMR from animal husbandry (Dibner & Richards, 2005). Although there is much debate about the total ban of antimicrobials as growth promoters and AMR prevalence, antimicrobials are still used as growth promoters outside of Europe. Therefore, there is a need to effectively control the dissemination of AMR off animal farms, and management and disposal of animal manure provide a critical control point in containing and reducing AMR arising from animal production systems.

5.1 Lagoons

In most swine and dairy farms, animal manure is typically collected from the barn into a pit and then pumped into an on-farm lagoon. The manure is stored in the waste lagoon for extended period of time (varying from weeks to months depending on seasons) until being applied to crop land. Such lagoons are large to ensure enough capacity to store the manure from large confined animal feeding operations (CAFOs). Quite a few studies have detected high levels of AMR in animal waste lagoons (Fox, 2004; Koike *et al.*, 2007; Macauley *et al.*, 2007; Mezriouia & Baleuxb, 1994). The bottom of animal waste lagoons is rarely lined by any impermeable material, and thus lagoon water, together with some compounds, bacteria, including antimicrobial-resistant ones, can seep into the aquifer underneath and be translocated into groundwater. Thus, this type of treatment, which is thought to be improper in many aspects, can lead to serious pollutions. Several studies have examined the impact of swine lagoons on AMR in groundwater. By comparing AMR profiles of *E. coli* in groundwater underneath swine waste lagoons with those in groundwater of crop farms, Anderson *et al.* showed that swine waste lagoon dramatically increased the prevalence *E. coli* and its multiple drug resistance (Anderson & Sobsey, 2006). Using PCR assays, AMR genes arising from swine waste lagoons were also found to be disseminated to groundwater (Chee-Sanford *et al.*, 2001; Koike *et al.*, 2007). Irrigation of crop land with the lagoon water and subsequent run off can disseminate AMR further to soil and surface water.

A number of studies have examined the potential of livestock waste lagoons to reduce AMR present in the animal manure. By analyzing fecal streptococci using a cultivation-based method, several *tet* gene classes by PCR, and methylation of 23S rRNA by probe hybridization, Jindal *et al.* found that swine waste lagoons had high prevalence of AMR (Jindal *et al.*, 2006). By comparing the abundance of both *tet* and *erm* genes, between swine manure and corresponding waste lagoons, swine waste lagoons were not found to be effective in reducing AMR appreciably (Chen *et al.*, 2008; Chen *et al.*, 2007; Wang *et al.*, 2011;

Yu *et al.*, 2005). Actually, some AMR can increase during lagoon storage (Wang *et al.*, 2011). This is consistent with the previous finding that AMR can increase in lagoons that store sewage (Mezriouia & Baleuxb, 1994).

Currently, there is no regulation on animal waste lagoons, but the potential risk posed by such lagoons is of great concern. Recognizing the potential risk, several research groups have investigated reduction of manure by tertiary treatments that have been used in municipal wastewater treatments. Macauley *et al.* (Macauley *et al.*, 2006) examined the effect of chlorine, ultraviolet light and ozone on swine lagoon bacteria. They found that these treatments at enough concentration or strengths dramatically decreased total bacteria present in swine lagoons, and a combination of chlorine and tetracycline killed all bacteria. Because antimicrobial resistant bacteria have similar ecological and physiological traits than as their susceptible peers, except for their AMR ability, these treatments should equally kill antimicrobial resistant bacteria and thereby reducing AMR present in lagoons. However, additional cost associated with these tertiary treatments probably prevents them from being applied in farms. Indeed, few farms have adopted these treatments.

5.2 Aerobic and anaerobic treatments

Intensive treatments have been implemented on a few animal farms, especially swine farms. These treatments use biological and/or chemical processes to reduce organic strength of the wastewater from CAFOs. The influent and the effluent of an Ekokan upflow biofilter system implemented at a swine farm were found to contain similar levels of both *erm* and *tet* genes (Chen *et al.*, 2010; Chen *et al.*, 2007). Based on a laboratory-scale study, Chenier *et al.* also concluded that aerobic treatments were ineffective in preventing AMR from being disseminated to the environments (Chenier & Juteau, 2009; Chenier & Juteau, 2009). The survival of aerobic and facultative anaerobic resistant bacteria and HGT were suggested as possible reasons for the persistence of AMR during aerobic treatments. It should be noted, however, that aerobic treatments can alter the prevalence of individual resistant bacteria as bacterial species can differ in AMR they carry and in survival during the same aerobic treatments.

Anaerobic digestion of animal manure is increasingly being implemented. The ability of an anaerobic sequencing batch reactor (ASBR) to decrease the AMR present in swine waste was assessed by Angenent *et al.* (Angenent *et al.*, 2008). Although the anaerobic treatment was effective in reducing the tylosin present in the swine manure, both the content and the effluent of the ASBR had substantially higher levels of AMR than that the waste stream fed to this system. In a full-scale anaerobic digester, Chen *et al.* (Chen *et al.*, 2010) also found that multiple classes of *erm* genes and *tet* genes present in swine manure did not reduce substantially during anaerobic digestion even though some classes of *erm* and *tet* genes reduced to some extent. Similar results were obtained by Ma *et al.* (Ma *et al.*, 2011) who used a laboratory-scale digester to digest municipal sludge at both mesophilic and thermophilic temperatures. The similar conditions (mesophilic temperature and anaerobic environments) in anaerobic digester might explain the inability to reduce AMR. However, anaerobic digesters differ in design (complete mixed, plug-flow, etc.) and operation (organic loading rate, hydraulic retention time, temperature, etc.). More studies are warranted to examine persistence of AMR in different anaerobic digesters operated under different conditions.

5.3 Composting

Composting has been used in management and treatment of livestock manure to produce fertilizer with reduced pest and disease incidence (Deluca & Deluca, 1997; Kashmanian & Rynk, 1995; Litterick *et al.*, 2004). Compost has been shown to be effective to kill pathogens and indicator bacteria present in livestock manure (Grewal *et al.*, 2007; Grewal *et al.*, 2006; Jiang *et al.*, 2003; Lemunier *et al.*, 2005; Tiquia, 2005). In surveying abundance of a large number of *tet* genes and *erm* genes, composted manure was found to contain much less AMR genes, up to seven orders of magnitude, than fresh manure or manure treated by other technologies, including lagoon, aerobic treatment, and anaerobic treatments (Chen *et al.*, 2010; Chen *et al.*, 2007; Yu *et al.*, 2005). In a filed study using windrows of beef cattle manure, *E. coli* resistant to ampicillin and tetracycline substantially reduced in the initial two weeks (Sharma *et al.*, 2009). Multiple classes of both *tet* and *erm* genes also exhibited significant reduction in abundance, however, the magnitude of the reduction was much smaller, even after 11 weeks. Nevertheless, the *tet* and *erm* genes differed in dynamics during the 18-week composting, with *tet*(A,C) and *erm*(A) increased marginally by week 11 relative to weeks 0 and 5, while *tet*(G), RPP *tet*, *erm*(B), *erm*(C), *erm*(F), *erm*(T), and *erm*(X)) decreasing at most time points analyzed. The relatively cold ambient temperature (September to November in Alberta, Canada) prevented the temperature from reaching 55°C inside of the windrows and might have contributed to the relatively small magnitudes of decrease in the *tet* and *erm* genes.

The intensity of composting management can affect the reduction of AMR and degradation of antimicrobials during composting because composting management can dramatically affect the microbial activities within composting windrows. This was exemplified in a pilot study using horse manure (Storteboom *et al.*, 2007) where high-intensity management (including amending with alfalfa and dried leaves, and regularly watering and turning) was found to degrade antimicrobials (i.e. chlortetracycline, tylosin, and monensin) and reduce *tet*(O) gene more rapidly than low-intensity management (no amendment or watering or turning). However, *tet*(W) increased in both the composting treatments after 141 days of treatment. More classes and types of AMR genes need to be examined to determine to what extent intensities of composting management affect AMR persistence during composting treatment. By comparing the dynamics of *tet*(W) and *tet*(O) genes between beef cattle manure containing high levels of AMR and dairy manure containing low level of AMR, this pilot study also showed that manure that contains high levels of AMR requires a longer time to achieve significant reduction of AMR. Increased HGT in the presence of high levels of AMR might be one of the explanations in the observed difference in the AMR dynamics.

The temporal changes in AMR carried by both cultivated and uncultivated bacteria present in swine manure during simulated composting at 55°C (the typical temperature achieved inside of large compost windrows) were compared to a simulated lagoon treatment at room temperature in a recent study (Wang *et al.*, 2011). Over a 48-day period cultivated aerobic heterotrophic tetracycline-resistant bacteria and erythromycin-resistant bacteria decreased by more than 7 and 4 logs, respectively, in the simulated composting treatment, while only 1 to 2 logs for both resistant bacterial groups in the simulated lagoon treatment. In the above study, the dynamics of six classes each of *erm* and *tet* genes, including *erm*(A), *erm*(B), *erm*(C), *erm*(F), *erm*(T), *erm*(X), *tet*(A/C), *tet*(G), *tet*(M), *tet*(O), *tet*(T), and *tet*(W), were also monitored. Except *erm*(B) and *tet*(A/C), all the resistance gene classes analyzed declined marginally during the first 17 days of the composting treatment, but dramatically thereafter within 31 days of the composting treatment. The observed decreases in AMR were not attributed to decrease in overall bacterial population, which did not decrease in the course of the composting treatment (Wang *et al.,* 2011). It remains to be determined why different AMR genes decreased at varying rates during composting. Two plausible explanations were offered to explain why cultured resistant bacteria decreased to a greater extent than the AMR genes analyzed: first, some resistant bacteria lost culturability or viability during composting, but their genetic materials, including the AMR genes, persisted. Second, not all the AMR genes were accounted for, as not all AMR genes could be detected by any existing real-time PCR assays. However, it is also possible that AMR might be more prevalent among culturable bacteria than among unculturable bacteria. Future studies are needed to test this hypothesis.

Different classes of *tet* or *erm* genes were found to have different persistence during composting treatment. For example, *tet*(W) was reduced slower than *tet*(O) irrespective of intensity of composting treatment of horse manure (Storteboom *et al.,* 2007). Wang *et al.* also showed that *erm*(B) and *tet*(A/C) were more persistent than *erm*(A), *erm*(B), *erm*(C), *erm*(F), *erm*(T), *erm*(X), *tet*(A/C), *tet*(G), *tet*(M), *tet*(O), *tet*(T), or *tet*(W). Difference in host ranges of AMR genes and ecology and physiology of resistant bacterial hosts are major factors contributing to the variations in persistence of AMR genes. However, more detailed investigation is needed to elucidate the mechanism that affecting persistence of different AMR.

The high efficacy of composting in reducing AMR was hypothesized to be attributed to several reasons (Chen *et al.,* 2010; Wang *et al.,* 2011). First, livestock manure is dominated by mesophilic anaerobic bacteria, which can be killed by the thermal aerobic conditions created in compost. Second, compost has relatively low water content and thus water activity. As such, proliferation of bacteria, including antimicrobial-resistant bacteria, can be greatly reduced within compost piles or windrows. Third, horizontal transfer of resistant genes is hindered because of the phylogenetic distance between aerobic thermophiles and the anaerobic mesophiles (Chenier & Juteau, 2009; Chenier & Juteau, 2009). Indeed, Guan *et al.* (Guan *et al.,* 2010; Guan *et al.,* 2007) showed that although resistant mobile plasmids carried by *E. coli* could survive and be transferred during chicken manure composting, higher temperature helped prevent spread of the plasmids in the environment. The relatively low water activity and the solid state within compost matrix should also reduce HGT (Wang *et al.,* 2011). Taken together, composting is an effective technology to reduce AMR and should help mitigate dissemination of AMR arising from animal production. .

6. Concluding remarks

Although the role(s) of AMR to bacteria is a matter of debate (Aminov, 2009; Davies, 2006; Yim *et al.,* 2007; Yim *et al.,* 2006), it is a fact that the widespread of AMR poses a risk to human health and livestock manure from CAFOs is a large source of AMR. Reduced use of antimicrobials in animal production is an option in decreasing development of AMR, but the perceived negative effects on productivity make it not likely, at least in the near future, to ban Antibiotic growth promoter (AGP) in many countries. Therefore, manure treatment and management should be considered as a critical control point to reduce dissemination of AMR off animal farms. Lagoon storage is probably the poorest in terms of reducing AMR present in animal manure, while compost is the most effective. Aerobic biological treatments do not effectively reduce total AMR, but shift the resistant bacterial populations. Anaerobic treatment operated at thermophilic temperature, but not at mesophilic temperature, is another option to mitigate AMR present in animal manure. However, because the current conclusions are based on studies on either a few select cultured bacteria (e.g. *E. coli, Enterococcus, Staphylococcus* and *Streptococcus*) or select AMR genes (mostly *tet* genes and *erm* genes), future studies are warranted to include more AMR so that the conclusions will be applicable to AMR in general.

Understanding the AMR genes and the corresponding resistant bacteria is essential to assess the risk posed to health of both humans and animals. DNA-based techniques (e.g. real-time PCR) enable measurement of AMR carried in both cultured and uncultured bacteria; however, these techniques typically do not allow identification of AMR-carrying bacteria. To complement this limitation cultivation-based studies are needed. Additionally, metagenomics empowered by massively parallel DNA sequencing provide an alternative in identifying the genes and bacteria in resistant populations.

No treatment technology is practical that can completely eliminate AMR present in animal manure. The surviving AMR will eventually find its way to the environments. In a recent study, we analyzed the cultured bacteria resistant to tetracyclines or erythromycin that were recovered from swine manure before and after composting treatment in a comparative manner. We observed considerable shifts in resistant bacterial populations, AMR genes (i.e. *tet* and *erm* genes), carriage of multiple AMR per isolate, and plasmids (unpublished data). This type of studies is needed to identify the surviving resistant bacteria and their ecology upon land application of composted manure.

7. References

Aarestrup, F. M., Oliver Duran, C. & Burch, D. G. (2008). Antimicrobial resistance in swine production. *Anim Health Res Rev*, 9(2), 135-148.

Agustin, A. I., Carraminana, J. J., Rota, C. & Herrera, A. (2005). Antimicrobial resistance of Salmonella spp. from pigs at slaughter in Spain in 1993 and 2001. *Letters in Applied Microbiology*, 41(1), 39-44.

Ahmad, A., Ghosh, A., Schal, C. & Zurek, L. (2011). Insects in confined swine operations carry a large antibiotic resistant and potentially virulent enterococcal community. *BMC Microbiology*, 11(1), 23.

Akwar, T. H., Poppe, C., Wilson, J., Reid-Smith, R. J., Dyck, M., Waddington, J., Shang, D., Dassie, N. & McEwen, S. A. (2007). Risk factors for antimicrobial resistance among fecal Escherichia coli from residents on forty-three swine farms. *Microb Drug Resist*, 13(1), 69-76.

Aminov, R. I. (2009). The role of antibiotics and antibiotic resistance in nature. *Environ Microbiol*, 11(12), 2970-2988.

Anderson, M. E. & Sobsey, M. D. (2006). Detection and occurrence of antimicrobially resistant E. coli in groundwater on or near swine farms in eastern North Carolina. *Water Sci Technol*, 54(3), 211-8.

Andremont, A. (2003). Commensal flora may play key role in spreading antibiotic resistance. *ASM News*, 69(12), 601-607.

Angenent, L. T., Mau, M., George, U., Zahn, J. A. & Raskin, L. (2008). Effect of the presence of the antimicrobial tylosin in swine waste on anaerobic treatment. *Water Res*, 42(10-11), 2377-84.

Barlow, M. (2009). What antimicrobial resistance has taught us about horizontal gene transfer. *Methods Mol Biol*, 532, 397-411.

Barlow, R. S., Fegan, N. & Gobius, K. S. (2008). A comparison of antibiotic resistance integrons in cattle from separate beef meat production systems at slaughter. *J Appl Microbiol*, 104(3), 651-8.

Barton, M. D. (2000). Antibiotic use in animal feed and its impact on human health. *Nutr. Res. Rev.*, 13, 279-299.

Binh, C. T., Heuer, H., Kaupenjohann, M. & Smalla, K. (2008). Piggery manure used for soil fertilization is a reservoir for transferable antibiotic resistance plasmids. *FEMS Microbiol Ecol*, 66(1), 25-37.

Boehme, S., Werner, G., Klare, I., Reissbrodt, R. & Witte, W. (2004). Occurrence of antibiotic-resistant enterobacteria in agricultural foodstuffs. *Mol Nutr Food Res*, 48(7), 522-31.

Brody, T., Yavatkar, A. S., Lin, Y., Ross, J., Kuzin, A., Kundu, M., Fann, Y. & Odenwald, W. F. (2008). Horizontal gene transfers link a human MRSA pathogen to contagious bovine mastitis bacteria. *PLoS ONE*, 3(8), e3074.

Buswell, C. M., Herlihy, Y. M., Lawrence, L. M., McGuiggan, J. T., Marsh, P. D., Keevil, C. W. & Leach, S. A. (1998). Extended survival and persistence of Campylobacter spp. in water and aquatic biofilms and their detection by immunofluorescent-antibody and -rRNA staining. *Appl Environ Microbiol*, 64(2), 733-41.

Campagnolo, E. R., Johnson, K. R., Karpati, A., Rubin, C. S., Kolpin, D. W., Meyer, M. T., Esteban, J. E., Currier, R. W., Smith, K., Thu, K. M. & McGeehin, M. (2002). Antimicrobial residues in animal waste and water resources proximal to large-scale swine and poultry feeding operations. *Sci Total Environ*, 299(1-3), 89-95.

Canton, R. (2009). Antibiotic resistance genes from the environment: a perspective through newly identified antibiotic resistance mechanisms in the clinical setting. *Clin Microbiol Infect*, 15 Suppl 1, 20-5.

Casewell, M., Friis, C., Marco, E., McMullin, P. & Phillips, I. (2003). The European ban on growth-promoting antibiotics and emerging consequences for human and animal health. *J Antimicrob Chemother*, 52(2), 159-61.

Chee-Sanford, J. C., Aminov, R. I., Krapac, I. J., Garrigues-Jeanjean, N. & Mackie, R. I. (2001). Occurrence and diversity of tetracycline resistance genes in lagoons and groundwater underlying two swine production facilities. *Appl. Environ. Microbiol.*, 67(4), 1494-1502.

Chee-Sanford, J. C., Mackie, R. I., Koike, S., Krapac, I. G., Lin, Y. F., Yannarell, A. C., Maxwell, S. & Aminov, R. I. (2009). Fate and transport of antibiotic residues and antibiotic resistance genes following land application of manure waste. *J Environ Qual*, 38(3), 1086-108.

Chen, J., Fluharty, F. L., St-Pierre, N., Morrison, M. & Yu, Z. (2008). Technical note: Occurrence in fecal microbiota of genes conferring resistance to both macrolide-lincosamide-streptogramin B and tetracyclines concomitant with feeding of beef cattle with tylosin. *J Anim Sci*, 86(9), 2385-2391.

Chen, J., Michel Jr., F. C., Sreevatsan, S., Morrison, M. & Yu, Z. (2010). Occurrence and persistence of erythromycin resistance genes (*erm*) and tetracycline resistance genes (*tet*) in waste treatment systems on swine farms. *Microbial Ecology*, 60, 479-486.

Chen, J., Yu, Z., Michel Jr., F. C., Wittum, T. & Morrison, M. (2007). Development and application of real-time PCR assays for quantification of *erm* genes conferring resistance to macrolides-lincosamides-streptogramin B in livestock manure and manure management systems. *Appl. Environ. Microbiol.*, 73(14), 4407-4416.

Chenier, M. R. & Juteau, P. (2009). Fate of chlortetracycline- and tylosin-resistant bacteria in an aerobic thermophilic sequencing batch reactor treating swine waste. *Microb Ecol*, 58(1), 86-97.

Chenier, M. R. & Juteau, P. (2009). Impact of an aerobic thermophilic sequencing batch reactor on antibiotic-resistant anaerobic bacteria in swine waste. *Microb Ecol*, 58(4), 773-85.

D'Lima, C. B., Miller, W. G., Mandrell, R. E., Wright, S. L., Siletzky, R. M., Carver, D. K. & Kathariou, S. (2007). Clonal Population Structure and Specific Genotypes of Multidrug-Resistant Campylobacter coli from Turkeys. *Appl. Environ. Microbiol.*, 73(7), 2156-2164.

Davies, J. (2006). Are antibiotics naturally antibiotics? *J Ind Microbiol Biotechnol*, 33(7), 496-9.

Deluca, T. H. & Deluca, D. K. (1997). Composting for feedlot manure management and soil quality. *Journal of Production Agriculture*, 10(2), 235-241.

Dibner, J. J. & Richards, J. D. (2005). Antibiotic growth promoters in agriculture: history and mode of action. *Poult Sci*, 84(4), 634-43.

Dubel, J. R., Zink, D. L., Kelley, L. M., Naqi, S. A. & Renshaw, H. W. (1982). Bacterial antibiotic resistance frequency of gentamicin resistant strains of *Escherichia coli* in the fecal microflora of commercial turkeys. *American Journal of Veterinary Research*, 43(10), 1786-1789.

Dunlop, R. H., McEwen, S. A., Meek, A. H., Black, W. D., Friendship, R. M. & Clarke, R. C. (1998). Prevalences of resistance to seven antimicrobials among fecal Escherichia coli of swine on thirty-four farrow-to-finish farms in Ontario, Canada. *Prev Vet Med*, 34(4), 265-82.

Egea, P., Lopez-Cerero, L., Navarro, M. D., Rodriguez-Bano, J. & Pascual, A. (2011). Assessment of the presence of extended-spectrum beta-lactamase-producing Escherichia coli in eggshells and ready-to-eat products. *Eur J Clin Microbiol Infect Dis*, 30(9), 1045-7.

Fox, J. (2004). Drug resistance at the community level and in swine lagoons, ground water. *ASM News*, 70(9), 392-393.

Gezon, H. M. & Cryst, E. E. (1948). Antibiotic studies on beta hemolytic streptococci; streptomycin resistance acquired by group A, B, and C organisms. *Proc Soc Exp Biol Med*, 68(3), 653-7.

Grewal, S., Sreevatsan, S. & Michel Jr., F. C. (2007). Persistence of *Listeria monocytogenes* and *Salmonella enterica* serovar typhimurium during simulated composting, pack storage, and aerated and unaerated liquid storage of swine manure. *Compost Sci. Util.* , 15(1), 53-62.

Grewal, S. K., Rajeev, S., Sreevatsan, S. & Michel, F. C., Jr. (2006). Persistence of Mycobacterium avium subsp. paratuberculosis and other zoonotic pathogens during simulated composting, manure packing, and liquid storage of dairy manure. *Appl Environ Microbiol*, 72(1), 565-74.

Guan, J., Chan, M. & Spencer, J. L. (2010). The fate of recombinant plasmids during composting of organic wastes. *J Environ Sci Health B*, 45(4), 279-84.

Guan, J., Wasty, A., Grenier, C. & Chan, M. (2007). Influence of temperature on survival and conjugative transfer of multiple antibiotic-resistant plasmids in chicken manure and compost microcosms. *Poult Sci*, 86(4), 610-3.

Guo, X., Chen, J., Brackett, R. E. & Beuchat, L. R. (2002). Survival of Salmonella on tomatoes stored at high relative humidity, in soil, and on tomatoes in contact with soil. *J Food Prot*, 65(2), 274-9.

Haack, B. J. & Andrews, R. E. J. (2000). Isolation of Tn916-like conjugal elements from swine lot effluent. *Canadian Journal of Microbiology*, 46(6), 542-549.

Hammerum, A. M. & Heuer, O. E. (2009). Human health hazards from antimicrobial-resistant *Escherichia coli* of animal origin. *Clin Infect Dis*, 48(7), 916-21.

Hanzawa, Y., Oka, C., Ishiguro, N. & Sato, G. (1984). Antibiotic-resistant coliforms in the waste of piggeries and dairy farms. *Japanese Journal of Veterinary Science*, 46, 363-372.

Hawkey, P. M. & Jones, A. M. (2009). The changing epidemiology of resistance. *J Antimicrob Chemother*, 64 Suppl 1, i3-10.

Hendriksen, R. S., Mevius, D. J., Schroeter, A., Teale, C., Jouy, E., Butaye, P., Franco, A., Utinane, A., Amado, A., Moreno, M., Greko, C., Stark, K. D., Berghold, C., Myllyniemi, A. L., Hoszowski, A., Sunde, M. & Aarestrup, F. M. (2008). Occurrence of antimicrobial resistance among bacterial pathogens and indicator bacteria in pigs in different European countries from year 2002 - 2004: the ARBAO-II study. *Acta Vet Scand*, 50, 19.

Hendriksen, R. S., Mevius, D. J., Schroeter, A., Teale, C., Meunier, D., Butaye, P., Franco, A., Utinane, A., Amado, A., Moreno, M., Greko, C., Stark, K., Berghold, C., Myllyniemi, A. L., Wasyl, D., Sunde, M. & Aarestrup, F. M. (2008). Prevalence of antimicrobial resistance among bacterial pathogens isolated from cattle in different European countries: 2002-2004. *Acta Vet Scand*, 50, 28.

Heuer, H. & Smalla, K. (2007). Manure and sulfadiazine synergistically increased bacterial antibiotic resistance in soil over at least two months. *Environmental Microbiology*, 9(3), 657-666.

Huang, T. M., Lin, T. L. & Wu, C. C. (2009). Antimicrobial susceptibility and resistance of chicken Escherichia coli, Salmonella spp., and Pasteurella multocida isolates. *Avian Dis*, 53(1), 89-93.

Jackson, C. R., Fedorka-Cray, P. J., Barrett, J. B. & Ladely, S. R. (2004). Effects of tylosin use on erythromycin resistance in enterococci isolated from swine. *Appl. Environ. Microbiol.*, 70(7), 4205-4210.

Jiang, X., Morgan, J. & Doyle, M. P. (2003). Fate of *Escherichia coli* O157:H7 during composting of bovine manure in a laboratory-scale bioreactor. *J. of Food Protection*, 66(1), 25-30.

Jindal, A., Kocherginskaya, S., Mehboob, A., Robert, M., Mackie, R. I., Raskin, L. & Zilles, J. L. (2006). Antimicrobial use and resistance in swine waste treatment systems. *Appl. Environ. Microbiol.*, 72(12), 7813-7820.

Kashmanian, R. M. & Rynk, R. F. (1995). Agricultural composting in the United States. *Compost Sci. & Utiliz.*, 3(3), 84-88.

Koike, S., Krapac, I. G., Oliver, H. D., Yannarell, A. C., Chee-Sanford, J. C., Aminov, R. I. & Mackie, R. I. (2007). Monitoring and source tracking of tetracycline resistance genes in lagoons and groundwater adjacent to swine production facilities over a 3-year period. *Appl. Environ. Microbiol.*, 73(15), 4813-4823.

Kong, W. D., Zhu, Y. G., Fu, B. J., Marschner, P. & He, J. Z. (2006). The veterinary antibiotic oxytetracycline and Cu influence functional diversity of the soil microbial community. *Environ Pollut*, 143(1), 129-137.

Lawley, T. D., Burland, V. & Taylor, D. E. (2000). Analysis of the complete nucleotide sequence of the tetracycline-resistance transposon Tn10. *Plasmid*, 43(3), 235-239.

Lemunier, M., Francou, C., Rousseaux, S., Houot, S., Dantigny, P., Piveteau, P. & Guzzo, J. (2005). Long-Term Survival of Pathogenic and Sanitation Indicator Bacteria in Experimental Biowaste Composts. *Appl. Environ. Microbiol.*, 71(10), 5779-5786.

Litterick, A. M., Harrier, L., Wallace, P., Watson, C. A. & Wood, M. (2004). The role of uncomposted materials, composts, manures, and compost extracts in reducing pest and disease incidence and severity in sustainable temperate agricultural and horticultural crop production - A review. *Critical Reviews in Plant Sciences*, 23(6), 453-479.

Luangtongkum, T., Jeon, B., Han, J., Plummer, P., Logue, C. M. & Zhang, Q. (2009). Antibiotic resistance in Campylobacter: emergence, transmission and persistence. *Future Microbiol*, 4(2), 189-200.

Luangtongkum, T., Morishita, T. Y., Ison, A. J., Huang, S., McDermott, P. F. & Zhang, Q. (2006). Effect of conventional and organic production practices on the prevalence and antimicrobial resistance of *Campylobacter* spp. in poultry. *Appl. Environ. Microbiol.*, 72(5), 3600-3607.

Lundin, J. I., Dargatz, D. A., Wagner, B. A., Lombard, J. E., Hill, A. E., Ladely, S. R. & Fedorka-Cray, P. J. (2008). Antimicrobial drug resistance of fecal Escherichia coli and Salmonella spp. isolates from United States dairy cows. *Foodborne Pathog Dis*, 5(1), 7-19.

Ma, Y., Wilson, C. A., Novak, J. T., Riffat, R., Aynur, S., Murthy, S. & Pruden, A. (2011). Effect of Various Sludge Digestion Conditions on Sulfonamide, Macrolide, and Tetracycline Resistance Genes and Class I Integrons. *Environ Sci Technol.*

Macauley, J. J., Adams, C. D. & Mormile, M. R. (2007). Diversity of tet resistance genes in tetracycline-resistant bacteria isolated from a swine lagoon with low antibiotic impact. *Can J Microbiol*, 53(12), 1307-15.

Macauley, J. J., Qiang, Z., Adams, C. D., Surampalli, R. & Mormile, M. R. (2006). Disinfection of swine wastewater using chlorine, ultraviolet light and ozone. *Water Res*, 40(10), 2017-26.

Martinez, J. L. (2009). Environmental pollution by antibiotics and by antibiotic resistance determinants. *Environ Pollut*, 157(11), 2893-2902.

Mathew, A. G., Cissell, R. & Liamthong, S. (2007). Antibiotic resistance in bacteria associated with food animals: a United States perspective of livestock production. *Foodborne Pathog Dis*, 4(2), 115-33.

Mellon, M., Benbrook, C. M. & Benbrook, K. L. (2001). *Hogging it: estimates of antimicrobial abuse in livestock*. UCS Publications., Cambridge, MA.

Mezriouia, N. & Baleuxb, B. (1994). Resistance patterns of *E. coli* strains isolated from domestic sewage before and after treatment in both aerobic lagoon and activated sludge. *Water Res.*, 28(11), 2399-2406.

Nandi, S., Maurer, J. J., Hofacre, C. & Summers, A. O. (2004). Gram-positive bacteria are a major reservoir of Class 1 antibiotic resistance integrons in poultry litter. *PNAS*, 101(18), 7118-7122.

Prescott, J. F. (2008). Antimicrobial use in food and companion animals. *Anim Health Res Rev*, 9(2), 127-33.

Rice, L. B. (1998). Tn916 family conjugative transposons and dissemination of antimicrobial resistance determinants. *Antimicrob Agents Chemother*, 42(8), 1871-7.

Rizek, C. F., Matte, M. H., Dropa, M., Mamizuka, E. M., de Almeida, L. M., Lincopan, N., Matte, G. R. & Germano, P. M. (2011). Identification of Staphylococcus aureus carrying the mecA gene in ready-to-eat food products sold in Brazil. *Foodborne Pathog Dis*, 8(4), 561-3.

Roe, M. T. & Pillai, S. D. (2003). Monitoring and identifying antibiotic resistance mechanisms in bacteria. *Poultry Science*, 82(4), 622-626.

Rutherford, R. H., Marquardt, G. H. & Van Ravenswaay, A. C. (1946). Resistance to antibiotic agents. *Mo Med*, 43(8), 535-8.

Santo Domingo, J. W., Harmon, S. & Bennett, J. (2000). Survival of Salmonella species in river water. *Curr Microbiol*, 40(6), 409-17.

Sengeløv, G., Agersø, Y., Halling-Sørensen, B., Baloda, S. B., Andersen, J. S. & Jensen, L. B. (2003). Bacterial antibiotic resistance levels in Danish farmland as a result of treatment with pig manure slurry. *Environment International*, 28(7), 587-595.

Sharma, R., Larney, F. J., Chen, J., Yanke, L. J., Morrison, M., Topp, E., McAllister, T. A. & Yu, Z. (2009). Selected antimicrobial resistance during composting of manure from cattle administered sub-therapeutic antimicrobials. *J Environ Qual*, 38(2), 567-75.

Smalla, K., Heuer, H., Gotz, A., Niemeyer, D., Krogerrecklenfort, E. & Tietze, E. (2000). Exogenous isolation of antibiotic resistance plasmids from piggery manure slurries reveals a high prevalence and diversity of IncQ-like plasmids. *Appl Environ Microbiol*, 66(11), 4854-62.

Smith, H. W. (1967). The effect of the use of antibacterial drugs, particularly as food additives, on the emergence of drug-resistant strains of bacteria in animals. *New Zealand Veterinary Journal*, 15(9), 153-166.

Stine, O. C., Johnson, J. A., Keefer-Norris, A., Perry, K. L., Tigno, J., Qaiyumi, S., Stine, M. S. & Morris, J. G., Jr. (2007). Widespread distribution of tetracycline resistance genes in a confined animal feeding facility. *Int J Antimicrob Agents*, 29(3), 348-52.

Storteboom, H. N., Kim, S. C., Doesken, K. C., Carlson, K. H., Davis, J. G. & Pruden, A. (2007). Response of antibiotics and resistance genes to high-intensity and low-intensity manure management. *J Environ Qual*, 36(6), 1695-703.

Tauxe, R. V. (1997). Emerging foodborne diseases: an evolving public health challenge. *Emerg Infect Dis*, 3(4), 425-34.

Teuber, M. (2001). Veterinary use and antibiotic resistance. *Curr. Opin. Microbiol.*, 4(5), 493-499.

Tiquia, S. M. (2005). Microbiological parameters as indicators of compost maturity. *Journal of Applied Microbiology*, 99(4), 816-828.

Torsvik, V., Goksoyr, J. & Daae, F. L. (1990). High diversity in DNA of soil bacteria. *Appl. Environ. Microbiol.*, 56(3), 782-787.

Walsh, C. & Fanning, S. (2008). Antimicrobial resistance in foodborne pathogens--a cause for concern? *Curr Drug Targets*, 9(9), 808-15.

Wang, G. & Doyle, M. P. (1998). Survival of enterohemorrhagic Escherichia coli O157:H7 in water. *J Food Prot*, 61(6), 662-7.

Wang, L., Oda, Y., Grewal, S., Morrison, M., F.C., M. J. & Yu, Z. (2011). Persistance of resistance to erythromycin and in swine manure during simulated composting and treatments. *Microbial Ecology*, online First.

Witte, W. (2000). Selective pressure by antibiotic use in livestock. *Int. J. Antimicrob. Agents*, 16(Sup 1), S19-S24.

Wright, G. D. (2010). Antibiotic resistance in the environment: a link to the clinic? *Curr Opin Microbiol*, 13(5), 589-94.

Yan, S. S. & Gilbert, J. M. (2004). Antimicrobial drug delivery in food animals and microbial food safety concerns: an overview of in vitro and in vivo factors potentially affecting the animal gut microflora. *Adv Drug Deliv Rev*, 56(10), 1497-521.

Yim, G., Wang, H. H. & Davies, J. (2007). Antibiotics as signalling molecules. *Philos Trans R Soc Lond B Biol Sci*, 362(1483), 1195-200.

Yim, G., Wang, H. H. & Davies, J. (2006). The truth about antibiotics. *Int J Med Microbiol*, 296(2-3), 163-70.

Yu, Z., Michel Jr., F. C., Hansen, G., Wittum, T. & Morrison, M. (2005). Development and application of real-time PCR assays for quantification of genes encoding tetracycline resistance. *Appl. Environ. Microbiol.*, 71(11), 6926-6933.

Zhao, S., Qaiyumi, S., Friedman, S., Singh, R., Foley, S. L., White, D. G., McDermott, P. F., Donkar, T., Bolin, C., Munro, S., Baron, E. J. & Walker, R. D. (2003). Characterization of *Salmonella enterica* serotype Newport isolated from humans and food animals. *J Clin Microbiol*, 41(12), 5366-71.

Zilles, J., Shimada, T., Jindal, A., Robert, M. & Raskin, L. (2005). Presence of macrolide-lincosamide-streptogramin B and tetracycline antimicrobials in swine waste treatment processes and amended soil. *Water Environ Res*, 77(1), 57-62.

Part 2

Synthesis of New Antibiotics and Probiotics: The Promise of the Next Decade

22

Design, Development and Synthesis of Novel Cephalosporin Group of Antibiotics

Kumar Gaurav, Sourish Karmakar, Kanika Kundu and Subir Kundu*
Institute of Technology & MMV, Banaras Hindu University, Varanasi, India

1. Introduction

Cephalosporins are β- lactam antibiotics. In cephalosporin C, four membered β- lactam ring (which is mainly responsible for the activity) is fused with six membered dihydrothiazine ring to form the basic nucleus, 7-aminocephalosporanic acid (7-ACA) and to which α-aminoadipic acid side chain is attached through an amide bond (Fig 1). (Mandell and Sande,1991)Although cephalosporin was found to be active against large number of pathogenic bacteria (Medeiros, 1997) but the main hindrance in its application is its low stability. Also, occurrence of bacterial strains that are resistant to already existing antibiotics such as methicillin resistant *Staphylococcus aureus* (MRSA) and vancomycin resistant *E. faecalis* (VRE) has led to the search of new semisynthetic cephalosporins with better solubility and new mechanism of action. Only cephalosporin C is found naturally, so it's chemical modification allowed production of a whole series of semisynthetic cephalosporins which can be used as therapeutics to fight organisms that have become penicillin resistant. Chemical modifications of cephalosporin C resulted in new cephalosporin derivatives. These semisynthetic cephalosporins are classified based on their activity profile, the antibacterial spectrum. Each newer generation of cephalosporin has significantly greater Gram -ve antimicrobial properties than the preceding generations, (Stan,2004; Jones,1994; Jacoby,2000; Babini and Livermore, 2000) in most cases with decreased activity against Gram +ve organism. Fourth generation cephalosporins are known to have true broad spectrum activity. (Wilson,1998; Tzouvelekis et al., 1998) In the past decade, even though the cephalosporin antibiotics have made remarkable progress and contribution in the treatment of acute diseases originated from pathogenic infection in clinics, many efforts still exist to achieve the well balanced broad spectrum and to improve beta-lactamase stability. 7α-formamido cephalosporins were isolated as fermentation product of various gram negative bacteria. The development of a new antibiotic focuses mainly with the study and characterization of its mechanism of its activity (Table 1). The β-lactam antibiotics like penicillin, cephalosporins, vancomycin, etc. are specific inhibitor working against bacterial cell wall (peptidoglycan) synthesis but newer strains have β-lactamase activity which destroys most of the β-lactam antibiotics and thus make them resistant to it. However, cephalosporins proved to be more stable to β-lactamase. Cephalosporin-C (CPC) shows similarity to in structure with the penicillin in having an acyl side chain attached to an

* Corresponding Author

amino group of a double ring nucleus (Figure 1). The side chain was identical to that of penicillin N, *i.e.* D-α-aminoadipic acid. Although both the types have the four membered β-lactam group, cephalosporin-C have a six membered dihydrothiazine ring in place of the five membered thiazolidine ring system which is a characteristic of penicillins. But these antibiotics are not that effective to be used for clinical purposes. The cephalosporin nucleus, 7-aminocephalosporanic acid (7-ACA) is derived from cephalosporin-C, prove to be more effective. Modification of 7-ACA side chains resulted in the development of newer generations of useful antibiotic agents, which leaded to various generations of cephalosporins.

Antibiotics	**Source**	**Mode of action**
Antibacterial antibiotics		
Bacitracin	*Bacillus subtilis*	Cell-wall synthesis
Cephalosporin	*Cephalosporium sp.*	Cell-wall synthesis
Chloramphenicol	*Streptomyces venezuelae*	Protein synthesis
Cycloserin	*Streptomyces leavendulae*	Cell-wall synthesis
Erythromycin	*Streptomyces erythraeus*	Protein synthesis
Kanamycin	*Streptomyces kanomycetoius*	Protein synthesis
Neomycin	*Streptomyces fradiae*	Protein synthesis
Novobiocin	*Streptomyces* sp.	DNA synthesis
Penicillin	*Penicillium* sp.	Cell-wall synthesis
Polymixin	*Bacillus polymyxa*	Cell membrane
Streptomycin	*Streptomyces griseus*	Protein synthesis
Tetracycline	*Streptomyces aureofaciens*	Protein synthesis
Vancomycin	*Streptomyces orientalis*	Cell-wall synthesis
Antiprotozoan antibiotics		
Fumagilin	*Aspergillus fumigatus*	Protein synthesis
Antifungal antibiotics		
Amphotericin B	*Streptomyces nodosus*	Membrane function
Cycloheximide	*Streptomyces griseus*	Protein synthesis
Griseofulvin	*Penicillium griseofulvum*	Cell-wall, microtubules
Nystatin	*Streptomyces noursei*	Damages cell-membrane

Table 1. Different mode of activity/ action of major antibiotics. (Gaurav *et al.*, 2011)

The β-lactam antibiotics like penicillin, cephalosporins, vancomycin, etc. are specific inhibitor working against bacterial cell wall (peptidoglycan) synthesis but newer strains have β-lactamase activity which destroys most of the β-lactam antibiotics and thus make them resistant to it. However, cephalosporins proved to be more stable to β-lactamase. Cephalosporin-C (CPC) shows similarity to in structure with the penicillins in having an acyl side chain attached to an amino group of a double ring nucleus (Figure 1). The side chain was identical to that of penicillin N, *i.e.* D-α-aminoadipic acid. Although both the types have the four membered β-lactam group, cephalosporin-C have a six membered dihydrothiazine ring in place of the five membered thiazolidine ring system which is a characteristic of penicillins. But these antibiotics are not that effective to be used for clinical purposes. The cephalosporin nucleus, 7- aminocephalosporanic acid (7-ACA) is derived from cephalosporin-C, prove to be more effective. Modification of 7-ACA side chains resulted in the development of newer generations of useful antibiotic agents, which leaded to various generations of cephalosporins.

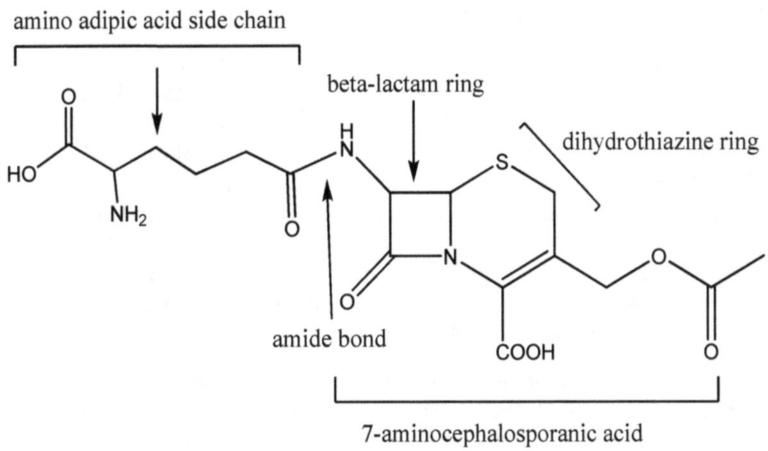

Cephalosporin C

Fig. 1. The structure of Cephalosporin

Cephalosporins are nowadays more suggested for the prophylaxis and treatment of bacterial infections caused by susceptible microorganisms. First generation cephalosporins are predominantly effective against gram positive bacteria and successive generations (Table 2) have further enhanced the activity against the gram negative bacteria too (Essack, 2001) However, the synthesis of different generations of cephalosporins are only possible either by microbial routes or by enzymatically converting cephalosporin-C. Hence, a brief discussion on microbial synthesis of cephalosporin-C is quite needed.

Various Generation	Example
First generation Cephalosporins	Cephalothin
	Cephaloridine
	Cephazolin
	Cephradine
	Cefroxadine
Second generation Cephalosporins	Cephamandole
	Cefuroime
	Ceforanide
	Cefotiam
Third generation Cephalosporins	Cefotaxime
	Ceftazidime
	Ceftizoxime
	Ceftriaxone
	Cefixime
	Ceftibuten
Fourth generation Cephalosporins	Cefipime
	Cefpirome

Table 2. Various Generations of Cephalosporin group of antibiotics

2. Microbial synthesis of cephalosporin-C

The biosynthesis of cephalosporin-C is carried only by few microorganisms, viz. fungi, *Streptomyces* sp. and bacteria. It can produced by free and immobilized microbial cells (Kundu *et al.*, 2000) using various cultivation modes of batch and continuous strategy (Mahapatra *et al.*, 2002). In batch mode of fermentation, Cephalosporin-C is produced in stirred tank bioreactors (Srivastava *et.al*, 1996) as well as in air lift bioreactor (Srivastava *et al.*, 1995; 1999).In continuous mode of fermentation, it can be produced both by packed bed bioreactor using different types of immobilization processes and in continuous stirred tank bioreactor. As it's a highly aerobic process in nature, cephalosporin-C is also produced by immobilized microbial cells utilizing symbiotic mode (*in-situ* oxygen production) in a packed bed bioreactor. (Kundu *et al.*, 1993)

In order to fulfill the need of large quantity of semi-synthetic cephalosporin, the key intermediates should be produced in large quantity through very efficient and cheap production routes. But the chemical production of the intermediates generates large quantities of wastes and requires expensive and hazardous chemicals and reaction conditions. In order to overcome these problems, enzymes are used to perform the required reactions. Cephalosporin C is converted to 7-ACA in a two step enzymatic process. First the side chain is deaminated by a D-amino oxidase, resulting in an α-keto acid that spontaneously loses carbon dioxide in the presence of hydrogen peroxide to form glutaryl-7-ACA. Subsequent enzymztic deacylation of the glutaryl side chain yields 7-ACA. The enzyme used, cephalosporin acylase, removes a charged aliphatic side chain without damaging the β- lactam nucleus. These enzymatic processes have the advantage of generating less waste and requiring less expensive chemicals. Thus, cephalosporin-C is directly converted to 7-ACA by cephalosporin-C acylase enzyme. (Zhang and Xu, 1993)

2.1 Production strategy of cephalosporin C (primary precursor)

Microbial production of Cephalosporin C, a secondary metabolite, occurs in late stationary phase (Idio-phase) of growth. So the main strategy of the production is to grow the culture to saturation level and then control the flow of nutrient to maintain the stationary phase. (Srivastava *et al.*, 2006) Cephalosporin C fermentation always requires highly aerobic condition to maintain uniform yield. Hence, maximum focus is given on oxygenation of the media. There are different processes involved using various modes of bioreactors, *viz.* conventional and non conventional Bioreactors. The conventional mode of bioreactors involves in batch or continuous stirred tank bioreactors whereas non conventional mode involves in packed bed bioreactors, airlift bioreactors and the like. (Srivastava *et al.*, 1996)

2.1.1 Cephalosporin C production by conventional mode of bioreactors

Conventional mode involves production by batch bioreactor or continuous stirred tank reactor (Kundu et al., 1993). Surface liquid culture and solid state fermentation are not very much favorable as there is high probability of oxygen limitation. There are some research occurring in the field but the stable process involved is the stirred tank batch bioreactors. They have special attachment for oxygen sparging and agitation for making the oxygen more available to microorganisms (Srivastava *et al.*, 1996).The morphological characteristics of the mold change under high agitation which in turn affects the yield of the Cephalosporin C. (Kundu et al., 1993)

Continuous mode involves various continuous stirred tank bioreactors. The first type is where the oxygen is being sparged in the reactor fitted with an agitator (Figure 2 A). The second process involves addition of highly oxygenated media in the bioreactor (Figure 2 B). The continuous processes have advantages but there are several parameters which are to be maintained. Due to the microorganism, being filamentous and taking long time to reach stationary phase microorganism are first allowed to grow under batch condition and then continuous mode of operation is started. (Srivastava *et al.*, 2006)

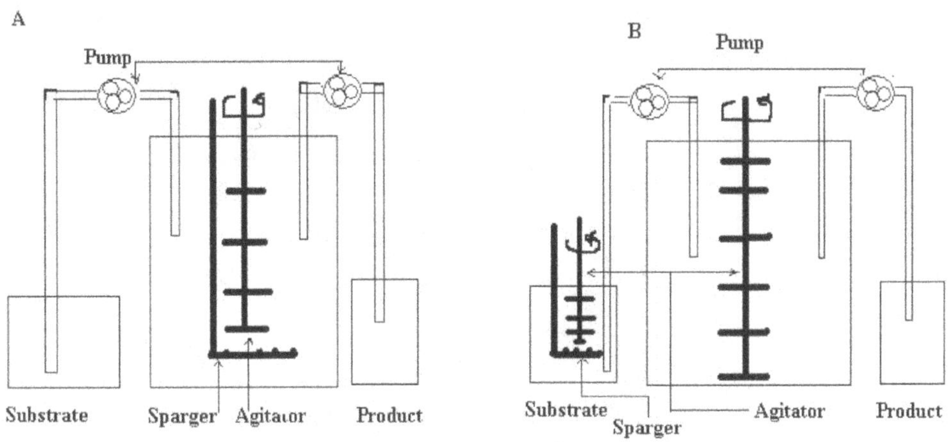

Fig. 2. A) Continuous Bioreactor with oxygen Sparger B) Continuous Bioreactor with oxygen enriched fresh substrate

2.1.2 Cephalosporin C production by Non conventional mode of bioreactors

The non conventional mode involves in either Packed bed bioreactor or Airlift bioreactor. Various modes of immobilized microorganisms are used in packed bed reactors. The main advantage of packed bed reactor is that it can be operated in batch or continuous mode. The residence time and microorganism reusability is high in case of packed bed reactors. There are reported studies involving silk sachets for holding the immobilized beads with significant increase in production. (Kundu et al., 2000)

Cephalosporin C fermentation is a highly aerobic process. The major problem which arises with aerobic fermentation are the mass transfer limitation of oxygen to immobilized cell. (Mishra *et al.*, 2005) Even with addition of highly oxygenated media, the beads packed in depth doesn't have enough oxygen to carry out cephalosporin C production, instead they produce Penicillin N, which is not desirable. There is a reported study where mixed culture technique for improving the oxygen supply to the immobilized cells. In such system, the products of metabolism of one microorganism are utilized by the second microorganism. Photoautotrophic algae (*Chlorella* sp.) which produce oxygen *in situ* are coupled with fungi (*Cephalosporium acremonium*) which in turn produce the Cephalosporin C. (Figure 3) (Kundu and Mahapatra, 1993; Kundu *et al.*, 2003) The algae absorb CO_2 from air and media producing free oxygen which not only removes the anaerobic condition prevailing in packed bed reactor but also adds up oxygen to the media. Co-immobilization of whole cells were reported to be carried out by using various immobilizing agents, *viz.* Bagasse, Silk sachets, calcium/Barium/strontium alginate and the same coated with poly-acrylamide resin.

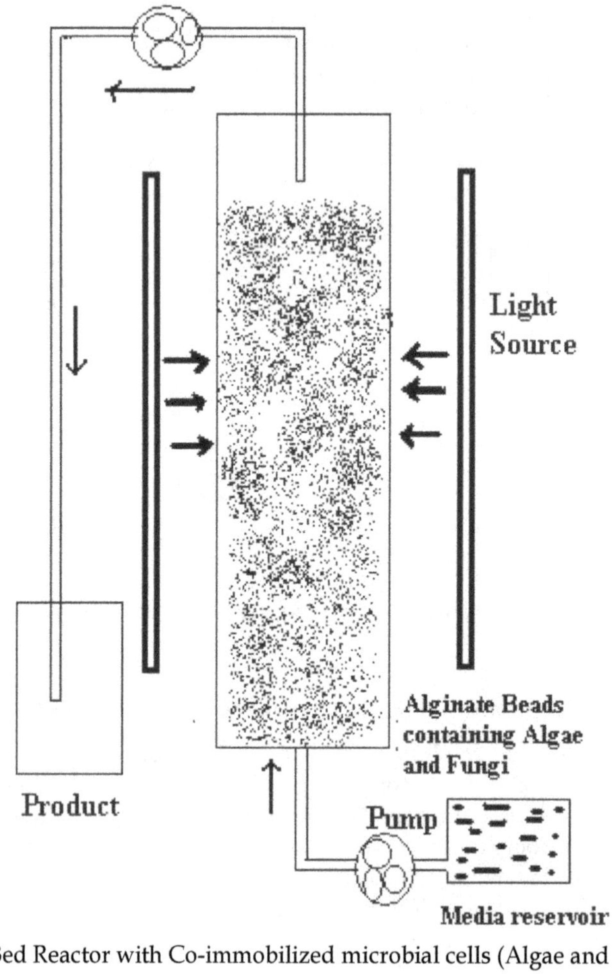

Fig. 3. Packed Bed Reactor with Co-immobilized microbial cells (Algae and Fungi) for enhanced oxygenation

Airlift Bioreactors are the most favorable reactors for production as it completely solve the oxygenation issue. There are two types of Airlift bioreactors. Internal air loop reactors have inner draft tube (Figure 4) while the external bioreactors have external tube as downcomer. They both have significant production values. (Srivastava and Kundu, 1999; Srivastava *et al.*, 1995)The air lift reactor ensures proper oxygenation and agitation. They are also gentle on filamentous fungi imparting low shear than any other conventional process agitator, improving production. Though, the process is costlier and tough but it ensures high cephalosporin C production. Figure 4 shows the airlift bioreactors involved in cephalosporin C production. The internal loop airlift reactors have better oxygenation and are preferred above external loop bioreactor.

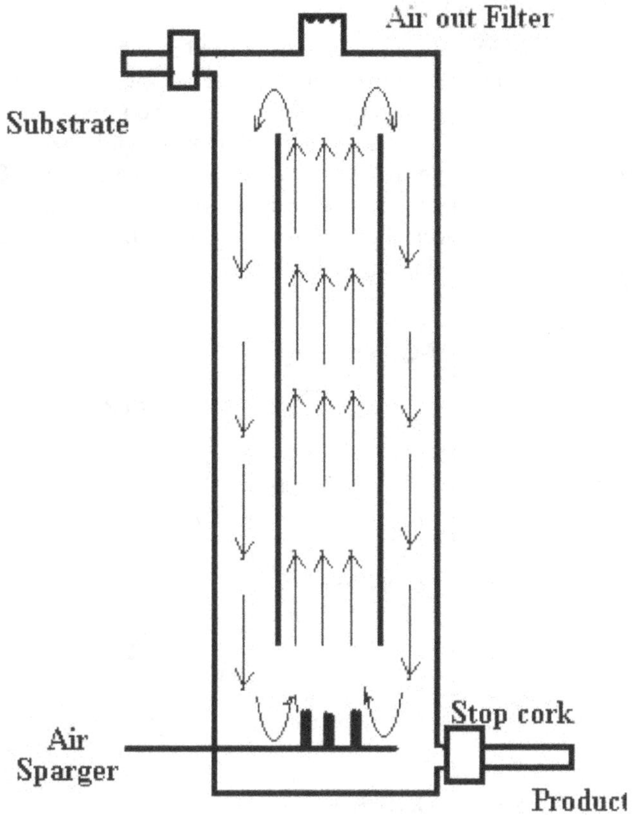

Fig. 4. Internal air-loop reactor for Cephalosporin C production

2.2 Production strategy of 7- amino cephalosporanic acid (secondary precursor)

Biosynthesis of 7- Amino cephalosporanic acid (7-ACA) is an important process which involves the use of free and immobilized microbial cells. This can be single step or multi-step microbial enzymatic process (Gaurav *et al.*, 2007). There are lots of advantages of single step over the multi-step process (Nigam *et al.*, 2005). Cephalosporin C acylase enzyme is involved in the conversion of Cephalosporin C to 7- ACA in single step mode of conversion. The microorganisms used for the synthesis of this enzyme are *Pseudomonas diminuta, Bacillus megaterium* and *E. coli* (Nigam and Kundu, 1999). There is also study on continuous production of 7-ACA by loading immobilized microbial cell in a packed bed bioreactor at optimum cells to carrier ratio and at an optimum flow rate (Nigam *et al.*, 2005).

3. Different generations Cephalosporins

Cephalosporins can usually be classified into four different generations though newer generations are in active research, developed in response to a specific clinical need for a drug with different characteristics than the previous generation. Table 2 narrates the examples of various generation of Cephalosporins group of antibiotics.

3.1 First generation cephalosporins

The first generation cephalosporins were first introduced in the mid-1960s and were stable to the β-lactamases known at that time. They permeated the outer membrane of gram-negative bacilli quicker than the penicillins. The first generation drugs include Cephalothin, Cephaloridine and Cefazolin (Figure 5). Cephalothin was synthesized by biochemically using different processing strategies [Gaurav et.al., 2007]. Cephalexin and Cefeclor are both used as oral treatment drugs, and have broad activity against both gram-positive and gram-negative microorganisms. However, they are inactive against *Enterococci* as they don't bind well to PBPs of the *Enterococci* having slight difference.

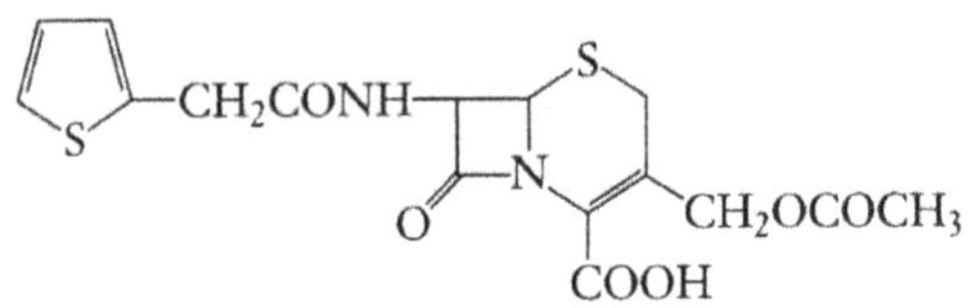

Cephalothin

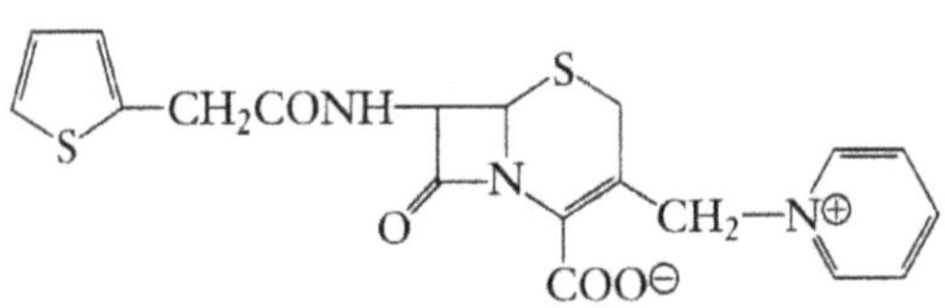

Cephaloridine

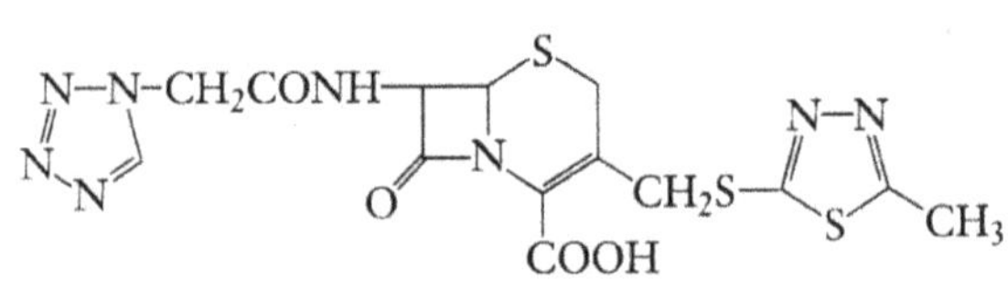

Cefazolin

Fig. 5. First generation Cephalosporins

3.2 Second generation cephalosporins

The second generation cephalosporins have enhanced activity against gram-negative microorganisms (Livermore 1987; Stan *et al.*, 2004). They are more stable to hydrolysis by plasmid-mediated β-lactamases when compared to cefoxitin, to the chromosomal class C cephalosporinase of several *Enterobacteriaceae.* (Medeiros 1997). The second generation cephalosporins include, Cefoxitin, Cefmetazole, Cefuroxime and Cefotetan (Figure 6). Cefuroxime is generally used for respiratory tract and community acquired infections. Cefoxitin has an extra methoxy-group that imparts protection against β-lactamase , but with an added disadvantage that it causes induction of the chromosomal β-lactamases in several bacterial organisms (which can be counterproductive). Cefoxitin (as well as Cefotetan) is well effective against *Bacteroides fragilis,* an enteric anaerobe but not against *Pseudomonas* or *Enterobacter* as it can't enter them.

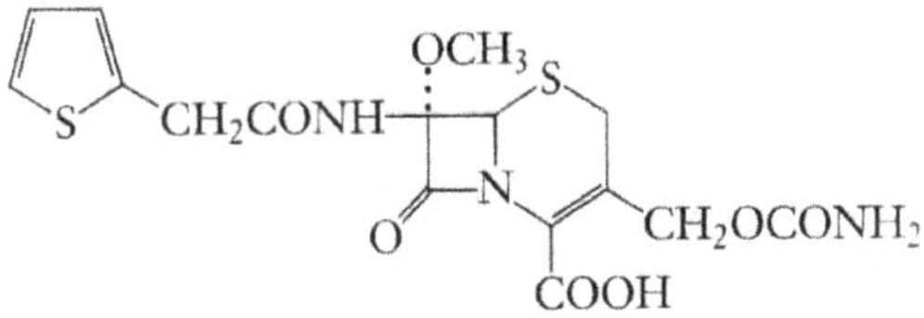

Cefoxitin

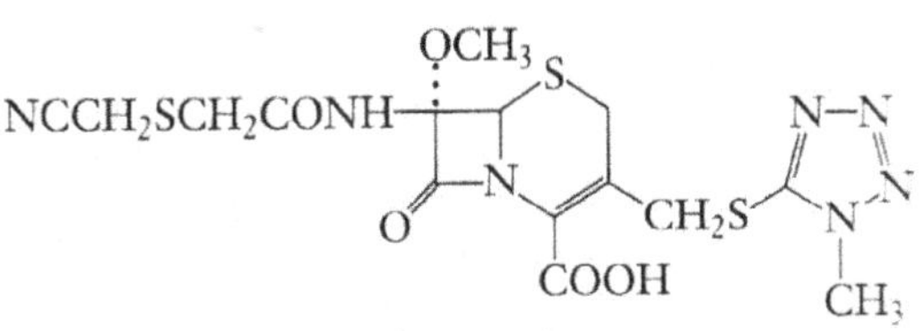

Cefmetazole

Fig. 6. Second generation Cephalosporins

3.3 Third generation cephalosporins

The third generation cephalosporins are less effective than the first generation cephalosporins against gram-positive cocci but are very much potent against *Enterobacteriaceae,* including the β-lactamase-producing strains (Mandell & Sande 1991). The aminothiazolyl and iminomethoxy groups are the substituents in third generation cephalosporins (Neu 1986), which imparted greater stability against the chromosomal class C β-lactamases and with an increased spectrum of activity.These cephalosporins include Cefotaxime, Ceftizoxime and Ceftazidime (Figure 7). The drugs are broad spectrum antibiotics that are effective against both gram-negative and gram-positive microorganisms. The sodium salts of these antibiotics also showed a greater potential.

Cefotaxime has an enhanced affinity to penicillin binding proteins (PBPs) of gram-negative bacteria and thus it could penetrate faster into bacterial cell as compared to older generation cephalosporins.

Also, cefotaxime is the main intermediary in the synthesis of cefpodoxime proxetil, a third generation oral cephalosporin, introduced recently into medical practice (Durckheimer *et al.,* 1985; Reynolds 1989). Third-generation cephalosporins have a broad spectrum of antimicrobial activity including Gram-positive, Gram-negative, and selected anaerobic species. (Neu 1991).

β -lactamase induction or resistant organism selections are an important issue, especially in nosocomial infections (Stratton *et al.,* 1992). Third generation cephalosporins vary in their ability to induce β-lactamases, but none is as effective inducers as the cephamycins, clavams, or carbapenems The discovery of *Klebsiella* isolates resistant to oxyiminocephalosporins imparted more difficulties to β-lactam antibiotics mediated by extended-spectrum β-lactamases (ESBLs). Mutation in the structural genes of plasmid-mediated TEM, SHV, and OXA β-lactamases and to a lesser extent in the PER and CTX enzymes enhanced their affinity for third generation cephalosporins and monobactams, but with varying degrees marking the pavement for newer generations.

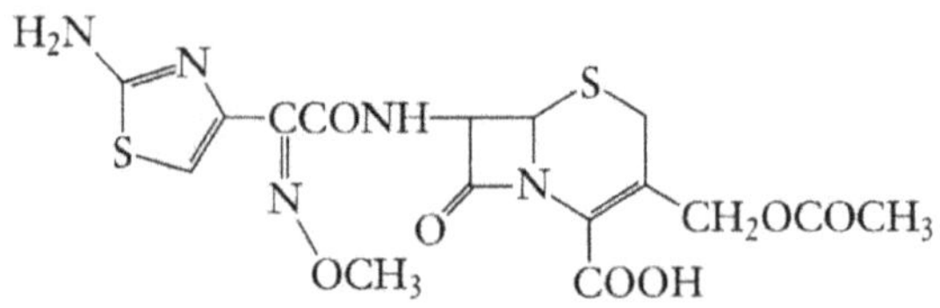

Cefotaxime

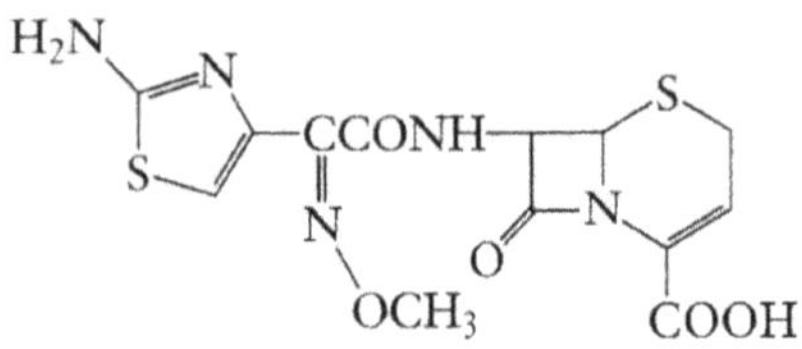

Ceftizoxime

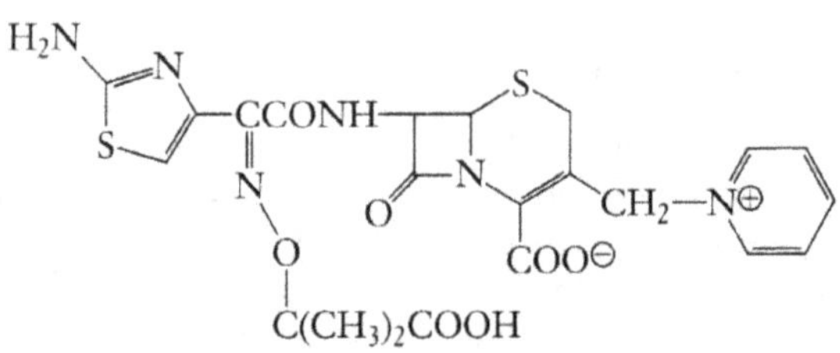

Ceftazidime

Fig. 7. Third generation cephalosporins

3.4 Fourth generation cephalosporins

The fourth generation cephalosporins contains a positively charged quaternary nitrogen atom at C-3, resulting in higher activity (compared to the third-generation cephalosporins) against β-lactamase derepressed mutants of *P. areuginosa* and other enteric bacteria (Georgopapdakau *et al.*, 1989). The fourth generation cephalosporins, Cefepime, Cefpirome and Cefclidin (Figure 8) have the 7-amino-thiazolyl groups [(Livermore & Williams 1996). Cefepime have good potency against gram-negative organisms such as *Pseudomonas aeruginosa,* and gram-positive organism such as *Staphylococcus aureus,* also exhibiting increased stability against β-lactamase-overproducing bacteria. Cefepime is [6 R – [6 α, 7 β (Z)]]-1-[[7-[[(2-amino-4-thiazolyl) (methoxyimino) acetyl] amino]-2-carboxy-8-oxo-5-thia-1-azabicyclo oct-2-en-3yl] methyl]-1-methylpyrrolidinium inner salt. It is synthesized from 7-aminocephalosporanic acid (7-ACA) with help of trimethylsilyl iodide and N-methylpyrrolidine. It is stable to hydrolysis by the more common chromosomal and plasmid-mediated β-lactamases, and it is quite stable against inducible chromosomally mediated cephalosporinases

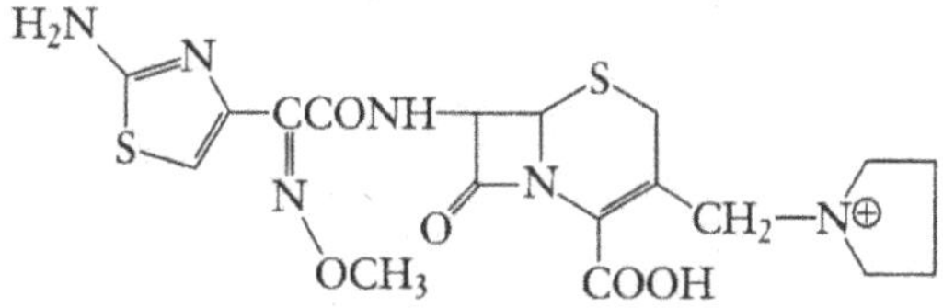

Cefepime

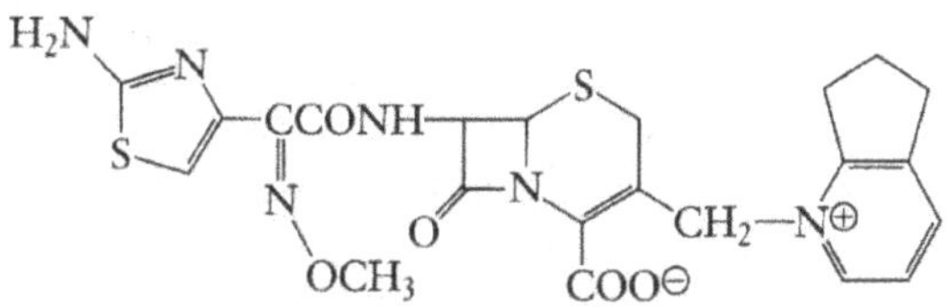

Cefpirome

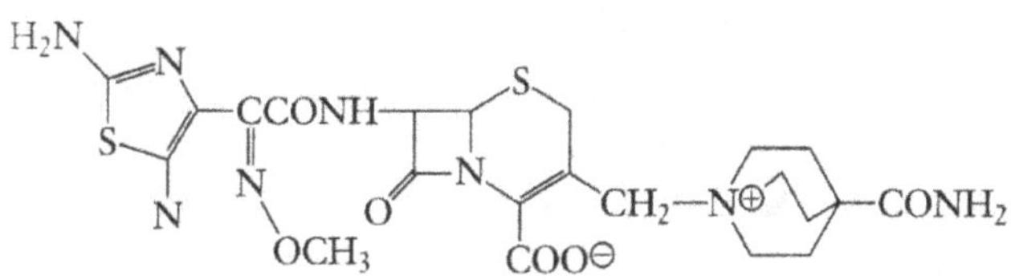

Cefclidin

Fig. 8. Fourth generation Cephalosporins

3.5 Fifth generation cephalosporins

The fifth generation cephalosporin is still an unclear picture with many new modified cephalosporins in the research sector. This generation antibiotic is specifically developed against nosocomial infections of MRSA and Pseudomonas based refractory infection in immuno-compromised patients. Drugs which are in immediate attention of FDA are Ceftobiprole, LB10522 (Kim et al., 1996) and RU-59863 (Figure 9). Ceftobiprole specifically attacks by binding to this penicillin-resistant target. Interactions with cephalosporin side chains occurs in the groove, closed in the free PBP 2a enzyme, binds to the 7-acyl amino side chain, and in another extended groove where it interacts with the 3'-cephem side chain through noncovalent interactions (Lim & Strynadka 2002). It is stable to class A penicillinases produced by *S. aureus* and enteric gram-negative microorganisms and is more stable to few class C beta-lactamases of enteric gram-negative microorganisms (Hebeisen *et al.*, 2001).

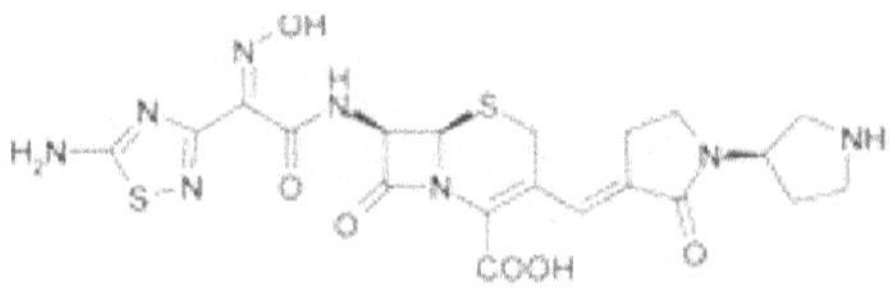

Ceftobiprole

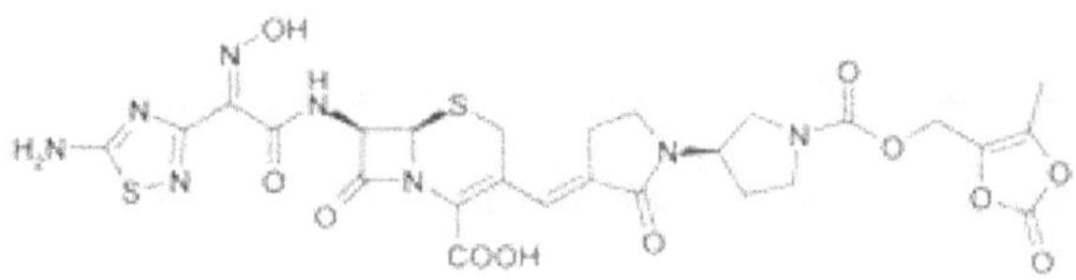

Ceftobiprole medocaril

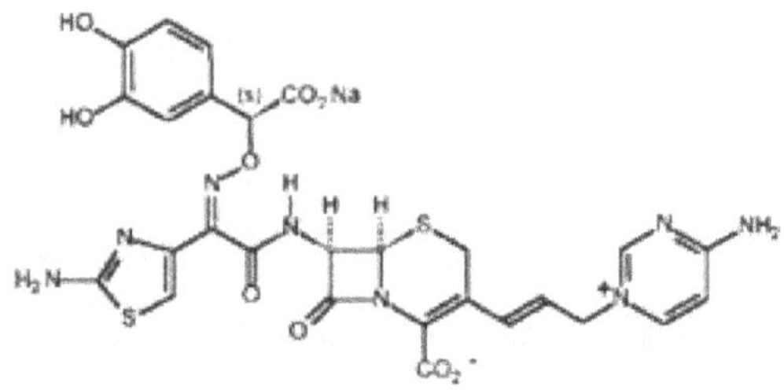

LB10522

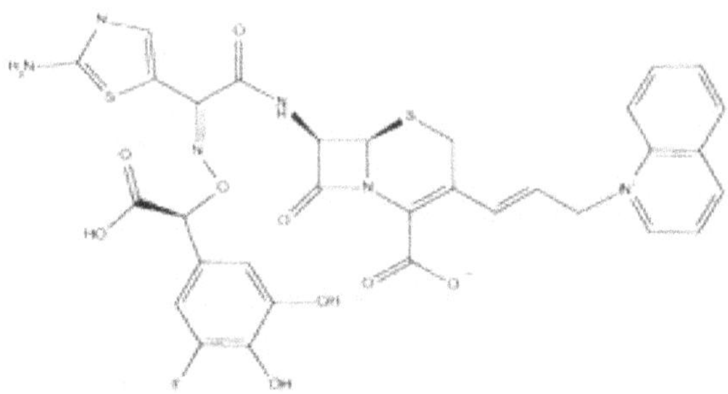

RU-59863

Fig. 9. Fifth generation Cephalosporins

4. Current research in new generation cephalosporins

It is also known that incorporation of a methoxy group in both cephalosporin and penicillin has led to a considerable increase in beta-lactamase stability. These findings prompted us to prepare methoxy and formamido derivatives of Cephalosporin and screen them for their antibacterial activity.

Our research team's current work is to attempt synthesizing some new semi-synthetic cephalosporins and some by modifying already existing semi-synthetic cephalosporins such as cefotaxime (third generation). It is broad spectrum antibiotic with high resistance against beta-lactamases. But the main problem is that it is poorly soluble in water. Hence, the efforts have been made to prepare cephalosporins having better solubility using cefotaxime. All these semi-synthetic cephalosporins are derived from the key intermediate 7- ACA, a product derived from cephalosporin C hydrolysis. They differ in the nature of the substitute attached at the 3 and/ or 7- position of the cephem ring and express various biological and pharmacological effects.

In the present work, enzymatic method has been employed to produce 7-ACA, the key intermediate and this 7-ACA is then utilized for the synthesis of new semi-synthetic cephalosporins. Nicotinic acid, benzimidazole, imidazole or substituted benzimidazole system has been shown to have different pharmacological effects including antifungal, antibacterial and antiviral effects. 2-substituted benzimidazoles, with various types of biological activity, have a close relationship to nucleic acid metabolism. Hence, semi-synthetic cephalosporins containing these nucleuses were prepared and the assessment of these molecules has been checked to interfere with various cellular and metabolic processes. (Figure 10)

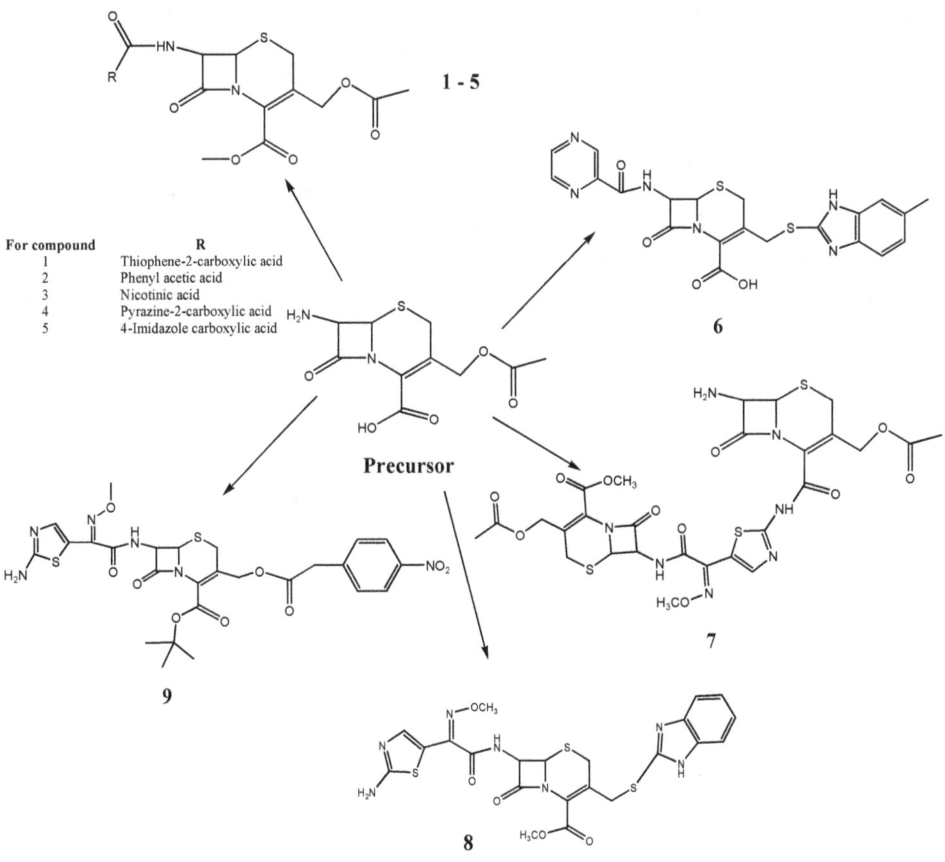

Fig. 10. Formation of new generation Cephalosporins.

In a search for unique and potent cephalosporin antibiotics, we have prepared new semi-synthetic cephalosporins. The motivation for synthesizing these semi-synthetic cephalosporins was to increase the availability of drug at the target site and their oral absorptivity and increased stability. Thus, recurring need for an easily cleaved blocking group for the carboxylic acid in the cephalosporin synthetic chemistry forms the basis of the research. All the synthesised cephalosporins were having easily hydrolysable esters for oral absorption studies; they were also having such suitable blocking groups for the carboxyl, which might be removed later without disruption of the beta-lactam ring. Although simple esters, like the methyl ester, are known to possess diminished antibiotic activity compared to the free acids, the possibility exists that more easily hydrolysable esters (by enzymatic or chemical means) might exhibit significant in vivo activity. A therapeutic advantage might be anticipated from derived compounds if the structural environment of the carboxyl group is a bar to absorption through the gastric or intestinal walls. Activity could be inherent in the derivative or be produced a result of enzymatic cleavage to the parent compound after absorption has occurred. Gastric acidity, often a negative influence in oral absorptibility of penicillins, would send to be an unlikely factor in cephalosporin absorption because of the relatively good acid stability of this class of antibiotics. For the synthesis of these analogues, the methods that are of general applicability are used. To form peptides from a cephalosporin required that the carboxyl at C-4 be appropriately activated for acylation of a protected amino acid. In synthetic organic chemistry, compound containing the carbodiimide functionality are dehydrating agents and are often used to activate carboxylic acids towards amide or ester formation. Additives, such as N-hydroxybenzotriazole are often added to increase yields and decrease side reactions. EDC (acronym for 1-ethyl-3-(3-dimethylaminopropyl) carbodiimide hydrochloride) is a water soluble carbodiimide which is used as a carboxyl activating agent for the coupling of primary amines to yield amide bonds. The possibility that amides derived from a cephalosporanic acid and an amino acid might cross the intestinal wall and be cleaved in the body.

5. Conclusion

In general, attempts to modify the β- lactam thiazolidine ring system of penicillin without loss of antibacterial activity had been unsuccessful. The discovery, structure elucidation and modification of cephalosporin C, which led to important new generations of Cephalosporin group of antibiotics and its large scale production and marketing. In the past decade, even though cephalosporin antibiotics have made remarkable progress and contribution in the treatment of acute disease, many efforts still exist to achieve the well-balanced broad-spectrum and to improve beta-lactamases stability. This work, lead to highly active, acid stable, penicillin resistant, nontoxic antibiotic with increased potency against a wide range of bacteria. Although the progress is in preliminary stage but significance of the work is enormous.

6. References

Babini, G.S. and D.M. Livermore , 2000. Antimicrobial resistance amongst Klebsiella spp. collected from intensive care units in southern and western europe in 1997–1998. *J Antimicrob Chemother.*, Vol. 45, pp. 183–189

Durckheimer, W., Blumbach, J., Lattrell, R. and Scheunemann, K.H. (1985). Recent developments in the field of b-Lactam antibiotics Angew. *Chem. Int. Ed. Engl.*, Vol. 24, pp. 180-182.

Essack, S.Y. (2001). The development of b-Lactam antibiotics in response to the Evolution of b-lactamases. *Pharmaceutical Res.*, Vol.18, pp. 1391-1399.

Gaurav, K., Kundu, K. and Kundu, S. (2007). Microbial Production of 7-aminocepahlosporanic acid and new generation cephalosporins (Cephalothin) by different processing strategies. *Artificial Cells, Blood SubstBiotechnol.*, Vol.35, pp. 345-358.

Gaurav, K., Kundu, K. , Karmakar, S. and Kundu, S. (2011). Development of New Generation Cephalosporins. In Recent advances in life sciences. A.K. Rai (ed.), pp. 173-186, I. K. Publishers, India

Georgopapdakau, N.H. and Bertasso, A. (1993). Mechanisms of action of cephalosporin 3'-quinolone esters,carbamates, and tertiary amines in *Escherichia coli*. *Antimicrob Agents Chemother.*, Vol.37, pp. 559-565.

Hebeisen, P., Heinze-Krauss, I., Angehrn, P., Hohl, P., Page, M.G.P. and Then, R.L. (2001). *In vitro* and *in vivo* Properties of Ro 63-9141, a novel broad-spectrum cephalosporin with activity against methicillin-resistant Staphylococci. *Antimicrob. Agents Chemother.*, Vol.45, pp. 825-836.

Jacoby, B. K. (2000). Amino acid sequences for TEM, SHV and OXA extended-spectrum and inhibitor resistant β-lactamases. Available from http://lahey.org/studies/webt.htm

Jones, R.N. (1994). Summation the injectable cephalosporins in the treatment of serious infections. *Infection*, Vol. 22, pp. S182-S183.

Kim, M.Y., Oh, J.I., Paek, K.S., Kim, Y.Z., Kim, I.C. and Kwak, J.H. (1996). *In vitro* and *in vivo* activities of LB10522, a new catecholic cephalosporin. *Antimicrob. Agents Chemother.*, Vol. 40, pp. 1825-1831.

Kundu, S., Gupta, S., Bihari, V. and Agrawal, S.C. (2000). Studies on free and immobilized cells of *C. acremonium* on the production of cephalosporins. *Indian J. Microbiol.*, Vol. 40, pp. 141-143.

Kundu, S. and A.C. Mahapatra (1993). Microbial Production of cephalosporin C using co cultures of *Cephalosporium acremonium* and *Chlorella pyrenoidosa* in a packed bed reactor. In: *Recent trends in Biotechnology*. C. Ayanna (ed.), pp. 31-35, Tata McGraw Hill, India,

Kundu, S., Mahapatra, A.C., Nigam, V.K. and Kundu, K. (2003). Continuous production of cephalosporin-C by immobilized microbial cells using symbiotic mode in a packed bed bioreactor. *Artificial Cells, Blood Substitutes and Biotechnology*, Vol. 31, pp. 313-327.

Kundu, S., Singh, S.K. and Nigam, V.K. (1993). Comparative studies of cephalosporin-C production in batch and continuous stirred tank bioreactor. *J. Microb. Biotech.*, Vol.8, pp. 76-84.

Lim, D. and Strynadka, N.C. (2002). Structural basis for the beta lactam resistance of PBP2a from methicillin resistant *Staphylococcus aureus*. *Nat. Struct. Biol.*, Vol.9, pp. 870-876.

Livermore, D.M. (1987). Mechanisms of resistance to cephalosporin antibiotics. *Drugs* , Vol.34, pp. 64.

Livermore, D.M. (1998). Beta-lactamase-mediated resistance and opportunities for its control. *J. Antimicrob. Chemother.*, Vol. 41, pp. 25-41.

Livermore, D.M. and Williams, J.D. (1996). Lactams: mode of action and mechanisms of bacterial resistance, In: *Antibiotics in laboratory medicine*, Lorian V (Ed.), 4th edn, pp. 502-578, Williams & Wilkins, Baltimore, Md..

Mahapatra, A.C., Kundu, K., Nigam, V.K., Mandava, M.V.P. and Kundu, S. (2002). Comparative studies of CPC production by free and immobilized cells of

Cephalosporium acremonium in different modes of bioreactors. *Indian J. Microbiol.*, Vol. 42, pp. 319-322.

Mandell, G.L. and Sande, M.A. (1991). *Goodman and Gilman's, The Pharmacological Basis of Therapeutics*, 8th Edition. pp. 1065, Pergamon Press, New York..

Medeiros, A. (1997). Evolution and dissemination of b-lactamases. *Clin. Infect. Dis.*, Vol. 24, pp. S19-S45.

Mishra, P., Srivastava, P. and Kundu, S., (2005). A Comparative evaluation of oxygen mass transfer and broth viscosity using cephalosporin C production as a case strategy. *World Journal of Microbiology & Biotechnology*, Vol. 21, pp. 525-530

Neu, H.C. (1986). beta-Lactam antibiotics: structural relationships affecting in vitro activity and pharmacologic properties. *Rev. Infect. Dis.*, Vol. 8, pp. S237–S259.

Neu, H.C. (1991). Cephalosporins-cefotaxime 10 years later, a major drug with continued use. *Infection*, Vol. 19: pp. 309-315.

Nigam,V.K., S. Kundu and P. Ghosh, (2005). Single step conversion of Cephalosporin- C acylase to 7- ACA by free and Immobilized cells of Pseudomonas diminuta. *Appl. Biochem. & Biotechnol*, Vol. 126,pp. 13-21

Nigam, V.K. and Kundu, S (1999). Batch Production of 7-ACA by Different Microorganisms - A Comparative Study. *Ind. Chemical Engg.*, Vol. 41, no. 1, pp. 5-9

Reynolds, J.E.F. (1989). *Martindale-The Extra Pharmacopoeia*, 29th edn, p. 151., Pharmaceutical Press, London.

Srivastava, P. and Kundu, S. (1990). A simple kinetic analysis of ephalosporin-C production using various carbon substrates. *J. Microb. Biotechnol.*, Vol. 5, pp. 34-41.

Srivastava, P. and Kundu, S. (1995). A laboratory air lift reactor for cephalosporin-C. *J. Ind. Chem Engg.* , Vol. 37, pp. 138-139.

Srivastava, P. and Kundu, S. (1999). Studies on cephalosporin-C production in an air lift reactor using different growth modes of *Cephalosporium acremonium. Process Biochem.* , Vol. 34, pp. 329-333.

Srivastava, P., Nigam, V.K. and Kundu, S. (1996). A comparative evaluation of Cephalosporin-C production in stirred-tank reactor and air lift reactor. *Ind. J. Chem Tech.*, Vol. 3, pp. 371-372.

Srivastava, P., Mishra, P. and Kundu, S., (2006). Process strategies for Cephalosporin-C Fermentation. *J. of Scientific and Industrial Research*, Vol. 65, pp. 599-602.

Stan, C., Dumitrache, M. and Diaconu, D.E. (2004). Means of purification of cephalexin with a view to therapeutic use. *Rev. Med. Chir. Soc. Med. Nat. Iasi*, Vol. 108, pp. 718-720.

Stratton, C.W., Ratner, H., Johnston, P.E. and Schaffner, W. (1992). Focused microbiologic surveillance by specific hospital unit as a sensitive means of defining antimicrobial resistance problems. *Diagn Microbiol Infect Dis.*, Vol. 15, pp. 11S-18S.

Tzouvelekis, L.S., Tzelepi, E., Prinarakis, E., Gazouli, M., Katrahoura, A., Giakkoupi, P., Paniara, O. and Legakis, (1998). Sporadic Emergence of Klebsiella pneumoniae Strains Resistant to Cefepime and Cefpirome in Greek Hospitals. *J. Clin. Microbiol*, Vol. 36, pp. 266-268

Wilson, W.R., 1998. The role of fourth-generation cephalosporins in the treatment of serious infectious diseases in hospitalized patients. *Diagn Microbiol Infect Dis.*, Vol. 31, pp. 473–477

Zhang, Q.J. and Xu, W.X. (1993). Morphological physiological and enzymatic characteristics of cephalosporin acylase producing *Arthrobacter* strain 45-A. *Arch. Microbiol.*, Vol. 159, pp. 392-395.

Assessment of Antibiotic Resistance in Probiotic Lactobacilli

Masanori Fukao and Nobuhiro Yajima
Research Institute, KAGOME Co., Ltd.
Japan

1. Introduction

Probiotics are live microorganisms that confer a health benefit on the host when administered in adequate amounts (Food and Agriculture Organization of the United Nations-World Health Organization Working Group, 2002). Many microbial species have probiotic properties, but those most commonly used are lactobacilli (Salminen et al, 1998; Caplice & Fitzgerald, 1999; Leroy & De Vuyst, 2004). Lactobacilli have a long history of safe use in the production and consumption of fermented foods and beverages. Over recent decades, as awareness of the beneficial effects of probiotic strains in promoting gut and general health has grown, the development and consumption of probiotic foods has increased worldwide (Saarela et al, 2002). Thus, it is essential to thoroughly investigate the safety of lactobacilli used in probiotic products (Salminen et al, 1998; Borriello et al, 2003).

The human gut is the natural habitat for a large and dynamic bacterial community that has a great relevance for health (Spor et al, 2011). The human gut microbiota is a complex ecosystem colonized by approximately 10^{14} bacterial cells with *Bacteroides, Eubacterium, Bifidobacterium, Ruminococcus,* and *Clostridium* as the pre-dominant genera (Kurokawa et al, 2007). The huge diversity of antibiotic resistance genes detected in the human gut microbiome suggests that antibiotic resistant bacteria in the gastrointestinal tract (GIT) function as reservoir of antibiotic resistance genes (Salyers et al, 2007; Sommer et al, 2009). When probiotic strains enter the gut, they interact with the native microbiota and gene transfer can occur (Teuber et al, 1999; Mathur & Singh, 2005; Salim Ammor et al, 2007). The dissemination of antibiotic resistance genes can reduce the therapeutic possibilities in infectious diseases. It is therefore relevant to look for the presence of transferable antibiotic resistance genes in lactobacilli that are or shall be used as probiotic strains for human consumption or as starter cultures of fermented food or feed products.

This article reviews the experiments to be performed and the criteria for assessment of antibiotic resistance in probiotic lactobacilli. Due to the growing availability of whole bacterial genome sequences, sequence-based identification approaches for antibiotic resistance are also discussed.

2. Antibiotic resistance of probiotic lactobacilli

Many food production is estimated to involve microbial fermentation processes by using lactic acid bacterial (LAB) strains (Food and Agriculture Organization of the United

Nations-World Health Organization Working Group, 2002), for example, sausage, ham, cheese, and dairy products. In addition, probiotics have become available on the market, containing a single strain or a combination of strains. The proposed problem is that probiotic strains might contain acquired resistance genes. From a point of safety, it is necessary to distinguish between intrinsic and acquired resistance genes.

Antibiotic resistance profiles have recently been reported for several lactobailli. These have been found susceptible to penicillins and ampicillin (cell wall synthesis inhibitor) (Danielsen & Wind, 2003; Coppola et al, 2005) in contrast to vancomycin. Most lactobacilli have been found to be resistant to glycopeptides types of antibiotics. However, the resistance towards vancomycin has been demonstrated being as intrinsic (Tynkkynen et al, 1998). Lactobacilli are usually susceptible to chloramphenicol, erythromycin and clindamycin (protein synthesis inhibitors) (Coppola et al, 2005; Klare et al, 2007). In addition, resistance against trimethoprim (nucleic acid synthesis inhibitor), seems to be intrinsic (Ammor et al, 2007). Resistance to tetracycline has been observed more often among lactobacilli (Roberts, 2005; Korhonen et al, 2008). Resistance against neomycin, kanamycin, streptomycin and gentamicin (aminoglycosides) has been observed more frequently among lactobacilli (Coppola et al, 2005; Danielsen, 2002; Zhou et al, 2005).

Acquired resistance genes which are potentially transferable have been detected in lactobailli. These have been described in multiple studies and have been reviewed (Ammor et al, 2007). Two of the most commonly observed resistance genes in lactobacilli found so far are *tet*(M) for tetracycline resistance and *erm*(B) for erythromycin resistance, followed with *cat* genes coding for chloramphenicol resistance (Danielsen, 2002; Lin et al, 1996; Gevers et al, 2003a; Cataloluk & Gogebakan, 2004).

Acquired resistance genes of probiotic lactobacilli have been reported previously (Table 1). In the PROSAFE project, probiotic lactobacilli possessed *erm*(B) and/or *tet*(W), *tet*(M) or unidentified members of the *tet*(M) group (Klare et al, 2007). In probiotic commercial *L. reuteri* ATCC 55730, *tet*(W) and the lincosamide resistance gene *lnu*(A) were detected (Kastner et al, 2006). Hummel et al determined antibiotic resistances of probiotic lactobacilli and to verify these at the genetic level. *L. salivarius* BFE 7441 possessed an *erm*(B) gene, which was encoded on the chromosome (Hummel et al, 2007). Probiotic lactobacilli of African and European origins were studied and compared for their susceptibility to antibiotics. Acquired resistance genes encoding aminoglycoside (*aph*(3')-III, *aadA*, *aadE*) and *tet*(S) and *erm*(B) were detected (Ouoba et al, 2008). The potentially probiotic strain *L. plantarum* CCUG 43738, which displayed atypical phenotypic resistance to tetracycline and minocycline, was found to contain a *tet*(S) gene located on a plasmid of approximately 14 kb (Huys et al, 2006).

3. Evidence of potential horizontal gene transfer of probiotic lactobacilli

When probiotic strains enter the gut, they interact with the native microbiota and gene transfer can occur. Probiotics might contribute to the transfer of antibiotic resistance genes to other commensal bacteria or pathogens present in the GIT. The occurrence of large numbers of transferable resistance genes within the intestinal microbiota is undesirable due to the potential risk of acquisition by pathogens present in the GIT and subsequent antibiotic treatment failure (Licht & Wilcks, 2005).

Probiotic strains	Antibiotic phenotype	Antibiotic genotype (gene location)	Transferability	Reference
L. rhamnosus GG (ATCC 53103)	Vm^r	Not detacted	No transconjugants in mating experiment	Tynkkynen et al, 1998
L. brevis KB290	Vm^r, Tc^r, Ci^r	Not detected	No transconjugants in mating experiment	Fukao et al, 2009
L. reuteri ATCC 55730	Tc^r, Lm^r	*tet*(W), *lnu*(A) (pLR581, pLR585)	Potentially transferable	Rosander et al, 2008
L. crispatus L-295	Em^r, Cm^r, Tc^r	*erm*(B), *tet*(W)	No transconjugants in mating experiment	Klare et al, 2007
L. crispatus L-296	Em^r, Cm^r, Tc^r	*erm*(B), *tet*(W)	No transconjugants in mating experiment	Klare et al, 2007
L. plantarum L-437	Tc^r	*tet*(M) group	No transconjugants in mating experiment	Klare et al, 2007
L. reuteri L-285	Tc^r	*tet*(W)	No transconjugants in mating experiment	Klare et al, 2007
L. reuteri L-285-2	Tc^r	*tet*(M) group	No transconjugants in mating experiment	Klare et al, 2007
L. salivarius BFE 7441	Em^r, Ci^r, Gm^r, Sm^r	*erm*(B) (chromosome)	No transconjugants in mating experiment	Hummel et al, 2007
L. reuteri L4: 12002	Ci^r, Em^r, Gm^r, Sm^r, Km^r, Nm^r, Tc^r, Vm^r	*erm*(B) (plasmid)	Transferable	Ouoba et al, 2008
L. paracasei L5	Am^r, Ci^r, Gm^r, Km^r, Sm^r, Vm^r	*aph*(3')-III, *aadA*	No transconjugants in mating experiment	Ouoba et al, 2008
L. plantarum L7	Am^r, Ci^r, Gm^r, Tc^r, Km^r, Sm^r, Vm^r	*aadE*	No transconjugants in mating experiment	Ouoba et al, 2008
L. casei L9	Am^r, Ci^r, Gm^r, Km^r, Sm^r, Vm^r	*aph*(3')-III, *aadA*, *aadE*	No transconjugants in mating experiment	Ouoba et al, 2008
L. paraplantarm L10	Am^r, Ci^r, Tc^r, Vm^r	*tet*(S)	No transconjugants in mating experiment	Ouoba et al, 2008

Vancomycin (Vm), ampicillin (Am), tetracycline (Tc), erythromycin (Em), clindamycin (Cm), gentamicin (Gm), ciprofloxacin (Ci), lincosamide (Lm), Kanamycin (Km), streptomycin (Sm) and chloramphenicol (Cl)

Table 1. Systematic assessment of antibiotic resistance in probiotic lactobacilli have been reported previously

Several of these genetic determinants in lactobacilli are harboured by extrachromosomal elements which are conjugative plasmids and transposons (Mathur & Singh, 2005; Danielsen, 2002; Gevers et al, 2003a; Axelsson et al, 1988; Gfeller et al, 2003). Transfer from lactobacilli to other commensal bacteria has been documented in vitro (Feld et al, 2008;

Gevers et al, 2003b; Jacobsen et al, 2007; Sasaki et al, 1988; Schlundt et al, 1994). Studying the board-host-range conjugative plasmid pAMβ1, transfer was observed in vitro from lactobacilli (*L. plantarum, L. reuteri, L. fermentum,* and *L. murinus*) to other commensal bacteria (Ouoba et al, 2008; Tannock, 1987; Gasson & Davies, 1980; Shrago et al, 1986; West & Warner, 1985). In the diassociated model pAMβ1 has been transferred from *L. reuteri* to *Enterococcus faecalis* (Morelli et al, 1988). Interspecies conjugative transfer of tetracycline and erythromycin resistance plasmids from lactobacilli has been demonstrated previously in vitro (Gevers et al, 2003a; Ouoba et al, 2008; Feld et al, 2008). Recently, tetracycline-resistant *L. paracasei* strains were identified in samples of milk and natural whey starter cultures. A transposon *Tn916* including *tet*(M) was transferred to *E. faecalis* in vitro (Devirgiliis et al, 2009).

Transfer has been demonstrated in the GIT of rodents, both gnotobiotic (Feld et al, 2008; Jacobsen et al, 2007; Morelli et al, 1988) and those having an indigenous gut microbiota (Feld et al, 2008; Jacobsen et al, 2007; Schlundt et al, 1994; McConnell et al, 1991; Gruzza et al, 1994; Igimi et al, 1996). In addition, the in vivo transfer of vancomycin resistance has recently been shown between enterococci and probiotic lactobacilli in gnotobiotic mice (Mater et al, 2008). Recent experiments of antibiotic resistance transferability in vivo were also conducted from *L. plantarum* to *E. faecalis* (Jacobsen et al, 2007). However, the potential contribution of lactobacilli to the acquisition and dissemination of antibiotic resistance genes in the human GIT is poorly addressed for both conjugative and non-conjugative resistance plasmids. Nevertheless, conclusive documentation of transfer in the GI from probiotic lactobacilli is lacking and therefore more studies need to be carried out.

4. Systematic assessment of antibiotic resistance in probiotic lactobacilli

Antibiotic-resistance screening for lactobacilli intended for use in dairy products such as probiotics or as starters is now tending to become systematic. The European Food Safety Authority (EFSA) has taken responsibility to launch the European initiative toward a "qualified presumption of safety" (QPS) concept which, similar to the GRAS system in the United States, is aimed to allow strains with an established history and safety status to enter the market without extensive testing requirements (European Commission, 2003). The QPS approach together with the recommendations of the FEEDAP panel of EFSA will give a framework for better decision making in safety assessments of antibiotic resistance (Figure 1) (European Commission, 2005; European Food Safety Authority, 2008).

In phenotypic methods, FEEDAP requires the determination of the MICs of the most relevant antibiotics for each bacterial strain that is used as a feed additive in order to eliminate the possibility of acquired resistances. Those microbiological breakpoints define a MICs which, if exceeded, triggers the need for a more extensive investigation to define the genetic basis of the observed resistance and to assess the risk for transfer of this resistance to other bacteria. In genotypic methods, the latest literature indicates that the search for acquired resistance genes using PCR-based techniques (Klare et al, 2007; Hummel et al, 2007; Ouoba et al, 2008; Ammor et al, 2008; Devirgiliis et al, 2008; Fukao et al, 2009; Rizzotti et al, 2009; Comunian et al, 2010) or micro-arrays (Ammor et al, 2008) is a powerful tool to identify resistant LAB strains.

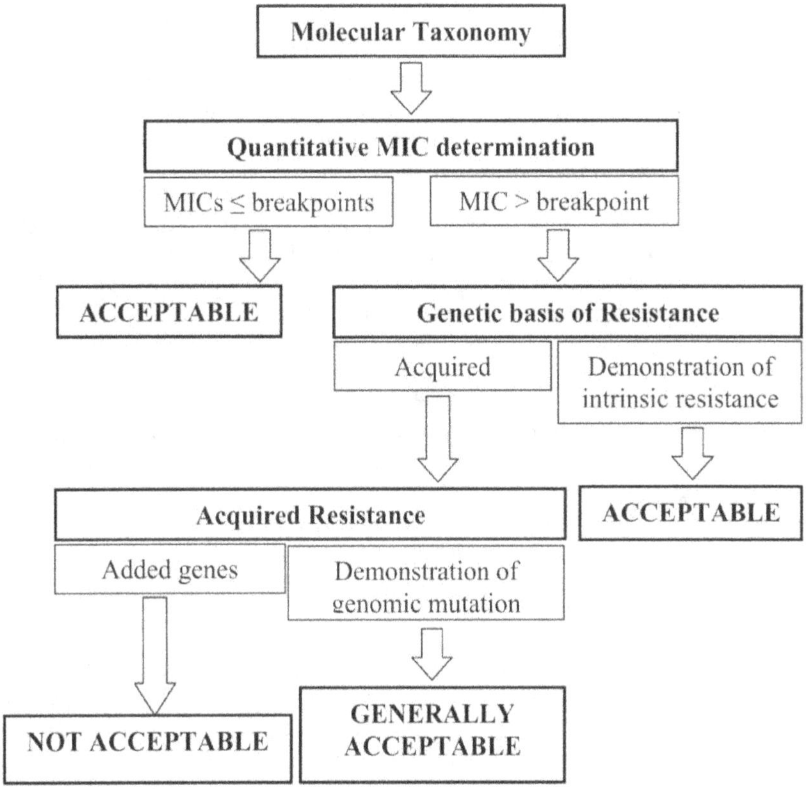

Fig. 1. Proposed scheme for the antibiotic resistance assessment of a bacterial strain (European Commission, 2005; European Food Safety Authority, 2008)

In case of suspected acquired resistance or intrinsic resistance, transferability tests are optional. Conjugation can be detected with bacterial mating experiments. The suspected donor with an antibiotic resistant phenotype is mixed with a recipient strain sensitive to the respective antibiotic, and the transfer of the resistance is subsequently checked. Frequencies of 10^{-6} to 10^{-5} of transconjugant cells are usually the highest experimentally obtainable. If transferability of the resistance is proven, then the strain will not be considered for use in microbial products and further tests are superfluous.

Systematic assessment of antibiotic resistance in some commercial probiotic lactobacilli have been reported previously (Table 1). *L. rhamnosus* GG (ATCC 53103) is a probiotic strain used in fermented dairy products in many countries. Studies have shown that the genes needed for vancomycin resistance in *L. rhamnosus* GG are not related to transferable enterococcal *van* genes and have not revealed any potential risks caused by the vancomycin resistance in this strain (Tynkkynen et al, 1998). The QPS approach was applied to determine the resistance of the probiotic strain *Lactobacillus brevis* KB290 that is used as a probiotic strain in fermented food products in Japan. The authors concluded from their investigation that the antibiotic resistance observed in *L. brevis* KB290 was due not to a potentially acquired mechanisms but to intrinsic resistance. It was concluded that according to the QPS criteria, these results provided safety assurance for the ongoing use of *L. brevis* KB290 as a probiotic (Fukao et al,

2009). In the PROSAFE project, probiotic lactobacilli displayed phenotypic resistance to tetracycline and/or erythromycin possessed *erm*(B) and/or *tet*(W), *tet*(M) or unidentified members of the *tet*(M) group. In vitro intra- and interspecies filter-mating experiments failed to show transfer of resistance determinants. *L. reuteri* ATCC 55730, a commercially available, well-documented a probiotic bacterium, has been shown to carry unusual resistances to tetracycline and lincosamides (Kastner et al, 2006). Deletion of the two plasmids was achieved by use of a protoplast-formation technique. BioGaia concluded that *L. reuteri* strain DSM 17938, except for the deletion of plasmids pLR581 and pLR585, was substantially equivalent to its parent strain *L. reuteri* ATCC 55730. Additionally, BioGaia concluded that the evidence demonstrating the safety of strain ATCC 55730 is equally applicable to strain DSM 17938 (Rosander et al, 2008). Hummel et al determined antibiotic resistances and to verify these at the genetic level according to the QPS system. *L. salivarius* BFE 7441 possessed an *erm*(B) gene, which was encoded on the chromosome and which could not be transferred in filter-mating experiments (Hummel et al, 2007). Probiotic lactobacilli of African and European origins were studied and compared for their susceptibility to antibiotics. Acquired antibiotic resistance genes encoding aminoglycoside (*aph*(3')-III, *aadA*, *aadE*) and *tet*(S) and *erm*(B) were detected. Only the *erm*(B) gene found in *L. reuteri* 12002 could be transferred in vitro to enterococci (Ouoba et al, 2008).

5. Whole genome based assessment of antibiotic resistance in probiotic lactobacilli

Due to the growing availability of whole bacterial genome sequences, sequence-based identification approaches have in recent years been intensively explored for safety evaluation such as antibiotic resistance in probiotic lactobacilli. Commercial probiotic *L. acidophilus* NCFM and *L. reuteri* DSM 17938 were assessed with whole genome and no known acquired resistance genes were detected (Agency Response Letter GRAS Notice No. GRN 000357; (Heimbach, 2008). Whole genome sequences were used to screen for acquired antibiotic resistance genes in lactobacilli strains which could be used in human nutrition (Bennedsen et al, 2011).

Moreover the overall NCBI clusters of orthologous groups (COGs) analysis is recommended (Heimbach, 2008). The COG category V (termed defense mechanisms) consists of many COGs that may have a potential safety interest, such as antibiotic resistance (Heimbach, 2008). Although it doesn't imply that these genes in COG category V are involved in antibiotic resistance, it is recommended to be assessed that there is nothing unusual about the number of COGs belonging to category V and none of the each gene was a part of a detectable mobile element such as predicted transposase genes (Heimbach, 2008). The overall COG analysis of *L. reuteri* DSM 17938 with complete genomes revealed that several COGs belonging to category V were found (Heimbach, 2008). The data indicated that there was nothing unusual about the number of COGs belonging to category V among these strains. Further analysis of each of the genes revealed that no gene was clustered with complete transposons or ISs. Thus none of the genes was a part of a detectable mobile element (Heimbach, 2008).

6. Conclusions

In this context, probiotic lactobacilli are considered to pool the resistant genes and might transfer these to pathogenic bacteria. In order to eliminate this possibility, resistance to the most relevant antibiotics for each strain used as probiotic lactobacilli, food or feed additives could be determined using the systematic QPS protocols. Moreover, due to the growing availability of whole bacterial genome sequences, sequence-based identification approaches have been enployed. These can be used to screen strains for unwanted genetic content such as antibiotic resistance. This screening supports normal safety assessment of probiotic lactobacilli.

7. References

Ammor MS, Florez AB, van Hoek AH, de Los Reyes-Gavilan CG, Aarts HJ, Margolles A, *et al.* (2008). Molecular characterization of intrinsic and acquired antibiotic resistance in lactic acid bacteria and bifidobacteria. J Mol Microbiol Biotechnol 14:6-15.

Ammor MS, Florez AB, Mayo B (2007). Antibiotic resistance in non-enterococcal lactic acid bacteria and bifidobacteria. Food Microbiol 24:559-570.

Axelsson LT, Ahrne SE, Andersson MC, Stahl SR (1988). Identification and cloning of a plasmid-encoded erythromycin resistance determinant from *Lactobacillus reuteri.* Plasmid 20:171-174.

Bennedsen M, Stuer-Lauridsen B, Danielsen M, Johansen E (2011). Screening for antimicrobial resistance genes and virulence factors via genome sequencing. Appl Environ Microbiol 77:2785-2787.

Borriello SP, Hammes WP, Holzapfel W, Marteau P, Schrezenmeir J, Vaara M, *et al.* (2003). Safety of probiotics that contain lactobacilli or bifidobacteria. Clin Infect Dis 36:775-780.

Caplice E, Fitzgerald GF (1999). Food fermentations: role of microorganisms in food production and preservation. Int J Food Microbiol 50:131-149.

Cataloluk O, Gogebakan B (2004). Presence of drug resistance in intestinal lactobacilli of dairy and human origin in Turkey. FEMS Microbiol Lett 236:7-12.

Comunian R, Daga E, Dupre I, Paba A, Devirgiliis C, Piccioni V, *et al.* (2010). Susceptibility to tetracycline and erythromycin of *Lactobacillus paracasei* strains isolated from traditional Italian fermented foods. Int J Food Microbiol 138:151-156.

Coppola R, Succi M, Tremonte P, Reale A, Salzano G, Sorrentino E (2005). Antibiotic susceptibility of *Lactobacillus rhamnosus* strains isolated from Parmigiano Reggiano cheese. Lait 85:193-204.

Danielsen M, Wind A (2003). Susceptibility of *Lactobacillus* spp. to antimicrobial agents. Int J Food Microbiol 82:1-11.

Danielsen M (2002). Characterization of the tetracycline resistance plasmid pMD5057 from *Lactobacillus plantarum* 5057 reveals a composite structure. Plasmid 48:98-103.

Devirgiliis C, Coppola D, Barile S, Colonna B, Perozzi G (2009). Characterization of the Tn*916* conjugative transposon in a food-borne strain of *Lactobacillus paracasei.* Appl Environ Microbiol 75:3866-3871.

Devirgiliis C, Caravelli A, Coppola D, Barile S, Perozzi G (2008). Antibiotic resistance and microbial composition along the manufacturing process of Mozzarella di Bufala Campana. Int J Food Microbiol 128:378-384.

European Commission (2005). Opinion of the Scientific Committee on Animal Nutrition on the criteria for assessing the safety of micro-organisms resistant to antibiotics of human clinical and veterinary importance. European Commission .

European Commission (2003). On a generic approach to the safety assessment of micro-organisms used in feed/food and feed/food production. European Commission .

European Food Safety Authority (2008). Update of the criteria used in the assessment of bacterial resistance to antibiotics of human or veterinary importance. EFSA J 732:1-15.

Feld L, Schjorring S, Hammer K, Licht TR, Danielsen M, Krogfelt K, *et al.* (2008). Selective pressure affects transfer and establishment of a *Lactobacillus plantarum* resistance plasmid in the gastrointestinal environment. J Antimicrob Chemother 61:845-852.

Food and Agriculture Organization of the United Nations-World Health Organization Working Group (2002). Guidelines for the evaluation of probiotics in foods, Report of a joint FAO/WHO working group on drafting guidelines for the evaluation of probiotics in food.

Fukao M, Tomita H, Yakabe T, Nomura T, Ike Y, Yajima N (2009). Assessment of antibiotic resistance in probiotic strain *Lactobacillus brevis* KB290. J Food Prot 72:1923-1929.

Gasson MJ, Davies FL (1980). Cnjugal transfer of the drug resistance plasmid pAMβ1 in the lactic streptococci. FEMS Microbiol Lett 7:51-53.

Gevers D, Danielsen M, Huys G, Swings J (2003a). Molecular characterization of *tet*(M) genes in *Lactobacillus* isolates from different types of fermented dry sausage. Appl Environ Microbiol 69:1270-1275.

Gevers D, Huys G, Swings J (2003b). In vitro conjugal transfer of tetracycline resistance from *Lactobacillus* isolates to other Gram-positive bacteria. FEMS Microbiol Lett 225:125-130.

Gfeller KY, Roth M, Meile L, Teuber M (2003). Sequence and genetic organization of the 19.3-kb erythromycin- and dalfopristin-resistance plasmid pLME300 from *Lactobacillus fermentum* ROT1. Plasmid 50:190-201.

Gruzza M, Fons M, Ouriet MF, Duval-Iflah Y, Ducluzeau R (1994). Study of gene transfer in vitro and in the digestive tract of gnotobiotic mice from *Lactococcus lactis* strains to various strains belonging to human intestinal flora. Microb Releases 2:183-189.

Heimbach J (2008). Generally Recognized as Safe (GRAS) determination of *Lactobacillus reuteri* strain DSM 17938. GRAS Notice (disclosable information) .

Hummel AS, Hertel C, Holzapfel WH, Franz CM (2007). Antibiotic resistances of starter and probiotic strains of lactic acid bacteria. Appl Environ Microbiol 73:730-739.

Huys G, D'Haene K, Swings J (2006). Genetic basis of tetracycline and minocycline resistance in potentially probiotic *Lactobacillus plantarum* strain CCUG 43738. Antimicrob Agents Chemother 50:1550-1551.

Igimi S, Ryu CH, Park SH, Sasaki Y, Sasaki T, Kumagai S (1996). Transfer of conjugative plasmid pAM beta 1 from *Lactococcus lactis* to mouse intestinal bacteria. Lett Appl Microbiol 23:31-35.

Jacobsen L, Wilcks A, Hammer K, Huys G, Gevers D, Andersen SR (2007). Horizontal transfer of *tet*(M) and *erm*(B) resistance plasmids from food strains of *Lactobacillus plantarum* to *Enterococcus faecalis* JH2-2 in the gastrointestinal tract of gnotobiotic rats. FEMS Microbiol Ecol 59:158-166.

Kastner S, Perreten V, Bleuler H, Hugenschmidt G, Lacroix C, Meile L (2006). Antibiotic susceptibility patterns and resistance genes of starter cultures and probiotic bacteria used in food. Syst Appl Microbiol 29:145-155.

Klare I, Konstabel C, Werner G, Huys G, Vankerckhoven V, Kahlmeter G, *et al.* (2007). Antimicrobial susceptibilities of *Lactobacillus, Pediococcus* and *Lactococcus* human isolates and cultures intended for probiotic or nutritional use. J Antimicrob Chemother 59:900-912.

Korhonen JM, Danielsen M, Mayo B, Egervärn M, Axelsson L, H uys G, *et al.* (2008). Antimicrobial susceptibility and proposed microbiological cut-off values of lactobacilli by phenotypic determination. Int J Prob Preb 3:257-268.

Kurokawa K, Itoh T, Kuwahara T, Oshima K, Toh H, Toyoda A, *et al.* (2007). Comparative metagenomics revealed commonly enriched gene sets in human gut microbiomes. DNA Res 14:169-181.

Leroy F, De Vuyst L (2004). Lactic acid bacteria as functional starter cultures for the food fermentation industry. Trends Food Sci Technol 15:67-78.

Licht TR, Wilcks A (2005). Conjugative Gene Transfer in the Gastrointestinal Environment. Adv Appl Microbiol 58C:77-95.

Lin CF, Fung ZF, Wu CL, Chung TC (1996). Molecular characterization of a plasmid-borne (pTC82) chloramphenicol resistance determinant (*cat*-TC) from *Lactobacillus reuteri* G4. Plasmid 36:116-124.

Mater DD, Langella P, Corthier G, Flores MJ (2008). A probiotic *Lactobacillus* strain can acquire vancomycin resistance during digestive transit in mice. J Mol Microbiol Biotechnol 14:123-127.

Mathur S, Singh R (2005). Antibiotic resistance in food lactic acid bacteria--a review. Int J Food Microbiol 105:281-295.

McConnell M, Mercer A, Tannock G (1991). Transfer of Plasmid pAMβ1 Between Members of the Normal Microflora Inhabiting the Murine Digestive Tract and Modification of the Plasmid in a *Lactobacillus reuteri* Host. Microbial Ecology in Health and Disease 4:343-355.

Morelli L, Sarra PG, Bottazzi V (1988). *In vivo* transfer of pAM beta 1 from *Lactobacillus reuteri* to *Enterococcus faecalis*. J Appl Bacteriol 65:371-375.

Ouoba LI, Lei V, Jensen LB (2008). Resistance of potential probiotic lactic acid bacteria and bifidobacteria of African and European origin to antimicrobials: determination and transferability of the resistance genes to other bacteria. Int J Food Microbiol 121:217-224.

Rizzotti L, La Gioia F, Dellaglio F, Torriani S (2009). Characterization of tetracycline-resistant *Streptococcus thermophilus* isolates from Italian soft cheeses. Appl Environ Microbiol 75:4224-4229.

Roberts MC (2005). Update on acquired tetracycline resistance genes. FEMS Microbiol Lett 245:195-203.

Rosander A, Connolly E, Roos S (2008). Removal of antibiotic resistance gene-carrying plasmids from *Lactobacillus reuteri* ATCC 55730 and characterization of the resulting daughter strain, *L. reuteri* DSM 17938. Appl Environ Microbiol 74:6032-6040.

Saarela M, Lahteenmaki L, Crittenden R, Salminen S, Mattila-Sandholm T (2002). Gut bacteria and health foods--the European perspective. Int J Food Microbiol 78:99-117.

Salim Ammor M, Belen Florez A, Mayo B (2007). Antibiotic resistance in non-enterococcal lactic acid bacteria and bifidobacteria. Food Microbiol 24:559-570.

Salminen S, von Wright A, Morelli L, Marteau P, Brassart D, de Vos WM, *et al.* (1998). Demonstration of safety of probiotics -- a review. Int J Food Microbiol 44:93-106.

Salyers A, Moon K, Schlesinger D (2007). The human intestinal tract - a hotbed of resistance gene transfer? Part I CM Newsletter 29:17-21.

Sasaki Y, Taketomo N, Sasaki T (1988). Factors affecting transfer frequency of pAM beta 1 from *Streptococcus faecalis* to *Lactobacillus plantarum.* J Bacteriol 170:5939-5942.

Schlundt J, Saadbye P, Lohmann B, Jacobsen BL, Nielsen EM (1994). Conjugal Transfer of Plasmid Dna between *Lactococcus-lactis* Strains and Distribution of Transconjugants in the Digestive-Tract of Gnotobiotic-Rats. Microb Ecol Health Dis 7:59-69.

Shrago AW, Chassy BM, Dobrogosz WJ (1986). Conjugal plasmid transfer (pAM beta 1) in *Lactobacillus plantarum.* Appl Environ Microbiol 52:574-576.

Sommer MO, Dantas G, Church GM (2009). Functional characterization of the antibiotic resistance reservoir in the human microflora. Science 325:1128-1131.

Spor A, Koren O, Ley R (2011). Unravelling the effects of the environment and host genotype on the gut microbiome. Nat Rev Microbiol 9:279-290.

Tannock GW (1987). Conjugal transfer of plasmid pAM beta 1 in *Lactobacillus reuteri* and between lactobacilli and *Enterococcus faecalis.* Appl Environ Microbiol 53:2693-2695.

Teuber M, Meile L, Schwarz F (1999). Acquired antibiotic resistance in lactic acid bacteria from food. Antonie Van Leeuwenhoek 76:115-137.

Tynkkynen S, Singh KV, Varmanen P (1998). Vancomycin resistance factor of *Lactobacillus rhamnosus* GG in relation to enterococcal vancomycin resistance (*van*) genes. Int J Food Microbiol 41:195-204.

West CA, Warner PJ (1985). Plasmid profiles and transfer of plasmid-encoded antibiotic resistance in *Lactobacillus plantarum.* Appl Environ Microbiol 50:1319-1321.

Zhou JS, Pillidge CJ, Gopal PK, Gill HS (2005). Antibiotic susceptibility profiles of new probiotic *Lactobacillus* and *Bifidobacterium* strains. Int J Food Microbiol 98:211-217.

Antimicrobial Resistance and Potential Probiotic Application of *Enterococcus* spp. in Sea Bass and Sea Bream Aquaculture

Ouissal Chahad Bourouni[1], Monia El Bour[1],
Pilar Calo-Mata[2] and Jorge Barros-Velàzquez[2]
[1]*Institut National des Sciences et Technologies de la Mer (INSTM), Tunis,*
[2]*Department of Analytical Chemistry, Nutrition and Food Science, LHICA,*
School of Veterinary Sciences, University of Santiago de Compostela,
[1]*Tunisia*
[2]*Spain*

1. Introduction

Microbial resistance to antibiotics is a world-wide problem in human and veterinary medicine. It is generally accepted that the main risk factor for the increase in the antibiotic resistance is an extensive use of antibiotics. In fact, for the last 50 years, high levels of antibiotics are commonly used for treatment and prevention of infectious diseases in humans and animals. This led to emergence and dissemination of resistant bacteria and resistance genes in wild populations (Bogaard & Stobberingh 2000). The antimicrobial agents used in animal care are also significant, both in increasing resistance in animal pathogens, and in transmission of resistant bacteria from animals to humans. In part, this is due to the transfer of antimicrobial-resistant normal or commensal microflora of animals, *via* the food chain to humans. Several recent papers reported link between antibiotic use in food producing animals, emergence of antibiotic resistance in *Salmonella, Escherichia coli,* enterococci or *Campylobacter* in treated animals and transfer of these resistances to humans (or their resistance genes to human pathogens) *via* the food chain (Barton 2000; Angulo et al. 2004). However, less attention was paid to potential for antibiotic use in aquaculture industries to compromise human health. In addition to transfer of resistant bacteria through consumption of contaminated fish and shellfish, there is substantial risk of environmental contamination due to practice of using medicated feeds to treat whole pens or cages.

2. Antibiotic resistance in aquaculture

Aquaculture around the Mediterranean basin has increased significantly to satisfy the demand for seafood, which cannot be met by wild fisheries harvesting as this is currently in a state of decline because of over-fishing, pollution and marine habitat destruction. Recent reports of the United Nations Food and Agriculture Organization (FAO), noted approximately more than 290.10^3 tons for the mainly species of marine fish farmed (sea bass and sea bream) and had previously estimated that half of the world's seafood demand will be met by aquaculture in 2020 (FAO, 2008). In Mediterranean aquaculture, the culture practices for most farmed fish species are mostly semi-intensive or intensive and a significant challenge to fish farming however is disease caused by bacteria such as *Aeromonas* sp., *Vibrio* sp., *Pseudomonas* sp. and *Flavobacterium* sp. Both prophylactic and therapeutic treatments utilize drug supplemented feeds to keep farmed fish free of diseases.

Antibiotics such as oxytetracycline (OTC) and quinolone such as oxolinic acid (OA) are the most widely used in Mediterranean aquaculture in feed (Rigos & Troisi, 2005) and treatments discharge drugs directly into the marine environment, where they are relatively resistant to biodegradation. Rigos et al., 2004 found that 60-73% of the OTC and 8-12% of the OA administered to farmed sea bream were excreted with the faeces. Also, the results of ARMed (Antibiotic Resistance in the south-eastern Mediterranean) suggest existence of high resistances of bacteria particularly in the eastern region where the resistance in *E. coli* appears to be more important than in other Mediterranean countries.

Previous reports noted that resistance emergence result directly from infections treatment with antibacterial drugs (Sorum 1998, 1999) and therefore limited their value in control of bacterial diseases of fish (Smith et al., 1994), apart from any public health concerns.

Further, antibacterial drugs were shown to persist in animal tissues and in the sea, including the aquatic food chain (CIESM, 2004) and development of antibiotic resistance is direct consequence of drug pollution. Chelossi et al., 2003 found that antibiotics discharged through faeces or undigested feed, contributed to high incidences of quinolone, tetracyclin and penicillin-resistant benthic bacteria and caused a shift in structure of the benthic microbial assemblage next to fish farms. Moreover, a considerable increase in resistance to several antimicrobial drugs has been discovered in some species of *Vibrio* and *Pseudomonas* recovered from diseased farmed sea bream of south-western Spain (Zorilla et al., 2003).

In Turkey, bacteria isolated from sea bass (*Dicentrarchus labrax*) showed a multidrug resistance to trimethoprim-sulfamethoxazole, cephalothin, tetracyclin and streptomycin suggesting that fish farms act as a reservoir of multidrug-resistant pathogenic bacteria such as *Pseudomonas* and *Vibrio* (Matyar, 2007). Considering the frequent usage of anti-bacterial drugs in Mediterranean fish farming, and serious problems of their rapid increase in resistance and transfer to non-target microflora including human and animal pathogens, there is an urgent need for monitoring drug contamination in aquatic environment and thus, the need for alternative techniques replacing drugs with effective and inexpensive probiotics which became increasingly evident and necessary to avoid resistance in fish farming sites and antibiotic residues in fish flesh destined for human consumption.

In Tunisia, aquaculture fish industry was developed since 1989 and has highly increased during these last ten years and national production passed from 1566 tons in 2000 to 4468 tons in 2009 with an increase in number of aquatic farms multiplied by about five. The production statistics in 2009 noted more than 2800 tons for marine fish farming. Regarded as a strategic activity that can support the fishing sector, aquaculture benefits in Tunisia of a particular interest mainly for the most two marine species farmed sea bass (*Dicentrarchus labrax*) and sea bream (*Sparus aurata*), which were undertaken in almost private farms.

The evolution of antibiotic resistance of the main bacterial species of medical interest is subject to increased surveillance in Tunisia. Since 1999, the research laboratory on antibiotic resistance (LAB MDT-03) established a system for monitoring bacterial resistance to antibiotics (L'Antibio - Résistance en Tunisie or LART). It includes four hospitals regularly monitoring the epidemiology of major bacterial species of medical importance and antibiotic resistance data collected are used in development of recommendations to antibiotic therapy (Boutiba et al., 2007). However, the problem of antibiotic resistance is underestimated in animal production including aquaculture and studies related are scarced. A study of pathogens vibrios isolated from sea bass showed a multi-resistance of *Vibrio alginolyticus* and *Vibrio parahaemolyticus* for almost antibiotics used and sensitivity was only demonstrated for furazolidone and chloramphenicol (Bakhrouf et al., 1995). Bouamama et al., 2001 isolated several multiresistant bacteria from mussel *Mytilus galloprovincialis* with resistance profiles to 12 different antibiotics in *Aeromonas hydrophila* and *Propioni acnes. Vibrio alginolyticus* was isolated from internal organs of sea bream and sea bass reared in two fish farms located in Tunisian coast. Multi-drug resistance to antimicrobial agents was detected, all the 34 strains tested were resistant to ampicillin, 31 strains were resistant to nitrofurantoïne and 12 were resistant to tetracycline (Ben Kahla-Nakbi et al., 2006). The most recent study of Rezgui et al., (2010) showed abundance of antibiotic resistant bacteria isolated mainly from gills and intestinal tract of sea bream and sea bass which belong to several species of the genus *Pseudomonas, Aeromonas, Vibrio* and *Enterobacteriaceae* and were resistant essentially to tetracyclin and penicillin (antibiotics commonly used respectively in veterinary and human clinical).

3. Probiotics as alternative to antibiotics in aquaculture

The increasing problems associated with infectious diseases in fish, the frequent usage of drugs for treatment and prevention of these diseases and the rapid increase in resistance to these antibiotics represent major challenges for this source of food production worldwide. Thus, replacing drugs with effective and inexpensive probiotics was became increasingly evident and necessary to avoid resistance in fish farming sites and antibiotic residues in fish flesh destined for human consumption (Vershuere et al., 2000; Balcazar et al., 2006; Rengpipat et al., 2008).

3.1 Probiotics: definition and principles

The term, probiotic, simply means "for life", originating from the Greek words "pro" and "bios" (Gismondo et al., 1999). The most widely quoted definition was made by Fuller (1989). He defined a probiotic as "a live microbial feed supplement which beneficially affects the host animal by improving its intestinal balance". This definition is still widely referred to, despite continual contention with regard to the correct definition of the term. Current probiotic applications and scientific data on mechanisms of action indicate that non-viable microbial components act in a beneficial manner and this benefit is not limited just to the intestinal region (Salminen et al., 1999). Besides, based on the intricate relationship an aquatic organism has with the external environment when compared with that of terrestrial animals, the definition of a probiotic for aquatic environments needs to be modified. Verschuere et al. (2000a) suggested the definition "a live microbial adjunct which has a beneficial effect on the host by modifying the host-associated or ambient microbial community, by ensuring improved use of the feed or enhancing its nutritional value, by enhancing the host response towards disease, or by improving the quality of its ambient environment".

3.2 Different modes of action

Several studies have demonstrated certain modes of probiotic action in effect in the aquatic environment. Bairagi et al. (2002) assessed aerobic bacteria associated with the gastrointestinal tract (GIT) of nine freshwater fish. They determined that selected strains produced digestive enzymes, thus facilitating feed utilization and digestion. Ramirez & Dixon (2003) reported on the enzymatic properties of anaerobic intestinal bacteria isolated from three fish species, showing the potential role a probiotic could play. In the paper of Bairagi et al. (2004) the benefit of adding *B. subtilis* and *B. circulans* to the diet of rohu, *Labeo rohita,* was shown. In the search to replace fish meal with leaf meal in fish feed, they found that addition of the two fish intestinal *Bacillus spp.* increased performance as judged by several factors (growth, feed conversion ratio, and protein efficiency ratio). They attributed this to the extracellular cellulolytic and amylolytic enzyme production by the bacteria. Although competition for adhesion sites has been widely suggested as a mode of action, there is little evidence in the literature to demonstrate this. Although for not direct attachment competition, Yan et al. (2002) demonstrated that production of antibiotic substances by two seaweed-associated *Bacillus* sp. was dependent on biofilm formation by the bacteria. This study highlighted a factor which might be important for some bacteria to be effective probiotics, i.e. surface attachment. Such observation concurred with Fuller's (1989) definition of a probiotic, i.e. the requirement for GIT colonization. It has been proposed that the mechanism of competitive exclusion for attachment sites could be given a distinct advantage via addition of probiotic bacteria during the initial egg fertilization steps of larviculture, thereby "getting in there first" (Irianto and Austin, 2002a).

Several studies have attributed a probiotic effect to competition for energy sources (Rico Mora et al., 1998; Verschuere et al., 1999; Verschuere et al., 2000b). Beneficial growth and survival was found in Artemia sp. pre-exposed to nine strains of bacteria before challenge with *V. proteolyticus* (Verschuere et al., 1999). It was concluded that the effect was not caused by extracellular products, but required the live bacterial cell. Although it was not specifically tested, they hypothesized that the protective effect probably resulted from competition for energy sources and for adhesion sites.

Itami et al. (1998) found that addition of *Bifidobacterium thermophilum* derived peptidoglycan to kuruma shrimp increased significantly their survival when they were challenged with *V. penaeicida.* They attributed this to an immunostimulatory effect, as the phagocytic activity of shrimp granulocytes was significantly higher in the treated shrimp compared with those of the control animals. Gullian et al. (2004) tested immunostimulation by a live *Vibrio sp.* (P62) and *Bacillus sp.* (P64), using *V. alginolyticus* as a positive control. They concluded that P64 and *V. alginolyticus* were immunostimulants. A review by Smith et al. (2003) provided important information on the potential problems associated with immunostimulants in crustacean aquaculture. They argued that the prolonged use of immunostimulants was in fact detrimental to the host and that much more research was needed before their use during critical periods could be considered safe.

Competition for iron has been reported as an important factor in marine bacteria (Verschuere et al., 2000a). Iron is needed by most bacteria for growth, but is generally limited in the tissues and body fluids of animals and in the insoluble ferric $Fe3+$ form (Verschuere et al., 2000a). Iron-binding agents, siderophores, allow acquisition of iron suitable for microbial growth. Siderophore production is a mechanism of virulence in some pathogens (Gram et al., 1999). Equally, a siderophore producing probiotic could deprive potential pathogens of iron under iron limiting conditions. This was shown by Gram et al. (1999), who found that a culture supernatant of *Pseudomonas fluorescens*, grown in iron-limited conditions, inhibited growth of *V. anguillarum*, whereas the supernatant from iron-available cultures did not.

Possibly the most studied mode of probiotic action in aquatic animals is the production of inhibitory substances. Currently, there are four methods commonly employed to screen for inhibitory substances *in vitro*; the double layer method, the well diffusion method, the cross-streak method, and the disc diffusion method. All methods are based on the principle that a bacterium produces extracellular substance inhibitor to itself or another bacterial strain (the indicator). The inhibitory activity is displayed by growth increase of the producer culture in agar medium.

This *in vitro* screening method has identified very good probiotics in aquaculture (Irianto & Austin, 2002b; Lategan and Gibson, 2003; Vaseeharan et al., 2004; Lategan et al., 2004a,b), with two major limitations for this approach. The first is that other modes of probiotic activity (e.g. immunostimulation, digestive enzymes production, competition for attachment site, or nutrients) will not be expressed in the laboratory on agar plate and, hence, a major source of potential beneficial action will be overlooked. The second drawback is that positive results *in vitro* fail to determine the real *in vivo* effect.

3.3 Developing probiotics for aquaculture

It has been widely published that a probiotic must possess certain properties (Verschuere et al., 2000a). These properties were proposed in order to aid in correct establishment of new, effective and safe products and included:

1. The probiotic should not be harmful to the host it is desired for,
2. It should be accepted by the host, e.g. through ingestion and potential colonization and replication within the host,
3. It should reach the location where the effect is required to take place,
4. It should actually work *in vivo* as opposed to *in vitro* findings,
5. It should preferably not contain virulence resistance genes or antibiotic resistance genes.

The future application for probiotics in aquaculture looks bright. There is an ever-increasing demand for aquaculture products and a similar increase in the search for alternatives to antibiotics. The field of probiotics intended for aquacultured animals is now attracting considerable attention and a number of commercial products are available.

3.4 Probiotic strains studied in aquaculture

Most probiotics proposed as biological control agents in aquaculture belong to the lactic acid bacteria (*Lactobacillus* and *Carnobacterium*), although other genera or species have also been studied, belonging to the genus *Vibrio*, to the genus *Bacillus*, or to the genus *Pseudomonas*, and also *Aeromonas* and *Flavobacterium* (Table 1).

Within probiotic group, lactic acid bacteria (LAB) have been recognized for their fermentative ability as well as their health and nutritional benefits since they exert strong antimicrobial activities against many pathogenic microorganisms and were considered as harmless bacteriocin-producing strains which may act antagonistic against fish pathogens (Maugin & Novel, 1994; Ringo & Gatesoupe, 1998). Moreover, LAB were signalled as competing for nutrients or space with spoiling microorganisms due to their ability to produce organic acids, hydrogen peroxide, diacetyl and bacteriocins and therefore should be of applied interest for marine fish and shellfish food bio-preservation (Franz C. et al., 2007).

Animals tested	**Potential probiotic**	**Pathogen tested or type of study conducted**	**Test method**
Gilthead sea bream	*Cytophaga sp., Roseobacter sp., Ruergeria sp., Paracoccus sp.,A. sp., Shewanella sp.*	Natural larval survival study	*In vivo*
Gilthead sea bream	*V. spp., Micrococcus sp.*	*L. anguillarum*	*In vitro and in vivo*
Atlantic cod	*Carnobacterium divergens*	*V. anguillarum*	*In vitro and in vivo*
Atlantic cod	*Carnobacterium divergens*	*V. anguillarum*	*In vitro and in vivo*
Atlantic salmon	*Lactobacillus plantarum*	*A. salmonicida*	*In vitro and in vivo*
Atlantic salmon	*Carnobacterium sp. (K1)*	*V. anguillarum, A. salmonicida*	*In vitro and in vivo*
Atlantic salmon	*Ps. fluorescens*	*A. salmonicida*	*In vitro and in vivo*
Atlantic salmon, rainbow trout	*Carnobacterium sp.*	*V. anguillarum, V. ordalii, Y. ruckeri, A. salmonicida*	*In vitro and in vivo*
Eel	*Commercial product: Cernivet® LBC (Ent. Faecium SF68), Toyocerin® (B. toyoi)*	*Ed. tarda*	*In vivo*
Eel.	*A. media*	*Saprolegnia sp*	*In vitro and in vivo*
Eel	*A. media*	*Saprolegnia parasitica*	*In vivo*
Goldfish	*Dead cells of A. hydrophila*	*A. salmonicida*	*In vivo*
Indian major carp	*B. subtilis*	*A. hydrophila*	*In vivo*
Nile tilapia	*Str. faecium, Lactobacillus acidophilus, Sacc. cerevisiae*	*Growth study*	*In vivo*
Pollack	*Commercial product: Bactocell (Pediococcus acidilactici), Levucell (Sacc. cerevisiae)*	*Pollack growth study using enriched Artemia*	*In vivo*
Rainbow trout	*Ps.fluorescens*	*V. anguillarum*	*In vitro and in vivo*
Rainbow trout	*Lactobacillus rhamnosus*	*A. salmonicida ssp. salmonicida*	-
Rainbow trout	*Ps. spp.*	*(furunculosis)*	
Rainbow trout	*A. hydrophila, V. fluvialis, Carnobacterium sp.*	*V. anguillarum*	*In vitro and in vivo*
Rainbow trout	*Dead cells of A. hydrophila, V. fluvialis,*	*A. salmonicida*	*In vitro and in vivo*
	Carnobacterium sp.	*A. salmonicida*	*In vivo*
Rainbow trout	*Lactobacillus rhamnosus*	*Immune enhancement paper*	*In vivo*
Rainbow trout	*Commercial product: BioPlus2B (B. subtilis, B. licheniformis)*	*Y. ruckeri* *Natural immunostimulation measured*	*In vivo*
Rainbow trout	*Lactobacillus rhamnosus*	*Prevention of vertebral column*	*In vivo*
Rainbow trout	*Pediococcus acidilactici, Sacc. boulardii*	*compression syndrome*	*In vivo*
Rainbow trout	*A. sobria*	*L. garvieae, Str. iniae*	*In vivo*
Rainbow trout	*Lactobacillus rhamnosus*	*Natural immunostimulation measured*	*In vivo*
Rohu	*B. circulans, B. subtilis*	*Digestive enzyme study*	*In vivo*
Sea bass	*Debaryomyces hansenii, Sacc. cerevisiae*	*Digestive enzyme study*	*In vivo*
Senegalese sole	*V. spp., Ps. spp., Micrococcus sp.*	*V. harveyi*	*In vitro and in vivo*
Silver perch	*A. media*	*Saprolegnia sp.*	*In vivo*
Tilapia	*Commercial product: Alchem Poseidon, Korea*	*Ed. tarda*	*In vivo*
Turbot	*2 unidentified marine bacteria*	*GIT colonization study*	*In vivo*
Turbot	*Marine bacteria*	*Natural survival study*	*In vivo*
Turbot	*Roseobacter spp., V. spp.*	*V. anguillarum, V. splendidus, Psalt. sp.*	*In vitro and in vivo*

Table 1. Summary of research towards probiotics for finfish

The LAB bacteriocin producer widespread in nature, and were isolated from several sources: dairy products, fermented sausages, vegetables, sillage, and mammalian gastro-intestinal tract (Laukova et al., 1993; Kato et al., 1994; Giraffa, 1995; Ennahar et al.,1998). Recently, bacteriocin producing LAB were efficiently tested in attempt to improve aquatic environment for both shrimp and fish aquaculture (Calo-Mata P et al., 2007; Chae-Woo et al., 2009). Among them, bacteria belonging to the genus *Enterococcus* are primarily associated with the indigenous human and animal gastrointestinal flora and are widely distributed, being found in air, water, sewage, soil and vegetation (J. Lukasova & A. sustackova, 2003). Although certain *Enterococcus* spp. have recently been associated with human nosocomial infections (Murray, 1998), a wide variety of enterococcal strains are increasingly being used as probiotics owing to their contribution to the healthy microflora of human mucosal surfaces. They have also been introduced into animal foods owing to their contribution to the health of farmed animals and as biological control agents in aquaculture (Calo-Mata P. et al., 2007).

4. Probiotic development in aquaculture farming in Tunisia

In Tunisia, fish farming of the two species sea bass (*Dicentrarchus labrax*) and gilthead sea bream (*Sparus aurata*) has significantly increased since a great benefit for such aquaculture which was threatened by microbial infections causing high mortalities at larval stages, and therefore decrease in farmed fish production. In addition, widespread use of antibiotics created an ecological problem for coastal ecosystems due to emergence of antibiotic resistant pathogen bacteria (Bouamama, 2001; Dellali, 2001; El Bour et al., 2001). Therefore, selection and use of probiotic bacteria capable of inhibiting pathogenic bacteria in sustainable way without ecosystem alteration would be a useful for specific farming problems. In this scope, for several years the INSTM team in Tunisia, in collaboration with the Department of Analytical Chemistry, Nutrition and Food Science, from the University of Santiago de Compostela in Spain were focusing in isolation and characterization of probiotic group, lactic acid bacteria (LAB) which were recognized for their fermentative ability as well as their health and nutritional benefits.

The study aimed to investigate the occurrence and antibiotic resistance profiles of *Enterococcus* spp. associated to the skin and the gastrointestinal tract of farmed sea bass and sea bream, the main fish species with high economic value cultured in Mediterranean aquaculture. This was accomplished by phenotypic and genotypic analysis, the latter including 16S rRNA sequencing and RAPD-PCR analysis. Besides, and with a view to perform a preliminary screening of potential probiotic LAB, the strains were investigated in their ability to produce antibacterial compounds against spoilage and pathogenic bacteria.

4.1 Methodology

Gilthead sea bream (*Sparus aurata*) and European sea bass (*Dicentrarchus labrax*) were collected from a fish farm in Hergla (Aquaculture Tunisiènne, Monastir, Tunisia). Skin patches were excised and the intestinal content was removed by dissecting the fish, removing the intestine and squeezing out the contents. Eighty four LAB strains were then isolated and investigated. The phenotypic characterization of bacterial isolates was studied to determine their colony morphology, cell morphology, motility, Gram stain and the production of cytochrome oxidase and catalase. The phenotypic identification of LAB strains was carried out by means of miniaturized API 50 CH biochemical tests (BioMérieux, Marcy L'Etoile, France). The results of the identification tests were interpreted using the APILAB PLUS software (BioMérieux).

Production of antibacterial activities was investigated, against a range of 39 pathogenic and spoilage microorganisms (Table2), to select potential producer strains. Detection of bacteriocin activity in LAB strains was screened by means of a standardized agar disk diffusion method.

Code	Genus	Species	Origin
AmH01	*Aeromonas*	*hydrophila*	ATCC 7966
BaC23	*Bacillus*	*cereus*	ATCC 14893
BaP31	*Bacillus*	*pumilus*	ATCC 7061
BaS05	*Bacillus*	*Subtilis ssp. Spizizenii*	ATCC 6633
BxT01	*Brochotrix*	*thermosphacta*	ATCC 11509
CbD21	*Carnobacterium*	*divergens*	ATCC 35677
CbM01	*Carnobacterium*	*maltaromaticum*	LHICA collection
EbA01	*Enterobacter*	*aerogenes*	ATCC 13048
EbC11	*Enterobacter*	*cloacae*	ATCC 13047
HaA02	*Hafnia*	*alvei*	ATCC 9760
KlOx11	*Klebsiella*	*oxytoca*	ATCC 13182
KlP02	*Klebsiella*	*planticola*	ATCC 33531
KlPn21	*Klebsiella*	*Pneumoniae* ssp. *pneumoniae*	ATCC 10031
Lb30A	*Lactobacillus*	*saerimneri*	LHICA collection
MoM02	*Morganella*	*morganii* ssp. *morganii*	ATCC 8076H
PhD11	*Photobacterium*	*damselae*	ATCC 33539
PrM01	*Proteus*	*mirabilis*	ATCC 14153
PrP11	*Proteus*	*penneri*	ATCC 33519
PrV21	*Proteus*	*vulgaris*	ATCC 9484
PsF12	*Pseudomonas*	*fluorescens*	ATCC 13525
PsFr51	*Pseudomonas*	*fragi*	ATCC 4973
PsG21	*Pseudomonas*	*gessardii*	LHICA collection
SrM53	*Serratia*	*marcescens* ssp. *marcescens*	ATCC 274
SyE21	*Staphylococcus*	*epidermidis*	ATCC 35983
SyX11	*Staphylococcus*	*xylosus*	ATCC 29971
StM03	*Stenotrophomonas*	*maltophilia*	ATCC 13637
59	*Staphylococcus*	*aureus*	ATCC 9144
4521	*Staphylococcus*	*aureus*	ATCC 35845
4032	*Lysteria*	*monocytogenes*	NCTC 11994
1112	*Lysteria*	*monocytogenes* 1112	LHICA collection
CI34.1	*Pseudomonas*	*anguilliseptica*	Seabream*
ACR5.1(AS)	*Aeromonas*	*salmonicida*	Turbot*
CI52.1(VCI)	*Vibrio*	*anguillarum*	Seabream*
ACC30.1	*Photobacterium*	*damselae* ssp. *piscida*	Sole*
V62	*Vibrio*	*anguillarum*	Seabream**
VF	*Vibrio*	*anguillarum*	Seabass***
AF	*Aeromonas*	*salmonicida*	Seabass***
V90.11.287(V287)	*Vibrio*	*anguillarum*	Seabass****
AH2	*Pseudomonas*	*fluorescens*	*Lates niloticus*****

* Strains provided by Pr. J. L. Romalde (Spain). ** Strain provided by Pr. G. Breuil (France).
*** Strains provided by Pr. J. C. Raymond (France). **** Strains provided by Pr. L. Gram (Denmark).

Table 2. Pathogenic and spoilage indicator microorganisms used to test the antibacterial activities of LAB isolates.

Genetic characterization of producer LAB strains was then performed by PCR targeted to the 16S rRNA gene using the universal set of primers: p8FPL (forward: 5′-AGTTTGATCCTGGCTCAG-3′) and p806R (reverse: 5′-GGACTACCAGGGTATCTAAT-3′), that yield a 800 bp PCR product of the 16S rRNA gene. The PCR products were purified and sequenced. The sequences were compared with others present in GenBank database.

Further genetic characterization of LAB isolates was performed by RAPD-PCR using primers M13 (5′-GAGGGTGGCGGTTCT-3′) (Andrighetto et al., 2004). To check reproducibility, all PCR assays were performed in triplicate. Each reaction we included a tube without template DNA as a negative control.

The antibacterial sensitivity was determined by the agar diffusion method according to Chabbert (1982), using 16 antibiotics that were selected as representative of different classes of antimicrobial agents relevant in human and animal medicine (Penicillin G, Amoxicillin, Oxacilin, Cefoxitin, Ceftriaxon, Streptomycin, Tobramycin, Neomycin, Chloramphenicol, Tetracyclin, Oleandomycin, Nitrofurantoin, Trimethoprim-Sulphonamid, Rifampicin, Oxolinic acid and also Vancomycin). Based on the zones of inhibition a qualitative report of "susceptible", "intermediate" or "resistant" can be determined for the tested bacteria according to French national guidelines (Comité de l'Antibiogramme de la Société Française de Microbiologie, 1996).

4.2 Results and discussion

Eighty four strains of LAB were isolated from both gastrointestinal content and skin of fish studied. All isolates were Gram-positive, catalase-negative, facultatively anaerobic and nonmotile chain-forming cocci. They were tested for assaying inhibitory production against 39 Gram-positives and Gram-negatives bacteria, including pathogenic bacteria in aquaculture and others spoilage bacteria. 58 strains (69%) exhibited inhibitory activity against a large number of the indicator organisms investigated. Greater inhibition was observed against *L. monocytogenes, S. aureus, A. hydrophila, A. salmonicida, V. anguillarum* and *Carnobacterium* strains in comparison with the remaining indicators. The diameters of the inhibition halos were within the 7.5–18 mm range. Thus, we selected 35 highly producing strains that generated inhibitory zones with diameters between 12 and 18 mm.

The results allowed the classification of the strains as belonging to the species *E. faecium* (29 strains) and *E. sanguinicola* (6 strains) (paper under process) (Table3). Other studies, previously mentioned, also showed that the skin and gastrointestinal tract of various fish species contains lactic acid bacteria which produce antibacterial compounds able to inhibit the growth of several micoorganisms (Ringo 1999; Spanggaard B. et al., 2001; Rengpipat S. et al., 2008; Vijayabaskar P & Somasundaram S. T., 2008; Ringo, 2008).

According to the results obtained, all the strains tested were resistant to at least three different antibiotics. The frequency of resistance to the various antimicrobials for all bacteria is presented in Fig. 1. Differences of resistance rates were noted for amoxicillin, oxacillin, cephalosporins (cefoxitin, ceftriaxon), aminosids (streptomycin, tobramycin and neomycin), macrolids (oleandomycin) and oxolinic acid. In contrast, phenicol, tetracyclin, rifampicin and trimethoprim-sulphamid were the most active antibiotics against the majority of the bacterial isolates (fig1).

In fact, more than half (64.8%) of all the isolates were found to be resistant to amoxicillin and 71.4% were resistant to oleandomycin, 78.1% to ceftriaxon, 80.1% to streptomycin and 85% to cefoxitin. Oxacillin resistance was found in 92.5% of the isolates and tobramycin and oxolinic acid resistance in 94.2%. Resistance to neomycin was found in 98.3% of the isolates. Resistance to chloramphenicol and trimethoprim-sulphamide was detected in 5.1% and 2.2% of the isolates respectively, 8% of the isolates were found to be resistant to tetracyclin. Resistance to rifampicin was seen in 16.9% of the isolates

Strains	Fish	Organ	Identification	Accession number
UPAA 1	Sea bass	GIT	*Enterococcus sanguinicola*	GU460379
UPAA 4	Sea bass	GIT	*Enterococcus faecium*	GU460381
UPAA 7	Sea bass	Skin	*Enterococcus faecium*	GU460383
UPAA 11	Sea bream	GIT	*Enterococcus faecium*	HQ450696
UPAA 15	Sea bass	Skin	*Enterococcus faecium*	GU460385
UPAA 23	Sea bass	GIT	*Enterococcus faecium*	GU460388
UPAA 24	Sea bass	GIT	*Enterococcus faecium*	GU460389
UPAA 25	Sea bass	GIT	*Enterococcus faecium*	GU460390
UPAA 31	Sea bass	Skin	*Enterococcus faecium*	GU460394
UPAA 32	Sea bass	GIT	*Enterococcus faecium*	GU460395
UPAA 33	Sea bass	GIT	*Enterococcus sanguinicola*	GU460396
UPAA 34	Sea bream	Skin	*Enterococcus faecium*	HQ450701
UPAA 35	Sea bream	GIT	*Enterococcus faecium*	HQ450702
UPAA 37	Sea bass	GIT	*Enterococcus faecium*	GU460398
UPAA 39	Sea bream	GIT	*Enterococcus faecium*	HQ450704
UPAA 40	Sea bream	GIT	*Enterococcus faecium*	HQ450705
UPAA 44	Sea bream	Skin	*Enterococcus faecuim*	HQ450706
UPAA 45	Sea bream	GIT	*Enterococcus faecuim*	HQ450707
UPAA 53	Sea bass	GIT	*Enterococcus faecium*	GU460402
UPAA 54	Sea bass	GIT	*Enterococcus faecium*	GU460403
UPAA 56	Sea bass	Skin	*Enterococcus faecium*	GU460404
UPAA 57	Sea bass	Skin	*Enterococcus sanguinicola*	GU460405
UPAA 58	Sea bass	Skin	*Enterococcus faecium*	GU460406
UPAA 63	Sea bass	GIT	*Enterococcus faecium*	GU460409
UPAA 71	Sea bream	GIT	*Enterococcus sanguinicola*	HQ450716
UPAA 80	Sea bass	GIT	*Enterococcus faecium*	GU460416
UPAA 83	Sea bass	Skin	*Enterococcus faecium*	GU460415
UPAA 85	Sea bream	GIT	*Enterococcus faecium*	HQ450721
UPAA 89	Sea bream	GIT	*Enterococcus faecium*	HQ450724
UPAA 105	Sea bass	GIT	*Enterococcus faecium*	GU460417
UPAA 110	Sea bream	GIT	*Enterococcus faecium*	HQ450730
UPAA 111	Sea bass	Skin	*Enterococcus faecium*	GU460420
UPAA 113	Sea bass	GIT	*Enterococcus sanguinicola*	GU460421
UPAA 114	Sea bass	GIT	*Enterococcus faecium*	GU460422
UPAA 116	Sea bass	Skin	*Enterococcus sanguinicola.*	GU460423

Table 3. Antibacterial producing isolates

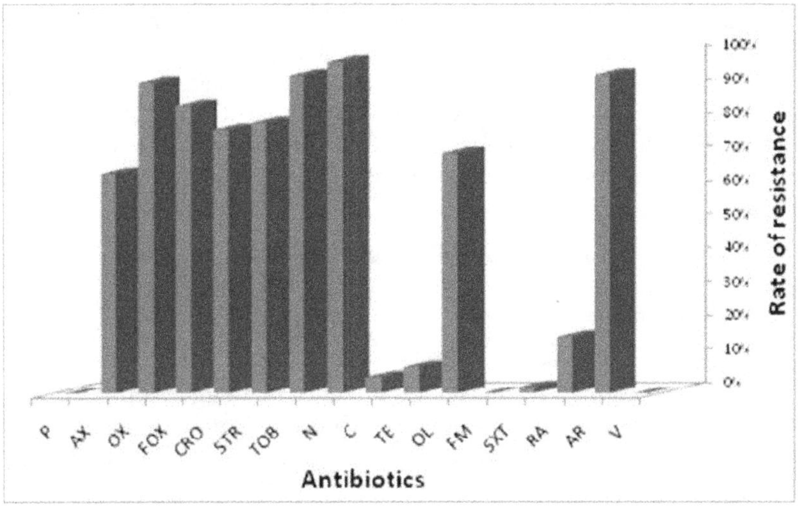

P: penicillin G; Ax: amoxicillin; Ox: oxacillin; Fox: cefoxitin; Cro: ceftriaxon; Str: streptomycin; Tob: tobramycin; N: neomycin; C: chloramphenicol; Te: tetracyclin; Ol: oleandomycin; Fm: furans; Sxt: trimethoprim-sulphamide; Ra: rifampicin; Ar: oxolinic acid; V: vancomycine.

Fig. 1. Profiles of resistance obtained for the different enterococci isolates against the 16 antimicrobial agents tested.

Interestingly, all the strains were sensitive to vancomycin, penicillin and furans and were not haemolytic.

Enterococci have been known to be resistant to most antibiotics used in clinical practice. Multidrug-resistant and vancomycin-resistant enterococci are commonly isolated from humans, animal sources, aquatic habitats, agricultural run-off which indicates their ability to enter the human food chain (Rice et al., 1995). They are naturally resistant to cephalosporins, aminoglycosides and clindamycin and may also be resistant to tetracyclins and erythromycin. They are intermediate sensitive to penicillin and ampicillin and glycopeptides. The strains that produce β-lactamase are rare and Vancomycin-resistant enterococci (VRE) are emerging as a global threat to public health.

Enterococci are known to acquire antibiotic resistance with relative ease and to be able to spread these resistance genes to other species (Kuhn et al., 2000). *Enterococcus faecalis* has been reported to transfer plasmids harbouring antibiotic-resistance traits to other enterococci and to *Listeria monocytogenes* in water treatment plants (Marcinek et al., 1998). *Enterococcus faecium* conjugative transposons can be transferred from animal bacteria to human ones. Such conjugative trasposons can also transfer vancomycin resistance to *Staphylococcus aureus*, streptococci and lactobacilli.

The extremely high level of antibiotic resistance observed in these bacteria has made them feared infectious agents in intensive care wards. Possible pathogenicity factors like hemolysins have been described. The most important species are *E. faecalis* and *E. faecium*, the first being more common in human illnesses, the second one (though less common in human infections) may pose a larger resistance threat (Huycke et al., 1998).

In both species, the evolutionary development of resistance has been attributed to the possession of broad host range and extremely mobile genetic elements like conjugative plasmids and transposons. The molecular details of the structures and functions of these elements are fairly well studied and becoming understood (Clewell et al., 1995; Marra & Scott 1999). It is noteworthy that transcription of the transfer functions of Tn*916* requiring excission of the element is dramatically increased in the presence of tetracyclin (Celli & Trieu-Cuot 1998).

Therefore, antibiotic resistance, notably to vancomycin, and the presence of haemolysins as an indicator of potential pathogenecity, must be evaluated in these microorganisms, before they can be used as probiotics and/or food additives.

The antimicrobial spectra observed for the *Enterococcus* species isolated included several genera indicating a broad spectrum of activity against Gram-positive but also Gram-negative pathogenic and spoilage organisms. A number of earlier studies have also shown that several marine bacteria produce inhibitory substances that inhibit bacterial pathogens in aquaculture systems (Nogami & Maeda, 1992; Austin et al., 1995; Rengpipat et al., 1998; Gram et al., 1999; Chahad et al., 2007). The use of such bacteria to inhibit pathogens by release of antimicrobial substances is now gaining importance in fish farming as a better and more effective alternative than administering antibiotics to manage the health of these organisms (Vijayan et al., 2006). Spanggaard et al. (2001) reported that this antagonism was the most influential factor preventing the establishment of the exogenous bacteria and indicates that the antagonistic part of an indigenous flora may offer a significant contribution to the control of unwanted (pathogenic) bacteria.

LAB isolated from the same environment on which they will be further used as bio-control cultures, ensure that these LAB strains are well ecological adapted. This fact is an important factor for their effectiveness as natural antimicrobial agents. The local results suggest the potential usefulness of the inhibitory-producing strains isolated from fish, as probiotics in aquaculture, in order to prevent bacterial infections caused by *A. salmonicida, A. hydrophila* and *V. anguillarum* which are the most common pathogenic bacteria isolated from the marine environment, causing high mortalities of fish and shellfish. Their inhibitory activities show some properties which make it potentially remarkable food preservatives.

5. Conclusion

In comparison with studies on impact of antibio-resistance on terrestrial food producing animals, those related to marine aquaculture enterprises still scarced. The present study supports the view that there is a risk of transfer of resistant bacteria to humans from consumption of aquaculture products. In Tunisian field, although there are no products registered for use in aquaculture, antimicrobial resistance resistance is present in isolates from aquaculture..

The extent of the resistance found and in particular the significant levels of multiple resistance are of concern. Follow-up studies are required to investigate the extent of antibiotic use in Tunisian aquaculture farms and environments and to determine the molecular basis of antimicrobial resistance to the different antibiotics, the potential for transfer of resistance genes from aquaculture isolates to human pathogens, some assessment of the risk of transfer of resistant organisms (or genes) to humans *via* food chain and the threats imposed by environmental contamination with antibiotic resistant bacteria.

The highly antibacterial producing *Enterococcus* strains isolated from both sea bream and sea bass which inhibit growth of pathogenic and spoiling bacteria should have a potential practical interest and offer a natural means for simultaneous application as probiotics and/or for preventing the development of *Listeria* in food stuffs.

6. References

Andrighetto, C.; Knijif E.; Lombardi, A.; Vancanneyt, M.; Kersters, K.; Swings, J. & Dellaglio F (2004). Phenotypic and genetic diversity of enterococci isolated from Italian cheeses. *Journal of Dairy Research*, Vol.68, pp.303-316

Angulo, F. J.; Nargund, V. N. & Chiller, T. C. (2004). Evidence of an Association Between Use of Anti-microbial Agents in Food Animals and Anti-microbial Resistance Among Bacteria Isolated from Humans and the Human Health Consequences of Such Resistance. *Journal of Veterinary Medecine*, Vol. 51, pp.374–379

Austin, B.; Stuckey, L.F.; Robertson, PAW.; Effendi, I. & Griffith, DRW. (1995). A probiotic strain of *Vibrio alginolyticus* effective in reducing diseases caused by *Aeromonas salmonicida, Vibrio anguillarum* and *Vibrio ordalii*. *Journal of Fish Diseases*, Vol.18, pp.93-96

Bairagi, A.; Sakar Ghosh; K., Sen; S.K. & Ray, A.K. (2002). Enzyme producing bacterial flora isolated from fish digestive tracts. *Aquaculture International*, Vol.10, pp.109–121

Bairagi, A.; Sarkar Ghosh, K.; Sen, S.K. & Ray, A.K. (2004). Evaluation of the nutritive value of Leucaena leucocephala leaf meal, inoculated with fish intestinal bacteria *Bacillus subtilis* and Bacillus circulans in formulated diets for rohu, Labeo rohita (Hamilton) fingerlings. *Aquaculture Research*, Vol. 35, pp. 436–446

Bakhrouf, A. ; Ben Ouada, H. & Oueslati, R. (1995). Essai de traitement des vibrioses du loup *Dicentrarchus labrax* dans une zone de pisciculture, à Monastir, Tunisie. *Marine Life*, Vol.5, pp. 47-54

Balcàzar, JL.; de Blas, I.; Ruiz-Zarzuela, I.; Cunningham, D., Vendrell, D. & Muuzquiz, JL. (2006). The role of probiotics in aquaculture. *Veterinary Microbiology*, Vol. 114, pp.173–186

Barton, M.D. (2000). Antibiotic use in animals feed and its impact on human health. *Nuritiont Research Reviews*, Vol.13, pp.79–299

Ben Kahla-Nakbi, A.; K., Chaieb; A., Besbes; T., Zmantar & A., Bakhrouf, (2006). Virulence and enterobacterial repetitive intergenic consensus PCR of *Vibrio alginolyticus* strains isolated from Tunisian cultured gilthead sea bream and sea bass outbreaks. *Veterinary Microbiology*, Vol.117, pp.321-327

Boggard van den, AE. & Stobberingh EE. (2000). Epidemiology of resistance to antibiotics-Links between animals and humans. *International Journal of Antimicrobial Agents*, Vol.**14**, pp.327-335

Bouamama, K. (2001). *Mytilus galloprovincialis* de la lagune de Bizerte : populations bactériennes et Biomarqueurs non spécifiques. Diplôme des études approfondies (DEA). Faculté des Sciences de Tunis, Institut des Sciences et Technologies de la Mer. Tunis, Tunisia

Boutiba, I.; Ghozzi, R.; Jouaihia, W.; Mahjoubi, F.; Thabet, L.. Smaoui, H.; Ben Hassen, A. Hàmmamí, A.; Kechrid, A. & Ben Redjeb, S. (2007). Résistance bactérienne aux antibiotiques en Tunisie : Données de 1999 A 2003, *Revue Tunisienne d'Infectiologie*, Vol. 1, pp. 5-11

Calo-Mata, P.; Arlindo, S.; Boehm. K. ; De Miguel, T. Pascoal A. & Barros-Velazquez, J. (2007). Current application and future trends of lactic acid bacteria and their bacteriocins for biopreservation of aquatic food products. *Food Bioprocess Technology*, Vol.1(1), pp.43-63

Celli, J. & Trieu-Cuot, P. (1998). Circularization of Tn916 is required for expression of the transposon-encoded transfer functions: characterization of long tetracycline-inducible transcripts reading through the attachment site. *Molecular Microbiology*, Vol. 28, pp.103–117

Chabbert Y.A (1982). L'antibiogramme. In : Bactériologie médicaleL. Le Miror, M. véron, (eds): Flammarion. Medecine Science. Paris, 205-212.

Chae-Woo, M.; Yun-Seok, C. & Kye-Heon, O. (2009). Removal of pathogenic bacteria and nitrogens by *Lactobacillus spp*. JK-8 and JK-11. *Aquaculture*, Vol.287, pp.266-270

Chahad Ouissal, B.; El Bour, M.; Mraouna, R.; Abdennaceur, H. & Boudabous, A. (2007). Preliminary selection study of potential probiotic bacteria from aquacultural areas in Tunisia. *Annals of Microbiology*, Vol.57 (2), pp.185-190

Chelossi, E. ; Vezzulli, L. ; Milano, A. ; Branzoni, M. ; Fabiano, M. ; Riccardi, G. & Banat, I.M., (2003). Antibiotic resistance of benthic bacteria in fish-farm and control sediments of the Western Mediterranean. *Aquaculture*, Vol. 219, pp.83–97

CIESM 2004. Novel contaminants and pathogens in coastal waters. CIESM Workshop Monograph N°26, Monaco "www.ciesm.org/online/monographs/Neuchatel.pdf"

Clewell, DB., Flannagan, SE. & Jaworsky. DD. (1995). Unconstrained bacterial promiscuity: the Tn*916*-Tn*1545* family of conjugative transposons. *Trends in Microbiology*, Vol.3, pp.229–236

Comité de l'Antibiogramme de la Société Française de Microbiologie, (1996). Statement 1996 CA-SFM. Zone sizes and MIC breakpoints for non-fastidious organisms. *Clinical Microbiology and Infecion*, Vol.2, Suppl. 1, pp.46-49

Dellali, M., (2001). Utilisation d'indicateurs microbiologiques et biochimiques chez *Ruditapes decussatus* et *Mytilus galloprovincialis* dans la biosurveillance de la lagune de Bizerte : Validation de certains biomarqueurs. Thèse de doctorat, Faculté des Sciences de Bizerte. Tunisia

El Bour, M.; Attia El Hilli, H.; Mraouna, R. & Ayari, W. (2001). Bacterial study of mesophilic Aeromonads distribution in shellfish. Proceeding of the fifth international conference on the Mediterranean coastal environment, *MEDCOAST*, pp.557- 565

Ennahar, S.; Aoude-Werner. D.; Assobhei, O. & Hasselmann, D. (1998). Antilisterial activity of enterocin 81, a bacteriocin produced by *Enterococcus faecium* WHE 81 isolated from cheese, *Journal of Applied Microbiology, Vol.*85, pp.521–526

Franz, CMAP; van Belkum, MJ.; Holzapfel, WH; Abriouel, H. & Galvez, A. (2007). Diversity of Enterococcal bacteriocins and their grouping in a new classification scheme. *FEMS Microbiology Review*, Vol.31, pp.293–310

Fuller, R. (1989). Probiotics in man and animals. *Journal of Applied Bacteriology*, Vol. 66, pp.365–378

Giraffa, G. (1995). Enterococcal bacteriocins: their potential as anti-*Listeria* factors in dairy technology. *Food Microbe,* Vol.12, pp.291-299

Gismondo, M.R.; Drago, L.; Lombardi, A. (1999). Review of probiotics available to modify gastrointestinal flora. *International Journal of Antimicrobial Agents,* Vol. 12, pp.287-292

Gram, L.; Melchiorsen, J.; Spanggaard, B.; Huber, I. & Nielsen, T.F. (1999). Inhibition of Vibrio anguillarum by Pseudomonas fluorescens AH2, a possible probiotic treatment of fish. *Applied and Environmental Microbiology, Vol.*65 (3), pp.969-973

Gullian, M.; Thompson, F. & Rodriguez, J. (2004). Selection of probiotic bacteria and study of their immunostimulatory effect in Penaeus vannamei. *Aquaculture,* Vol.233, pp.1-14

Huycke, MM.; Sahm, DF. & Gilmore, MS. (1998). Multiple-drug resistant enterococci: the nature of the problem and an agenda for the future. *Emerging Infectious Diseases,* Vol.4(2), pp.239-249

Irianto, A. & Austin, B. (2002a). Probiotics in aquaculture. *Journal of Fish Diseases,* Vol.25, pp.633-642

Irianto, A. & Austin, B. (2002b). Use of probiotics to control furunculosis in rainbow trout, Oncorhynchus mykiss (Walbaum). *Journal of Fish Diseases,* Vol.25, pp.333-342

Itami, T.; Asano, M.; Tokushige, K.; Kubono, K.; Nakagawa, A.; Noboru, T.; Nishimura, H.; Maeda, M.; Kondo, M. & Takahashi, Y. (1998). Enhancement of disease resistance of kuruma shrimp, *Penaeus japonicus,* after oral administration of peptidoglycan derived from Bifidobacterium thermophilum. *Aquaculture,* Vol.164, pp.277-288

Murray, BE. (1998). Diversity among multidrug-resistant enterococci. *Emerging Infectious Diseases, Vol.* 4, pp.37-47

Kato, T.; Matsuda, T.; Ogawa, E.; Ogawa, H.; Kato, H.; Doi, U. & Nakamura, R. (1994). Plantaricin-149, a bacteriocin produced by *Lactobacillus pluntarum* NRIC 149. *Journal of Fermentution and Bioengineering,* Vol.77, pp.277-282

Kuhn, I.; Iversen, A.; Burman, L.G.; Olsson-Liljequist, B.; Franklin, A.; Finn, M.; Aarestrup, F.; Seyfarth, A.M.; Blanch, A.R., Taylor, H.; Caplin, J.; Moreno, M.A.; Dominguez, L. & Mollby, R. (2000). Epidemiology and ecology of enterococci, with special reference to antibiotic resistant strains, in animals, humans and the environment. Example of an ongoing project within the European research programme. *International Journal of Antimicrobial Agents.* Vol.14, pp.337-342

Lategan, M.J. & Gibson, L.F. (2003). Antagonistic activity of *Aeromonas media* strain A199 against Saprolegnia sp., an opportunistic pathogen of the eel, *Anguilla australis* Richardson. *Journal of Fish Diseases,* Vol.26, pp.147-153

Lategan, M.J.; Torpy, F.R. & Gibson, L.F. (2004a). Biocontrol of saprolegniosis in silver perch Bidyanus bidyanus (Mitchell) by Aeromonas media strain A199. *Aquaculture,* Vol.235, pp.77-88

Lategan, M.J.; Torpy, F.R. & Gibson, L.F. (2004b). Control of saprolegniosis in the eel *Anguilla australis* Richardson, by *Aeromonas media* strain A199. *Aquaculture,* Vol.240, pp.19-27

Laukova, A.; M., Marekova & P. Javorsky. (1993). Detection and antimicrobial spectrum of a bacteriocin like substances produced by Enterococcus faecium CCM4231. *J. Letters in Applied Microbiology, Vol.*16, pp.257-260

Lukàsova, J. & Sustàckovà, A. (2003). Enterococci and Antibiotic Resistance: Review Article. *Acta. Veterinaria Brno.*, Vol.72, pp.315-323

Marcinek, H.; Wirth, R.; Muscholl-Silberhorn, A. & Gauer, M. (1998). Enterococcus faecalis gene transfer under natural conditions in municipal sewage water treatment plants. *Applied and Environmental Microbiology*, Vol.64, pp.626-632

Mauguin, S. & Novel, G. (1994). Characterization of lactic acid bacteria isolated from seafood. *Journal of Applied Bacteriology*, Vol.76, pp.616–625

Marra, D. & Scott. JR. (1999). Regulation of excision of the conjugative transposon Tn916. *Molecular Microbio*logy, Vol.31, pp.609–621

Matyar, F. (2007). Distribution and antimicrobial multiresistance in Gram-negative bacteria isolated from Turkish sea bass (*Dicentrarchus labrax* L., 1781) farm. *Annals of Microbiology*, Vol.**57**, pp.35–38

Nogami, K. & Maeda, M. (1992). Bacteria as biocontrol agents for rearing larvae of the Crab *Portunus trituberculatus*. *Canadian Journal of Fish. and Aquatic Sciences*, pp.2373-2376

Ramirez, R.F. & Dixon, B.A. (2003). Enzyme production by obligate intestinal anaerobic bacteria isolated from Oscars (*Astronotus ocellatus*), angelfish (*Pterophyllum scalare*) and southern flounder (*Paralichthys lethostigma*). *Aquaculture* , Vol.227, pp.417–426

Rengpipat, S.; Phianphak, W.; Piyatiratitivorakul, S. & Menasveta, P. (1998). Effects of a probiotic bacterium on black tiger shrimp *Penaeus monodon* survival and growth. *Aquaculture* Vol.167, pp.301-313

Rengpipat, S., Rueangruklikhit, T. & Piyatiratitivorakul, S. (2008). Evaluations of lactic acid bacteria as probiotics for juvenile sea bass *Lates calcarifer*. *Aquaculture Research*, Vol.39, pp.134-143

Rezgui, I. (2010). Etude de l'antibioresistance chez deux espèces de poisons aquacoles en Tunisie: le loup (*Dicentrarchus labrax*) et la daurade (*Sparus aurata*). Master of Biology. University of Sciences of Tunis. Institut des Sciences et Technologies de la Mer. Tunis, Tunisia

Rice, E.W.; Messer, J.W.; Johnson, C.H. & Reasoner, D.J. (1995). Occurrence of high-level aminoglycoside resistance in environmental isolates of enterococci. *Applied and Environmental Microbiology*. Vol.61, pp.374–376

Rico-Mora, R.; Voltolina, D. & Villaescusa-Celaya, J.A. (1998). Biological control of Vibrio alginolyticus in Skeletonema costatum (Bacillariophyceae) cultures. *Aquacultural Engineering* Vol.19, pp.1–6

Rigos, G.; Nengas, I.; Alexis, M. & Troisi, G. (2004). Potential drug (oxytetracycline & oxolinic acid) pollution from Mediterranean sparid fish farms. *Aquatic Toxicology*, Vol.69, pp.281-288

Rigos, G. & Troisi, G. (2005). Antibacterial agents in Mediterranean finfish farming: a synopsis of drug pharmacokinetics in important euryhaline fish species and possible environmental implications. *Reviews in Fish Biology and Fisheries*, Vol.15, pp.53-73

Ringo, E. (1999). Lactic acid bacteria in fish: antibacterial effect against fish pathogens.In effects of Anti nutrients on the Nutritional Value of Legume Diets, Vol.8, ed.

Krogdahl, Mathiesen, SD. And Pryme, I. COST 98. 70-75, Luxembourg: EEC Publication.

Ringø, E. & Gatesoupe, F.-J. (1998). Lactic acid bacteria in fish: a review. *Aquaculture*, Vol.160, pp.177–203

Ringo, E. (2008). The ability of *Carnobacteria* isolated from fish intestine to inhibit growth of fish pathogenic bacteria: a screening study. *Aquaculture Research*, Vol.39, pp.171-180

Salminen, S.; Ouwehand, A.; Benno, Y. & Lee, Y.K. (1999). Probiotics: how should they be defined. *Trends in Food Science and Technology*, Vol.10, pp.107–110

Smith, P.; Hiney, M. & Samuelson, O. (1994). Bacterialresistance to antimicrobial agents used in fish farming: a critical evaluation of method and meaning. *Annual Review of Fish Diseases*, Vol.4, pp.273–313

Smith, V.J.; Brown, J.H. & Hauton, C. (2003). Immunostimulation in crustaceans: does it really protect against infection?. *Fish and Shellfish Immunology*, Vol.15, pp.71–90

Sorum, H. (1998). Mobile drug resistance genes among fish bacteria. *APMIS Suppl.*, Vol.106, pp.74–76

Sorum, H. (1999). Antibiotic resistance in aquaculture. *Acta Veterinaria Scandinavica Suppl.*, Vol.92, pp.29–36

Spanggaard, B.; Huber, I., Nielsen, J.; Sick. E.B.; Pipper, C.B.; Martinussen, T.; Slierendrecht, W.J. & Gram, L. (2001). The probiotic potential against vibriosis of the indigenous microflora of rainbow trout. *Environmental Microbiology*, Vol.3(12), pp.755-765

Vaseeharan, B.; Lin, J. & Ramasamy, P. (2004). Effect of probiotics, antibiotic sensitivity, pathogenicity, and plasmid profiles of *Listonella anguillarum* like bacteria isolated from Penaeus monodon culture systems. *Aquaculture*, Vol.241, pp.77–91

Verschuere, L. ; Rombaut, G. ; Huys, G. ; Dhont, J. ; Sorgeloos, P. & Verstraete, W. (1999). Microbial control of the culture of Artemia juveniles through preemptive colonization by selected bacterial strains. *Applied and Environmental Microbiology*, Vol.65, pp.2527–2533

Verschuere, L.; Rombaut, G.; Sorgeloos, P. & Verstraete, W. (2000a). Probiotic bacteria as biological control agents in aquaculture. *Microbiology and Molecular Biology Review*, Vol.64, pp.655–671

Verschuere, L.; Heang, H.; Criel, G.; Sorgeloos, P. & Verstraete,W. (2000b). Selected bacterial strains protect Artemia spp. from the pathogenic effects of Vibrio proteolyticus CW8T2. *Applied and Environmental Microbiology*, Vol.66(3), pp.1139–1146

Vijayabaskar, P. & Somasundaram, S. T. (2008). Isolation of bacteriocin producing lactic acid bacteria from fish gut and probiotic activity against common fresh water fish pathogen *Aeromonas hydrophila*. *Biotechnology*, Vol.7, pp.124-128

Vijayan, K.K.; Bright Singh, I.S.; Jayaprakash, N.S.; Alavandi, S.V.; Somnath Pai, S., Preetha, R.; Rajan, J.J.S. & Santiago, T.C. (2006). A brackish water isolate of *Pseudomonas* PS-102, a potential antagonistic bacterium against pathogenic vibrios in penaeid and non-penaeid rearing systems. *Aquaculture*, Vol.251, pp.192-200

Yan, L.; Boyd, K.G. & Burgess, J.G. (2002). Surface attachment induced production of antimicrobial compounds by marine epiphytic bacteria using modified roller bottle cultivation. *Marine Biotechnology*, Vol.4, pp.356–366

Zorrilla, I.; M., Chabrillón; S., Arijo; P., Díaz Rosales; E., Martínez-Manzanares; M.C., Balebona & M.A., Moriñigo, (2003). Bacteria recovered from diseased cultured gilthead sea bream (*Sparus aurata* L.) in southwestern Spain. *Aquaculture*, Vol.218, pp.11-20

25

Antibiotic-Free Selection for Bio-Production: Moving Towards a New „Gold Standard"

Régis Sodoyer, Virginie Courtois, Isabelle Peubez and Charlotte Mignon
Sanofi Pasteur,
France

1. Introduction

Antibiotics have shown a proven efficiency profile in therapy against some infectious agents for several decades. Nevertheless, a large-scale spreading of antibiotics in the environment, and emergence of resistant or even multi-resistant pathogenic bacterial strains has become a general concern promise to even further increase. Besides therapeutic applications, antibiotics are often used as a selection pressure to avoid bio-contamination in production processes such as fermentation. In this particular context the problem can show two distinct facets: the antibiotic molecule itself, seen as a contaminant product in a given biological and the antibiotic resistance gene used as a selection marker.

The increasing regulatory requirements to which biological agents are subjected will hopefully have a great impact in the field of industrial protein expression and production. There is an expectation that in a near future, there may be "zero tolerance" towards antibiotic-based selection and production systems. Besides the antibiotic itself, the antibiotic resistance gene is a major subject of consideration. The complete absence of antibiotic-resistance gene being the only way to ensure that propagation in the environment or transfer of resistance to pathogenic strains will not happen.

In order to address these issues, different and complementary approaches can be applied. The first would be to design more stable host/vector couples allowing to set-up and conduct fermentation processes in complete absence of antibiotics. A more achieved strategy would be to substitute the antibiotic-based selection by an alternative mean such as the complementation of an essential gene product, not expressed by the host or sophisticated post-segregational killing mechanism.

For specific therapeutic agents or fields of application such as DNA vaccination or gene therapy the presence of an antibiotic resistance gene in the vector backbone is seen as undesirable to health authorities. In that case the problem is the possibility of horizontal transfer of antibiotic resistance to circulating microbial population.

2. Current selection methods

2.1 Different antibiotic-based systems

Most commercialized vectors use antibiotic-based selection markers. Ampicillin and kanamycin resistance genes are two widely used selection markers.

Ampicillin resistance gene, Amp^R also known as bla_{TEM1}, is derived from *Salmonella paratyphi*. It allows the synthesis of the beta-lactamase enzyme, which neutralizes antibiotics of the penicillin group, such as ampicillin. Surprisingly, ampicillin that is the most popular selection marker used in research laboratories is in fact a very inefficient selection mean in liquid cultures. The antibiotic-resistance gene product, β-lactamase, efficiently secreted into the culture supernatant rapidly eliminates the antibiotic, even if used at high concentration.

Chloramphenicol is more rarely used, or for some specific applications, for instance, large plasmid or cosmid DNA amplification. The spectra of activity of this antibiotic being variable between true bactericidal and bacteriostatic effect according to the gram character or nature of the bacterial strain considered (Rahal and Simberkoff 1979).

Kanamycin resistance gene, Kan^R also know as *ntpII* (neomycin phosphotransferase II) was initially isolated from the transposon Tn5 that was present in the bacterium strain *Escherichia coli* K12. The gene encodes the aminoglycoside 3'-phosphotransferase enzyme, which inactivates by phosphorylation a range of aminoglycoside antibiotics such as neomycin and kanamycin.

2.2 Advantages and drawbacks

Even if antibiotic resistance gene are widely use for DNA production and recombinant protein expression in bacteria, regulatory agencies tend to restrict their use because of potential horizontal transfer to environmental bacteria. Indeed, due to several mechanisms of gene transfer between bacteria, a potential risk of antibiotic resistance spread exists.

3. Potential concern

3.1 Safety issue

Antibiotic resistance genes are the most commonly used selectable markers for plasmid production (i.e. for vaccine or therapeutic DNA or for production of recombinant proteins as biotherapeutics).To date, kanamycin resistance gene is the most commonly used as selectable antibiotic marker. Ampicillin resistance gene is not acceptable due to concerns for patients which have reactivity to β-lactam antibiotics. Tetracyclin resistance gene is toxic for *E.coli* (Williams et al., 2009)

The major issue is the horizontal genetic transfer of antibiotic resistance gene to prokaryotic organisms present in the environment for biotherapeutic production or in commensal flora.

3.2 Horizontal transfer

Horizontal genetic transfer (HGT) is the passage of genetic elements between organisms (Tuller et al., 2011). This HGT is a major driving force in bacterial evolution by facilitating the diversity of bacteria. An essential element in HGT is to determine which factors influence the fixation of transferred genes. Some of these factors have already been identified (Tuller et al., 2011) and correspond to the advantage conferred by the transferred gene, the toxicity of its product, the ability of the transferred gene to be integrated into the host genome and to be stabilized, the number of interactions of the transferred gene product and the compatibility of codon usage between the transferred gene and the host. Tuller et al., 2011, have shown a correlation between the number of horizontally transferred gene with different organisms and the similarity between their tRNA pools. Moreover, organisms present in a same ecological environment have similar tRNA pools. These two points increase the probability of integration and fixation of a HTG into a new host genome.

Acquisition of antibiotic resistance is one element of this evolution by HTG. For example, Datta and Kontomichalou in 1965 have shown the importance of the penicillin resistance transfer across the *Enterobacteriaceae*. More recently, acquisition of the virulence factors that distinguish *Salmonella* from *Escherichia coli* has been shown as the result of HTG (Wiedenbeck & Cohan, 2011).

Moreover, one element favoring HTG is the length of DNA and this is the case with plasmid harboring antibiotic resistance gene used in recombinant protein (biotherapeutic) expression.

These elements are potential concerns that have to be taken into account in production of therapeutics or vaccine plasmid products and of biotherapeutics to restrict safety issues.

4. Regulatory point of view

A large number of guidance for industry, have been released by the FDA. Among these some are directly applied to the use of antibiotic resistance marker genes in different contexts such as transgenic plants at large or crops for animal feed. Here we have deliberately decided to restrict our focus on vaccines and biological therapeutics.

The market of "biotherapeutics", derived from recombinant DNA technologies, is entering an exponential growing phase. As much as 34 monoclonal antibodies have been, to date, approved by the FDA for various therapeutic applications. Besides antibodies, other products such as next generation recombinant vaccines and gene therapy constructs are progressively invading new therapeutic areas. As a result of growth in existing markets and the opening of new opportunities, the global demand is largely projected to further increase. A direct consequence is a progressive adaptation and strengthening of the existing regulation. A reasonable expectation is a move towards a "zero tolerance" for antibiotic based selection in production systems.

4.1 North American & European regulation

As soon as in July 1993, the FDA drafted some points to consider in the characterization of cell lines used to produce biological products.

> *'Penicillin or other beta lactam antibiotics should not be present in production cell cultures. Minimal concentrations of other antibiotics or inducing agents may be acceptable [21 CFR 610.15(c)]. However, the presence of any antibiotic or inducing agent in the product is discouraged.'*

The WHO technical report series N° 878: "Requirements for the use of animal cells as *in vitro* substrates for the production of biologicals", published in 1998 goes exactly in the same direction.

> *'Penicillin or other β-lactam antibiotics shall not be present in production cell cultures.*

> *Minimal concentration of other antibiotics may be acceptable. However the presence of any antibiotic in a biological process or product is discouraged.'*

Over the years the recommendation became more precise or specific to some categories of biological products such as DNA vaccines. The potential issue of allergic responses to some classes of antibiotics is evoked, the necessity to document the trace amount of antibiotics in the final product clearly seen as mandatory. And finally appears an interesting allusion to novel strategies to replace antibiotic-based selection.

In December 1996 FDA issued a draft guidance entitled - Points to Consider on Plasmid DNA Vaccines for Preventive Infectious Disease Indications

> *'Antibiotic resistance is commonly employed as a selection marker. In considering the use of an antibiotic resistance marker, CBER is advising manufacturers against the use of penicillin or other beta-lactam antibiotics as these antibiotics can, in certain individuals, result in allergic reactions ranging in severity from skin rashes to immediate anaphylaxis. When an antibiotic resistance marker is required in a plasmid DNA vaccine construct, CBER advises the use of an antibiotic such as kanamycin or neomycin. These aminoglycoside antibiotics are not extensively used in the treatment of clinical infections due to their low activity spectrum, prevalence of kanamycin-resistant bacteria, and their problematic therapeutic index with toxicities including irreversible ototoxicity and nephrotoxicity. Specifications for the level of antibiotic present in the final container should be established and should consider the minimum level of antibiotic that will give an unintentional clinical effect. The use of alternative antibiotic resistance markers or the use of suppressor tRNA genes in a plasmid construct intended as plasmid DNA vaccine should be discussed with CBER prior to full scale development of a new vaccine product.'*

Several updates (2006 and 2009) of this guidance are accessible on the web.

The EMEA is perfectly in line with its North American counterpart, as a matter of example, a 2001 guidance indicates:

> *'lack of expression in mammalian cells should be verified due to regulatory concerns'*

This comment is an illustration of the concern applied to the antibiotic-resistance gene itself.

In a draft review, released from the FDA in November 2004, it is clearly specified that the use of beta-lactams should be avoided or at least very clearly documented in terms of safety for the patient. This recommendation, even if not prohibitive, appears as extremely dissuasive.

Content and Review of Chemistry, Manufacturing and Control (CMC) Information for Human Gene Therapy Investigational New Drug Application (INDs)

> *'Because some patients may be sensitive to penicillin, we recommend that you, a sponsor, do not use beta-lactam antibiotics during the manufacturing of a therapeutic product for humans. If beta-lactam antibiotics are used, we recommend that you take and describe precautions to prevent hypersensitivity reactions.'*

In a recent release from the FDA (October 23, 2009) dedicated to Vaccines, Blood & Biologics, entitled: Common Ingredients in U.S. Licensed Vaccines: Why are antibiotics in some vaccines?

> *'Certain antibiotics may be used in some vaccine production to help prevent bacterial contamination during manufacturing. As a result, small amounts of antibiotics may be present in some vaccines. Because some antibiotics can cause severe allergic reactions in those children*

allergic to them (like hives, swelling at the back of the throat, and low blood pressure), some parents are concerned that antibiotics contained in vaccines might be harmful. However, antibiotics most likely to cause severe allergic reactions (e.g., penicillins, cephalosporins and sulfa drugs) are not used in vaccine production, and therefore are not contained in vaccines.'

In the issue of july 7th 2011 of: Common Ingredients in U.S. Licensed Vaccines, some comments on antibiotics used in vaccine manufacturing processes are somewhat moderated.

'Examples of antibiotics used during vaccine manufacture include neomycin, polymyxin B, streptomycin and gentamicin. Some antibiotics used in vaccine production are present in the vaccine, either in very small amounts or they are undetectable. For example, antibiotics are used in some production methods for making inactivated influenza virus vaccines. They are used to reduce bacterial growth in eggs during processing steps, because eggs are not sterile products. The antibiotics that are used are reduced to very small or undetectable amounts during subsequent purification steps. The very small amounts of antibiotics contained in vaccines have not been clearly associated with severe allergic reactions.'

4.2 Conclusion and future rules

According to the above mentioned information:

- It is not yet prohibited but strongly advised to avoid or minimize the use of any kind of antibiotics in cell or bacterial culture,
- If antibiotics are used, it is mandatory to minimize their amount and to control for the presence of traces in the final product,
- The rationale for the use of antibiotics must be clearly documented in the CTD
- Penicillin, more generally β-lactams and streptomycin must not be used in reason of potential concerns with hyper reactivity of some patients to antibiotics of the β-lactam family
- Kanamycin and neomycin are the preferred choice and still tolerated.

The use of antibiotic resistance markers is generally discouraged, and if used the *in vivo* effect needs to be evaluated.

There are specific mentions for the nature of the gene encoding resistance to kanamycin, as reviewed by Williams et al., (2009). The gene neomycin phosphotransferase III [npt-III, *aph* (3')-III] should be avoided, since it also confers resistance to amikacin, a reserve antibiotic (EMEA, 2008).

As a final comment it is easy to anticipate, what might be the future requirements from health authorities: constructs have to be completely devoid of antibiotic resistance genes in their final structure, even if in use at early stages of construction. Alternative solutions would be available and validated soon.

5. Alternatives to antibiotics in bio-production

5.1 Vector stabilization

One aspect to be considered during recombinant biopharmaceutical expression is the stability of the plasmid used. More than 20 years ago, several studies on natural plasmids have highlighted that some plasmids naturally display regions necessary for their stability.

Ogura & Higara,, 1983a, have shown that plasmid F, that exists only as one to two copies per chromosome and is stably inherited to daughter cells during cell growth, contains stabilization sequences. They did show that these sequences were independent from plasmid replication function. They first identify 3 regions essential for plasmid maintenance: *SopA* and *SopB* that acts in trans and *SopC* that acts in *cis* to stabilize the plasmid by probably interacting with cellular components. These authors also put in evidence that *SopA*, *SopB* and *SopC* were not sufficient for full stability of mini-F plasmid, and identified the *ccd* (control of cell death) region that seemed to control cell division when copy number carrying *ccd* segment decreases (Ogura & Higara, 1983b). The so-called *ccd* region is divided into two functional regions: *ccdB*, which product inhibits the host cell division and *ccdA*, which product is able to inhibit the *ccdB* function. Two years after, Jaffé et al., 1985, demonstrated that cell division is not immediately inhibited and that residual division could take place in the plasmid free-cells before finally being inhibited. Authors concluded that *ccd* region guarantees that plasmid carrying cells could grow preferentially in a population by killing plasmid free daughter cells, introducing the concept of post-segregational killing.

Plasmid R1 has also been shown to contain a stabilization system (Gerdes et al., 1985). As for plamid F, the stabilization system is based on post segregational killing du to the *parAB+* locus. This locus is composed of two genes *Hok* (Host killing) and *Sok* (suppression of killing). The translation of the Hok messenger, encoding a toxin lethal to the bacteria, is completely blocked by the anti-messenger Sok. In the absence of plasmid, Sok, which is less stable than Hok, is lost first, allowing the translation of the Hok mRNA and expression of the toxin lethal to the cell.

Concerning plasmid maintenance, it has been shown that factors reducing mutlimerization of plasmid could increase plasmid stability (Summers & Sherratt, 1984). ColE1 plasmid contains a region, *cer* that seems to be necessary for a recombination event converting multimers to monomers, allowing the plasmid to be more stable. Multimer resolution is achieved through action of the XerCD site-specific recombinase at the *cer* site (see Figure 1). Cloning of the *cer* locus into various expression vectors has been extensively documented and the proof of principle largely established in high-cell density cultures.

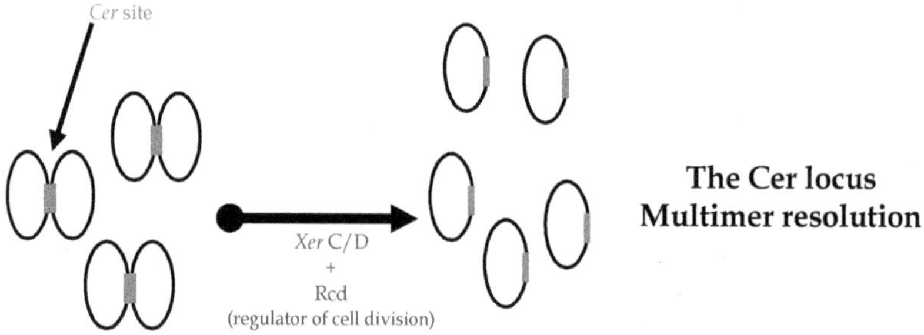

Fig. 1. Multimers resolution of high copy plasmids by XerC/D recombinase at *cer* locus.

5.2 Genomic integration

If mutation and deletion into *E.coli* genome are now widely used, it seems that genomic integration is not the preferred way to express a recombinant protein without antibiotic selection. However, some plasmid-free system have been described (see Figure 2).

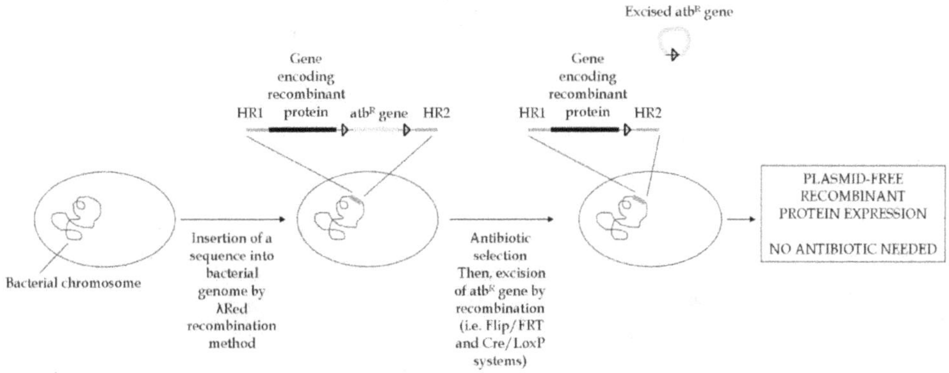

Fig. 2. Establishment of a plasmid-free expression system, illustration adapted from Striedner et al., 2010.

In 2009, a "plasmid-free T7-based *E.coli* expression system" has been developed by inserting a region of a pET plasmid into bacterial genome by λ Red recombination and P1 transduction (Datsenko & Wanner, 2000, as cited in Striedner et al., 2010). The study compared protein expression between plasmid-based and plasmid-free expression system showing an improved protein production with chromosome-based system. This system also conferred a high stability and simple upstream processing as well as high flexibility in process design.(Striedner et al., 2010).

More recently, Lemuth et al., 2011, reported the construction of the first plasmid-free *E. coli* strain that produces astaxanthin. This engineered *E. coli* strain harbors 5 heterologous biosynthetic genes from *P. ananatis* and one from *N. punctiforme* that are required for the formation of astaxanthin. Furthermore, a plasmid-free *E.coli* strain that accumulated astaxanthin as the exclusive carotenoid was engineered. This system presents many advantages compared to a plasmid-based strategy: a reduced metabolic burden, a better stability and obviously the absence of selection markers such as antibiotic resistance genes.

5.3 Complementation of essential gene product and auxotrophy markers

Essential gene complementation requires the engineering of a bacterial strain lacking an essential gene. The activity of the lacking gene product can be complemented by the culture medium or by transforming the bacteria with a plasmid having this gene as selection marker (see Figure 3).

Several antibiotic-free selection systems are based on gene complementation. One of the first systems was based on *dapD* gene (Degryse, 1991). The *dapD* gene, which has a role in the lysine biosynthetic pathway as well as cell wall assembly, has been selected as a preferred candidate by several authors, knowing that mutations in the DAP pathway are lethal. The limitations, in that case, are the intrinsic difficulty in construction of a *dapD* mutant strain and the dependence towards defined culture media composition.

Based on the same gene, a more elaborated strategy called "operator repressor titration" emerged in 2001. In this system, *dapD* gene is engineered in order to be under the control of lac Operon. When not supplemented with IPTG or DAP, *dapD* gene is not expressed

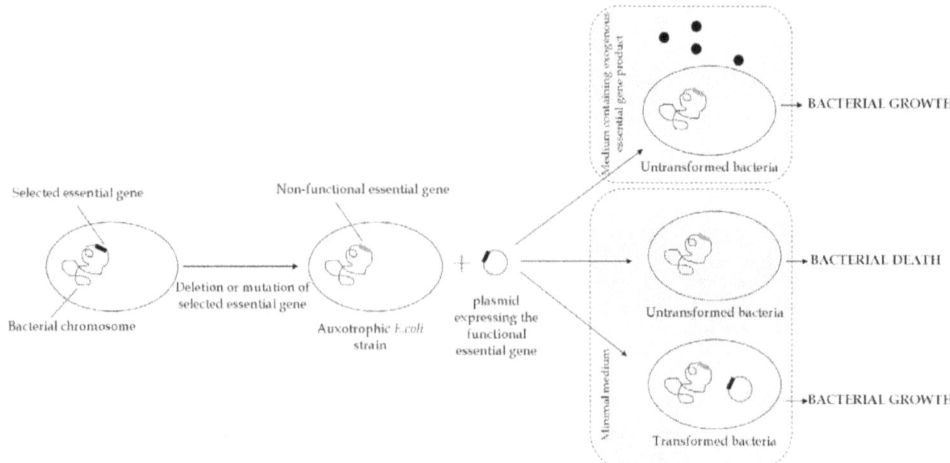

Fig. 3. Antibiotic-free selection system based on essential gene complementation.

inducing bacterial death. When the strain is transformed by a lac operator containing multi copy plasmid, the operator competitively titrates the Lac I repressor and allows the expression of *dapD* from the lac promoter allowing bacterial growth. (Cranenburgh et al., 2001 & 2004)

Other essential genes have been selected for the same purpose, such as *infA*, coding for translation initiation factor 1 (IF1), an essential protein for cell viability. In 2004, Hägg et al. generated a strain in which the *infA* gene has been deleted by a plasmid-based gene replacement method. They used a plasmid encoding a functional IF1 as selection marker and show that the system is tightly regulated and that no cross feeding is observed since initiation factors released into the media from lysed cells are not absorbed by plasmid-free cells.

The *fabl* essential gene has been used in an original way because of its property to reduce the *E.coli* susceptibility to triclosan when overexpressed. In this system, only plasmid containing cells overexpress *fabl* gene and can grow in presence of triclosan. Even if triclosan is a biocide, it is considered as non-antibiotic and regulatory agencies approve the use of triclosan for clinical use (Goh & Good, 2008).

More recently, Dong et al., 2010, developed a novel antibiotic-free selection system based on complementation of host auxotrophy in the NAD synthesis pathway. NAD can be *de novo* synthesized from tryptophan and aspartate with the quinolinic acid phosphoribosyltransferase (QAPRTase) or synthesized using the salvage pathway according to different substrates such as nicotinamide. Authors constructed a bacterial strain depleted for QAPRTase gene that can only grow if the NAD synthesis pathway is complemented by addition of salvage pathway substrate or QAPRTase gene present on a plasmid. The results obtained with this novel selection system show that the QAPRTase seletion marker does not represent a metabolic burden for bacterial growth and the stability of all plasmid harboring this system were 100% in the ΔQAPRTase strain even after 6 days of continuous growth. In this study, reserchers went further by complementing for the first time in an antibiotic-free selection system a bacterial strain by a mammalian QAPRTase gene with success.

A strain is auxotrophic for one amino-acid if it carries a genetic mutation that renders it unable to synthesize the amino-acid. Such a strain will be able to grow only if the amino-acid is present in the environment or if the functional gene product is expressed from a plasmid. Amino-acid auxotrophy markers had been investigated as novel antibiotic-free selection markers.

In 2001, Fiedler & Skerra developed expression vectors containing the *proAB* gene, in order to complement their proline-auxotrophic K12 strain. Their aim was not to develop an antibiotic-free selection system but to use their strain to obtain a better expression of recombinant antibody Fab fragment. For this reason, the plasmid-mediated complementation is used simultaneously with beta-lactamase selection to completely abolish plasmid loss during high scale fermentation.

In 2008, Vidal et al. described a plasmid selection system, devoid of antibiotic resistance gene and based on glycine auxotrophy. Researchers generated an *E.coli* strain that contains a deletion in the *glyA* gene, which encode for serine hydroxymethyl transferase, an enzyme involved in glycine biosynthesis pathway in *E.coli*. This strain can grow fast on a defined media only if glycine is added to the culture medium or if the bacteria harbor a plasmid expressing a functional *glyA* gene. They show comparable amount of recombinant protein with their system compared to a classical beta-lactamase selection system.

5.4 RNA-based antibiotic-free selection systems

Several antibiotic-free selection strategies are based on RNA, using antisense or anti-messenger properties or using suppressor tRNA.

The principle of down regulating an essential gene upon plasmid loss has been exploited in a very original way for the design of new vectors for gene therapy (Mairhofer et al., 2008). The expression of the essential gene *murA* encoding an enzyme essential for the biosynthesis of cell wall is under control of the Tet repressor, TetR expression is inhibited by an RNA-RNA antisense interaction with RNAI derived from plasmid origin of replication ColE1 (see Figure 4A). The major advantage of this system is that no additional sequence is required on the plasmid. (Pfaffenzeller et al., 2006; see figure 4B)

In a recent paper, RNA based selectable marker, not restricted to ColE1 containing vectors is described (Luke et al., 2009). Briefly, a counter-selectable marker (*sacB)* levansucrase from *Bacillus subtilis*, under control of the RNA-IN promoter is integrated into the bacterial chromosome induces cell death in presence of sucrose. Plasmid maintenance is ensured by the presence of the plasmid-borne regulator RNA-OUT anti-messenger acting as a down regulator of the expression of levansucrase (see Figure 4C).

Another vector system so-called pCOR, based on the complementation of an amber mutation using a suppressor tRNA, and conditional origin of replication has also been established (Soubrier et al., 1999). The original feature of the model is that an additional degree of refinement was introduced, since the dependence created between the host and the vector has become bilateral (see Figure 4D).

Nevertheless, the requirement for a minimal medium for culture means these systems are more likely to be used for DNA production rather than recombinant protein over expression.

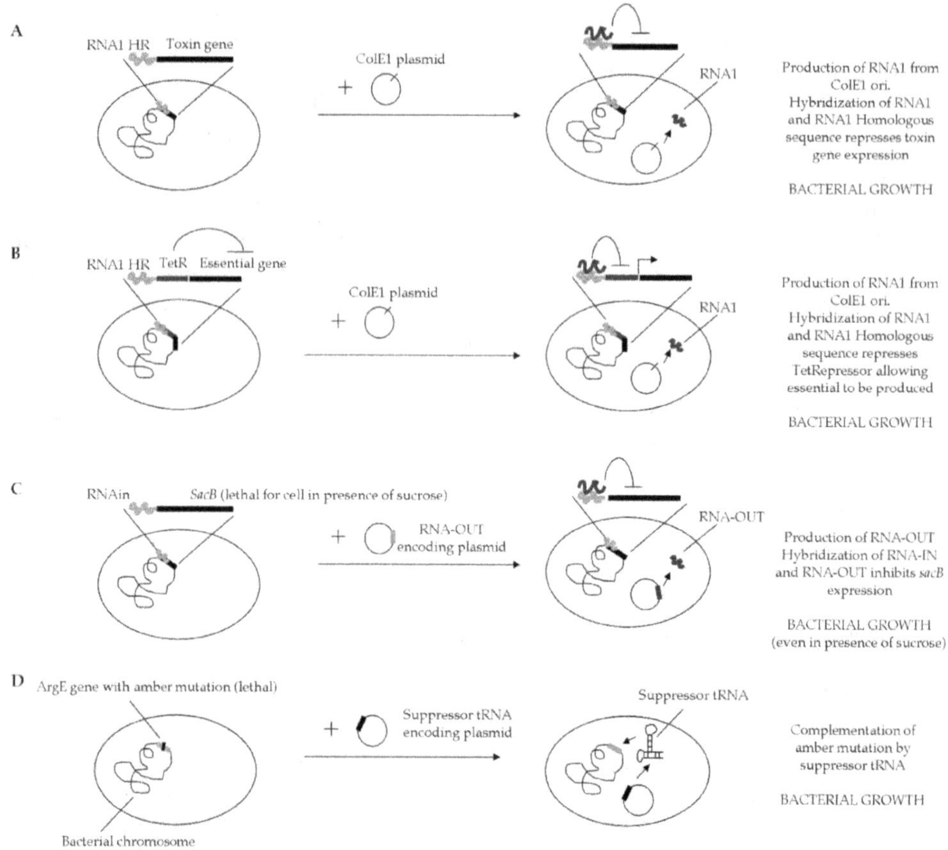

Fig. 4. RNA-based antibiotic-free systems. Illustration adapted from Pfaffenzeller et al., 2006; Luke et al., 2009 & Soubrier et al., 1999.

5.5 Post-segregational killing

Post-segregational killing is a mechanism by which plasmids are stably maintained by expressing a gene product that would be toxic to cells becoming plasmid-free upon division (see Figure 5). This mechanism, discovered on natural plasmid, has been used as selection system devoid of antibiotic.

One of these systems, based on *ccdA/ccdB* genes has been proposed by Szpirer & Milinkovitch, 2005, and is commercialized by the Delphigenetics Company. *ccdB* gene is inserted into the bacterial genome of the *E. coli* strain BL21 (DE3) and encodes a stable protein (100 aa), binding gyrase, essential for cell division. Upon binding gyrase, the *ccdB* gene product impairs DNA replication and induces cell death. *ccdA* gene, plasmid-born, encodes an instable protein (90 aa) under control of the mob promoter, acting as a natural inhibitor of *ccdB*. It has been shown that after 20 generations on a non-selective medium 100% of the bacteria still contain the plasmid. Two hours after induction, the plasmid is still present into all bacteria, which is not the case with a standard pET/BL21λDE3 system.

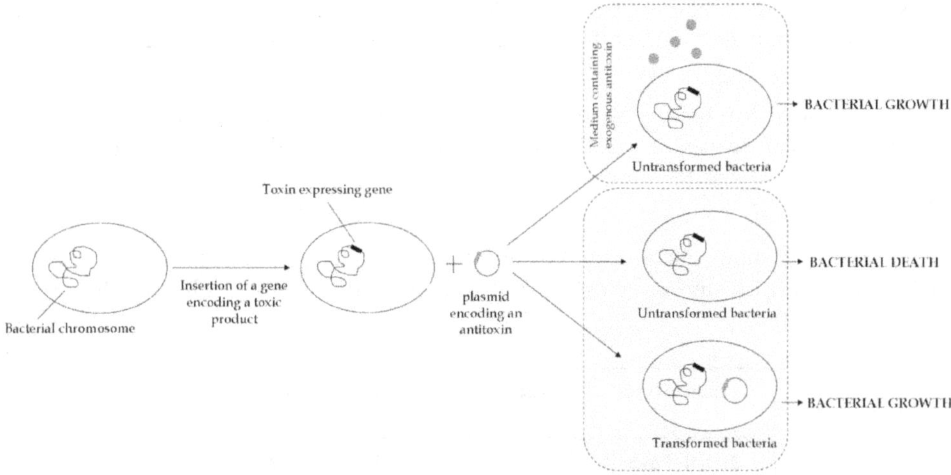

Fig. 5. Antibiotic-free selection system based on Toxin/antitoxin post-segragational killing. Illustration adapted from Szpirer & Milinkovitch, 2005.

To go further, Peubez et al. proposed in 2010 a system combining the *ccdA/ccdB* selection marker to the *cer* fragment to increase plasmid stability among long-term fermentation.

Different toxin/antitoxin (TA) systems have been described and could allow the generation of novel antibiotic-free systems. In order to detect putative TA systems, Milinkovitch's team had developed an algorithm based on predefined similarities and TA-specific structural constraints (Guglielmini et al., 2008).

Interestingly, this TA-based antibiotic-free selection system is starting to be adapted to mammalian cells selection. The toxin Kid (Killing determinant) and its antidote Kis (killing suppressor) have been used to control cell proliferation during expression of a recombinant protein in CHO-K1 cells (Nehlsen et al., 2010). If antibiotics are still used in this study, authors show that the TA strategy can significantly increase the recombinant protein expression level and could be a benefit for "difficult" to produce proteins.

6. Additional benefits

6.1 Recombinant protein production

In many cases, especially for "difficult proteins" the yield of protein production has proven to be higher with antibiotic-free system compared to a conventional one. The presence of an antibiotic resistance gene can indirectly reduce the amount of expressed protein, since even in absence of selection pressure the gene would be transcribed and account for an additional stress for the host during the fermentation process. However, even if the yield of protein is not superior to a conventional system, the antibiotic-free systems remain interesting due to their biosafety.

6.1.1 Plasmid stabilisation cer locus

Most commonly used multicopy plasmids are unstable and are lost during culture. Plasmid stabilization and increased maintenance during a fermentation process can be considered as a first step towards antibiotic starvation. Genetic elements allowing plasmid maintenance during cell division and limiting the probability of plasmid loss over generations should be considered.

To stabilize the plasmid, the well-studied mechanism of site specific recombination of *E.Coli* plasmid ColE1 can be used. The 380 bp *Cer* fragment was inserted into the plasmid carrying the gene of interest and the multimers are resolved to monomers by the Xer recombinase. (Described in 5.1, see Figure 1)

Tables 1 and 2 show the contribution of the cer fragment in increasing the plasmid maintenance over time is clearly established. The plasmid loss is dependant on the antigen expressed.

Culture time	Plasmid without *cer*	With *cer*
2h(IPTG added)	97%	100%
4h	25%	100%
6h	20%	75%
23h	3%	79%

Table 1. Example of *Helicobacter pylori* AlpA protein produced in erlen flask in absence of Kanamycin.

Culture time	Plasmid without *cer*	With *cer*
1h	87%	100%
2h	IPTG addition	
3h	67%	100%
5h	1%	50%
25h	0%	9%

Table 2. Example of *Helicobacter pylori* Urease produced in erlen flask in absence of kanamycin.

6.1.2 ccdA/ccdB

The combination of different genetic elements can allow an increased stability and antibiotic-free selection. In this case, the kanamycin resistant gene present on the vector backbone was eliminated by a restriction enzyme digestion and self-relegation.

The selection system based on the couple poison (gene *ccdB*)/antidote:(gene *ccdA*), proposed by Szpirer & Milinkovitch, 2005, combined with the stabilizing element, the *cer* locus, was tested to express different recombinant proteins.

- the poison gene (*ccdB*), inserted into the bacterial genome, encodes a stable protein (100 aa), which is an inhibitor of the DNA replication capable to bind to the gyrase (an essential protein for cell division). This interaction induces the cell death.

- the antidote gene (*ccdA*), localized on the plasmid under the control of a constitutive promoter, encodes for a small unstable protein (90aa) which neutralizes the effect of ccdB protein action.

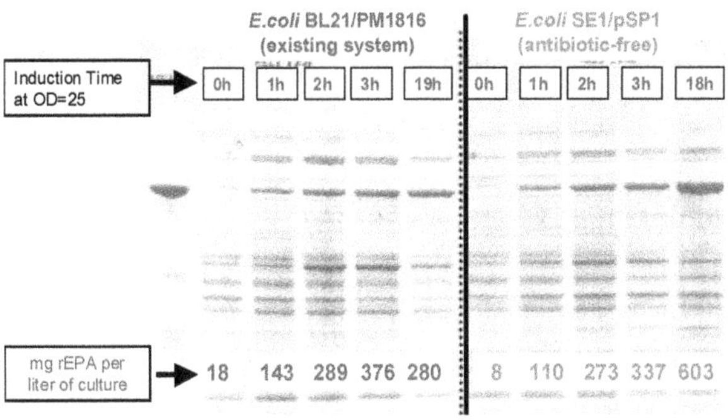

Fig. 6. Protein production evaluation in 1 liter fermenter.

Figure 6 shows a comparison of expression of the same protein with the kanamycin resistant gene (E. coli BL21/pM1816) and the antibiotic-free system (E. coli SE1/pSP1) without the kanamycin resistant gene and with the *ccdA* gene. Both have the *cer* element. Upon induction, the behavior of both systems is comparable but a clear increase in protein production is observed with the antibiotic-free system at the end of fermentation.

6.1.3 Antibiotic resistance gene elimination

Antibiotic-based selection, convenient for cloning steps, must be removed for production.

Even if antibiotic selection pressure is not used during the fermentation process, removal of this antibiotic resistance marker is of major importance to prevent horizontal transfer in the environment. This is particularly true for vectors to be used in gene therapy or DNA vaccination protocols

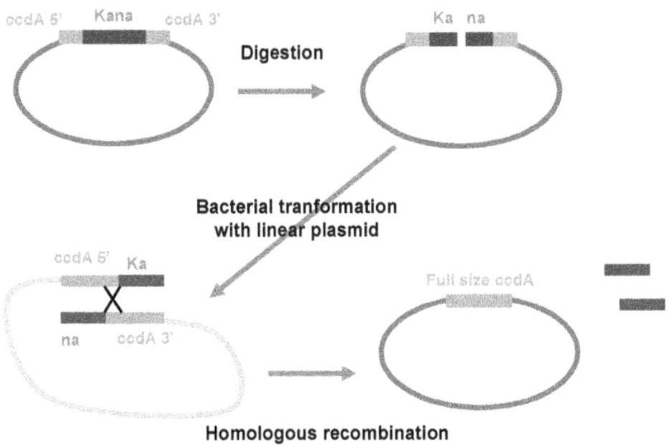

Fig. 7. Homologous recombination process allowing assembly of a functional *ccdA* encoding gene.

In order to overcome the problem of positive pressure of selection, a new apporach has been developed ensuring the elimination of the antibiotic-resistance gene through homologous recombination. In this model the *ccdA* locus is split into 2 parts, containing a common sequence, and cloned at the 5′ and 3′ regions flanking the antibiotic resistance gene (figure 7). After digestion at a unique restriction site located inside the antibiotic selection marker and transformation of ccdB expressing cells with linear DNA, a fully functional *ccdA* would assemble through homologous recombination. Only bacteria containing a recombinant plasmid with a functional *ccdA* can grow upon transformation.

6.1.4 Summary of different antibiotic-free systems

System developed	Mode of action	Protein expressed	Comments/ potential drawbacks	Ref article
Plasmid-free system	Chromosome based expression system	GFP Human superoxide dismutase(SOD)	Modified *E coli* strain, required	Striedner et al., 2010
Fabl-triclosan	Endogenous essential gene	None	Chemical Biocid utilisation	Goh & Good, 2008
***E. coli* strain ΔQAPRTase gene**	Complementation	EGFP	Modified *E coli* strain, required	Dong et al., 2010
Pro BA	Complementation	Fab fragment	Modified *E coli* strain, required Presence of antibiotic	Fiedler & Skerra, 2001
***E coli* strain ΔglyA**	Glycine auxotrophy	RhuA	Modified *E coli* strain, required. Comparable to the conventional system	Vidal et al., 2008
RNA/RNA interference	RNA/RNA interaction	EGFP	Modified *E coli* strain, required	Pfaffenzeller et al., 2006
RNA out	RNA/RNA interaction	EGFP HA vaccine candidate		Luke et al., 2009
pCOr	Complementation of amber mutation tRNA suppressor	Luciferase	Modified *E coli* strain, and minimum medium required	Soubrier et al., 1999
ccdA/ccdB	Toxin/antitoxin	AlpA/rEPA vaccine candidates	Modified *E coli* strain required	Peubez et al., 2010
Kid/Kis	Toxin/antitoxin	EGFP	Presence of antibiotic	Nehlsen et al., 2010

6.2 DNA immunization and gene therapy

Requirement can also be variable according to the nature of the therapeutic product, the presence of an antibiotic resistance gene, tolerated on a vector expressing a recombinant biopharmaceutical, will be totally undesirable on a gene therapy plasmid.

Among systems described in paragraph 5, some have been developed especially for DNA vaccine production such as pCOR (Soubrier et al., 1989), RNA/RNA interference (Pfaffenzeller et al., 2006) and RNA out (Luke et al., 2009).

To go further, Carnes et al., 2009, have proposed a combination of antibiotic-free selection system and an autolytic *E.coli* strain to improve both upstream and downstream processes. The antibiotic-free selection is based on RNA selectable marker described by Luke et al., 2009 and the autolytic plasmid DNA extraction method uses integrated bacteriophage endolysin gene (λR), encoding a peptidoglycan hydrolase (lysozyme) enzyme to permeabilize the bacterial cell wall, and to selectively extract the plasmid DNA from the cells in an acetate buffer. Authors found that their autolytic strain allowed efficient plasmid DNA recovery, similar to alkaline lysis plasmid DNA purification.

7. Conclusion and perspectives

Antibiotic-free selection is a general and ultimate goal that can be reached by the implementation of various and combined approaches. An increasing knowledge of bacterial physiology will give access to comprehensive information on essential genes or pathways that would be an unlimited source of inspiration for the design of novel selection means.

The major driver for the definition of antibiotic-free systems is an anticipation of fulfilling future recommendations from health authorities to overcome safety concerns. It is easy to imagine that, upon availability and functional validation, these alternative selection means will progressively gain the status of "preferred", "strongly recommended" and finally "mandatory".

In addition to their safety profile, some antibiotic-free systems can give access to unexpected properties such as a marked increase in recombinant protein production or plasmid recovery.

The complete elimination of any antibiotic resistance gene is, for different reasons, of critical importance for recombinant protein production, DNA immunization and gene therapy vectors.

It is likely to think that upon validation at industrial scale, antibiotic-free selection might be an added value for biotherapeutics in terms of safety profile of the product and become an important element of the marketing strategy as well. A direct consequence would be the emergence of a new "gold standard".

8. References

Carnes, A.E.; Hodgson, C.P.; Luke, J.M.; Vincent, J.M. & Williams, J.A. (2009). Plasmid DNA production combining antibiotic-free selection, inducible high yield fermentation, and novel autolytic purification. *Biotechnol Bioeng.*, Vol.104, No.3, (Oct 2009), pp.505-515

Cranenburgh, R.M.; Hanak, J.A.; Williams, S.G. & Sherratt, D.J. (2001). Escherichia coli strains that allow antibiotic-free plasmid selection and maintenance by repressor titration. *Nucleic Acids Res.*, Vol. 29, No.5, (Mar 2001), E26

Cranenburgh, R.M.; Lewis, K.S. & Hanak, J.A. (2004). Effect of plasmid copy number and lac operator sequence on antibiotic-free plasmid selection by operator-repressor titration in Escherichia coli. *J Mol Microbiol Biotechnol.*, Vol.7, No.4, (2004), pp.197-203

Datsenko, K.A. & Wanner, B.L. (2000). One-step inactivation of chromosomal genes in Escherichia coli K-12 using PCR products. *Proc Natl Acad Sci U S A.*, Vol.97, No.12, (Jun 2000), pp.6640-6645

Datta, N. & Kontomichalou, P.(1965). Penicillinase synthesis controlled by infectious R factors in Enterobacteriaceae. *Nature. Vol.208, No.5007,* (Oct 1965), pp.239-241

Degryse, E. (1985). Stability of a host-vector system based on complementation of an essential gene in Escherichia coli. *J Biotechnol.*, Vol.18, No.1-2, (Apr 1991), pp.29-39

Dong, W.R.; Xiang, L.X. & Shao, J.Z. (2010). Novel antibiotic-free plasmid selection system based on complementation of host auxotrophy in the NAD de novo synthesis pathway. *Appl Environ Microbiol.*, Vol.76, No.7, (Apr 2010), pp.2295-2303. Epub 2010 Jan 29

Durany, O.; Bassett, P.; Weiss, A.M.; Cranenburgh, R.M.; Ferrer, P.; López-Santín, J.; de Mas, C. & Hanak, J.A. (2005). Production of fuculose-1-phosphate aldolase using operator-repressor titration for plasmid maintenance in high cell density Escherichia coli fermentations. *Biotechnol Bioeng.*, Vol. 91, No.4, (Aug 2005), pp.460-467

Fiedler, M. & Skerra, A. (2001). proBA complementation of an auxotrophic E. coli strain improves plasmid stability and expression yield during fermenter production of a recombinant antibody fragment. *Gene*, Vol.274, No.1-2, (Aug 2001), pp.111-118

Gerdes, K.; Larsen, J.E. & Molin, S. (1985). Stable inheritance of plasmid R1 requires two different loci. *J Bacteriol.* Vol.161, No.1, (Jan 1985), pp.292-298

Goh, S. & Good, L. (2008). Plasmid selection in Escherichia coli using an endogenous essential gene marker. *BMC Biotechnol.*, Vol.11, No. 8, (Aug 2008), pp.61

Guglielmini, J.; Szpirer, C.Y. & Milinkovitch, M.C. (2008). Automated discovery and phylogenetic analysis of new toxin-antitoxin systems. *BMC Microbiol.* Vol.25; No.8, (Jun 2008), pp.104

Hägg, P.; de Pohl, J.W.; Abdulkarim, F. & Isaksson, L.A. (2004). A host/plasmid system that is not dependent on antibiotics and antibiotic resistance genes for stable plasmid maintenance in Escherichia coli. *J Biotechnol.*, Vol.111, No.1, (Jul 2004), pp.17-30

Jaffé, A.; Ogura, T. & Hiraga, S. (1985). Effects of the ccd function of the F plasmid on bacterial growth. *J Bacteriol.*, Vol.163, No.3, (Sep 1985), pp.841-849

Lemuth, K.; Steuer, K. & Albermann, C. (2011). Engineering of a plasmid-free Escherichia coli strain for improved in vivo biosynthesis of astaxanthin. *Microb Cell Fact.*, Vol.26, No.10, (Apr 2011), pp.29

Luke, J.; Carnes, A.E.; Hodgson, C.P. & Williams, J.A. (2009). Improved antibiotic-free DNA vaccine vectors utilizing a novel RNA based plasmid selection system. *Vaccine.*, Vol.27, No.46, (Oct 2009), pp.6454-6459. Epub 2009 Jun 24

Mairhofer, J.; Pfaffenzeller, I.; Merz, D. & Grabherr, R. (2008). A novel antibiotic free plasmid selection system: advances in safe and efficient DNA therapy. *Biotechnol J.*, Vol.3, No.1, (Jan 2008), pp.83-89

Nehlsen, K.; Herrmann, S.; Zauers, J.; Hauser, H. & Wirth, D. (2010). Toxin-antitoxin based transgene expression in mammalian cells. *Nucleic Acids Res.*, Vol.38, No.5, (Mar 2010), e32.

Ogura, T. & Hiraga, S. (1983). Partition mechanism of F plasmid: two plasmid gene-encoded products and a cis-acting region are involved in partition. *Cell.* Vol.32, No.2, (Feb 1983), pp.351-360

Ogura, T. & Hiraga, S. (1983). Mini-F plasmid genes that couple host cell division to plasmid proliferation. *Proc Natl Acad Sci U S A*, Vol.80, No.15, (Aug 1983), pp.4784-4788

Peubez, I.; Chaudet, N.; Mignon, C.; Hild, G.; Husson, S.; Courtois, V.; De Luca, K.; Speck, D. & Sodoyer, R. (2010). Antibiotic-free selection in E. coli: new considerations for optimal design and improved production. *Microb Cell Fact.*, Vol.7, No.9, (Sep 2010), pp.65.

Pfaffenzeller, I.; Mairhofer, J.; Striedner, G.; Bayer, K. & Grabherr, R. (2006). Using ColE1-derived RNA I for suppression of a bacterially encoded gene: implication for a novel plasmid addiction system. *Biotechnol J.*, Vol. 1, No.6, (Jun 2006), pp.675-681.

Rahal, J.J. Jr.& Simberkoff, M.S. (1979). Bactericidal and bacteriostatic action of chloramphenicol against memingeal pathogens. *Antimicrob Agents Chemother.* Vol.16, No.1, (Jul 1979), pp.13-18

Soubrier, F.; Cameron, B.; Manse, B.; Somarriba, S.; Dubertret, C.; Jaslin, G.; Jung, G.; Caer, C.L.; Dang, D.; Mouvault, J.M.; Scherman, D.; Mayaux, J.F. & Crouzet, J. (1999). pCOR: a new design of plasmid vectors for nonviral gene therapy. *Gene Ther.*, Vol.6, No.8, (Aug 1999), pp.1482-1488

Summers, D.K. & Sherratt, D.J. (1984). Multimerization of high copy number plasmids causes instability: ColE1 encodes a determinant essential for plasmid monomerization and stability., *Cell.*, Vol. 36, No.4, (Apr 1984), pp.1097-1103

Striedner, G.; Pfaffenzeller, I.; Markus, L.; Nemecek, S.; Grabherr, R. & Bayer, K. (2010). Plasmid-free T7-based Escherichia coli expression systems. *Biotechnol Bioeng.*, Vol. 105, No.4, (Mar 2010), pp.786-794

Szpirer, C.Y. & Milinkovitch, M.C. (2005). Separate-component-stabilization system for protein and DNA production without the use of antibiotics. *Biotechniques.*, Vol.38, No.5, (May 2005), pp.775-781

Tuller, T.; Girshovich, Y.; Sella, Y.; Kreimer, A.; Freilich, S.; Kupiec, M.; Gophna, U. & Ruppin, E. (2011). Association between translation efficiency and horizontal gene transfer within microbial communities. *Nucleic Acids Res.* Vol.39, No.11, (Jun 2011), pp.4743-4755

Vidal, L.; Pinsach, J.; Striedner, G.; Caminal, G. & Ferrer, P. (2008). Development of an antibiotic-free plasmid selection system based on glycine auxotrophy for recombinant protein overproduction in Escherichia coli. *J Biotechnol*, Vol.134, No.1-2, (Mar 2008), pp.127-136

Wiedenbeck, J. & Cohan, F.M. (2011), Origins of bacterial diversity through horizontal genetic transfer and adaptation to new ecological niches. *FEMS Microbiol Rev.* doi: 10.1111/j.1574-6976.2011.00292.x. (Jun 2011), [Ahead of print]

Williams, J.A.; Carnes, A.E. & Hodgson, C.P. (2009). Plasmid DNA vaccine vector design: impact on efficacy, safety and upstream production. *Biotechnol Adv.* Vol.27, No.4, (Jul-Aug 2009), pp.353-370

26

Antibiotic Susceptibility of Probiotic Bacteria

Zorica Radulović[1], Tanja Petrović[1] and Snežana Bulajić[2]
[1]*University of Belgrade, Faculty of Agriculture*
[2]*University of Belgrade, Faculty of Veterinary Medicine*
Republic of Serbia

1. Introduction

Lactic acid bacteria (LAB) are a heterogeneous group of bacteria widely distributed in nature. These bacteria are found in gastrointestinal (GI) and urogenital tract of humans and animals; they are present on plant material, in milk and meat, and numerous fermented foods. Lactic acid bacteria have been associated with traditional dairy products, cereals, vegetable and meat fermented foods, due to their natural presence leading to spontaneous fermentation. They are also used as starter cultures in industrial food production, as well as in the production of probiotic products due to their potential health benefits to consumer. Milk and dairy products are the most examined food system for the delivery of probiotic bacteria to the human gut. The probiotic concept has progressed and is now in the focus of different research. Significant improvements have been made in selection and characterization of new cultures and their application in food production.

The food products, which are produced by traditional methods, exhibit a rich biodiversity with the respect to bacterial contents. From these products, new probiotic strains with the potential functional properties can been isolated and selected. The selected strains have to be further characterized in order to be used in the food industry. Before the probiotics can benefit human health, they must fulfill several criteria including: a) scientifically validated health properties; b) good technological properties meaning that they can be manufactured and incorporated into food products without loosing viability, functionality and technological performance; c) high survival through the upper gastrointestinal tract and high viability at its site of action; d) antagonistic activity to pathogens; e) antibiotic susceptibility; and f) to be able to function in the gut environment. Bearing in mind importance of antibiotic resistance of LAB in food chain, antibiotic susceptibility of potential probiotic strains is a very important criteria for their selection.

In the recent decade, releasing of antibiotics in biosphere seriously increased, leading to a strong selective pressure for the emergence and persistence of resistant LAB strains. Since LAB are naturally present in traditionally made fermented food and GI tract and are also added as starter culture or probiotic bacteria in industrial food production, concerns have been raised about the antibiotic resistance of these beneficial bacteria strains. Probiotic bacteria can help maintaining balance in gastrointestinal tract in cases of diarrhea caused by antibiotic treatment. However, there is high risk associated with the ability of these resistant strains to transmit the resistance gene to pathogenic bacteria in gut microbiota. This can complicate the treatment of a patient with an antibiotic resistant bacterial infection or disease. The circulation of genes coding for antibiotic resistance from beneficial LAB in the food chain via animals to humans is a complex problem. Therefore, there is a need to evaluate the safety of potential probitic strains regarding their ability to acquire and disseminate antibiotic resistance determinants in selection of LAB.

In this study, importance of LAB in the food chain will be reviewed. Morphological and biochemical characteristics of lactobacilli, bifidobactera and enterococci, as well as criteria for probiotic selection and role of probiotics in health benefit will be discussed. Antibiotic susceptibility as criteria for potential probiotic bacteria selection and mechanisms of gene transfers will be considered.

2. Lactic acid bacteria in the GI tract

The human GI tract represents a complex ecosystem in which interactions between food, microbes and the host cells occur. The bacterial population of normal gut of an adult comprise of more than 500 different species. The quantity of microbes present in the intestine (about 10^{14}) exceeds 10-fold the total number of all human cells (Backhed et al., 2005). The most important function of this intestinal microbiota is to act as a microbial barrier against pathogens, by so-called competitive exclusion mechanisms, but also influence the humoral and cellular mucosal immune responses during the neonatal phase of life, and thereafter to maintain a physiologically-normal steady-state condition throughout life (Tancrede, 1992). The gut microflora profoundly influences nutritional, physiologic and protective processes. Both direct and indirect defensive functions are provided by the normal microbiota. Specifically, gut bacteria directly prevent colonization by pathogenic organisms by competing for essential nutrients or for epithelial attachment sites. By producing antimicrobial compounds, volatile fatty acids, and chemically modified bile acids, indigenous gut bacteria also create a local environment that is generally unfavourable for the growth of enteric pathogens. This phenomenon is called Colonization Resistance, which can be defined as the ability of microorganisms belonging to the normal gut microflora to impede the implantation of pathogens (van der Waaij, 1988). This function of the microflora is also known as the barrier effect. While probiotic bacteria improve colonization resistance, consensus thinking is that the importance of LAB as probiotic agents lies more in the indirect mechanisms such as immunomodulation. When the genetic repertoire of these bacteria is considered, the GI tract translates into a reservoir of genes encoding numerous physiological functions from which the human GI tract can benefit. Bacteria represent the most extensively investigated group of microorganisms. Which species of bacteria will be long-term colonized in GI tract depends on the biochemical capability of the microorganisms, the microenvironment determined by the host cells and the available foodstuffs. Lactobacilli are probably the most well known representative of favourable microorganisms in GI tract. There is a number of species of lactobacilli reside in the human intestine in a symbiotic relationship with each other and with other microorganisms (Claesson et al., 2007). They are generally considered essential for maintaining gut microfloral health; however, it is the overall balance of the various microorganisms which is ultimately of most importance.

2.1 The composition of the GI tract

The composition of the GI microflora undergoes considerable changes from the day of birth until adulthood. The GI tract of a normal fetus is sterile, but colonization begins immediately after birth and is influenced by the mode of delivery, the infant diet, hygiene levels and medication (Benett et al., 1986; Gronlund et al., 1999). During the first months of life diet has a significant influence on the development of the intestinal flora (Heavey & Rowland, 1999; Stark & Lee, 1982). Within one to two days facultative anaerobes predominate and create a reduced environment that allows the growth of strict anaerobes. Within three to four days, bifidobacteria appear and become predominant. The average number of bifidobacteria in breast-fed infants is 10^{10}–10^{11} cfu/g. In formula fed infants, bifidobacteria have also been demonstrated to be a numerically important species, but they generally occur in lower numbers than in breastfed infants of the same age (Mountzouris et al., 2002). The predominance of beneficial bacteria in the gut microbiota of breast-fed infants is thought to result from the fermentation of oligosaccharides-non-digestible carbohydrates consisting of several linked monosaccharides (typically 3-10 simple sugars) in breastmilk (Agostoni et al., 2004). Oligosaccharides pass unabsorbed through the small intestine into the colon, where they are fermented by resident bifidobacteria to short-chain fatty acids and lactic acid, reducing the gut pH to approximately 5.7, thus providing the protection against enteric infections (Newburg, 2000, Coppa et al., 2004). In contrast, the gut microflora of formula-fed infants produces a different profile of short-chain fatty acids and a pH in the local microenvironment of approximately 7.0 (Ogawa et al., 1992). Infant faecal flora appears to be stabilized at 4 weeks of age and until weaning when introduction of solid foods takes place (Mountzouris et al., 2002). During weaning, bifidobacteria decrease by 1 log, the microbiota alters from infant-type to adult-type, and a remarkable proliferation of bacteroides, eubacteria, peptostreptococcaceae, and clostridia occur. The faecal flora of children closely resembles that of adults, where the numbers of bacteroidaceae, eubacteria, peptococcaceae, and usually clostridia outnumbered bifidobacteria, which constitute 5-10% of the total flora.

An adult individual's GI tract is extremely stable and it is very difficult to introduce new species. There are several factors that can alter the composition of the GI flora such as medications (especially antibiotics), diet, climate, aging, illness, stress, pH, infections, geographic location, and even race (Murphy et al., 2009). Thus it is not surprising to find out that the composition of the GI flora not only differs among individuals, but also differs during the life within the same individual. Furthermore, indigenous bacteria are not distributed randomly throughout the gastrointestinal tract but instead are found at population levels and in species distributions that are characteristic of specific regions of the tract.

As shown in Figure 1, there are three main regions that offer very different conditions for the survival of various microorganisms in the GI environment. In the stomach, microbial growth is greatly reduced by the high acidity and presence of oxygen provided by the swallowing. As a result, in the stomach acidotolerant microorganisms and facultative anaerobes such as lactobacilli, streptococci, yeasts, etc. are present. In the second region (small intestine), the microflora consists mainly of facultative anaerobic bacteria such as lactobacilli, streptococci and enterobacteria, and anaerobes such as bifidobacteria, bacteroides and clostridia. In the last region (colon), the number of bacteria is considerably high, due to the low redox potential and relatively high concentration of short-chain fatty acid, and counts 10^9–10^{12} cfu/ml (Cummings et al. 1989). The colon has an important role in food digestion, and microflora in this region participates in the transformation of many carbohydrates, proteins and amino acids. The microflora of the colon is very complex and dominated by anaerobic bacteria (*Bacteroides* spp., *Clostridium* spp, *Bifidobacterium* spp., etc), while the facultative anaerobic bacteria are less numerous and represented by lactobacilli, enterococci, streptococci and *Enterobacteriaceae*. Yeasts (eg., *Candida albicans*) are relatively poorly represented.

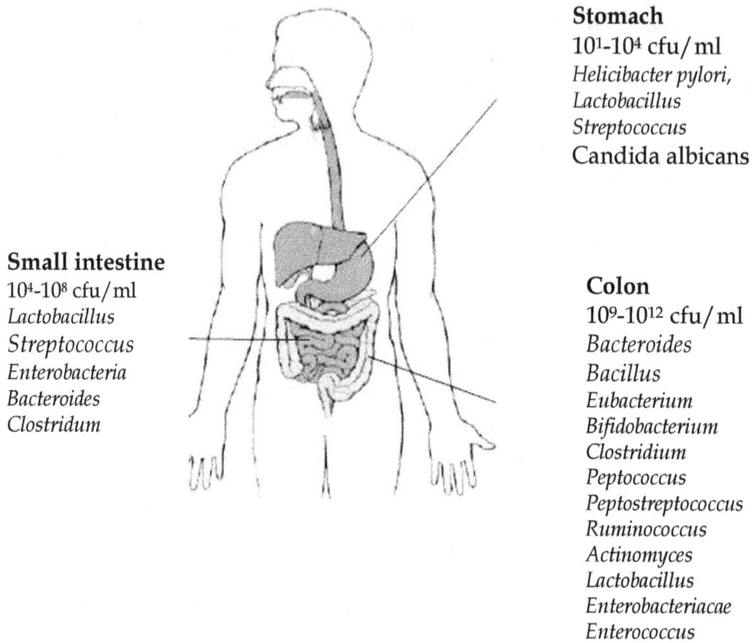

Fig. 1. The average concentration of microorganisms in the GI tract (adapted from Ouwehand & Vesterlund, 2003)

As part of gut microbiota, it is estimated that lactobacilli are present in following concentrations: 10^3–10^6 cfu/ml in the oral cavity; 10^3 cfu/ml in the stomach; 10^4 cfu /ml in the duodenum and jejunum; 10^8 cfu /ml in the ileum and 10^9 cfu /ml in the colon (Reuter, 2001; Koll et al., 2008; Ryan et al., 2008). An overview of lactobacilli commonly found in the GI tract microbiota is shown in Table 1.

Considering that lactobacilli and bifidobacteria constitute a significant population in the GI tract, this environment represents a good source for the isolation of new strains of LAB.

3. Lactic acid bacteria as probiotic bacteria

By definition probiotics are described as „living microorganisms, which upon ingestion in certain numbers, exert health benefits beyond inherent basic nutrition" (Guarner & Schaafsma, 1998). Regarding the probiotics, the majority of research is focused on bacterial genera *Lactobacillus* and *Bifidobacterium* (Table 2).

Oral cavity	Stomach	Small intestine	Faeces	Colon epithelial biopsies
L. paracasei	*L. gasseri*	*L. gasseri*	*L. gasseri*	*L. plantarum*
L. rhamnosus	*L. reuteri*	*L. reuteri*	*L. paracasei*	*L. rhamnosus*
L. fermentum	*L. ruminis*	*L. rhamnosus*	*L. ruminis*	*L. paracasei*
L. plantarum			*L. reuteri*	
L. gasseri			*L. plantarum*	
			L. salivarius	
			L. sakei	

Table 1. *Lactobacillus* species distribution in different parts of the GI tract (Lönnermark, 2010)

Lactobacillus sp.	*Bifidobacteriim sp.*	*Enterococcus sp.*	*Others*
L. acidophilus	*B. bifidum*	*E. faecium*	*Lactococcus lactis ssp. lactis*
L.plantarum	*B. infantis*	*E. faecalis*	*Lactococcus lactis ssp. cremoris*
L. casei	*B. adolescentis*		*Leuconostoc mesenteroides*
L. rhamnosus	*B. longum*		*Pediococcus acidilactici*
L. delbrueckii ssp. bulgaricus	*B. breve*		*Propionibacterium freudenreichii*
L. fermentum	*B. lactis*		*Streptococcus thermophilus*
L. johnsonii			
L. gasseri			
L. salivarius			
L. reuteri			

Table 2. Lactic acid bacteria used as probiotics (adapted from Gardnier et al., 2002)

They have a reputation of health promoters and they have a significant role as probiotic bacteria in the production of different foods, particularly in the production of fermented dairy products. Central position of lactobacilli and bifidobacteria in probiotic formulation is argumented due to (a) the association of these bacteria with human health, (b) the fact that they possess the Generally Regarded As Safe (GRAS) status. Enterococci, although not GRAS organisms, have been used as probiotics too. Some other LAB such as lactococci, pediococci, *Leuconostoc*, propionibacteria have also received attention as potential probiotic cultures (Table 2).

3.1 *Lactobacillus*

The genus *Lactobacillus* is large heterogeneous group of microorganisms, which lacks catalase and cytochromes and is usually microaerophilic, with growth improved under anaerobic conditions (Kandler & Weiss, 1989). They are Gram-positive nonmotile rods, often in pairs or chains, coccobacilli to long rods. They have a strictly fermentative metabolism and convert glucose solely or partly to lactic acid. They are classified as homofermentative (producing mainly lactic acid) or heterofermentative (producing carbon dioxide, ethanol, acetic acid and lactic acid). The optimum growth temperature is in the mesophilic range (30-40°C), but some strains can grow below 15°C and some at temperatures up to 55°C. Differentiation of *Lactobacillus* species depends on physiological criteria, carbohydrate fermentation, biochemical and molecular characterization (Petrovic et al., 2006). Lactobacilli play crucial role in the production of fermented foods: vegetables, meats and dairy products. Non starter lactic acid bacteria (NSLAB) are lactobacilli which form significant proportion of the microflora of most cheese varieties during ripening. Many species of mesophilic *Lactobacillus* have been isolated from cheese; the ones most frequently encountered are *L. casei, L. paracasei, L. pantarum, L. rhamnosus* and *L. curvatus* (Beresford et al., 2001). For example, *L. plantarum, L. casei* ssp. *casei* and *L. brevis* have been isolated from Armada cheese, a Spanish goat milk cheese (Herreros et al., 2003), *L. plantarum, L. paraplantarum, L. paracasei* ssp. *tolerans, L. sake, L. curvaus* and *L. pentosus* from Batzos, a traditional Greek cheese made from raw goat' s milk (Psoni et al., 2003) and *L. para.paracasei, L. plantarum, L. curvatus* and *L. brevis* from Sjenica cheese, traditional Serbian white brined cheese (Radulović, 2010). Traditional homemade dairy products have great potential for isolation of new strains, which could be used as starter cultures in food industry, as adjunct cultures for improving flavour of cheeses, or as probiotic in production of functional foods.

3.2 *Bifidobacterium*

Species from the genus *Bifidobacterium* are generally characterized as Gram-positive, non-spore forming, nonmotile and catalase negative. They are strict anaerobes, although some species and strains may tolerate oxygen in the presence of carbon dioxide. Within the genus *Bifidobacterium* pleomorphism exists and it is described as short regular, thin cells with pointed ends, long cells with slight bends with a large variety of branching; single or in chains of many elements; in star-like clusters or disposed in "V" or palisade arrangements (Scardovi, 1986). In bifidobacteria, glucose catabolism occurs through the fructose 6-phosphate phodphoketolase pathway, which can be used as distinguishing feature of bifidobacteria. During fermentation, acetic and lactic acids are produced in molar ratios 3:2. The optimum temperature for growth is 31-41°C within the range 25-45°C. Bifidobacteria are less acid tolerant than lactobacilli and no growth occurs at pH values less than 4.5 (Scardovi, 1986). Nutritional requirements for growth of bifidobacteria are less complex than those of lactobacilli, but in some cases bifidobacteria do require specific factors for optimal growth (Modler et al., 1990). Bifidobacteria are natural habitants of GI tract and strains with probiotic properties are mainly of human origin. *Bifidobacterium* species constitute a significant portion of probiotic cultures used in functional food production.

3.3 *Enterococcus*

Although lactobacilli and bifidobacteria are most commonly used as probiotics, some enterococci can also be used as health-promoting bacteria. Species *E. faecium* and *E. faecalis* have been used as probiotic bacteria, although they are not recognized as GRAS organisms. All species of genus *Enterococcus* are Gram-positive, non-spore forming, catalasa negative, facultative anaerobes. They are spherical or ovoid cocci in pairs or short chains. Their properties, such as the ability to grow at 10°C and 45°C in 6.5%NaCl and at pH 9.6 and their survival heating to 60°C for 30 min, are used to differentiate enterococci from other Gram-positive catalase-negative cocci (Franz et al., 1999). Enterococci are homofermentative with respect to glucose metabolism, although some amounts of formic and lactic acid may be produced in some media. As the other LAB, enterococci do require B vitamins, amino acids, purine and pyramidine bases for optimal growth (Garg & Mital, 1991).

3.4 LAB associated with therapeutic properties

In recent years an increasing number of probiotic pharmaceutical preparations as well as food supplements are being promoted with health claims. The application of LAB has been more developed for the production of functional foods, where probiotic bacteria have an important role. The commercial probiotic strains, used in functional food production, must be well-substantiated with scientific evidence.

The health benefits of probiotic bacteria can be considered as nutritional or therapeutic/prophylactic. Nutritional benefits are mainly connected with their role in enhancing the bioavailability of vitamins and minerals, and an increase of the digestibility of protein (Tamime et al., 2003). Many researchers (Begley et al., 2006; Ouwehand et al., 2003; Rodrigeuz et al., 2010) investigated the therapeutic/prophylactic benefits of probiotics and confirmed their effects:

- Prevention of diarrhoea caused by certain pathogenic bacteria and viruses;
- Regulation of intestinal microflora after an antibiotic therapy;
- Treating the infection with *Helicobacter pylori*, responsible for the development of gastritis, ulcers and gastric cancer;
- Improvement of digestion in "lactose-intolerant" individuals, who have reduced capability for lactose digestion;
- Anticancer effect, as a result of the production of certain compounds during its growth;
- Reducing cholesterol levels;
- Stimulation of γ-interferon production, which contributes to increased resistance to some infections;
- Increasing antibody titar (IgG immunoglobulins), which enhances the immune response of an organism;

Health effects are related to microflora modification and strengthening of the gut mucosal barrier. Some scientific data indicated that probiotic strains have potential in the prevention and treatment of intestinal and urogenital infections and these cultures may be useful as an alternatives to antibiotic therapy. The World Health Organization (WHO) has recommended the reconsideration of microbial interference therapy for infection control (Bengmark, 1998). Certain probiotic strains have been shown multiple effects including prevention of pathogen attachment and invasion in cell culture, inhibiting of the growth of enteropatogens *in vitro* and enhancement the immune response. Considering thee effects, the usage of probiotics may decrease antibiotics dependence. Fooks et al., (1999) have suggested that probiotic bacteria can control the infection in several ways such as the competition for nutrients, secretion of antimicrobial substances, reduction of pH, blocking of adhesion sites, reduction of virulence, blocking of toxin receptor sites, immune stimulation and suppression of toxin production.

Infections by bacterial or viral agents most frequently result in diarrhea. One of the most investigated probiotic, *L.rhamnosus* GG, has been very effective in the treatment of viral diarrhea in children, most cases of which were caused by rotavirus. Other probiotic strains such as *Lactocacillus casei Shirota, B. bifidum* and *S. thermophillus* have also been shown to be effective in the treatment and prevention of rotavirus diarrhea in children (Korhonen, et al., 2007; Saavedra et al., 1994).

Antibiotic-associated diarrhea (AAD) is a major clinical problem that occurs following antibiotic use. The most serious form of this kind is pseudomembranous colitis. Diarrhea is caused by pathogen overgrowth and in 20% cases the etiological agent is *Clostridium difficile*, a pathogen that is especially persistent and difficult to treat (Lewis & Freedman, 1998). Antibiotics are often used to treat for pseudomembranous colitis or other AAD, although the relapse may occurs when the probiotic therapy may be especially useful. Oral therapy with *L. rhamnosus* GG was effective in the prevention of AAD, in treatment of colitis, as well as in traveller's diarrhea (Shah, 2007). A combination of *B. bifidum, S. thermophilus, L. delbrueckii spp. bulgaricus* and *L. acidophilus* have been also effective in the prevention of traveller's diarrhea (Black et al., 1989).

On the other hand, many studies have shown no effect of probiotic treatment (Lewis & Freedman, 1998). There is still some doubts regaring the quality and efficacy of probiotic products. Nevertheless, the probiotic food industry is flourishing. In many European counties the market is expanding resulting in sell of probiotic yogurts that account for over 10% of all yogurts sold in Europe (Stanton et al., 2001).

4. Criteria associated with probiotic bacteria

Consortium of LAB constitute a major part of the natural microflora of human intestine and when present in sufficient numbers create a healthy equilibrium between beneficial and potentially harmful microflora in the gut (Dune et al., 2001). For some positive effects on human health, a probiotic strain has to reach the large intestine at a concentration of about 10^7 viable cells/g (Stanton et al., 2001). Microorganisms ingested with food begin their journey to the lower intestinal tract via the mouth and are exposed during their transit through the GI tract to successive stress factors that influence their survival. The time from entrance to release from the stomach is about 90 min, but further digestive processes have longer residence times (Berrada et al., 1991). Probiotic bacteria must overcome physical and chemical barriers in the GI tract, especially acidic environment of the stomach, and then the activity of hydrolytic enzymes and bile salts in the small intestine. In a typical acid tolerance tests, the viability of potential probiotic organisms is determined by exposing them to low pH in a buffer solution or medium for a certain period of time, during which the number of surviving probiotic bacteria is determined. The generally requirements for probiotics are shown in Table 3.

Acid and bile stability
Adherence to human intestinal cells
Ability to reduce the adhesion of pathogens to surfaces
Colonization of human GI tract
Antagonism against carcinogenic and pathogenic bacteria
Production of anti-microbial substances
Survive the various technological processes of production
Safety evaluation: nonpathogenic, nontoxic, nonallergic, nonmutagenic
Desirable metabolic activity and antibiotic resistance/sensitivity
Clinically validated and documented health effects

Table 3. The desired properties of probiotic strains (adapted from Mattila & Sarraela, 2000)

Bile plays an essential role in lipid digestion; it emulsifies and solubilizes lipids and functions as biological detergent. Prior to secretion into the duodenum, bile acids, which are synthesized from cholesterol, are conjugated to either glycine or taurine in liver (Begley et al., 2006). In the colon conjugated bile undergoes to the various chemical changes including deconjugation, dehydroxylation, dehydrogenation, and deglucuronidation, almost solely by microbial activity (Begley et al., 2006). Bile reduces the survival of bacteria by destroying their cell membranes, whose major components are lipids and fatty acids and these modifications may affect not only the cell permeability and viability, but also the interactions between the membranes and the environment. Bile salt hydrolases (BSHs) are generally intracellular, oxygeninsensitive enzymes that catalyze the hydrolysis of bile salts (Liong & Shah, 2005). A number of BSHs have been identified and characterized in probiotic bacteria (Franz et al., 2001a).

The adhesion ability as well as interaction with pathohens is regarded as important selection criteria for potential probiotic strains (Salminen et al. 2010). Adhesive properties of LAB depend on a variety of factors, including non-specifc adhesion determined by electrostatic or hydrophobic forces and specific binding dependent on particular molecules. To examine the adhesive property of LAB, several models have been developed. These include binding to tissue culture cells (Tuomola & Salminen, 1998), radiolabelling (Bernet et al., 1993), intestinal mucus (Ouwehand et al., 2001), extracellular matrix proteins (de Leeuw et al., 2006) and resected colonic tissue (Vesterlund et al., 2005). Although none of these models reflect the complex interactions occurring in the mucosal layer of the digestive tract, they represent a rapid method for the screening of potential probiotic strains.

Other functional property used to characterize probiotics is the production of antimicrobial compounds. Several antimicrobial substances that have considerable advantages in competition with pathogens and other harmful bacteria are produced by LAB (Klare et al., 2007; Radulović et al., 2010a). These substances include fatty acids, organic acids, hydrogen peroxide, and diacetyl, acetoin and the most studied inhibitory peptides called 'bacteriocins' (Todorov et al., 2011). The ability of probiotics to establish in the GI tract is enhanced by their ability to eliminate competitors. Some examples of antimicrobial substances produced by probiotic bacteria are presented in Table 4.

Probiotic	Compaund
Lactobacillus GG	Wide spread antibiotic
L. acidophilus	Acidolin,Acidophilin, Lactocidin
L. delbrueckii ssp. bulgaricus	Bulgarican
L. plantarum	Lactolin
L. brevis	Lactobacillin,Lactobrevin
L. reuteri	Reuterin

Table 4. Antimicrobial substances (Fuller, 1992)

Antibiotic susceptibility of potential probiotic strains is also considered as an important selection criterion for potential probiotic status (Hummel et al., 2007). Some LAB may carry potentially transmissible plasmid-encoded antibiotic resistance genes. The transmission of antibiotic resistance genes to unrelated pathogenic or potentially pathogenic bacteria in the gut is a major health concern related with the probiotic application (see detailed information in paragraph 6).

Along with above mentioned criteria, selected probiotic strains have to be able to survive well in the food and to have the appropriate technological properties (e.g. acidification during fermentation if required). In addition, it is important that the added probiotic does not adversely affect the taste, smell, and texture of the food or beverage.

In vitro tests based on these selection criteria, although not a definite means of strain selection, may provide an useful initial information. A validation model system, such as a Simulator of the Human Intestinal Microbial Ecosystem (SHIME), which aims to mimic complex physiological and physiochemical in vivo reactions, may also be of value in strain selection. However, the ultimate proof of probiotic effects requires validation in well designed statistically sound clinical trails. Generally, tools that may be employed in such an assessment include *in vitro* studies, studies of strain properties, pharmacokinetic studies, animal studies, use of intestinal models, human studies and epidemiological surveillance. Each strain needs to be tested separately.

It is evident that the selection of new potential probiotic bacteria is an enormous and time-consuming task with uncertain results.

5. Antibiotic resistance of LAB in the food chain

During the recent years, there has been great concern about the possibility of spreading the antibiotic resistance in the environment. According to the European Commission (2005), it has been estimated that one to ten million tons of antibiotics has been released into the biosphere over the last 60 years. This has lead to very strong selective pressure for the emergence of resistant bacterial strains. Since LAB are present in the GI tract in large amounts, LAB resistant to certain antibiotics could benefit the host organism. Nevertheless, there is a risk associated with the ability of these resistant strains to transmit the resistance gene to pathogenic bacteria. Literature data pointed out that some LAB, the predominant microbiota in fermented dairy and meat products, may serve as reservoirs of antibiotic resistance genes potentially transferable to human pathogens (Mathur & Singh, 2005).

The food chain could be regarded as one of the main pathways for the transmission of antibiotic resistant bacteria from animals to humans (Singer et al., 2003). Molecular analysis of resistance genes localized on transferable genetic elements showed they are identical in humans and animals, which confirm that food of animal origin, particularly sausages and cheeses made from raw milk, serve as a vehicle for the transmission of resistant bacteria and antibiotic resistance determinants. The antibiotics application in sub-therapeutic levels in animal's drinking water and feed increases the selective pressure and amplify the transfer of antibiotic resistance between bacterial species. Thus there is a direct correlation between the indigenous microflora of the GI tract of animals with the GI tract of humans. Although many species of LAB used as starter and probiotic cultures possess GRAS status, potential risk to human health caused by the genes transfer of antibiotic resistance has not yet been fully defined. To address this aspect, the safety of LAB should be verified with the respect of their ability to acquire and disseminate resistance determinants (Kastner et al., 2006). Particular concern is due to the evidence of a widespread occurrence in this bacterial group of conjugative plasmids and transposons. The presence of transmissible antibiotic resistance markers in the safety evaluation of LAB strains is a very important task since genes conferring resistance to several antimicrobials (e.g. chloramphenicol, erythromycin, streptomycin, tetracycline, and vancomycin) located on transferable genetic elements (plasmids or transposons) have already been characterized in lactococci (Perreten et al., 1997), lactobacilli (Axelsson et al., 1988; Danielsen, 2002) and enterococci (Eaton & Gasson, 2001; Huys et al., 2002) isolated from food. However, the transfer of antibiotic resistance genes from LAB reservoir strains to bacteria in the resident microflora of human GI tract and hence to pathogenic bacteria, has not been fully addressed.

Irrespective of the antibiotic resistance mechanisms and the bacterial taxon involved, the possibility of spreading an antibiotic resistance determinant through horizontal transfer relies on its genetic basis. Therefore, a distinction between intrinsic and acquired resistance has to be made. Antibiotic resistance may be intrinsic for bacterial species or a genus, and it is characterized by the ability of an organism to survive in the presence of certain antimicrobial agents, due to its inherent characteristics of resistance. Intrinsic or "natural" resistance mechanisms involve the absence of the target, low cell permeability, antibiotic inactivation and the presence of efflux mechanisms. Enterococci are intrinsically resistant to cephalosporins and low levels of aminoglycoside and clindamycin (Teuber et al., 1999). Lactobacilli, pediococci and *Leuconostoc* spp. have been reported to have a high natural resistance to vancomycin, a property that is useful to separate them from other Gram-positive bacteria (Hamilton- Miller & Shah, 1998; Simpson et al., 1988). Some lactobacilli have a high natural resistance to bacitracin, cefoxitin, ciprofloxacin, fusidic acid, kanamycin, gentamicin, metronidazole, nitrofurantoin, norfloxacin, streptomycin, sulphadiazine, teicoplanin, trimethoprim/sulphamethoxazole, and vancomycin (Danielsen & Wind, 2003). For a number of lactobacilli a very high frequency of spontaneous mutation to nitrofurazone (10^{-5}), kanamycin and streptomycin was found (Curragh & Collins, 1992). From these data it is clear that inter-genus and inter-species differences exist, and consequently identification at species level is required in order to interpret phenotypic susceptibility data. Acquired resistance is a characteristic of some strains within a species usually susceptible to certain antibiotics and can be horizontally spread among the bacteria. The acquisition of antibiotic resistance occurs via the mutation of pre-existing genes or by horizontal transmission of resistance determinants. With some exception, intrinsic resistance and resistance by mutation are unlikely to be disseminated, although any gene responsible for intrinsic resistance may spread provided that it is flanked by insertion sequences (European Commissions); horizontally transferred genes, particularly those carried on mobile genetic elements, are those most likely to be transmitted (Normark & Normark, 2002). Among the three well-known mechanisms for horizontal gene exchange between bacteria, namely free DNA mediated transformation, bacteriophage induced transduction, and conjugation, the last is acknowledged to be the most relevant for antibiotic resistance gene transfer (Salyers, 1995). Resistance genes are frequently carried by the mobile genetic elements involved in these mechanisms, such as plasmids and conjugative transposons, which can be freely exchanged irrespective of genus or species barriers, resulting in resistance transfer or co-transfer (Levy, 1986). Recently it has been discovered that the so-called "mobilome" also involves other genetic elements: the transposon can carry integrons, which are not self-transmissible but carry a gene encoding an integrase, which in turn mobilises resistance genes borne on the integron as cassettes (Clementi & Aquilanti, 2011). This mechanism seems to be active only in the context of resistance gene exchange and it surely determines a substantial increase in the horizontal mobility of these genes.

5.1 Procedure for antimicrobial susceptibility/resistance patterns of LAB

As mentioned above, an intrinsic resistance and resistance by mutation are unlikely to be disseminated, so the risk is mainly characterized by horizontally transferred genes. Therefore, distinction between natural and acquired antibiotic resistance among the population of LAB is of a great importance. Analysis of Minimal Inhibitory Concentration (MIC) and their distributions in defined species/antibiotic combinations helps to differentiate between these two resistance mechanisms. When a bacterial strain demonstrates higher resistance to a specific antibiotic than the other strains of the same taxonomical unit, the presence of acquired resistance is indicated and there is a need for further analysis to confirm the genetic basis of resistance.

According to Murray et al., (2003) the MIC distribution of a given antibiotic for a single bacterial species in the absence of resistance mechanisms should approach statistical normality while bimodal distribution of MIC values suggest acquired resistance. For the purpose of identifying bacterial strains with acquired and potentially transferable antibiotic resistance, microbiological breakpoints have been defined. Microbiological breakpoints are set by studying the MIC distribution in the bacterial population and the part of population that clearly deviates from a susceptible majority is considered resistant (Olsson-Liljequist et al., 1997).

The data used for the definition of microbiological breakpoints, as reported in Table 5, were derived from the published body of research and from national and European monitoring procedures. The antibiotics listed: ampicillin, vancomycin, gentamicin, kanamycin, streptomycin, erythromycin, clindamycin, quinupristin+dalfopristin, tetracycline and chloramphenicol were chosen to maximise the identification of resistance genotypes by assessing the resistance phenotypes.

In Gram-positive, bacteria acquired trimethoprim resistance, although occasionally detected is relatively rare. The data available (Korhonen et al., 2007) indicate that within species of lactobacilli the range of apparent trimethoprim resistances can be wide with no clear breakpoint values. Therefore, the MIC testing of trimethoprim for LAB was not considered relevant. Furthermore, testing for linezolid and neomycin is no longer considered necessary. The extremely rare non-mutational resistance to linezolid is due to the acquisition of the *cfr* gene, which also confers resistance to chloramphenicol (Arias et al., 2008; Toh et al., 2007). Testing for chloramphenicol resistance will efficiently cover for the hazard of acquiring resistance to linezolid. Neomycin is removed from the list since testing for the remaining three aminoglycosides efficiently covers the hazard of acquiring resistance to aminoglycosides.

Antibiotic susceptibility testing may be performed using different phenotypic test methods. In Clinical and Laboratory Standards Institute (CLSI), formerly National Committee on Clinical Laboratory Standards (NCCLS), the approved standards state that the methods of choice are agar dilution and broth microdilution (Anonym, 2007). Other widely used methods include the agar gradient method and commercial methods, such as Etest, which consists of a predefined gradient of antibiotic concentrations on a plastic strip (AbBiomerieux, Sweden). In addition to phenotypic antibiotic resistance determinations, also genotypic detection of particular genes causing resistance may be performed. These genotypic methods include different PCR -based methods, southern hybridization, plasmid profiling and microarray (Ammor et al., 2008; Aquilanti et al., 2007). The situation is clearest

Lactic acid bacteria	ampicillin	vancomycin	gentamicin**	Kanamycin**	streptomycin**	erythromycin	clindamycin	quinupristin+ dalphopristin	tetracycline	chloramphenicol
Lactobacillus obligate homofermentative	1	2	16	16	16	1	1	4	4	4
Lactobacillus helveticus	1	2	16	16	16	1	1	4	4	4
Lactobacillus acidophilus group	1	2	16	16	16	1	1	4	4	4
Lactobacillus delbrueckii	1	2	16	16	16	1	1	4	4	4
Lactobacillus obligate heterofermentative	2	n.r.	16	16	64	1	1	4	8	4
Lactobacillus reuteri	2	n.r.	8	16	64	1	1	4	16	4
Lactobacillus fermentum	1	n.r.	16	32	64	1	1	4	8	4
*Lactobacillus facultative heterofermentative**	4	n.r.	16	64	64	1	1	4	8	4
Lactobacillus plantarum	2	n.r.	16	64	n.r.	1	1	4	32	8
Lactobacillus rhamnosus	4	n.r.	16	64	32	1	1	4	8	4
Lactobacillus paracasei	2	n.r.	32	64	n.r.	1	1	4	4	4
Bifidobacterium	2	2	64	n.r.	128	0.5	0.25	1	8	4
Enterococcus	4	4	32	512	128	4	4	4	2	8
Pediococcus	4	n.r.	16	64	64	1	1	4	8	4
Leuconostoc	2	n.r.	16	16	64	1	1	4	8	4
Lactococcus lactis	2	4	32	64	64	2	4	4	4	8
Streptococcus thermophilus	2	4	32	64	64	2	2	4	4	4
Bacillus spp.	n.r.	4	4	8	8	4	4	4	8	8
Propionibacterium	2	4	64	64	64	0.5	0.25	0.5	2	2
Other Gram (-)	1	2	4	16	8	0.5	0.25	0.5	2	2

n.r. not required;
*including *Lactobacillus salivarius*;
**possible interference of the growth medium

Table 5. Microbiological breakpoints categorizing bacteria as resistant (mg L^{-1}). Strains with MIC higher than the breakpoints below are considered as resistant.

when the phenotypic and genotypic resistance patterns are in agreement. However, a phenotypically resistant strain may be genotypically "susceptible". This is usually due to the fact that appropriate genes are not included in the test patterns, or there might be unknown resistance genes. Tetracycline, for example, has more than 40 different genes conferring antibiotic resistance discovered at the moment, and the number of tetracycline resistance genes continues to increase (Roberts, 2005). In contrast, a susceptible phenotype may also carry silent genes, which are observed with genotyping.

However, there is still a lack of agreement on the resistance-susceptibility breakpoints for most antibiotics in LAB (Charteris et al., 1998; Danielsen & Wind, 2003; Katla et al., 2001). Generally, the choice of medium has been shown to have a profound impact on the MICs of

LAB. The recommended growth media by the National Committee for Clinical Laboratory Standards (Mueller-Hinton agar) (NCCLS, 2002) and by the British Society for Antimicrobial Chemotherapy (Iso-Sensitest agar) (Andrews, 2001) do not support growth of all LAB. MRS medium, that generally supports the growth of LAB much better, is not always compatible to the Iso-Sensitest medium for the use in susceptibility testing, as was reported for various classes of antibiotics (Huys et al., 2002). Furthermore, there are still no guidelines available for the interpretation of susceptibility test results of commensal or food-associated bacteria. Additionally, MIC breakpoints values have been shown to be species specific and thus vary between species of the same genera (Danielsen & Wind, 2003). Also, distinguishing between intrinsic, non-specific and acquired resistance is difficult and requires, besides the evaluation of genetic base of resistance, that the antimicrobial-resistance patterns of many LAB species from different sources may be compared (Teuber et al., 1999).

5.2 Mobile genetic elements in LAB

A prerequisite for LAB to acquire antibiotic resistance genes from other bacteria is their ability to communicate actively and passively with these bacteria with the aid of conjugative plasmids and transposons. Conjugative plasmids and transposons are common in LAB, and due to their wide environmental distribution, it is possible that these commensal bacteria act as vectors for the dissemination of antibiotic resistance determinants to the consumer via the food chain. Plasmids are found in many genera of LAB, characterized by different size, function and distribution (Davidson et al., 1996; Wang & Lee, 1997). The functions related to the plasmids include hydrolysis of proteins, metabolism of carbohydrates, amino acids and citrate, production of bacteriocins and exopolysaccharides, and resistance to antibiotics, heavy metals and phages. At least 25 species of lactobacilli contain native plasmids (Wang & Lee, 1997), and often appear to contain multiple (from 1 to 16) different plasmids in a single strain. R-plasmids encoding tetracycline, erythromycin, chloramphenicol, or macrolide-lincomycin-streptogramin resistance have been reported in *L. reuteri* (Lin et al., 1996; Tannock et al., 1994), *L. fermentum* (Fons et al., 1997; Ishiwa & Iwata, 1980), *L. acidophilus* (Vescovo et al., 1982), and *L. plantarum* (Danielsen, 2002) isolated from raw meat, silage and faeces. The reported prevalence of antibiotic resistance genes such as erythromycin, vancomycin, tetracycline, chloramphenicol, and gentamicin resistance genes, on transferable genetic elements in enterococci is more extensive, both on plasmids (Murray et al., 1988) and transposons (Clewell et al., 1995; Perreten et al., 1997a; Rice & Marshall, 1994;). A multiple antibiotic resistance plasmid was reported in a *L. lactis* strain isolated from cheese (Perreten et al., 1997b), encoding streptomycin, tetracycline and chloramphenicol resistance.

Conjugative transposons are the major vehicle regarding antibiotic resistance transport in LAB. They have been discovered in *E.faecalis* (Tn*916*, Tn*918*, Tn*920*, Tn*925*, Tn*2702*), *E. faecium* (Tn*5233*) and *L. lactis* (Tn*5276*, Tn*5301*). In enterococci and streptococci, resistances to tetracycline (tet (M)), erythromycin (ermAM, erm), chloramphenicol (cat) and kanamycin (aphA-3) have been determined. In lactococci, code for nisin (nis) production and sucrose fermentation (sac) has been observed. These transposons vary in size between 16 and 70 kb and may be inserted into plasmids or the chromosome in one or multiple copies. They may mobilize plasmids or chromosomal genes. The most remarkable observation is the extreme host range, which is the property of the Tn*916*/Tn*1545* family.

5.3 Horizontal transferability of antibiotic resistance from LAB in food chain

The possible transfer of antibiotic resistance genes between bacterial species have been studied mostly in harmful or pathogenic species, but also recently in LAB. The vast majority of the experiments have been made *in vitro*, using methods such as filter-mating (Klare et al., 2007, Ouoba et al.,2008), although these *in vitro* methods do not mimic the circumstances in nature, and results obtained cannot be compared with the results achieved or expected using *in vivo* methods. The transferability of antibiotic resistance genes in the GI tract from LAB is not straightforward, since the GI tract is a hostile environment to many allochthonous bacteria. Moreover, studies made *in vivo* usually are based on "worst-case scenario", simulating very high daily intake of food products containing the resistant bacteria (Jacobsen et al., 2007). The potentially transferable genes in LAB have been described in multiple studies and have been reviewed in Ammor et al. (2007). Two of the most commonly observed resistance genes in LAB found so far are *tet*(M) for tetracycline resistance and *erm*(B) for erythromycin, followed with *cat* genes coding for chloramphenicol resistance (Cataloluk & Gogebakan 2004; Danielsen, 2002).

Enterococci are known to be very well receptive for conjugation (Clewell & Weaver, 1989), but are also successful donor organisms for the transfer of antibiotic resistance genes to unrelated enterococci (Rice et al., 1998), lactobacilli (Shrago & Dobrogosz, 1988), other Gram-positives including *Bacillus subtilis* (Christie et al., 1987), *Staphylococcus* (Young et al., 1987) and *Listeria* spp. (Charpentier et al., 1997; Perreten et al., 1997b), and even Gram-negative bacteria (Courvalin, 1994). Moreover, the transfer of conjugative elements, including a plasmid-encoded kanamycin resistance and a transposon-encoded tetracycline and erythromycin resistance (Doucet-Populaire et al., 1991), were shown to be transferable from *E. faecalis* to *Escherichia coli* and *Listeria monocytogenes*, respectively, in the digestive tract of mice. In contrast, reports of conjugative transfer of antibiotic resistance genes in other LAB are rare. Two *in vivo* studies were performed, to examine the possibility of conjugative transfer between native Gram-positive members of the gut. Therefore, the broad host range conjugative plasmid pAMβ1 was transferred in vitro to *L. reuteri* (Morelli et al., 1988) and *L. lactis* (Igimi et al., 1996) and administered orally or using gastric intubation to mice. By analysis of faecal content, plasmid transfer to *E. faecalis* was observed in both studies.

In order to fully understand the extent to which LAB strains transfer resistance genes in the natural environment, it is essential to study genetic exchange in this context. Toomey et al., (2009) reported on the ability of wild-type antibiotic resistance determinants [*erm*(B) and *tet*(M)], present in LAB strains isolated from food sources, to be transferred to recipient strains. In vitro mating, using a traditional filter mating technique, showed that all four LAB mating pairs transferred their resistance determinants at high frequencies. By employing two in vivo models, an alfalfa sprout plant and an animal rumen model Toomey et al.., (2009) demonstrated the transfer of resistance determinants between all four LAB mating pairs in these models. Previously, in vivo transfer between LAB has only been shown in the gastrointestinal tracts of gnotobiotic rats (Jacobsen et al., 2007) and mice (McConnell et al., 1991; Morelli et al., 1988). The transfer frequencies have been observed to increase when the animals have received the antibiotic in question at subtherapeutic levels (Igimi et al., 1996; Licht et al., 2003; Salyers & Shoemaker 1996) in their drinking water or feed, suggesting that increasing the antibiotic pressure can amplify the transfer of antibiotic resistance between bacterial species. All of these above studies indicate that antibiotic resistant factors may be transferred from food related bacterium species (LAB) to other, potentially pathogenic species. The risks associated need to be considered, in light of the increasing concerns related to food as a potential reservoir for antibiotic resistance determinants.

6. Antibiotic resistance/susceptibility patterns of specific LAB genera applicable as probiotics

Some features appeared to be shared by the majority of LAB; in particular, it was reported that most LAB species are resistant to metronidazole and that they are all intrinsically resistant to sulphonamides and trimethoprim, while they are usually susceptible to piperacillin and piperacillin plus tazobactam. On the other hand, clear differences were highlighted among different LAB genera, although well-defined species-specific profiles were not always identifiable. A high resistance to cefoxitin was acknowledged for *Lactococcus*, *Leuconostoc*, and *Lactobacillus*, whereas, as regards vancomycin, *Leuconostoc*, *Pediococcus* and most lactobacilli species were recognised as intrinsically resistant and most *Lactococcus* isolates as highly susceptible.

Lactobacilli widely used in starter cultures or as probiotics in dairy products enter human intestines in large numbers and there interact with the intestinal microbiota (Teuber et al., 1999). Therefore they have the potential to serve as hosts for antibiotic-resistance genes, with the risk of transferring the genes to opportunistic or pathogenic bacteria. Routine antibiotic susceptibility testing has been advocated as an essential selection criterion for potentially starter or probiotic *Lactobacillus* cultures (Charteris & Kelly, 1993). The *Lactobacillus* species have been found susceptible to many cell wall synthesis inhibitors, like penicillins and ampicillin (Danielsen & Wind 2003, Coppola et al., 2005), in contrast to glycopeptides such as vancomycin, most *Lactobacillus* species, excluding obligate heterofermentative species, have been found to be resistant to these types of antibiotics. However, the resistance towards vancomycin has been demonstrated being as intrinsic (Tynkkynen et al., 1998) due the presence of D-alanine: D-alanine ligase-related enzymes (Elisha & Courvalin, 1995) and should not be compared with transmissible, plasmid-mediated resistance found in enterococci (Leclercq et al., 1992). As a general rule, lactobacilli have a high natural resistance to bacitracin, cefoxitin, ciprofloxacin, fusidic acid, kanamycin, gentamicin, metronidazole, nitrofurantoin, norfloxacin, streptomycin, sulphadiazine, teicoplanin (Danielsen & Wind, 2003). In addition, resistance against inhibitors of nucleic acid synthesis, such as trimethoprim, seems to be intrinsic, although further characterizations are required on this topic (Ammor et al., 2007). Resistance to tetracycline has been observed more often among *Lactobacillus* species, and it has been shown to have a wide range of MICs (Korhonen et al., 2008), also with a multimodal distribution of MICs, probably due to the extensive variability of tetracycline resistance mechanisms conferring diverse levels of susceptibility (Roberts, 2005). Especially with tetracycline, molecular methods should be applied in order to reveal the nature of resistance, i.e. is it due to intrinsic mechanisms, mutation or added, mobile genes.

Screening of antibiotic-resistance profile among *Lactobacillus* strains used in dairy products such as probiotics or as starters is now tending to become systematic. Coppola et al., (2005) pointed out that all of 63 *L. rhamnosus* strains isolated from Parmigiano Reggiano cheese showed resistance to six antibiotics (cefixime, vancomycin, neomycin, enoxacin, peflxacin, and sulphamethoxazole plus trimetoprim). Investigating the current antibiotic-resistance situation in microbial food additives in Switzerland, Kastner et al., (2006) determined that among 74 *Lactobacillus* isolates applicable as starter or probiotic cultures, two antibiotic resistances were detected in probiotic cultures. The genetic base of those resistances was confirmed; the tetracycline resistance gene tet(W) in *L. reuteri* SD 2112 (residing on a plasmid) and the lincosamide resistance gene lnu(A) in *L. reuteri* SD 2112. The similar trend was noticed in study of Katla et al., (2001). Only one of the 189 *Lactobacillus* strains isolated from Norwegian dairy products such as yoghurt, sour cream, fermented milk and cheese was classified as high level resistant to streptomycin. In contrast, a study conducted on "home-made" spanish cheese (Serena, Gamonedo, Cabrales) revealed the presence of lactobacilli resistant to penicillin G, cloxacillin, streptomycin, gentamycin, tetracycline, erythromycin and chloramphenicol (Herrero et al., 1996).

L. lactis strains were sensitive to amikacin, ampicillin, 1st generation cephalosporin, chloramphenicol, erythromycin, gentamicin, imipenem, oxacillin, penicillin, pipericillin, sulphonamide, tetracycline, trimethoprim/sulfomethoxazole, and vancomycin (de Fabrizio et al., 1994). A slightly lowered susceptibility was observed towards carbenicillin, ciprofloxacin, dicloxacillin and norfloxacin. Intrinsic resistances were recorded towards colistin, fosfomycin, pipemidic acid and rifamycin. Orberg & Sandine (1985) demonstrated that investigated strains of *L. lactis* subsp. *cremoris* and subsp. *lactis* were all resistant to thrimethoprim and almost all to sulphathiazole. Resistance to gentamicin, kanamycin, lincomycin, neomycin, rifampin and streptomycin varied.

The enterococcal strains are naturally tolerant to β-lactams, cephalosporins, lincosamides and polymyxins. A specific cause for concern and a factor contributing to the pathogenesis of enterococci is the resistance they acquire to aminoglycosides, tetracyclines, macrolides, chloramphenicol, penicillin, and ampicillin (Gray et al., 1991) and their capacity to exchange genetic information by conjugation. Enterococcal food isolates (mainly *E. faecalis* and *E. faecium*) were analysed for resistances to a broader range of different antibiotics using phenotypic susceptibility testing, both in raw meat (Knudtson & Hartman, 1993; Quednau et al., 1998) and fermented milk and meat products (Franz et al., 2001; Teuber & Perreten, 2000). Their data suggest a high prevalence of (multiple) antibiotic resistant enterococci in foods, which nevertheless were mostly susceptible to the clinically relevant antibiotics ampicillin and vancomycin. Enterococci from European cheeses, mainly belonging to *E. feacalis* and *E. faecium*, are susceptible to different antibiotics in different proportions (Teuber et al., 1999; Franz et al., 2001). From the study of European cheeses Teuber et al. (1999) ascertained that the incidence for vancomycin resistance among enterococcal isolates was as low as 4%. When Franz et al. (2001) tested 47 *E. faecalis* strains, isolated mostly from cheeses, they were all susceptible to vancomycin. Bulajić & Mijačević (2011) pointed out that among enterococcal strains isolated from autochthonous Sombor cheese, only one strain showed vancomycin resistance. In contrast, Citak et al. (2004) have shown resistance to vancomycin among the population of enterococci isolated from Turkish white cheeses and was found in 96.8% of *E. faecalis* isolates, and 76% of *E. faecium* strains. The susceptibility to vancomycin is of great importance as this glycopeptide antibiotic is one of the last therapeutic options in clinical therapy.

Bifidobacteria are generally considered to be food-grade organisms that do not impose health risks on the consumer or the environment. Nevertheless, it should be noted that rare cases of *Bifidobacterium*-associated gastrointestinal and extra-intestinal infections have been described. In contrast to susceptibility testing of clinically important bacteria, no standard procedures are specifically dedicated to the determination of resistance phenotypes in *Bifidobacterium* strains. To date, a large variety of methods and protocols have been described for antimicrobial susceptibility testing of bifidobacteria, including agar (overlay) disc diffusion, broth dilution and agar dilution. In addition, various growth media have been used primarily on the basis that they meet the complex growth requirements of bifidobacteria. As opposed to conventional susceptibility test media such as Mueller-Hinton and Iso-Sensitest medium none of these *Bifidobacterium*-specific media are well defined in terms of minimal interaction between specific antimicrobial agents and growth medium components. Recently, a newly defined medium formulation referred to as the Lactic acid bacteria Susceptibility test Medium supplemented with cysteine (LSM + cysteine) was proposed for susceptibility testing of bifidobacteria.

Moubareck et al., (2005) were tested the fifty bifidobacterial strains, isolated from humans, animals or probiotic products for susceptibility to 30 antibiotics by disc diffusion test on *Brucella* agar supplemented with 5% laked sheep blood and vitamin K (1mg/L). All strains were sensitive to penicilins: penicillin G, amoxicillin, piperacillin, ticarcillin, imipenem, and usually anti-Gram-positive antibiotics (macrolides, clindamycin, vancomycin and teicoplanin). Most isolates (70%) were resistant to fusidic acid and, as expected, high resistance profile were observed for aminoglycosides. Potentially acquired resistance was only observed against tetracycline and minocycline, in 14% of the tested strains. For the first time, Moubareck et al., (2005) identified *tet*(W) as the gene responsible for tetracycline resistance in *Bifidobacterium pseudocatenulatum* and *B. bifidum*. Interestingly, the tet(W) gene was previously found in human *B. longum* and three genera of rumen obligate anaerobes, suggesting intergenic transfer of this resistance gene between anaerobic bacteria (Scott et al., 2000). In the study of Masco et al., (2006), the LSM + cysteine medium was used to determine the susceptibility profile of 100 bifidobacterial isolates (strains of animal and human origin, isolates from probiotic products and strains from clinical sources) to 15 common antimicrobial agents. All strains tested were susceptible to amoxicillin, chloramphenicol, erythromycin, quinupristin/dalfopristin, rifampicin and vancomycin. The date from this study (Masco et al., 2006) also reinforce earlier observations indicating that bifidobacteria are intrinsically resistant to gentamicin, sulfamethoxazole and polymyxin B. Susceptibility to trimethoprim, trimethoprim/sulfamethoxazole, ciprofloxacin, clindamycin, tetracycline and minocycline was variable. The tet(W) gene was responsible for tetracycline resistance in 15 strains including 7 probiotic isolates belonging to the taxa *Bifidobacterium animalis* subsp. *lactis* and *B. bifidum*. This gene was present in a single copy on the chromosome and did not appear to be associated with the conjugative transposon TnB1230 previously found in tet(W)-containing *Butyrivibrio fibrisolvens*.

7. Conclusion

The selective pressure imposed by the use of antimicrobial agents plays a key role in the emergence of resistant bacteria. Under selective pressure, the numbers of these bacteria increase and some may transmit their resistance genes to other members of the population.. The food chain was considered as the main route of transmission of antibiotic resistant lactic acid bacteria between the animals and human population. Fermented dairy products and fermented meats, which are not heat-treated before consumption, provide a vehicle for antibiotic resistant LAB with a direct link between the animal indigenous microflora and the human gastrointestinal tract. There is the potential health risk, due to the transfer of antibiotic resistance genes from LAB to bacteria in the human gastrointestinal tract, especially to pathogenic bacteria.

Lactic acid bacteria used as starter cultures or probiotic bacteria, enter into human intestines in large number where they interact with the intestinal microflora. Since there has been a significant rise in the consumption of probiotic products, it is important that probiotics are well documented regarding antibiotic resistance profile. The ability to transfer antibiotic resistance genes must be considered as an important parameter for the selection of the probiotic strains. Continuous attention should be paid to the selection of probiotic strains free of transferable antibiotic-resistance determinants. Without doubt, the uncontrolled use of antimicrobial agents in farming practice has assisted the spread of resistant organisms. Therefore a much stricter control over the use of these drugs is essential.

8. Acknowledgment

This work was supported by Ministry of Education and Science of Republic of Serbia (Project No. 46010).

9. References

Agostoni, C., Axelsson, I., Goulet, O., Koletzko, B., Michaelsen, K.F. & Puntis, J. W., (2004). Prebiotic Oligosaccharides in Dietetic Products for Infants: A Commentary by the ESPGHAN Committee on Nutrition. *Journal of Pediatric Gastroenterology Nutrition,* Vol. 39, pp. 465-473.

Ammor, M. S., Florez, A. B. & Mayo, B. (2007). Antibiotic Resistance in Nonenterococcal Lactic Acid Bacteria and Bifidobacteria. *Food Microbiology,* Vol. 24, pp. 559-570.

Ammor, M. S., Florez, A. B., van Hoek, A. H., de Los Reyes-Gavilan, C. G., Aarts, H. J., Margolles, A. & Mayo, B. (2008). Molecular Characterization of Intrinsic and Acquired Antibiotic Resistance in Lactic Acid Bacteria and Bifidobacteria. *Journal of Molecular Microbiology and Biotechnology,* Vol. 14, pp. 6-15.

Andrews, J. M. (2001). BSAC Standardized Disc Susceptibility Testing Method. *Journal of Antimicrobial Chemotherapy,* Vol. 48 Suppl .1, pp. 43-57.

Anonym (2007). Methods for Antimicrobial Susceptibility Testing of Anaerobic Bacteria. Approved Standard. CLSI document M11-A7. *Applied and Environmental Microbiology,* 72, pp. 1729-1738.

Aquilanti, L., Silvestri, G., Zannini, E., Osimani, A., Santarelli, S. & Clementi, F. (2007). Phenotypic, Genotypic and Technological Characterization of Predominant Lactic Acid Bacteria in Pecorino Cheese from Central Italy. *Journal of Applied Microbiology,* Vol. 103, pp. 948-960.

Arias, C. A., Vallejo, M., Reyes, J., Panesso, D., Moreno, J., Castaneda, E., Villegas, M. V., Murray, B. E. & Quinn, J. P. (2008). Clinical and Microbiological Aspects of Linezolid Resistance Mediated by the *cfr* Gene Encoding a 23S rRNA Methyltransferaze. *Journal of Clinical Microbiology,* Vol. 46, pp. 892-896.

Axelsson, L.T., Ahrne, S., Andersson, M.C. & Stahl, S.R. (1988). Identification and Cloning of a Plasmid-Encoded Erythromycin Resistance Determinant from *Lactobacillus reuteri* G4. *Plasmid*, Vol. 20, pp. 171-174.

Backhed, F.; Ley, R.E.; Sonnenburg, J.L.; Peterson, D.A. & Gordon, J.I. (2005). Host-Bacterial Mutualism in the Hhuman Intestine. *Science*, Vol. 307, pp. 1915–1920.

Begley, M, Hill, C., & Gahan, C. G. M., (2006). Bile Salt Hydrolase Activity in Probiotics. *Applied and Environmental Microbiology*, Vol. 72, No. 3, pp. 1729-1738.

Bengmark, S. (1998). Ecological Control of the Gastrointestinal Tract. Rhe Role of Probiotic Flora. *Gut*, Vol. 27, pp. 2-7.

Bennet, R., Eriksson, M., Nord, C.E. & Zetterström, R. (1986). Fecal Bacterial Microflora of Newborn Infants During Intensive Care Management and Treatment with Five Antibiotic Regimens. *Pediatric Infectious Disease*, Vol. 5, pp. 533-539.

Beresford, T. P., Fitzimons, N. A., Brenan, N. L. & Cogan, T. M. (2001). Recent Advances in Cheese Microbiology. *International Dairy Journal*, Vol. 11, pp. 256-274.

Bernet, M. F., Brassart, D., Neeser, J. R. & Servin, A. L. (1994). *Lactobacillus acidophillus* LA 1 Binds to Cultured Human Intestinal Cell Lines and Inhibits Cell Attachment and Cell Invasion by Enterovirulent Bacteria. *Gut*, Vol. 35, pp. 483-489.

Bernet, M. F., Brassart, D., Neeser, J.R. & Servin, A.L. (1993). Adhesion of Human Bifidobacterial Strains to Cultured Human Intestinal Epithelial Cells and Inhibition of Enteropathogen–Cell Interactions. *Applied and Enviromental Microbiology.*, Vol. 59, pp. 4121–4128.

Berrada, N., Lemeland, J.F., Laroche, G., Thovenot P. & Piaia,M. (1991). *Bifidobactrium* from Fermented Milk: Survival During Gastic Transit. *Journal of Dairy Science*, Vol. 74, pp. 409-413.

Black, F. T. Anderson, P.L., Oeskov, J., Gaarskev, K. & Laulund, S. (1989). Prophylactic Efficacy of Lactobacilli on Traveler's Diarrhea. *Travel Medicine*, Vol. 7, pp. 333-335.

Bulajić, S. & Mijačević, Z. (2011). Antimicrobial Susceptibility of Lactic Acid Bacteria Isolated from Sombor Cheese. *Acta Veterinaria*, Vol. 61, No. 2-3, pp. 247-258.

Cataloluk, O. & Gogebakan, B. (2004). Presence of Drug Resistance in Intestinal Lactobacilli of Dairy and Human Origin in Turkey. *FEMS Microbiology Letters*, Vol. 236, pp. 7-12.

Charpentier, E. & Courvalin, P. (1997). Emergence of the Trimethoprim Resistance gene *dfr*D in *Listeria monocytogenes* BM4293. *Antimicrobial Agents and Chemoterapy*, Vol. 41, pp. 1134-1136.

Charteris, W. P., Kelly, P. M., Morelli, L. & Collins, J. K. (1998). Antibiotic Susceptibility of Potentially Probiotic *Lactobacillus* Species. *Journal of Food Protection*, Vol. 61, pp. 1636-1643.

Charteris, W. P. & Kelly, P. M. (1993). In Vitro Antibiotic Susceptibility of Potentially Probiotic Lactobacilli and Bifidobacteria. In *Second Annual Report, EU FLAIR Project No. AGRF-CT91-0053* ed. Morelli, L. Brussels: Commission of the European Communities.

Christie, P. J., Korman, R. Z., Zahler, S. A., Adsit, J. C. & Dunny, G. M. (1987). Two Conjugation Systems Associated with *Streptococcus faecalis* plasmid pCF10: Identification of a Conjugative Transposon that Transfers Between *S. facealis* and *Bacillus subtilis*. *Journal of Bacteriology*, Vol. 169, pp. 2529-2536.

Citak, S., Yucel, N. & Orhan, S. (2004). Antibiotic Resistance and Incidence of *Enterococcus* Species in Turkish White Cheese. *International Journal of Dairy Technology*, Vol. 57, pp. 27-31.

Claesson, M. J., van Sinderen, D. & O'Toole, P. W. (2007). The genus *Lactobacillus* - A Genomic Basis of Understanding its Diversity. *FEMS Microbiology Letters*, Vol. 269, No.1, pp. 22-28.

Clementi, F. & Aquilanti, F. A. (2011). Recent Investigations and Updated Criteria for the Assessment of Antibiotic Resistance in Food Lactic Acid Bacteria. *Anaerobe* (2011) 1-5, *Article in Press.*

Clewell, D. B. Weaver, K. E. (1989). Sex Pheromones and Plasmid Transfer in *Enterococcus faecalis*. *Plasmid*, Vol. 21, pp. 175-184.

Coppa, G., Bruni, S., Morelli, L., Soldi, S. & Gabrielli, O. (2004). The First Prebiotics in Humans: Human Milk Oligosaccharides. *Journal of Clinical Gastroenterology*, Vol. 38, pp. 80-83.

Coppola, R., Succi, M., Tremonte, P., Reale, A., Salzano, G. & Sorrentino, E. (2005). Antibiotic Susceptibility of *Lactobacillus rhamnosus* Strains Isolated from Parmigiano Reggiano Cheese. *Lait*, Vol. 85, pp. 193-204.

Courvalin, P. (1994). Transfer of Antibiotic Resistance Genes Between Gram-positive and Gram-negative Bacteria. *Antimicrobial Agents and Chemotherapy*, Vol. 38, pp. 1447-1451.

Cummings, J. H., Gibson, G. R. & Macfarlane, G. T. (1989). Qualitative Estimates of Fermentation in the Hind Gut of Man. *Acta Veterinaria Scandinavica* Suppl. Vol. 86, pp. 76-82.

Curragh, H. J. & Collins, M. A. (1992). High-levels of Spontaneous Drug-Resistance in *Lactobacillus*. *Journal of Applied Bacteriology*, Vol. 73, pp. 31-36.

Danielsen, M. & Wind, A. A. (2003). Susceptibility of *Lactobacillus* spp. to Antimicrobial Agents. *International Journal of Food Microbiology*, Vol. 82, pp. 1-11.

Danielsen, M. (2002). Characterization of the Tetracycline Resistance Plasmid pMD5057 from *Lactobacillus plantarum* 5057 Reveals a Composite Structure. *Plasmid*, Vol. 48, pp. 98-103.

Davidson, B. E., Kordias, N., Dobos, M. & Hillier, A. J. (1996). Genomic Organization of Lactic Acid Bacteria. *Antonie Van Leeuwenhoek International Journal of General and Molecular Microbiology*, Vol. 70, pp. 161-183.

de Leeuw, E., Li, X. & Lu, W. (2006). Binding Characteristics of the *Lactobacillus brevis* ATCC 8287 Surface Layer to Extracellular Matrix Proteins. *FEMS Microbiology Letters*, Vol. 260, pp. 210-215.

deFabrizio, S. V., Parada, J. L. & Torriani, S. (1994). Antibiotic Resistance of *Lactococcus lactis* - an Approach of Genetic Determinants Location through the Model System. *Microbiologie-Aliments-Nutritions*, Vol. 12, pp. 307-315.

Doucet-Populaire, F., Trieu-Cuot, P., Dosbaa, I., Andremont, A. & Courvalin, P. (1991). Inducible transfer of conjugative transposon Tn*1545* from *Enterococcus faecalis* to *Listeria monocytogenes* in the digestive tracts of gnotobiotic mice. *Antimicrobial Agents and Chemotherapy*, Vol. 35, pp. 185-187.

Dunne, C., O'Mahony, L., Murphy, L., Thornton, G., Morrissey, D., O'Halloran, S., Feeney, M., Flynn, S., Fitzgerald G., Daly, C., Kiely, B., O 'Sullivan, G.C., Shanahan, F. & Collins, J.K. (2001). *In vitro* Selection Criteria for Probiotic Bacteria of Human

Origin: Correlation with *In vivo* Findings. *American Journal of Clinical Nutrition,* Vol. 73, pp. 386-392.

Eaton, T. J. & Gasson, M. J. (2001). Molecular Screening of *Enterococcus* Virulence Determinants and Potential for Genetic Exchange between Food and Medical Isolates. *Applied and Environmental Microbiology,* Vol. 67, pp. 1628-1635.

EFSA. (2008). Technical Guidance Prepared by the Panel on Additives and Products or Substances used in Animal Feed (FEEDAP) on the Update of the Criteria Used in the Assessment of Bacterial Resistance to Antibiotics of Human and Veterinary Importance. *The EFSA Journal,* pp. 1-15.

Elisha, B. G. & Courvalin, P. (1995). Analysis of Genes Encoding Dalanine: d-Alanine Ligase-Related Enzymes in *Leuconostoc mesenteroides* and *Lactobacillus* spp. *Gene,* Vol. 152, pp. 79-83.

European Commissions (2005). Opinion of the Scientific Committee on Animal Nutrition on the Criteria for Assessing the Safety of Micro-organisms Resistant to Antibiotics of Human Clinical and Veterinary Importance. European Commissions, Health and Consmer protection Directorate General, Directorate C, Scientific Opinions, Brussels, Belgium.

Fons, M., Hege, T., Lafire, M., Raibaud, P., Ducluzeau, R. & Maguin, E. (1997). Isolation and Characterization pf a Plasmid from *Lactobacillus fermentum* Connferring Erythromycin Resistance. *Plasmid,* Vol. 37, pp. 199-203.

Fooks, L. J., Fuller, R. & Gibson, G. R. (1999). Prebiotics, Probiotic and Human Gut Microbiology. *International Dairy Journal,* Vol. 9, pp. 53-61.

Franz, C. M. A. P., Holzapfel, W. H. & Stiles, M. E. (1999). Enterococci at the Crossroads of Food Safety. *International Journal of Food Microbiology,* Vol. 47, pp. 193-197.

Franz, C. M., Muscholl-Silberhorn, A. B., Yousif, N.M.K., Vancanneyt, M., Swings, J. & Holzapfel, W. H. (2001). Incidence of Virulence Factors and Antibiotic Resistance among Enterococci Isolated from Food. *Applied and Environmental Microbiology,* Vol. 67, pp. 4385-4389.

Franz, C.M.A.P., Specht I., Haberer P. & Holzapfel W. H. (2001a). Bile Salt Hydrolase Activity of Enterococci Isolated from Food: Screening and Quantitative Determination. *Journal of Food Protection,* Vol. 64, No 5, pp. 725-729.

Fuller, R. (1992). *Probiotics: The scientific basis,* ISBN 0-412-40850-3, Chapman & Hall, London,

Gardnier, E. G., Ross, P. R., Kellz, M. P., Stanton, K., Collins, K. K. & Fitzgerald, G. (2002). Microbiology of Therapeutic Milks, In: *Dairy Microbiology Handbook, Third Edition,* R. K. Robinson (Ed.), Wiley-Interscience, Inc., 431-478, ISBN 0-471-38596-4, New York, USA.

Garg, S. K. & Mital, B. K. (1991). Enterococci i n Milk and Milk Products. *Critical Reviews in Microbiology,* Vol. 18, pp. 15-45.

Gevers, D., Huys, G. & Swings, J. (2003). In Vitro Conjugal Transfer of Tetracycline Resistance from Lactobacillus Isolates to Other Gram-positive Bacteria. *FEMS Microbiology Letters,* Vol. 225, pp. 125-130.

Gray, C. M., Stewart, D. & Pedler, S. J. (1991). Species Identification and Antibiotic Susceptibility Testing of Enterococci Isolated from Hospitalized Patients. *Antimicrobial Agents and Chemotherapy,* Vol 35, pp. 1943-1945.

Gronlund, M. M., Lehtonen, O. P., Erola, E.& Kero, P. (1999). Fecal Microflora in Healthy Infants Born by Different Methods of Delivery: Permenent Changes in Intestinal

Flora after Cesarean Delivery. *Journal of Pediatric Gastroeneterological Nutrition*, Vol. 28, pp. 19-25.

Guarner, F. & Schaafsma, G. J. (1998). Probiotics. *International Journal of Food Microbiology*, Vol. 39, pp. 237-238.

Hamilton-Miller, J. M. T & Shah, S. (1998). Vancomycin Susceptibility as an Aid to the Identification of Lactobacilli. *Letters in Applied Microbiology*, Vol. 26, pp. 153-154.

Herrero, M., Mayo, B. Ganzales, B. & Suarez, J.E. (1996). Evaluation of Technologically Important Traits in Lactic Acid Bacteria Isolated from Spontaneous Fermentations. *Journal of Applied Bacteriology*, Vol. 81, pp. 567-570.

Herreros, M. A., Fresno, J.M., Gonzalez Prieto, M. J. & Tornadijo, M. E. (2003). Technological Characterization of Lactic Acid Bacteria Isolated from Armada Cheese (a Spanish Goat 's milk Cheese). *International Dairy Journal*, Vol.13, pp. 469-479.

Hevey, P. & Rowland, I. (1999). The Gut Microflora of The Developing Infant: Microbiology and Metabolism. *Microbial Ecology in Health and Disease*. Vol. 11, pp. 75-83.

Hummel, A.S.; Hertel, C.; Holzapfel, W.H. & Franz, C. (2007). Antibiotic Resistances of Starter and Probiotic Strains of Lactic Acid Bacteria. *Applied and Enviromental Microbiology*, Vol.73, pp. 730-739.

Huys, G., D'Haene, K. & Swings, J. (2002). Influence of the Culture Medium on Antibiotic Susceptibility Testing of Food-Associated Lactic Acid Bacteria with the Agar Overlay Disc Diffusion Method. *Letters in Applied Microbiology*, Vol. 34, pp. 402-406.

Igimi, S., Ryu, C.H., Park, S.H., Sasaki, Y., Sasaki, T. & Kumagai, S.. (1996). Transfer of Conjugative Plasmid pAM beta 1 from *Lactococcus lactis* to Mouse Intestinal Bacteria. *Letters of Applied Microbiology*, Vol. 23, pp. 31-35.

Ishiwa, H & Iwata, S. (1980). Drug Resistance in *Lactobacillus fermentum*. *Journal of General and Applied Microbiology*, Vol. 26, pp. 71-74.

Jacobsen, I., Wicks, A., Hammer, K., Huys, G., Gevers, D. & Andersen, S.R. (2007). Horizontal Transfer of tet(M) and erm(B) Resistance Plasmids from Food Strains of *Lactobacillus plantarum* to *Enterococcus faecalis* JH2-2 in The Gastrointestinal Tract of Gnotobiotic Rats. *FEMS Microbiology Ecology*, Vol. 59, pp. 158-166.

Kandler, O. & Weiss, N. (1989). Genus *Lactobacillus*, In: *Bergeys Manual of Systematic Bacteriology*, P. H. Snearh, N. S. Mair, M. E. Sharpe, J. G. Holt (Ed.), Vol. 2, 1418-1434, ISBN 0-683-07893-3, Williams & Wilkins Baltimore, USA.

Kastner, S., Parreten, V., Bleuler, H., Hugenschmidt, G., Lacroix, C & Meile, L. (2006) Antibiotic Susceptibility Patterns and Resistance Genes of Starter Culture and Probiotic bacteria Used in Food. *Systematic and Applied Microbiology*, Vol. 29, pp. 145-55.

Katla, A. K., Kruse, H., Johnsen, G. & Herikstad, H. (2001). Antimicrobial Susceptibility of Starter Culture Bacteria Used in Norwegian Dairy Products. *International Journal of Food Microbiology*, Vol. 67, pp. 147-152.

Klare, I., Konstabel, C., Werner, G., Huys, G., Vankerckhoven, V., Kahlmetrr, G., Hildebrandt, B., Muller Bertling , S., Witte, W & Goossens, H. (2007). Antimicrobial Susceptibilities of *Lactobacillus, Pediococcus* and *Lactococcus* Human Isolates and Culture Intended for Probiotic or Nutritional Use. *Journal of Antimicrobial Chemotherapy*, Vol. 59, pp. 900-912.

Knudtson, L. M. & Hartman, P.A. (1993). Antibiotic Resistance among Enterococcal Isolates from Environmental and Clinical Sources. *Journal of Food Protection,* Vol. 56, pp. 489-492.

Koll, P., Mandar, R.., Marcotte, H., Leibur, E., Mikelsaar, M. & Hammarstrom, L. (2008). Characterization of Oral Lactobacilli as Potential Probiotics for Oral Health. *Oral Microbiol Immunol.,* Vol. 23, No 2, pp. 139-147.

Korhonen, J. M. Sclivagnotis, Y. & von Wright, A. (2007). Characterization of Dominant Cultivable Lactobacilli and their Antibiotic Resistance Profiles from Fecal Samples of Weaning Piglets. *Journal of Applied Microbiology,* Vol. 103, pp. 2496-2503.

Leclercq, R., Dutka-Malen, S., Brisson-Noel, A., Molinas, C., Derlot, E., Arthur, M., Duval, J. & Courvalin, P. (1992). Resistance of Enterococci to Aminoglycosides and Glycopeptides. *Clinical Infectious Diseases,* Vol. 15, pp. 495-501.

Levy, S. B. (1986). Ecology of Antibiotic Resistance Determinants. In:Levy, SB, Novick, RP (eds) *Antibiotic resistance genes: ecology, transfer and expression.* Cold Spring Harbor Press, New York, pp. 17-29.

Lewis, S. J. & Freedman, A. R. (1998). The Use of Biotherapeutic Agents in the Prevention and Treatment of Gastrointestinal Disease. *Alimentary Pharmacology and Therapeutics,* Vol. 12, pp. 807-822.

Licht, T. R., Struve, C., Christensen, B. B., Poulsen, R. L., Molin, S. & Krogfelt, K. A. (2003). Evidence of Increased Spread and Establishment of Plasmid RP4 In The Intestine Under Sub-inhibitory Tetracycline concentrations. *FEMS Microbiology Ecology,* Vol. 44, pp. 217-233.

Lin, C. F., Fung, Z .F, Wu, C. L. & Chung, T. C. (1996). Molecular Characterization of a Plasmidborne (pTC82) Chloramphenicol Resistance Determinant (cat-Tc) from *Lactobacillus reuteri. Plasmid,* Vol. 36, pp. 116-124.

Liong, M.T. & Shah, N.P. (2005). Bile Salt Deconjugation Ability, Bile Salt Hhydrolase Activity and Cholesterol Co-precipitation Ability of Lactobacilli Strains. *International Dairy Jounal,* Vol. 15, No 4, pp. 391-398.

Lönnermark, E. (2010). Lactobacilli in the Normal Microbiota and Probiotic Effects of *Lactobacillus plantarum. PhD Thesis,* Department of Infectious medicine, Sahlgrenska Academy, University of Gothenburg, Sweden.

Masco, I., Van Hoorde, De Brandt, E., Swings, J. & Huys, G. (2006). Antimicrobial Susceptibility of *Bifidobacterium* Strains from Humans, Animals and Probiotic Products. *Journal of Antimicrobial Chemotherapy,* Vol. 58, pp. 85-94

Mathur, S. & Singh, R. (2005). Antibiotic Resistance in Lactic Acid Bacteria-a review. *International Journal of Food Microbiology,* Vol. 105, pp. 281-95.

Mattila, T. & Saarela, M. (2000). Probiotic Functional Foods. In: *Functional foods,* Williams and Gibson R.G. (Ed), 287-313. CRC Press LLC. Boca Raton, Boston, New York, Washington, DC.

McConnell, M. A., Mercer, A. A. & Tannock, G. W. (1991). Transfer of Plasmid pAM-1 between Members of Microflora Inhabiting the Murine Digestive Tract and Modification of the Plasmid in a *Lactobacillus reuteri* Host. *Microbial Ecology in Health and Disease,* Vol. 4, pp. 343-355.

Modler, H. V., McKellar, R. C. & Yaguchi, M. (1990). Bifidobacteria and Bifidogenic Factors. *Canadian Institute of Food Science and Technology Journal,* Vol. 23, pp. 29-41.

Morelli, L., Sarra, P.G. & Bottazzi, V. (1988). In Vivo Transfer of pAM-beta-1 from *Lactobacillus reuteri* to *Enterococcus faecalis*. *Journal of Applied Bacteriology*, Vol. 65, pp. 371-375.

Moubareck, C., Gavini, F., Vaugien, L., Butel, M. J. & Doucet-Populaire, F. (2005). Antimicrobial Susceptibility of Bifidobacteria. *Journal of Antimicrobial Chemotherapy*, Vol. 55, pp. 38-44.

Mountzouris, K.C; McCartney, A.L; & Gibson, G.R. (2002). Intestinal Microflora of Human Infants and Current Trends for its Nutritional Modulation. *British Journal of Nutrition*, Vol. 87, pp. 405–420.

Murphy, E., Murphy, C. & O'Mahony, L. (2009). Influence of the Gut Microbiota with Aging. In: *Microbiology and Aging: Clinical Manifestations*, S.L. Percival, (Ed.), Springer-Verlag, ISBN 1588296407, New York, USA.

Murray, B. E., An, F. Y. & Clewell, D. B. (1988). Plasmid and Pheromone Response of the Betalactamase Producer *Streptococcus (Enterococcus) faecalis* HH22. *Antimicrobial Agents and Chemotherapy*, Vol. 32, pp. 547-551.

Murray, P. R., Baron, E. J., Jorgensen, J. H., Pfaller, M. A. & Yolken R. H. (2003). *Manual of Clinical Microbiology*, American Society for Microbiology, Washington.

National Committee for Clinical Laboratory Standards (NCCLS). (2002). Performance Standards for Antimicrobial Susceptibility Testing, *Twelfth informational supplement* (M100-S12)

Newburg, D.S. (2000). Oligosaccharides in Human Milk and Bacterial Colonization. *Journal of Pediatric Gastroenterological Nutrition*, Vol. 30, 2, pp. 8-17.

Normark, B. H. & Normark, S. (2002). Evolution and Spread of Antibiotic Resistance. *Journal of International Medicine*, Vol. 252, pp. 91-106

Ogawa, K., Ben, R.A., Pons, S., de Paolo, M. I. & Bustos Fernández, L. (1992). Volatile Fatty Acids, Lactic Acid, and pH in the Stools of Breast-fed and Bottlefed infants. *Journal of Pediatric Gastroenterological Nutrition*, Vol. 15, pp. 248-252.

Olsson-Liljequist, B., Larsson, P., Walder, M. & Miorner, H. (1997). Antimicrobial Susceptibility Testing in Sweden, III. Methodology for Susceptibility Testing in Sweden. *Scandinavian Journal of Infectious Disease*, 105S, pp. 13-23

Orberg, P. K. & Sandine, W.E. (1985). Survey of Antimicrobial Resistance in Lactic Streptococci. *Applied and Environmental Microbiology*, Vol. 49, pp. 538-542

Ouoba, L. I., Lei, V. & Jensen, L. B. (2008). Resistance of Potential Probiotic Lactic Acid Bacteria and Bifidobacteria of African and European Origin to Antimicrobials: Determination and Transferability of the Resistance Genes to Other Bacteria. *International Journal of Food Microbiology*, Vol. 121, pp. 217-224

Ouwehand, A. C. & Vesterlund, S. (2003). Health Aspects of Probiotics. *Drugs*, Vol. 6, pp. 573-580.

Ouwehand, A. C., Bianchi, Salvadori, B., Fonden, R., Mogensen, G., Salminen, S. & Sellara, R. (2003). Health Effects of Probiotics and Culture-Containing Dairy Products in Humans. *Bulliten of the International Dairy Federation*, Vol. 380, pp. 4-19.

Ouwehand, A. C., Tuomola, E. M., Tolkko, S. & Salminen, S. (2001). Assessment of Adhesion Properties of Novel Probiotic Strains to Human Intestinal Mucus. *International Journal of Food Microbiology*, Vol. 64, pp. 119-126.

Perreten, V., Schwarz, F., Cresta, L., Boeglin, M., Dasen, G. & Teuber, M. (1997a). Antibiotic Resistance Spread in Food. *Nature*, Vol. 389, pp. 801-802.

Perreten, V., Kolloffel, B. & Teuber, M. (1997b). Conjugal Transfer of the Tn*916*-like Transposon Tn*FO1* from *Enterococcus faecalis* Isolated from Cheese to Other Gram-positive Bacteria. *Systematic and Applied Microbiology*, Vol. 20, pp. 27-38.

Petrovic, T., Niksic, M. & Bringel, F. (2006). Strain Typing with ISLpl1 in Lactobacilli. *FEMS Microbiology Letters*, Vol.255, pp. 1-10.

Psoni, L., Tzanetakis, N. & Litopoulou-Tzanetaki, E. (2005). Microbiological Characteristics of Batzos, a Traditional Greek Cheese from Raw Goat's Milk. *Food Microbiology* Vol. 20, No. 5, pp. 575-582.

Quednau, M., Ahrne, S., Petersson, A.C. & Molin, G. (1998). Antibiotic-Resistant Strains of *Enterococcus* Isolated from Swedish and Danish Retailed Chicken and Pork. *Journal of Applied Microbiology*, Vol. 84, pp. 1163-1170

Radulović, Z. (2010). *Autochthonous Lactic Acid Bacteria as Starter Cultures*. Faculty of Agriculture University of Belgrade, ISBN 978-86-7843-081-9, Belgrade, Serbia.

Radulović, Z., Petrović, T., Nedović, V., Dimitrijević, S., Mirković, N., Petrušić, M. & Paunović, D. (2010a). Characterization of autochthonous *Lactobacillus paracasei* strains on potential probiotic ability. *Mljekarstvo*, Vol. 60, No.2, pp. 86-93.

Reuter, G. (2001). The *Lactobacillus* and *Bifidobacterium* Microflora of The Human Intestine: Composition and Succession. *Current Issues Intestinal Microbiology*, Vol. 2, pp. 43-53.

Rice, L. & Marshall, S. H. (1994). Insertions of IS256-like Element Flanking the Chromosomal Beta-lactamase Gene of *Enterococcus faecalis* CX19. *Antimicrobial Agents and Chemotherapy*, Vol. 38, pp. 693-701

Rice, L.B., Carias, L.L., Donskey, C.L. & Rudin, S.D. (1998). Transferable, Plasmid-Mediated VanB-type Glycopeptide Resistance in *Enterococcus faecium*. *Antimicrobial Agents and Chemotherapy*, Vol. 42, pp. 963-964

Roberts, M.C. (2005). Update on Acquired Tetracycline Resistance Genes. *FEMS Microbiology Letters*, Vol. 245, pp. 195-203

Rodriguez, C., Medici, M., Mozzi, F. & de Valdez, G. F. (2010). Therapeutic Effect of *Streptpcoccus thermophilus* CRL 1190 - Fermented Milk on Chronic Gastritis. *World Journal of Gastroenerology*, Vol. 16, pp. 1622-1630.

Ryan, K.A.; Jayaraman, T.; Daly, P.; Canchaya, C.; Curran, S.; Fang, F.; Quigley, E.M. & O'Toole, P.W. (2008) Isolation of Lactobacilli with Probiotic Properties from the Human Stomach. *Letters of Applied Microbiology*, Vol.47, pp. 269-274.

Saavedra, J. M., Bauman, N., Oung, I., Perman, J. & Yolken, R. (1994). Feeding of *Bifidobacterium bifidum* and *Streptococcus thermophilus* to Infants in Hospital for Prevention of Diarrhoea and Shedding of Rotavirus, *The Lancet*, Vol. 344, pp. 1046-1049.

Salminen, S., Nybom, S., Meriluoto, J., Carmen Collado, M., Vesterlund, S. & El-Nezami, H. 2010. Interaction of Probiotics and Pathogens—Benefits to Human Health? *Current Opinion in Biotehnology*, Vol. 21, pp. 157-167.

Salyers, A. A. & Shoemaker, N.B. (1996). Resistance Gene transfer in Anaerobes: New Insights, New problems. *Clinical Infectious Diseases*, Vol. 23 Suppl. 1, S36-43

Salyers, A. A. (1995). Antibiotic Resistance Transfer in the Mammalian Intestinal Tract: Implications for Human Health, *Food Safety and Biotechnology*, Heidelberg:Springer-Verlag, New York, USA.

Scardovi, V. (1986). Genus *Bifidobacterium*, In: *Bergeys Manual of Systematic Bacteriology*, P. H. Snearh, N. S. Mair, M. E. Sharpe, J. G. Holt (Ed.), Vol. 2, 1418-1434, ISBN 0-683-07893-3, Williams & Wilkins Baltimore, USA.

Scott, K. P., Melville, C.M., Barbosa, T.M. et al. (2000). Occurrence of the New Tetracycline Resistance Gene tet(W) in Bacteria from the Human Gut. *Antimicrobial Agents and Chemotherapy*, Vol. 44, pp. 775-777.

Shah, P. N. (2007). Functional Cultures and Health Benefits. *International Dairy Journal*, Vol. 17, pp. 1262-1277.

Shrago, A.W. & Dobrogosz, W.J. (1988). Conjugal Transfer of Group-B Streptococcal Plasmids and Comobilization of *Escherichia coli-Streptococcus* Shuttle Plasmids to *Lactobacillus plantarum*. *Applied and Environmental Microbiology*, Vol. 54, pp. 824-826.

Simpson, W. J., Hammond, J.R.M. & Miller, R.B. (1988). Avoparcin and Vancomycin-Useful Antibiotics for the Isolation of Brewery Lactic Acid Bacteria. *Journal of Applied Bacteriology*, Vol. 64, pp. 299-309.

Singer, R. S., Finch, R., Wegener, H.C., Bywater, R., Walters, J. & Lipstich, M. (2003). Antibiotic resistance - The Interplay Between antibiotic use in Animals and Human Beings. *Lancet Infectious Diseases*, Vol. 3, pp. 47-51.

Stanton, C., Gardiner, G., Meehan, H., Collins, J. K., Fitzgerald, G., Lynch, P. B. & Ross, R. P. (2001). Market Potential for Probiotics. *The American Journal of Clinical Nutrition*, Vol. 73 (suppl.), pp. 4765-4835.

Stark, P.L., & Lee, A. (1982). The Microbial Ecology of the Large Bowel of Breast-fed and Formula-fed Infants During the First Year of Life. *Journal of Medical Microbiology*, Vol. 15, pp. 189-203.

Tamime, A., Božanić, R., Rogelj, I. (2003). Probiotički fermentirani mliječni proizvodi. *Mljekarstvo*, Vol. 53, pp. 111-134.

Tancrede, C. (1992). Role of Human Microflora in Health and Disease. *European Journal of Clinical Microbiology Infection Disease*, 11, pp. 1012–1015.

Tannock, G.W., Luchansky, J.B., Miller, L., Connell, H., Thodeandersen, S., Mercer, A.A. & Kalenhammer, T.R. (1994). Molecular Characterization of a Plasmid Borne (pGT633) Erythromycin Resistance Determinant (ermGT) from *Lactobacillus reuteri* 100-63. *Plasmid*, Vol. 31, pp. 60-71

Teuber, M & Perreten, V. (2000). Role of Milk and Meat Products as Vehicles for Antibiotic Resistant Bacteria. *Acta Veterinaria Scandinavica*, pp. 75-87.

Teuber, M., Meile, L. & Schwarz, F. (1999). Acquired Antibiotic Resistance in Lactic Acid Bacteria from Food. *Antonie van Leeuvenhoek*, Vol. 76, pp. 115-137.

Todorov, S.D., Furtado, D.N., Saad, S. M. I. & Tome, E. (2011). Potential Beneficial Properties of Bacteriocin-Producing Lactic Acid Bacteria Isolated from Smoked Salmon. *Journal of Applied Microbiology*, 110, No 4, pp. 971-986.

Toh, S. M., Xiong, L., Arias, C. A., Villegas, M. V., Lolans, K., Quinn, J. & Mankin, A. S. (2007). Acquisition of a Natural Resistance Gene Renders a Clinical Strains of Methicilllin Resistant *Staphylococcus aureus* Resistant to the Synthetic Antibiotic Linezolid. *Molecular Microbiology*, Vol. 64, pp. 1506-1514.

Toomey, N., Monaghan, A., Fanning, S. & Bolton, D. (2009). Transfer of Antibiotic Resistance Marker Genes Between Lactic Acid Bacteria in Model Rumen and Plant Environments. *Applied and Environmental Microbiology*, Vol. 75, No. 10, pp. 346-3152.

Tuomola, E.M. & Salminen, S.J. (1998). Adhesion of Some Probiotic and Dairy Lactobacillus Strains to Caco-2 Cell Cultures. *International Journal of Food Microbiology*, Vol.41, pp. 45–51.

Tynkkynen, S., Singh, K. V. & Varmanen, P. (1998). Vancomycin Resistance Factor of *Lactobacillus rhamnosus* GG in Relation to Enterococcal Vancomycin Resistance (van) Genes. *International Journal of Food Microbiology*, Vol. 41, pp.195-204. UK.

van der Waaij, D. (1988). Evidence of Imunoregulation of the Composition of Intestinal Microflora and Its Practical Consequences. *European Journal Clinical Microbiology Infectious Diseases*, Vol. 7, pp. 103-106.

Vescovo, M., Morelli, L. & Botazzi, V. (1982). Drug resistance plasmids in *Lactobacillus acidophilus* and *Lactobacillus reuteri*. *Applied and Environmental Microbiology*, Vol. 43, pp. 50-56.

Vesterlund, S., Paltta, J., Karp, M. & Ouwehand, A. C. (2005). Adhesion of Bacteria to Resected Human Colonic Tissue: Quantitative Analysis of Bacterial Adhesion and Viability. *Research in Microbiology*, Vol. 156, pp. 238–244.

Wang, T.T. & Lee, B.H. (1997). Plasmids in *Lactobacillus*. *Critical Reviews in Biotechnology*, Vol. 17, pp. 227-272.

Young, H.K., Skurray, K.A. & Amyes, S.K. (1987). Plasmid-Mediated Trimethoprim-Resistance in *Staphylococcus aureus*. Characterization of the First Gram-Positive Plasmid Dihydrofolate Reductase (type S1). *Biochemistry Journal*, Vol. 243, No. 1, pp. 309-312.

www.ingramcontent.com/pod-product-compliance
Lightning Source LLC
Chambersburg PA
CBHW080803020925
31944CB00006B/276
9789535104728